Adolescent Medicine

A Practical Guide

Second Edition

Adolescent Medicine

A Practical Guide

Second Edition

Victor C. Strasburger, M.D.
Associate Professor of Pediatrics and Family Practice
Chief, Division of Adolescent Medicine
University of New Mexico School of Medicine
Albuquerque, New Mexico

Robert T. Brown, M.D.
Professor of Clinical Pediatrics and Clinical Obstetrics and Gynecology
Director of Adolescent Medicine
Ohio State University College of Medicine
Chief, Section of Adolescent Health
Children's Hospital
Columbus, Ohio

Foreword by
William A. Daniel, Jr., M.D.
Professor Emeritus of Pediatrics
Former Chief, Division of Adolescent Medicine
University of Alabama School of Medicine
Birmingham, Alabama

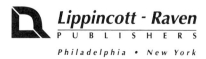

Lippincott - Raven
P U B L I S H E R S
Philadelphia • New York

Acquisitions Editor: Paula Callaghan
Coordinating Editorial Assistant: Julia Benson
Manufacturing Manager: Dennis Teston
Production Manager: Jodi Borgenicht
Production Editor: Jeff Somers
Cover Designer: Wanda Lubelska Design
Indexer: Alexandria Nickerson
Compositor: Compset, Inc.
Printer: Maple Press

Printed in the United States of America

9 8 7 6 5 4 3 2 1

Library of Congress Cataloging-in-Publication Data
Strasburger, Victor C., 1949–
 Adolescent medicine : a practical guide / Victor C. Strasburger.
 Robert T. Brown : foreword by William A. Daniel, Jr.—2nd ed.
  p. cm.
 Includes bibliographical references and index.
 ISBN 0-316-81875-5 (alk. paper)
 1. Adolescent medicine—Handbooks, manuals, etc. I. Brown,
Robert T. (Robert Theodore), 1945–   . II. Title.
 [DNLM: 1. Adolescent Medicine. WS 460 S897a 1997]
RJ550.S82 1997
616′.00835—DC21
DNLM/DLC
for Library of Congress

To Alya, Max, and Katya, with love.
And, in honor of Marge Strasburger and Stan Goldberg.

V.C.S.

To Joanna, Billy, and Megan—thanks for demonstrating the finest in adolescents. I love you dearly.

R.T.B.

Contents

Foreword

Adolescent Medicine: A Practical Guide is a small, concise, and highly informative book about adolescents and their health problems that will be useful to physicians and many other health professionals. It is a source of practical information by two physicians who have much experience in caring for teenagers. Doctors Strasburger and Brown have distinguished themselves as directors of adolescent medicine programs and are to be congratulated for clearly presenting so much useful information. The book is much more than an outline, less than an exhaustive source of medical information, and contains excellent references for further study. Its ultimate value will depend on who uses it and how it is utilized.

Physicians who have few adolescents in their practice can use the book to obtain practical information quickly about common, important physical and psychosocial problems. More experienced doctors will find the book a time-saving review of adolescent medicine that will increase proficiency in diagnosis and current treatment. For another category of physicians and health professionals, the book can be the beginning of a major educational endeavor.

Many practicing physicians who have had little, if any, formal training in adolescent medicine may now find increasing numbers of teenaged patients consulting them for more complex problems. Adolescents are interesting patients who provide a new stimulus in a practice of medicine that may have become routine. These doctors need and want to learn more about the growth, development, and biopsychosocial problems of teenagers. Learning more, coupled with experience in practice, will bring increased competence in caring for many complicated problems of adolescents and will also afford greater personal satisfaction. This book is especially valuable for the doctor who has infrequent adolescent patients or who has had limited experience with the presenting complaint and needs to be able to find accurate information quickly about the condition and recommended methods of treatment.

Any unused book is of little practical value. I encourage physicians and other health care providers to read *Adolescent Medicine: A Practical Guide* and learn from it. The authors are to be commended for preparing a source of information needed by many physicians who care for adolescents.

William A. Daniel, Jr., M.D.

Preface

"The best way to become acquainted with a subject is to write a book about it."
Benjamin Disraeli

As a specialty, adolescent medicine is at the age when it should be having its first mid-life crisis. Now 45 years old, adolescent medicine began when an internist, J. Roswell Gallagher, established the first Adolescent Unit at Boston Children's Hospital in 1952. His rationale was that such a unit would ensure "a physician's tendency to consider his patient" and "diminish the likelihood that he will focus upon disease alone (1)."

Since 1952, the American Academy of Pediatrics, the Society for Adolescent Medicine, The Task Force on Pediatric Education, the American Medical Association, and several foundations have all become interested in the health and welfare of adolescents. However, adolescents remain a seriously underserved population, and their exploits continue to endanger their lives (suicide, homicide, automobile accidents, and drugs) and their future well-being (sexually transmitted diseases, chronic illness, acne, and sports injuries). Where have we gone wrong? Or, to post the question in a slightly different way: What should we be doing that we are not currently doing (2,3)?

We hope that this book will stand as one small answer to this rather large question. This book starts small and works toward global issues. It is intended to be a concise, practical manual for those who want to treat adolescents. Perhaps this is the only method by which adolescent medicine can become universally recognized and accepted within the medical community—for physicians and nurses to actually be practicing it. Although adolescent medicine was begun by an internist and has settled largely in the academic realm of pediatrics, it is well known that family practitioners see more teenagers than any other group of health specialists. Who sees teenagers is not nearly as important as whether or not they *enjoy* seeing teenagers as patients and whether or not they are sufficiently trained to do so. Again, we hope that this small manual will provide a service to those practitioners who want to see teenagers but may be hesitant because practical information and guidance is not readily at hand.

Polonius, Ophelia's doddering old father in *Hamlet*, was famous for his "brevity is the soul of wit" speech, because he then carried on, long-winded, in his usual manner. We have tried to avoid that. Therefore, long and laborious lists or discussions of differential diagnoses, unusual treatments, and rare diseases generally have been omitted from this text. What is commonly encountered in a practice or clinic, what can be done for it easily, why it occurs, and where more information can be found—this is what we are most interested in; and the uncommon or obscure we will leave to the large textbooks. There are a steadily increasing number of excellent general adolescent medicine texts (4–7) and adolescent gynecology texts (8–10), and we do not aim (nor dare) to compete with either. Rather, we hope that pediatricians, family practitioners, internists, gynecologists, nurse practitioners, residents, and medical students will turn to this volume first when they are in the middle of their office or clinic practice and need a quick overview and treatment plan.

REFERENCES

1. Gallagher JR. A clinic for adolescents. *Children* 1954;1:165.
2. Irwin CE, Jr. Why adolescent medicine? *J Adolesc Health* 1986;Case 7:1S.
3. Strasburger VC. Adolescent medicine in the 1990s: no more excuses. *Clin Pediatr* 1997;36:87.
4. McAnarney E, Kriepe R, Orr D, and Comerci G, eds. *Textbook of Adolescent Medicine.* Philadelphia: W.B. Saunders, 1992.
5. Neinstein LS. *Adolescent Heath Care: A Practical Guide, 3/e.* Baltimore: Williams & Wilkins, 1996.
6. Hofmann AD and Greydanus DE. *Adolescent Medicine, 3/e.* Stamford, CT: Appleton & Lange, 1997.
7. Friedman SB, Fisher M, Schonberg SK, Alderman EM, eds. *Comprehensive Adolescent Health Care, 2/e.* St. Louis, MO: Mosby, 1997.
8. Pokorny S, ed. *Pediatric and Adolescent Gynecology.* New York: Chapman & Hall, 1996.
9. Goldfarb AF, ed. *Clinical Problems in Pediatric and Adolescent Gynecology.* New York: Chapman & Hall, 1996.
10. Emans SJH and Goldstein DP. *Pediatric and Adolescent Gynecology, 4/e.* Philadelphia: Lippincott-Raven Publishers, 1997.

Acknowledgments

I would like to thank several individuals at the University of New Mexico Health Sciences Center who made work on this second edition possible: Drs. Shirley Murphy (Chairperson, Pediatrics), Paul Roth (Dean, School of Medicine), and Jane Henney (Vice President, Health Sciences), who allowed and encouraged me to take a 6-month sabbatical which facilitated this extensive revision. Thanks also to my colleague, Dr. Jane McGrath, who graciously substituted during my sabbatical.

V.C.S.

I would like to thank Harold E. Regan, Jr., M.A., for his skillful and indefatigable efforts in the completion of this edition. I also appreciate the review supplied by Dr. John Mahan and the support and encouragement provided by Dr. Barbara Cromer, my professional alter ego. Thanks also to Dr. Tom Hansen for his understanding in making available the time needed to get this job done.

R.T.B.

1

Growth and Development

NORMAL GROWTH AND DEVELOPMENT

The ultimate goal of child and adolescent health care is to help children become functioning and competent adults. Children and adolescents reach that goal by proceeding through the various stages of development.

To assess whether a patient is proceeding along that normal road, a clinician must have more than a passing knowledge of normal growth and development. All primary care providers caring for children are aware of the developmental tasks that an infant must master to be considered normal, but knowledge of the components of adolescent growth and development is not so universal. This knowledge, however, is essential to any practitioner who cares for adolescents. Only with a sure grasp of the principles of adolescent growth and development can the clinician spot deviations from the path of normality and help to correct them.

In this chapter, we review the essential tenets of adolescent growth and development. Although these principles are presented sequentially (i.e., first physical, then cognitive, and then psychosocial), all the changes occur simultaneously in any one adolescent, albeit at different rates, and each has considerable impact on the others.

Physical Growth and Development

All adolescents go through the same processes and stages to reach the goal of physical maturity. The range of time over which these changes occur can be considerable. This process is called *puberty*.

Puberty is the period during which the adolescent experiences more physical changes than in any other life stage except as a fetus, and these changes occur rapidly. An adolescent can go from a child's body to that of an adult in as little as 2 to 3 years, or the process can take up to as many as 6 or 7 years. Yet adolescents who are at each of these extremes all may be normal. In general, the change from the body of a child to the body of an adult takes anywhere from 2 1/2 to 4 years, with the rate of growth during the pubertal growth spurt being faster than during any other period in extrauterine life (Fig. 1).

The Endocrinology of Puberty

The precise mechanism that initiates puberty remains unknown. It is known, however, that with the onset of puberty, the hypothalamic nuclei that produce gonadotropin-releasing hormone or luteinizing hormone-releasing hormone (LHRH) become progressively less sensitive to circulating gonadal steroids, leading, in a negative feedback system, to increased levels of those gonadal steroids (i.e., estrogen in girls and testosterone in boys). The levels of these hormones rise until they are high enough to initiate the changes in secondary sex characteristics that we call puberty. The levels of estrogen or testosterone continue to increase throughout puberty until adult levels are reached. In girls, a positive feedback mechanism between estrogen and LH/LHRH leads to monthly ovulation. In the meantime, the rising levels of sex steroids in the blood cause increases in growth hormone production, with a consequent increase in production of insulin-like growth factors. This process leads to an increase in linear growth and to changes in body configuration [1–3].

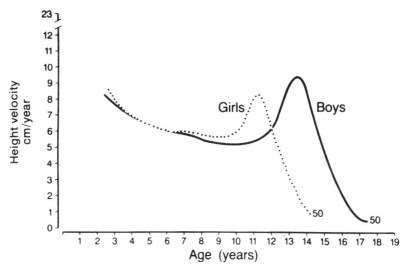

FIG. 1. Fiftieth-percentile height velocity curve for American boys and girls (Reprinted with permission from Slap GB. Normal physiological and psychosocial growth in the adolescent. *J Adolesc Health* 1986;7:135.)

Assessment of adequacy of pubertal maturation is most easily accomplished by judging the configuration of pubic hair and genitalia, a system known as *Tanner staging*. J. M. Tanner, an eminent English endocrinologist, was the first to elucidate this system for assessment of pubertal development [4]. In this system, stage 1 is childlike and stage 5 is adult configuration. Figures 2 and 3 show the whole gradation of Tanner stages, or sex maturity ratings.

In boys, puberty usually begins at approximately 12 years of age, but it can start as early as 9 years or as late as 13 1/2 years of age [5]. The later it starts, the longer it seems to take, a fact that highlights nature's sometimes cruel whimsy. The usual first sign of puberty in a boy is testicular enlargement, and measurement of testicular size (i.e., volume) is the most accurate, nontechnical method of assessing the stage of male pubertal development [6] (Table 1). Another method of assessing testicular volume uses a string of model testicles of increasing size to which the patient's testicles are compared. Enlargement of the testicles is followed by lengthening of the penis and, subsequently, by the appearance of pubic hair. During this early part of puberty, other parts of a boy's body are beginning to change. Adolescents grow from the outside in. In other words, the feet and hands enlarge first, followed by the rest of the limbs, and then the trunk. It is apparent, at times, that certain children have begun puberty because they have bright new sneakers on feet much too large for their bodies. At the end of the growth spurt, the typical boy is all elbows and knees. It is only after most of adult height is achieved that increase in muscle mass occurs. In other words, it is then that the boy "fills out." This process occurs in Tanner stage 4.

Girls begin to develop approximately 2 years, on average, before boys. Normal puberty can begin in girls between the ages of 8 and 13 years. The first sign of development in a girl [5] usually is the appearance of a firm nubbin of tissue under the areola, the "breast bud" [7] (Table 2). The appearance of this tissue is followed by the appearance of pubic hair. Occasionally, pubic hair, responsive to adrenal androgens rather than estrogen, appears before the breast buds. The growth spurt occurs in stage 2, always before menarche, which usually occurs by late stage 3. Five percent of girls wait until stage 5 for this event [7]. Girls do not experience the same muscle mass increase that boys do. Instead, fat, which is not lost in puberty as it is in boys, is rearranged into the typical pattern of the adult woman.

Tanner stages have many more uses than just assessing level of pubertal development. Many types of laboratory data are uninterpretable without knowledge of the subject's Tanner stage. For example, hematocrit and hemoglobin vary directly with Tanner stage, especially in boys (Fig. 4). Similarly, alkaline phosphatase also varies with sex maturity ratings rather than with age (Fig. 5). This blood com-

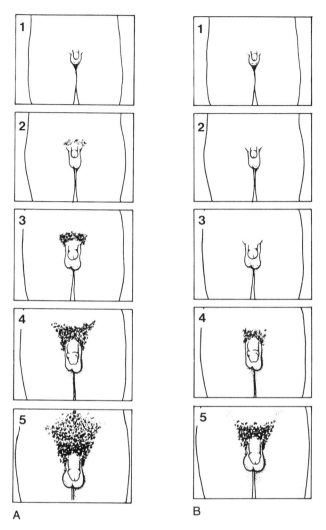

FIG. 2. Sex maturity stages. **A:** Boys' pubic hair. **B:** Boys' genitalia

ponent, which reflects bone metabolic activity, rises to a peak with the period of peak height velocity in height in both boys and girls. (Peak height velocity, also known as the *growth spurt*, is that period during puberty in which an adolescent's growth rate accelerates and in which 4 to 6 inches in height may be gained in a year or less.) Peak height velocity occurs in girls at Tanner pubic hair stage 2 to 3 and in boys at pubic hair stage 3 to 4. Figure 6 shows this and other milestones of puberty vis-à-vis Tanner stages.

Tanner stages can be helpful in the process of physical diagnosis. For example, an obese teenager who presents with pain in the upper thigh and with a limp could be a diagnostic puzzle, but if the Tanner rating is between stage 2 and early stage 4, then the likely diagnosis is slipped capital femoral epiphysis (SCFE). SCFE is actually a fracture of the head of the femur through the epiphyseal growth line. This epiphysis calcifies in stage 4 to 5. There are other causes of hip problems in stage 3 or 4 adolescents, but SCFE remains the prime consideration (see Chapter 3).

Preventive and therapeutic counseling efforts are also enhanced by knowledge of Tanner stages. A girl presenting with the complaint of primary amenorrhea when she is in stage 3 or 4 can be examined and, if the examination is normal, can be counseled with little need for more extensive studies. This is

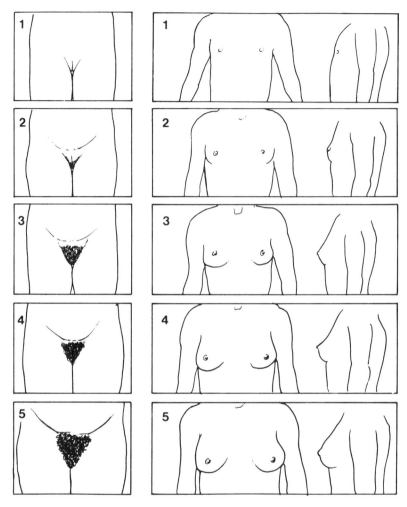

FIG. 3. Sex maturity stages. **A:** Girls' pubic hair. **B:** Girls' breasts

TABLE 1. *Classification of genital maturity stages in boys (Tanner ratings)*

Stage	Pubic hair	Penis	Testes
1	None	Preadolescent	Preadolescent
2	Scanty, long, slightly pig-mented	Slight enlargement	Enlarged scrotum, pink, texture changed
3	Darker, begins to curl, small amount	Longer	Larger
4	Resembles adult type, but less in quantity; coarse, curly	Larger, glans and breadth increase in size	Larger, scrotum darker
5	Adult distribution, spread to medial thighs	Adult	Adult

Adapted from Daniel WA Jr. *Adolescents in health and disease.* St. Louis: Mosby, 1977.

TABLE 2. *Classification of genital maturity stages in girls (Tanner ratings)*

Stage	Pubic hair	Breasts
1	Preadolescent	Preadolescent
2	Sparse, slightly pigmented, straight, at medial border of labia	Breast and papilla elevated as small mound, areolar diameter increased
3	Darker, beginning to curl, increased amount	Breast and areola enlarged, without contour separation
4	Coarse, curly, abundant, but amount less than in adult	Areola and papilla form secondary mound
5	Adult feminine triangle, spread to medial surface of thighs	Mature, nipple projects, areola part of general breast contour

Adapted from Daniel WA Jr. *Adolescents in health and disease.* St. Louis: Mosby, 1977.

because menarche may not occur until stage 5. However, if the girl began puberty more than 4 years before she presents to the physician and if she is in full stage 5, a diagnostic evaluation is most certainly indicated. Similarly, a boy may present to a physician's office with the complaint of failure to grow or mature. An assessment of his Tanner stage is critical to diagnosing his problem. If he is in stage 2 and has just begun puberty within the past year, he can be reassured that he is normal and will probably continue to develop without mishap. This point is more completely elucidated in the second part of this chapter.

Clearly, a thorough knowledge of the principles of pubertal development greatly simplifies and enhances the physician's ability to care for the adolescent patient.

Cognitive Development

In modern industrial society, the ability to think abstractly is the hallmark of adult cognitive activity. Piaget [8], the Swiss psychologist, proposed the most commonly accepted theory of cognitive development. He postulated that each person goes through four primary stages of cognitive development: sensorimotor (birth to 2 years old); preoperational (2 to 7 years old); concrete (7 to 12 years old); and formal operational (older than 12 years). Piaget proposed that children begin to have the capacity to

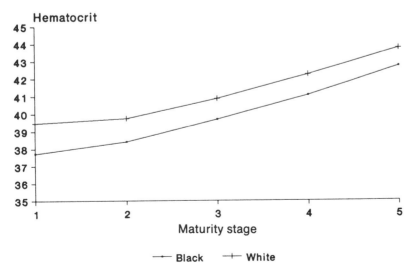

FIG. 4. Hematocrit–maturity correlation in boys. (Data from Daniel WA. Hematocrit: maturity relationship in adolescence. *Pediatrics* 1973;52:388.)

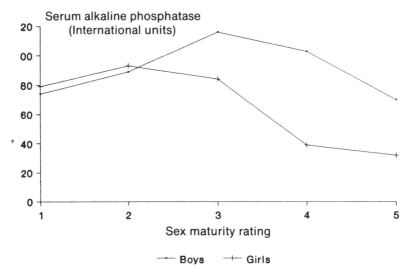

FIG. 5. Serum alkaline phosphatase–maturity correlation in adolescents. (Data from Bennett DM, et al. The relationship of serum alkaline phosphatase concentrations to sex maturity ratings in adolescents. *J Pediatr* 1976;88:633.)

think abstractly at approximately the age of 12 years. The more intelligent the child, the faster the ability develops, but the onset is not fully related to intelligence. Full abstract thought, however, is not achieved until an adolescent is 15 or 16 years of age, and there are gaps even then. Indeed, many adults do not use abstract thinking effectively. The main characteristics of formal operational thought are the abilities to

- Generate abstractions
- Generate hypotheses
- Consider contrary-to-fact situations
- Generate all possibilities from a specific situation
- Approach a problem in a systematic fashion
- Use combinatory logic

Early in the development of formal operational thought, the adolescent has not yet achieved mastery. This produces several qualities in the adolescent's thinking, including pseudostupidity, imaginary audience (or "on-stage" phenomenon), apparent hypocrisy, and personal fable [9] (see also Chapter 8). The early formal thinker can create but not prioritize many possible solutions to problems that really are simple or accidental (i.e., pseudostupidity). Adolescents are so egocentric that they assume that what they think is so important to them is automatically important to everyone else (i.e., the imaginary audience). This quality also leads to the feeling that everyone is aware of all of the adolescent's personal and intimate details, the feeling of being on stage. Apparent hypocrisy occurs when the adolescent can conceptualize abstract rules but is unable to apply them consistently to himself or herself. Last, the personal fable is the feeling of "specialness" that generates from adolescent egocentrism. This feeling allows the adolescent to believe that he or she is immune to the risks and consequences that affect others. Risk-taking behaviors frequently are the result [10].

In the medical setting, early and early middle adolescents (i.e., adolescents of 15 years or younger) cannot, therefore, be expected to use adult thought processes. They should be expected to be concrete thinkers. As a result, the physician must alter his or her usual history-taking format. Instead of asking open-ended questions and instead of being nondirective, the clinician must be very specific and directive in history taking to ferret out all the necessary facts about an adolescent's problems. For example, just a simple "How are you?" may generate an entire history from an adult but not from an adolescent. The most likely response to such a question from an early (10- to 13-year-old) adolescent would be

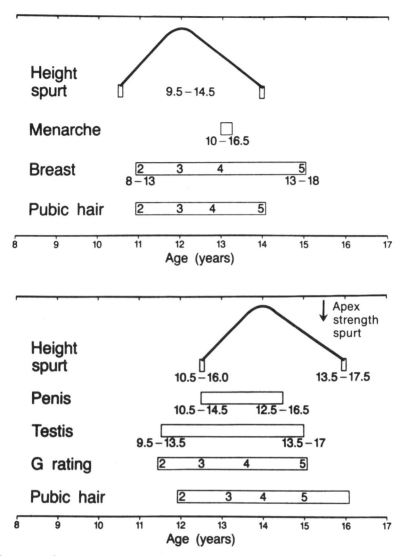

FIG. 6. Sequence of events in puberty—girls and boys. (Reprinted with permission from Slap GB. Normal physiological and psychosocial growth in the adolescent. *J Adolesc Health* 1986;7:135.)

"Fine." The practitioner must then ask why the adolescent has come to the office and must lead the adolescent step by step through the history to get the same information that an adult would reveal spontaneously.

In addition to history taking, the adolescent's lack of conceptual thinking ability must be taken into consideration when explaining findings and giving instructions. An adolescent with chest pain, for instance, must be told explicitly that the pain is not due to a heart attack, because that is the question that the adolescent is really asking. An adult could extrapolate that his or her heart was normal just from hearing the physician say, "Nothing is wrong" or "Everything is fine." The adolescent could not. The adolescent's cognitive immaturity forces the physician to work through the explanations in a step-by-step fashion.

When the clinician sees an older adolescent (i.e., older than 16 years), there is the chance that the patient will understand things in an adult fashion. People tend, in stressful situations, to regress in their cognitive capacities. The safest course is to be as concrete with an older adolescent as one would be with a younger one. The major point to be derived from this knowledge of adolescent cognitive development is that it usually is not the adolescent who is responsible for a less-than-adequate history or misunderstood diagnostic explanations or home-going instructions. The fault lies with the practitioner for not appreciating the way his, or her, information can best be presented to be understood.

Psychosocial Development

The third area of adolescent development is psychosocial development, or that which encompasses an adolescent's ability to view himself or herself and to relate to others, including both those with whom he or she is intimate and society at large. This type of development can be divided into four tasks that adolescents must be well on their way to completing before they can be said to have entered adulthood effectively [11]. These four tasks are:

- The achievement of effective separation or *independence* from parents and family
- The achievement of a realistic *vocational* goal
- The achievement of a mature level of *sexuality*
- Progress toward achievement of a realistic and positive *self-image*

To better understand development in this area, it is convenient to divide adolescence into an early stage (10 through 13 years of age), a middle stage (14 through 16 years of age), and a late stage (17 through 18 to 22 years of age, depending on the social situation after the high school years).

Independence

The achievement of effective separation from the home and the parents is a lifelong process beginning in infancy. The reason it is considered so significant during adolescence is that it is during this period that the major break is made. Adolescence is a time of individuation, a period in which the youth seeks to establish himself as an independent entity from his parents.

Early adolescents demonstrate the desire to separate from the parents in mostly ineffectual but highly annoying ways. In effect, they throw temper tantrums. They insist that they can function without parental assistance, yet a few minutes later they are clinging infants who want parents to protect them and to fend for them against a world that is not fair. Twelve- and 13-year-olds have been called the *terrible twos* of adolescence. In this phase, the budding teenager tries to separate from the family as a whole. Hence, when the parents say that it is time to go visit the grandparents, the 13-year-old throws a fit and refuses to go. Usually, if forced to go, he or she will sulk in the car all the way to grandma's but, within a half hour of arriving there, will have joined in the family fun.

Early adolescence is also the time of wanting to be alone. The bedroom and bathroom become havens, and minutes stretch into hours as parents anxiously await the reemergence of the nymph from its cocoon. At this stage, the adolescent is usually going through the major changes of puberty and is extremely preoccupied with physical stigmata, real or self-perceived. When this preoccupation with physical stigmata is combined with feelings of being "on stage," then each pimple takes on the proportion of Mt. Everest. Because of this obsession with physical appearance, the telephone assumes extreme importance at this stage. The phone provides early adolescents with the ability to communicate with peers without the need to be seen. Therefore, they can hide all the imperfections that they are sure others would see in face-to-face conversation. If early adolescents do mix in a peer group, the group almost always consists of peers of the same gender.

The drive to achieve independence in the middle adolescent is demonstrated best by the need of the youth to be in a mixed-gender peer group. The *peer group* can be defined, in adolescence, as a group of similarly aged teenagers with similar interests and similar needs, the members of which prefer to spend time with one another rather than with their parents or family. Is the peer group a negative influence on an adolescent? Perhaps, but only because the adolescent was looking for that kind of experience in the first place. In other words, teenagers join a peer group that fills their needs rather than one that forces them to do what they ordinarily would not feel inclined to do. Thus, if the adolescent has the need to participate in high-risk behaviors, he will seek like-minded peers to gain group support. If another adolescent shuns that type of behavior and instead feels the need for intellectual stimulation and companionship, she will tend to congregate with youths with similar needs and interests. Another view of the purpose served by the peer group is that it is an entity in which adolescents can try out different ways of being adults until they discover one with which they are comfortable.

The middle adolescent also demonstrates the need to separate by intense intellectual testing of parents. Parental beliefs and opinions are challenged constantly. When the parents want to go to church, for example, the middle adolescent is likely to say that she no longer believes in God and sees no reason to participate in such meaningless rituals. It is not that the teenager has truly lost faith so much as that she wants to learn how the parents react to the challenge and defend their beliefs. Similar intellectual attacks occur in areas of political opinion and clothing choices.

By late adolescence, the young adult usually arrives at some early conclusions as to the best way of being an adult. The need for the peer group, therefore, is no longer acute. The youth begins to make choices regarding behavior, recreational activities, and friends. Being within the protective group of peers is no longer necessary; adolescents are ready to begin to strike out on their own.

Vocation

Our society mandates that each adolescent choose a vocation by the time he or she reaches adulthood, and very few of those choices are dictated by the vocation of our parents, such as might be the case in a more traditional society. Therefore, the choosing of a vocation is a major task of adolescence.

To select a future vocation with insight and intelligence requires a measure of cognitive maturity found only in the later adolescent. It is only a very fortunate few who know when they are early adolescents (and who always have known) what they want to do vocationally. For the great majority of us, this task remains unresolved until late adolescence at the earliest.

Asking an adolescent what he or she wants to do when grown up is a simple way of assessing cognitive maturity. The typical early adolescent answers with a career choice that may have nothing to do with an objective assessment of his or her own abilities. It is not at all unusual to ask a short, thin 13-year-old boy about future career goals and be told that he wants to be a professional basketball or football player. The middle adolescent, on the other hand, will likely answer, "I don't know." This reflects a transfer from the fantasy of the idealized self-image of early adolescence to the more realistic image of late adolescence. By late adolescence, the answer to the question is much more likely to reflect the true abilities or interests of the adolescent.

Sexuality

The development of a mature level of sexuality is a prerequisite of effective adult functioning. *Sexuality* in this context means much more than just physical sex. It refers, instead, to how a person views himself, or herself, as a man, or woman, in our society and how that person relates to other men and women, in general, and to one particular person, specifically. It refers to the ability of a person to enter into and to maintain an intimate relationship on a giving basis.

Sexuality begins with XX or XY chromosomes modified by other hormonal factors. Family and culture teach us how men and women behave as well as how they interrelate with each other. Modifying those influences is the influence of society as a whole, expressed most effectively through media such as television and movies (Fig. 7).

The early adolescent expresses sexuality in what, to adults, appear to be very funny ways but, to the adolescent, are very painful. Fantasies of the ideal partner abound. Any real contact with the other sex occurs in social situations that are usually structured by adults, such as the seventh-grade dance. This event is a classic venue for the study of the expression of early adolescent sexuality behavior. The girls huddle in the middle of the room and bounce in unison to the beat of the music, while the boys, averaging a head shorter than the girls, circle around the perimeter. The girls resemble an amoeboid creature that occasionally pinches off a pseudopod of at least four girls who dash to the bathroom. There is something about 13-year-old girls that prevents them, in this situation, from going to the bathroom alone.

As the boy or girl grows into middle adolescence, efforts at relating to those to whom the adolescent is romantically inclined center more on group dating and social activities. Teenagers at this period of psychosocial development are more secure in their physical self-image and are, therefore, more prone to spend time with others of both genders in their peer groups. Any romantic involvement is normally with a partner within 1 or 2 years of their own age and is characterized not by the giving

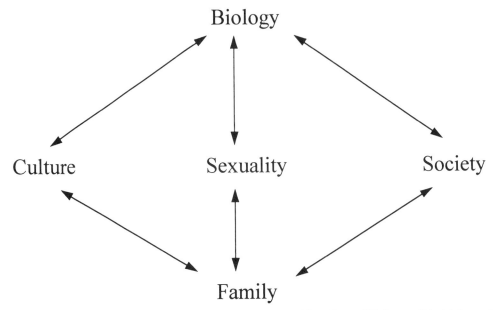

FIG. 7. Factors influencing development of sexuality. (Adapted from Brown RT, Cromer BA. Adolescent sexuality. In: Sanfilippo JS, Muram D, Lee PA, et al, eds. *Pediatric and adolescent gynecology*. Philadelphia: WB Saunders; 1994: 278.)

nature of a mature relationship but by more selfish motivations. The girl is preoccupied with how her partner matches up to her image of the ideal boy. The boy is frequently preoccupied with how far he can go sexually with this girl. Feelings are intense and, to the teenager involved in this romance, all-encompassing. However, the partner can never really match up to the image that the teenager has created; so, the relationships have, by adult standards, fairly short lives.

It is not normal for a middle-adolescent girl to date boys who are 4 or more years older than she. When that happens, the girl usually has a poor father figure in her life and can be said to be "looking for daddy." She is at great risk of becoming emotionally hurt, if not pregnant, and encountering all the problems of being an adolescent parent.

By late adolescence, the young person usually has grown to the point where he or she can enter into a relationship in a more adult fashion. These relationships are usually characterized by more concern by the participants for the feelings and welfare of their partners. The capacity for true intimacy has begun to develop, and the adolescents are capable of adult-type relationships.

Self-Image

The problem with early adolescents and self-image is that, basically, they do not have one. So many things are changing in their bodies, their thought processes, and their emotions that there is nothing definite available on which to hang an image. In other words, their image does not hold still long enough to hang a self on it. Teenagers at this stage, however, feel naked to the world. They are sure that every intimate fact about them and every thought that they have is immediately evident to anyone who looks at them. They are preoccupied with their fantasies of how they should look and be, and they do all they can to match up to these wraiths.

The middle adolescent has come to grips with his or her external appearance and is now trying on ways to be an adult. The self-image at this stage is centered on being different from the image that the adolescent has of parents. Teenagers look to the peer group to help define the image that they should have.

By late adolescence, it is hoped, teenagers realize that they will never match up to the image they have been trying to achieve; they begin to learn how to play the hand nature has dealt them. By now, they should be somewhat reconciled to their physical, emotional, and cognitive realities, as well as preoccupied with using their actual talents and abilities. They also are learning to deal with the realization that they are not so different from their parents and that being similar to their parents is not so bad.

Knowledge of normal adolescent growth and development is essential for the practitioner who is to care for these young people. Only by being familiar with the physical, cognitive, and psychosocial changes young people are experiencing can the practitioner help adolescents achieve a competent and functional adulthood.

REFERENCES

1. Kulin HE, Müller J. The biological aspects of puberty. *Pediatr Rev* 1996;17:75.
2. Styne DM. Physiology of puberty. *Adolescent Medicine: State of the Art Reviews* 1995;5:171.
3. Cara JF. Growth hormone in adolescence: normal and abnormal. *Endocrinol Metab Clin North Am* 1993;22: 533.
4. Tanner JM. *Growth at adolescence.* 2nd ed. Oxford: Blackwell Scientific; 1962.
5. Sizonenko PC. Normal sexual maturation. *Pediatrician* 1987;14:191.
6. Daniel WA Jr, Feinstein RA, Howard-Peebles P, et al. Testicular volume of adolescents. *J Pediatr* 1982;101: 1010.
7. Rosenfeld RG. Evaluation of growth and maturation in adolescence. *Pediatr Rev* 1982;4:175.
8. Piaget J. *Science of education and the psychology of the child* (Coltman D, transl). New York: Orion Press; 1970:30–33.
9. Elkind D. Understanding the young adolescent. *Adolescence* 1978;13:127.
10. Rosenthal SL, Biro FM. Communication with adolescents and their families. *Adolescent and Pediatric Gynecology* 1991;4:57.
11. Brown RT. Assessing adolescent development. *Pediatr Ann* 1982;7:587.

PROBLEMS OF GROWTH AND DEVELOPMENT

The range of normal adolescent physical growth and development is wide. Girls can begin puberty as early as 8 years or as late as 13 years of age and be normal. The limits for the normal beginning of puberty in boys are 8 1/2 years and 13 1/2 years. Once begun, the process of puberty should be concluded within 4 to 5 years, although some very late developers can take even longer. Late or slow development can have many causes that must be investigated. In addition to the onset and pace of puberty, the absolute height of an adolescent is of considerable importance. Any teen who is below the third percentile for age on standard growth charts, or who is more than two standard deviations below the mean, is considered to have short stature. Again, this condition can cause considerable consternation and must be investigated.

Short Stature

The adolescent who is significantly shorter than his (it is usually a boy) peers can have considerable problems, especially psychosocial ones [1–3]. Our society seems to favor taller people. There are correlations of success, power, athletic prowess, and social stature with height [4]. Girls who have isolated short stature do not seem to have the same problems. Most often, short stature is a function either of genetics (i.e., the members of the family to which the patient belongs are also short) or of an idiopathic delay in growth and development (i.e., constitutional short stature [along with delayed puberty]). Many other pathologic conditions can cause short stature (Table 3).

Determination of Abnormal Growth

Before we discuss the various causes of, and possible remedies for, short stature, the issue of how one decides whether a child is growing abnormally needs clarification. The best way to decide if an

TABLE 3. *Causes of short stature*

Intrinsic factors
Familial short stature
Genetic defects involving bone growth (osteochondrodystrophy, osteogenesis imperfecta)
Mucopolysaccharidoses and other storage disease
Chromosomal abnormalities (trisomy 15, 18, 21; gonadal dysgenesis [45 X mosaicism or structural
    anomaly of the X chromosome])
Intrauterine growth retardation (in utero infection, exposure to toxic agent such as alcohol or anticonvul-
    sant drug, placental insufficiency)
Miscellaneous syndromes (Seckel's, Noonan's)

Constitutional delay in linear growth and sexual development
Often reflects familial growth pattern. Occurs in some nutritionally deprived children

Nutritional deprivation
Anorexia nervosa
Abnormalities of digestion, absorption, utilization, or retention of calories
Specific nutrient deficiency (zinc)
Nutritional dwarfism

Disease-related (attenuated) short stature
Central nervous system (diencephalic syndrome, central nervous system insult)
Cardiac (congenital or acquired heart disease)
Respiratory (cystic fibrosis, obstructive sleep apnea)
Gastrointestinal (celiac disease, cystic fibrosis, chronic inflammatory bowel disease, chronic hepatic
    failure)
Renal (chronic insufficiency, tubular acidosis)
Hematologic (chronic anemia)
Skeletal (rickets, pseudohypoparathyroidism)
Metabolic (glycogen storage disease)
Endocrinologic (hypopituitarism, hypothyroidism, hyperadrenocorticism)

Psychosocial deprivation

Adapted from Root AW, et al. Short stature: when is growth hormone indicated? *Contemp Pediatr* 1987;4:26.

adolescent is significantly shorter than he or she ought to be is by accurately measuring his or her height and then plotting it on a standardized growth chart. Measurement of height should be done carefully and in a consistent manner using proper technique [5] (Fig. 8). Some DO's and DON'Ts are listed in Table 4. It is best to have some idea of which population was used to formulate the chart, because some ethnic groups are shorter than American whites and African Americans. If the height of the teen falls below the third percentile for his age on the standardized chart, he, by definition, has short stature [6]. About 50% of the children referred to an endocrinologist for short stature do not fit this definition [4]. The clinician should look at the shape of the curve formed by plots of height at various times in the past to decide whether, in addition to being short, the youth is growing abnormally slowly (Figs. 9 through 11). Of those 50 children who are short, only 12 or 13 will have an abnormally slow height velocity [4].

The other information that the clinician must have, to begin with, is the bone age as determined by radiographs of the wrists and knees. In addition, an assessment of whether pubertal development (Tanner stage) is consonant with the height age (the age at which the patient's height falls at the 50th percentile) or with the chronologic age is essential. If the slope of the growth curve is not abnormal and pubertal development is consonant with the height age, it may not be necessary to obtain bone age radiographs at that time. Along with these specific explorations of growth, a general physical examination is necessary to detect conditions that may have caused or contributed to the short stature. In girls, for example, the physician should look for signs of Turner's syndrome (Table 5). Aphthous ulcers in the mouth and rectal fissures along with lack of growth might indicate Crohn's disease. Alternatively, the history might reveal a familial obsession with weight; a calorie count could show insufficient caloric intake that has led to nutritional dwarfism [7].

When the initial evaluation suggests an endocrinologic cause of growth delay, such as growth hormone (GH) deficiency, referral to a pediatric endocrinologist is necessary. Despite the fact that the

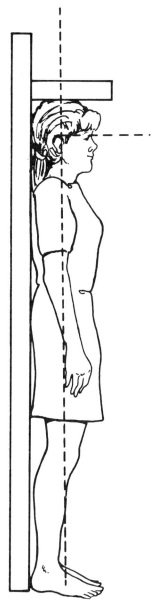

FIG. 8. Proper technique for measurement of height.

primary practitioner will not be carrying out intensive evaluations of growth problems, he or she should be familiar with what the endocrinologist will be doing. A basic knowledge of the processes involved in growth is necessary.

Causes of Short Stature

Factors that influence growth include genetic ones such as chromosomal abnormalities and skeletal dysplasias. Nutritional factors (as in nutritional dwarfism and Crohn's disease) can have considerable

TABLE 4. *DOs and DON'Ts*

Do	Don't
Measure the child's height and weight at least once annually, twice if possible.	Measure with a combined height/weight scale with a swinging arm.
Place a tape measure against the wall or the back of a door. The child should stand with shoulders, buttocks, and heels against the tape. To read the measurement, position a right-angled object on the child's head and against the tape.	Determine short stature solely on the basis of height. A physiologic disorder is indicated by poor growth velocity.
Calculate and plot the midparental height (MPH) and the target height (MPH ± 10 cm).	Underestimate the psychosocial implications of short stature in your evaluation of a child.
Determine the percentile ranking for age and plot all measurements on a standard growth chart.	

Adapted from Allen DB, Blizzard RM, Rosenfeld RG. The use—and misuse—of growth hormone *Contemp Pediatr* 1995;12:45.

impact. Chronic illnesses such as renal, cardiac, and pulmonary diseases can affect growth negatively. Mass lesions in the region of the hypophysis, such as craniopharyngiomas, also can cause growth failure. Finally, one must consider such endocrine problems as GH-related conditions and thyroid disease.

Growth hormone-releasing factor (GRF) is produced by the hypothalamus and stimulates the anterior pituitary gland to produce GH. GRF (and somatotropin release-inhibiting hormone) are modulated by a variety of other factors, including adrenergic, cholinergic, and dopaminergic stimuli and nutritional and emotional factors [8]. GRF appears to modulate the amount of GH secreted, and somatostatin secretion appears to control the frequency and duration of the GH secretory pulse [9]. GH exerts at least part of its growth-enhancing effect through the somatomedins, also known as *insulin-like growth factors* (IGF). The IGFs stimulate protein synthesis and cell proliferation at the tissue level.

There is considerable evidence that the pubertal rise in GH secretion is sex steroid dependent. First, the pubertal rise in IGF-1 and GH suggests that increasing sex steroid production may be the cause [10,11]. In addition, testosterone administration and low doses of estrogen both increase IGF-1 levels [12,13].

The child or adolescent with classic GH deficiency is usually short, normally proportioned, slightly overweight, and has a cherubic facial appearance. With evidence of a height velocity of less than 5 cm per year and of GH deficiency on overnight measurement or on provocative testing, the diagnosis can be made (assuming other causes have been ruled out) [13]. With GH deficiency and a normal growth rate, it is impossible to tell whether a child is growing too slowly. Patients with classic GH deficiency usually have no detectable cause (i.e., idiopathic), although a minority have tumors or other causes. Normal serum concentrations of IGF-1 and IGF binding protein-3 argue against GH deficiency [4].

Other short children can have neurosecretory GH deficiency (NGHD). These children have short stature, decreased growth velocity, low or normal somatomedin levels, bone age delay of more than 2 years, and abnormally low spontaneous secretion of GH. However, they have normal levels of GH secretion on provocative testing. NGHD may occur more frequently than classic GH deficiency [14]. Whether GH treatment will benefit these children with ultimate increase in adult height is still not clear [8]. Some suggest that children who receive GH, but who are not GH deficient, should be part of a controlled study [15,16]. Some children who have undergone cranial irradiation for leukemia have been found to have this variant [17,18].

In addition to the aforementioned syndromes, a child may also present with GRF deficiency, end-organ unresponsiveness to GH, or with somatomedin deficiency.

Familial short stature is characterized by a child with short parents, a bone age consonant with the chronologic age, and by a growth curve that follows the normal pattern even though it is significantly below the third percentile. Constitutional delay of growth and development is suggested by a child who is growing at a normal or mildly decreased rate, but who is delayed in pubertal development, and whose bone age significantly lags behind the chronologic age. The key here is the delay in puberty vis-à-vis chronologic age but not compared to bone age. These children achieve normal adult heights.

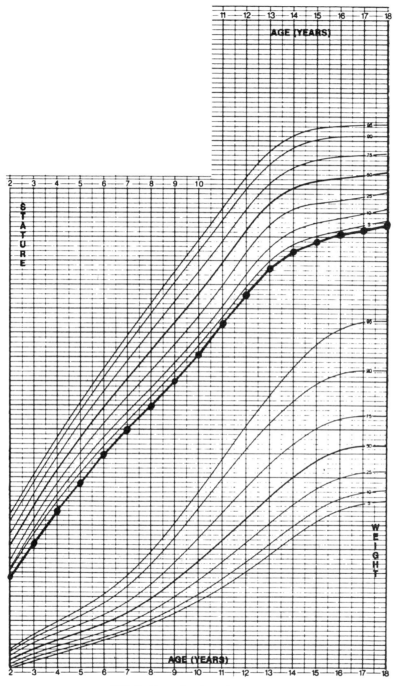

FIG. 9. Normal variant short stature.

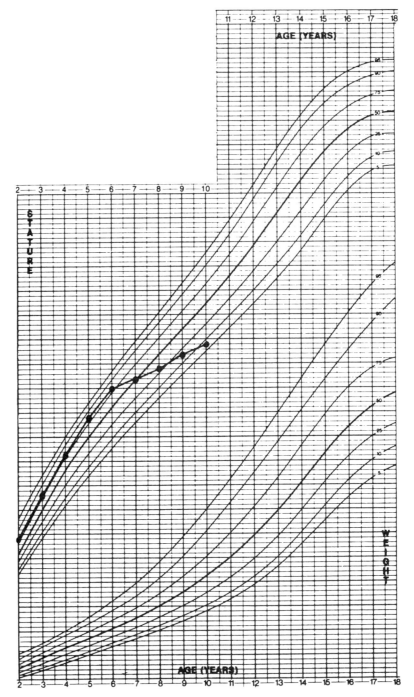

FIG. 10. Acquired growth hormone deficiency.

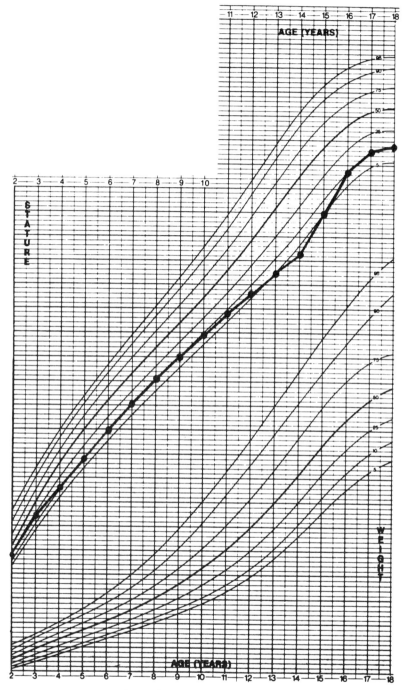

FIG. 11. Constitutional delay of growth.

TABLE 5. *Clinical features of Turner's syndrome*

Short stature	Extremity abnormalities
Gonadal failure	Wide carrying angle
Neck abnormalities	Short fourth and fifth metacarpals
Short neck	Congenital lymphedema
Webbing	Nail dysplasia
Low posterior hairline	Clinodactyly
Chest abnormalities	Cardiovascular abnormalities
Shield chest	Abnormal renal arteries
Hypoplastic nipples	Abnormal collecting systems
Facial abnormalities	Horseshoe kidney, etc.
Micrognathia	Miscellaneous
Rotated ears	Hashimoto's thyroiditis
Narrow, high-arched palate	Glucose intolerance
Ptosis	Multiple pigmented nevi
Epicanthal folds	Recurrent otitis media

Adapted from Underwood LE, et al. *Human growth and growth disorders: an update* (monograph). San Francisco: Genentech, Inc., 1989.

Treatment of Short Stature

Growth hormone deficiency is treated with biosynthetic human GH. With the ready availability of GH, there is much controversy over who should receive treatment other than those children with definite classic GH deficiency. GH has been used for many years to treat classic GH deficiency. Until biosynthetic GH became available, the only source of GH was pituitary glands from human cadavers. GH from 20 to 50 pituitary glands was needed to treat 1 patient for 1 year. This limited supply and the fact that it was controlled almost entirely by a government agency ensured that only those patients who absolutely needed it received the drug. However, with the discovery in the middle 1980s that human GH might be linked to a degenerative brain disease similar to Creutzfeldt-Jakob disease, and with the advent of the ability to manufacture biosynthetic GH, a potentially unlimited supply of GH became available.

With adolescents, the cardinal principle is that, to have any effect, there must be potential for growth. If the teenager is already a Tanner stage 4 or 5, there is little room for more growth, and the short teenager at this stage is destined to be a short adult. For the adolescent who is not only short but is in early puberty, or is prepubertal, there may be hope.

As stated earlier, the patient with classic GH deficiency needs to be treated with biosynthetic human GH. Which others should be treated with GH is still open to question [19]. GH administered under experimental protocols to several groups of slowly-growing children can increase growth velocity over the short term. These groups include children with Turner's syndrome [20], intrauterine growth retardation, chronic renal failure, and non–GH-deficient short stature [8,19,21]. Whether this treatment will ultimately help these children achieve their true potential height is unknown because no long-term data are yet available. Growth past the child's calculated genetic height potential has not been reported.

Prospective candidates for treatment must be informed that treatment involves daily injections given for years—in some cases, many years, because the earlier a problem is diagnosed and treated, the better the results. GH treatment should continue until growth is finished; height can continue to be gained up to the end of puberty [22]. In addition, treatment is expensive, $200 or more per month. Third-party payors may balk at covering this expense if there is no documentable need for the therapy.

Those children, or adolescents, who have secondary short stature benefit from treatment of their primary problem. They usually demonstrate catch-up growth and, if their previous debility was not too great, come close to achieving their potential height.

To summarize the guidelines for use of GH: 1) GH is safe and effective in treating growth failure due to GH deficiency; 2) GH also appears to be helpful in children with renal insufficiency or with Turner's syndrome; 3) GH does not help to increase height in constitutional delay of growth, nor is it helpful in children with other growth disorders; and 4) GH administration should be carried out by an experienced pediatric endocrinologist, and decisions on who should receive GH should be individualized, considering all aspects of the child's life [23].

Pubertal Delay

Delay of the onset or progression of puberty may accompany short stature or may be independent of it. Lists of possible causes are given in Tables 6 and 7. In girls, Turner's syndrome and its variants must be considered. This is true when there is no sexual development as well as when there is no progression after the onset of puberty. Nutritional causes of delay, as in anorexia nervosa, must also be considered. Athletes involved in gymnastics, long-distance running, and ballet also may have delayed onset of pubertal development. Boys must be investigated for Klinefelter's syndrome, although here, puberty usually has a normal onset [24]. As with short stature, pubertal delay can be a result of chronic illness, such as hypothyroidism and Crohn's disease.

The most common cause in boys is constitutional delay in growth and development. As stated earlier, these adolescents have delayed onset of puberty, slow progression through puberty, and, generally, short stature. Height can be normal for age but without pubertal development. They should have normal nutrition, no history or evidence of systemic illness, normal body proportions, and a normal physical examination [25,26]. Bone age is significantly delayed compared with the chronologic age. All laboratory data, including thyroid hormone and GH levels, should be normal, with gonadal hormones and gonadotropins appropriate for the bone age (Table 8). Constitutional delay does occur in both sexes, but societal bias leads to few girls being brought to medical attention. Therefore, more than 90% of the patients referred to endocrinologists are male [25].

The morbidity from constitutional delay is primarily psychosocial. A disproportionate number of children with this problem have behavioral difficulties and social withdrawal. They have low self-

TABLE 6. *Classification of hypogonadism in girls*

Hypergonadotropic hypogonadism (primary ovarian failure)
Congenital
   Turner's syndrome (XO) and its genetic variants
   Variant gonadal dygenesis (XO, SY, with sex ambiguity)
   Ovarian dysgenesis with 46, XX karyotype
   Dysmorphic syndrome association (Noonan's syndrome, XX)
Acquired
   Surgical or traumatic castration
   Postradiotherapy or postimmunosuppressive therapy
   Oophoritis associated with autoimmune diseases, thyroiditis, Addison's disease, lupus erythematosus
   Chronic infections (tuberculosis)
   Premature ovarian failure of unknown origin

Hypogonadotropic hypogonadism (secondary ovarian failure)
Hypothalamic
   Sporadic or familial gonadotropin deficiency
   Gonadotropin deficiency with anosmia
   Isolated deficiency of luteinizing hormone or follicle-stimulating hormone
   Suprasellar tumor
   Congenital anomaly of the hypothalamus
   Associated with dysmorphic syndromes (e.g., Prader-Willi-Labhart syndrome, Laurence-Moon-Biedl syndrome)
   Posttraumatic
Pituitary
   Panhypopituitarism
   Pituitary tumors (prolactinoma)
   Associated with growth hormone deficiency
   Posttraumatic

Delayed puberty
Sporadic
Familial (+++)
Associated with a chronic disease

Adapted from Sizonenko PC. Delayed sexual maturation. *Pediatrician* 1987;14:202.

TABLE 7. *Classification of hypogonadism in boys*

Hypergonadotropic Hypogonadism (primary testicular deficiency)
Congenital
    Klinefelter's syndrome and chromatin-negative syndromes
    XYY syndrome
    Various forms with sexual ambiguity and XO/XY, SY karyotype
    Congenital anorchism
    Noonan's syndrome (male Turner's syndrome)
    Enzymatic deficiency of testosterone synthesis
    Absent Sertoli cells
    Hereditary degenerative and polymalformation syndromes: Steinert's disease (myotonic dystrophy),
        ataxia telangiectasia, Werner's syndrome, Smith-Lemli-Opitz syndrome, leopard syndrome,
        Bloom's syndrome
    Kallman's syndrome (some rare cases)
Acquired
    Traumatic or surgical castration
    Rudimentary testes syndrome
    Bilateral orchitis
    Leydig cell hypoplasia
    Azoospermia
    Postradiotherapy or postimmnunosuppressive therapy

Hypogonadotropic hypogonadism (secondary testicular deficiency)
Hypothalamic
    Sporadic or familial gonadotropin deficiency
    Gonadotropin deficiency and anosmia (Kallman's syndrome)
    Isolated luteinizing hormone deficiency (fertile eunuch syndrome) or follicle-stimulating hormone defi-
        ciency
    Suprasellar tumors
    Congenital anomaly of the hypothalamus
    Association with a malformative syndrome: Prader-Willi-Labhart syndrome, Laurence-Moon-Biedl
        syndrome, congenital ichthyosis, etc.
    Posttraumatic

Delayed puberty
Sporadic
Familial
Associated with a chronic disease

Adapted from Sizonenko PC. Delayed sexual maturation. *Pediatrician* 1987;14:202.

TABLE 8. *Criteria for presumptive diagnosis of normal variant constitutional delay*

No history of systemic illness
Normal nutrition
Normal physical examination, including body proportions
Normal thyroid and growth hormone levels
Normal CBC, sedimentation rate, electrolytes, BUN
Height below the third percentile, but with a growth rate of at least 3.5 cm/yr
Delayed puberty
    Boys: Failure to achieve G2 (testicular volume of 4 ml) by 13 1/2 years of age or P2 by 14 years
    Girls: Failure to achieve B2 by 13 years of age
Delayed bone age (1–4 yr retarded)
Normal predicted adult height
    Boys: At least 64 inches
    Girls: At least 59 inches

CBC, complete blood count; BUN, blood urea nitrogen; G2, Tanner genital stage 2; P2, Tanner pubic hair stage 2; B2, Tanner breast stage 2.
From Rosenfeld RG. Constitutional delay in growth and development. *Semin Adolesc Med* 1987;3:267.

esteem, feel that they are unpopular, and are less satisfied with life in general than are their normal-stature peers [1,27]. Although these young adolescents have no physical abnormalities, they definitely have reason for medical attention and for treatment. The question is what the treatment should be.

Three studies confirmed previous reports that monthly administration of testosterone intramuscularly for 4 to 12 months significantly accelerates both height growth and pubertal development [27–29]. After treatment, growth and development proceeded normally, and final height attainment was close to, or at, pretreatment predicted heights. Pubertal development kept pace with height advancement. The dose of testosterone enanthate used was 50 mg in one study and 100 mg in the other. Because the results were similar, 50 mg can be recommended as the dose to use in most situations. The indication for treatment is a young teenager who fits the criteria for constitutional delay and is suffering significant psychological effects from this problem. Human GH does not seem to be necessary for successful enhancement of growth and development in these patients.

Girls with delayed puberty and no other hormonal or physical abnormalities pose a therapeutic dilemma. It has been suggested that they receive oral oxandrolone for 6 months until they attain a bone age of 10 years. If, at 13 years of age, puberty has yet to begin, girls may be treated with low-dose estrogen for 6 months [26].

REFERENCES

1. Gordon M, Crouthamel C, Post EM, et al. Psychosocial aspects of constitutional short stature: social competence, behavior problems, self-esteem, and family functioning. *J Pediatr* 1982;101:477.
2. Crawford JD. Meat, potatoes, and growth hormone. *N Engl J Med* 1981;305:164.
3. McDaid A, Finkelstein J. Psychosocial issues associated with short stature. *Adolescent Medicine: State of the Art Reviews* 1994;5:57.
4. Allen DB, Blizzard RM, Rosenfeld RG. The use—and misuse—of growth hormone. *Contemp Pediatr* 1995;12:45.
5. Preece M. Assessment of physical growth and pubertal development. *Adolescent Medicine: State of the Art Reviews* 1994;5:1.
6. Penney R. Growth retardation [Editorial]. *American Journal of Diseases of Children* 1989;143:1269.
7. Lifshitz F, Moses N, Cervantes C, et al. Nutritional dwarfing in adolescents. *Seminars in Adolescent Medicine* 1987;3:255.
8. Cara JF. Growth hormone in adolescence: normal and abnormal. *Endocrinol Metab Clin North Am* 1993;22:533.
9. Devesha J, Lima L, Tresguerres JAF. Neruoendocrine control of growth hormone secretion in humans. *Trends in Endocrinology and Metabolism* 1992;3:175.
10. Cara JF, Rosenfield RL, Furlanetto RW. A longitudinal study of the relationship of plasma somatomedin-C concentration to the pubertal growth spurt. *American Journal of Diseases of Children* 1987;141:562.
11. Luna AM, Wilson DM, Wibbelsman CJ, et al. Somatomedins in adolescence: a cross-sectional study of the effect of puberty on plasma insulin-like growth factor-1 and -2 levels. *J Clin Endocrinol Metab* 1983;57:268.
12. Rosenfield Rl, Furlanetto R. Physiologic testosterone or estradiol induction of puberty increases plasma somatomedin-C. *J Pediatr* 1985;107:415.
13. Ross JL, Cassorla FG, Skerda MC, et al. A preliminary study of the effect of estrogen dose on growth in Turner syndrome. *N Engl J Med* 1983;309:1104.
14. Bercu BB, Shulman DS, Root AW, et al. Growth hormone (GH) provocative testing frequently does not reflect endogenous GH secretion. *J Clin Endocrinol Metab* 1986;63:709.
15. Loche S, Cambiaso P, Setzu S, et al. Final height after growth hormone therapy in non-growth-hormone-deficient children with short statures. *J Pediatr* 1994;125:196.
16. Hopwood NJ, Hintz RL, Gernter JM, et al. Growth response of children with non-growth-hormone deficiency and marked short stature during three years of growth hormone therapy. *J Pediatr* 1993;123:125.
17. Kirk JA, Stevens MM, Menser MA, et al. Growth failure and growth-hormone deficiency after treatment for acute lymphoblastic leukemia. *Lancet* 1987;1:190.
18. Romshe CA, Zipf WB, Miser A, et al. Evaluation of growth hormone release and human growth hormone treatment in children with cranial irradiation-associated short stature. *J Pediatr* 1984;104:177.
19. Lippe B, Frasier SD. How should we test for growth hormone deficiency, and whom should we treat? *J Pediatr* 1989;115:585.
20. Hintz RL. New approaches to growth failure in Turner syndrome. *Adolescent and Pediatric Gynecology* 1989;2:172.
21. Kulin HE, Müller J. The biological aspects of puberty. *Pediatr Rev* 1996;17:75.
22. Cara JF, Kirschner B, Rosenfield RL. Growth response to growth hormone (GH) treatment (Rx) initiated in late adolescence. *Pediatr Res* 1989;25:3A.
23. Drug and Therapeutics Committee of the Lawson Wilkins Pediatric Endocrine Society. Guidelines for the use of growth hormone in children with short stature. *J Pediatr* 1995;127:857.

24. Klinefelter HF Jr, Reifenstein EC Jr, Albright F. Syndrome characterized by gynecomastia, aspermatogenesis without aleydigsm and increased excretion of follicle-stimulating hormone. *J Clin Endocrinol Metab* 1942;2:615.
25. Rosenfeld RG. Constitutional delay in growth and development. *Seminars in Adolescent Medicine* 1987;3: 267.
26. Ghai K, Rosenfield RL. Disorders of pubertal development: too early, too much, too late, or too little. *Adolescent Medicine: State of the Art Reviews* 1994;5:19.
27. Richman RA, Kirsch LR. Testosterone treatment in adolescent boys with constitutional delay in growth and development. *N Engl J Med* 1988;319:1563.
28. Kaplowitz PB. Diagnostic value of testosterone therapy in boys with delayed puberty. *American Journal of Diseases of Children* 1989;143:116.
29. Rosenfield RL. Diagnosis and management of delayed puberty. *J Clin Endocrinol Metab* 1990;70:559.

SUGGESTED READING

Brown RT. Assessing adolescent development. *Pediatr Ann* 1982;7:587.
Drug and Therapeutics Committee of the Lawson Wilkins Pediatric Endocrine Society. Guidelines for the use of growth hormone in children with short stature. *J Pediatr* 1995;127:857.
Kulin H, Müller J. The biological basis of puberty. *Pediatr Rev* 1996;17:75.
Layman L, Reindollar R. Diagnosis and treatment of pubertal disorder. *Adolescent Medicine: State of the Art Reviews* 1994;5:37.
Litt IF. Pubertal and psychosocial development: implications for pediatricians. *Pediatr Rev* 1995;16:243.
Rosenfeld RG. Is growth hormone just a tall story? *Pediatrics* 1977;130:1720.
Rosenthal SL, Biro F. Communication with adolescents and their families. *Adolescent and Pediatric Gynecology* 1991;4:57.
Styne D. Physiology of puberty. *Adolescent Medicine: State of the Art Reviews* 1994;5:171.

2

The Office Visit

AMBULATORY CARE FOR ADOLESCENTS AND THE OFFICE ENCOUNTER

The majority of health care delivery occurs in the ambulatory setting, and this is no less true for adolescents than it is for other age groups. To maximize the health of adolescents, it is generally agreed that adolescents need periodic visits to health care providers [1]. Many factors influence the system of health care provision for adolescents, and many factors affect adolescents' desire and ability to avail themselves of available health care services. In this chapter, we discuss these factors and attempt to provide the clinician with helpful guidelines to use in their care of adolescent patients.

Access to Care

It is particularly important for adolescents to have easy access to health care services. Adolescence, although a time of relative freedom from de novo organic disease, is a time of increased morbidity and mortality from causes such as violence, sexual behavior, and psychosocial factors such as family or learning problems. If the onset or consequences of these factors are to be prevented or ameliorated, the adolescent must be able to see a health care provider promptly with as little impediment as possible.

Today, that is not always the case. Factors such as lack of, or inadequate, insurance, ethnicity, lack of assurance of confidentiality, and unprepared or inhospitable providers limit adolescents' access to health care services. Other limiting factors include inadequate transportation and inconvenient office hours.

Adolescents and young adults have the lowest rate of primary care use and have lower rates of insurance coverage than any other American age cohort [2–3]. More African-American youths and Hispanic youths are uninsured compared with white adolescents [4]. Not being insured leads to not seeking preventive health services. Instead, uninsured youths do not seek care altogether or seek care only in emergencies. Even if uninsured adolescents do access health care, frequently they may not follow instructions to obtain further services or prescriptions because of the expense. Having a usual source of care and having insurance are strong predictors of routine use of medical care, whereas medical need, in conjunction with factors such as age and gender, are more predictive of seeking illness-related care [5]. A study of what adolescents find desirable in a health care provider concluded that the most important characteristics were:

- Provider hand-washing
- Clean instruments
- Honesty
- Respect toward teens
- Cleanliness
- Know-how
- Carefulness
- Experience
- Seronegativity for human immunodeficiency virus
- Equal treatment of all patients
- Confidentiality [6]

Clearly then, cleanliness, respect for the adolescent, and confidentiality are critical factors for provision of adolescent health care.

The Society for Adolescent Medicine stated in its position paper on "Access to Health Care for Adolescents" that health services for adolescents be evaluated by the following criteria:

- Availability
- Visibility (recognizable and convenient)
- Quality
- Confidentiality
- Affordability
- Flexibility
- Coordination (assurance that services must be comprehensive) [7]

Availability means that the practitioner should be able to see adolescents at somewhat nontraditional times such as evenings or weekends. Practitioners should make it known, such as by listings in local medical directories, that they want to see adolescents. Clinicians need to convey that they understand and have knowledge of adolescent issues. Services must be provided confidentially when it is in the best interest of the adolescent, and the provider must be accepting of teens with different life-styles. Finally, the clinicians should be aware of and have relationships with resources in the community that can provide consultative services to adolescents with varying needs.

The Health Encounter

Each visit by an adolescent to a clinician is a critical one. Whether the visit is for general reasons, such as a health maintenance examination, or for a more specific reason (i.e., an acute illness), each visit provides the clinician with an opportunity to explore potential problem areas in the adolescent's life. Certain principles should govern each health care encounter with an adolescent. Some of these have been mentioned in the previous section, but they are worth emphasizing.

The first visit by an adolescent to a practitioner, or the first visit as an adolescent to a practitioner who has provided child health care to this patient, can be critical to effective, ongoing health care for the adolescent.

It is at the initial visit that the physician garners all the crucial background information necessary to deliver comprehensive care to the adolescent, and it is at this time that the physician begins to establish, with the adolescent, the rapport that is essential to an effective therapeutic relationship. The first visit is also the physician's opportunity to define clearly to the teenager's parents the ground rules for future care of their child. Even if the physician has cared for this patient since birth, the first visit as an adolescent can be viewed as a new beginning and can be treated as a true initial visit.

One reason for obtaining a comprehensive picture of an adolescent at the first visit is that the physician may not see the teenager for a long while after that visit. Adolescents are notorious for not going to the doctor. The only time they may be seen again is for a camp or sports physical examination. This avoidance of medical contact necessitates what has been called the "one-stop shopping" approach to adolescent health care, which means getting as much done during one visit as is humanly possible. Another reason for obtaining comprehensive information from the start is that most adolescent health problems fall into the classification of the *new morbidity* [8] that is, problems not due to acute organic derangements but rather to social, psychological, or economic causes. A narrow medical workup misses problems such as these. For true health care, a comprehensive approach such as that recommended in the American Medical Association Guidelines for Adolescent Preventive Services is necessary [1].

OBTAINING INFORMATION

Written Forms

A convenient and time-saving method to help achieve a comprehensive examination is to use printed forms that the patient and his, or her, parents can complete before the visit or while they are waiting to be seen. In addition, a nurse or another office assistant can get the initial history from the adolescent and enter it on a preprinted form, which the physician can then use. These methods save time and make it possible to obtain the most information in a single visit.

In one of our clinics, three forms are used for the initial visit. One is a structured history form filled out by the nurse, or physician, while the patient is being interviewed. The form contains questions that address issues in each of the so-called "five boxes" (Fig. 1). The next half of that form contains information to be obtained from the physical examination. The second form is a questionnaire for the parents to complete while they are waiting for their teenager to be seen. It elicits information about the adolescent's history, the family history, and any concerns the parents might have about their child. It also asks for the reason for this visit; this is helpful, because, at times, the parents' reason for having their teenager seen and the teenager's reason for being seen are not the same. The third form is our so-called "worry form" (Fig. 2). This is a check-off form with a Likert scale that asks the adolescent to grade things, both medical and otherwise, that worry him or her. The worry form is very helpful in eliciting a true picture of each adolescent's concerns, so that we may address those worries and also engage in topic-oriented education.

The Interview

When all the paperwork is finished, the most important component of the visit—the interview—begins. The attitude of the interviewer and the method of asking questions are crucial both to effective history taking and to establishing rapport with the adolescent. The interviewer should find ways of putting the adolescent at ease quickly. Each person has his or her own style. One that works for many clinicians is to find an area in which the teenager has demonstrated interest, as gleaned from the complete forms. For example, if the physician notes that extracurricular activities include cheerleading, then that is a good topic with which to open. When at a loss for an opening, the interviewer can always ask the reason for the visit. Follow that up with an inquiry as to whether the visit was the adolescent's idea or that of the parents. If the patient and parents differ on this, explore the reason for the discrepancy.

To ensure that the history is as complete as possible, a system is needed. One of the authors has developed the five-box system [9] (see Fig. 1). The idea is that each adolescent's life involves five fairly

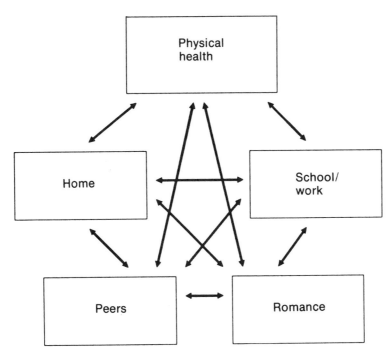

FIG. 1. The five boxes. (Reprinted with permission from Brown RT, et al. Treating the adolescent: the initial meeting. *Semin Adolesc Med* 3:79, 1987.)

			1	2	3	4	5	6	7	8	9	10	11	12	13	14	15	16
P	P	P	P	P	P	P	P	P	P	P	P	P	P	P	P	P
8	8	8	8	8	8	8	8	8	8	8	8	8	8	8	8
4	4	4	4	4	4	4	(4)	(4)	(4)	4	4	4	4	4	4
2	2	2	2	2	2	2	2	2	2	2	2	2	2	2	2
1	1	1	1	1	1	1	1	1	1	1	1	1	1	1	1

THINGS THAT WORRY ME   MR # _____

Instructions: We are interested in your worries or concerns. That is why we call this survey **THINGS THAT WORRY ME**. Please rate only worries that you actually have now or have had in the past. Remember, there aren't any right or wrong answers to this survey5 ____ and all of your answers are confidential. Fill in the circle under the number4 ____ that best describes the amount of worry that you have for each of the   3 ____ statements on the computer form: 1 - not a worry, 2 - little worry, 2 ____ 3 - medium worry, 4 - big worry, 5 - huge worry.   1 ____

		1	2	3	4	5
1.	Going to a new school	1	2	3	4	5
2.	Thoughts of killing myself	1	2	3	4	5
3.	Having a sick relative at home	1	2	3	4	5
4.	Will I get AIDS?	1	2	3	4	5
5.	Getting my feelings hurt	1	2	3	4	5
6.	The possibility of nuclear war	1	2	3	4	5
7.	Handling stress and anger	1	2	3	4	5
8.	Eating too much	1	2	3	4	5
9.	Being made fun of	1	2	3	4	5
10.	Parent away from home too much	1	2	3	4	5
11.	Getting pregnant or getting someone pregnant	1	2	3	4	5
12.	World hunger	1	2	3	4	5
13.	My face	1	2	3	4	5
14.	Making friends	1	2	3	4	5
15.	My periods	1	2	3	4	5
16.	Getting bad grades	1	2	3	4	5
17.	My friends' use of drugs and/or alcohol	1	2	3	4	5
18.	My parents' mental health/physical health	1	2	3	4	5
19.	Popularity with friends and/or classmates	1	2	3	4	5
20.	My parents' divorce	1	2	3	4	5
21.	My physical health	1	2	3	4	5
22.	Getting hurt physically	1	2	3	4	5
23.	Using drugs	1	2	3	4	5
24.	How I do in sports	1	2	3	4	5
25.	Problems with teachers	1	2	3	4	5
26.	Terrorism	1	2	3	4	5
27.	Having an abortion	1	2	3	4	5
28.	New stepfather or stepmother	1	2	3	4	5
29.	My weight	1	2	3	4	5
30.	Getting cancer	1	2	3	4	5
31.	The effect of AIDS on the world	1	2	3	4	5
32.	Crying without a good reason	1	2	3	4	5
33.	Sexually transmitted disease/VD	1	2	3	4	5
34.	Whether I am homosexual	1	2	3	4	5
35.	Feeling that I am a bad person	1	2	3	4	5
36.	People not listening to me	1	2	3	4	5
37.	Feeling depressed or sad most or all of the time	1	2	3	4	5
38.	Going to church	1	2	3	4	5
39.	Being shy	1	2	3	4	5
40.	My body	1	2	3	4	5

FIG. 2. Worry form

distinct areas and that questions pertaining to each are needed for a complete interview. The first is the *medical box*. Here the key questions involve the standard medical history. Second is the *home box*, for which the key questions involve the patient's relationships with parents and siblings, the parents' marital status and its implications, the family's financial situation, and so forth. The third box is the *school and work box*. Key questions here are geared to detecting areas of scholastic difficulty and what implications the adolescent's employment, or lack thereof, might have. Fourth is the *peer box*, with questions centering around best friends (each adolescent has friends, but each should also have a best friend; the absence of a best friend may indicate problems), peer group activities, and high-risk behaviors such as drug or alcohol misuse. For sensitive issues such as substance use, it is best to open the topic with nonthreatening questions such as, "Lots of kids are getting into trouble these days because they're experimenting with alcohol or drugs. Are any of your friends having these kinds of problems?" This type of questioning avoids direct confrontation with the patient and decreases anxiety about discussing this topic. The fifth box is the *romance box*, which is where inquiries about sex-

Fill in the circle under the number that best describes the amount of worry that you have nor or have had for each of the statements on the computer form: 1 - not a worry, 2 - little worry, 3 - medium worry, 4 - big worry, 5 - huge worry.

		1	2	3	4	5
41.	Being sexually abused	1	2	3	4	5
42.	Eating too little	1	2	3	4	5
43.	Arguments with my parents	1	2	3	4	5
44.	The environment	1	2	3	4	5
45.	Breaking up with boyfriend/girlfriend	1	2	3	4	5
46.	Job/career	1	2	3	4	5
47.	Not being treated my age	1	2	3	4	5
48.	Trouble with the law	1	2	3	4	5
49.	My parents use of alcohol or drugs	1	2	3	4	5
50.	Getting along with someone of the same sex	1	2	3	4	5
51.	My mental health	1	2	3	4	5
52.	Moving out on my own	1	2	3	4	5
53.	Using alcohol	1	2	3	4	5
54.	Taking tests at school	1	2	3	4	5
55.	Not having enough money	1	2	3	4	5
56.	Feeling out of control	1	2	3	4	5
57.	Vomiting after I eat	1	2	3	4	5
58.	Mother/father loss of a job	1	2	3	4	5
59.	Not seeing or hearing from my father/mother	1	2	3	4	5
60.	Working at a job while I go to school	1	2	3	4	5
61.	Getting along with someone of the opposite sex	1	2	3	4	5
62.	Pressure to try drugs and/or alcohol	1	2	3	4	5
63.	Getting raped	1	2	3	4	5
64.	My own illness	1	2	3	4	5
65.	My appearance	1	2	3	4	5
66.	Being hit by my parents	1	2	3	4	5
67.	Going crazy	1	2	3	4	5
68.	Thoughts about sex or having sex	1	2	3	4	5
69.	Whether I am like other people	1	2	3	4	5
70.	Being alone	1	2	3	4	5
71.	Wanting to live somewhere else	1	2	3	4	5
72.	My parents fighting	1	2	3	4	5
73.	Being in a car crash	1	2	3	4	5
74.	Having no friends	1	2	3	4	5
75.	My own death	1	2	3	4	5
76.	Feeling guilty	1	2	3	4	5
77.	Going to school	1	2	3	4	5
78.	Running Away	1	2	3	4	5
79.	Sleeping too little or too much	1	2	3	4	5
80.	My girlfriend having an abortion	1	2	3	4	5

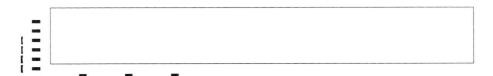

FIG. 2. *Continued.*

ual activity belong. Again, a nonthreatening approach to this topic is best to ensure gathering the most information. Try questions such as, "Are many of your friends sexually active? Tell me how you feel about that" or "Sexually transmitted diseases such as AIDS or herpes are big problems today. Do you ever worry that you could get one of these diseases?" Questions about sexual assault and sexual abuse best fit in this box also, although exploration of sexual abuse may fit better in inquiries about the home situation. Key questions for each of the five boxes are listed in Table 1.

Another technique that facilitates information gathering is the obtaining of history by more than one person, if possible. Adolescents may find it easier to discuss problem topics with one interviewer

TABLE 1. *Questions designed to detect possible problems in the five boxes*

Box	Questions
Physical health	(Usual medical history)
Home	With whom do you live?
School	(Age versus grade)
	What are your school grades now compared with this time last year?
Peers	Who is your best friend?
	Do any of your friends use drugs or alcohol frequently?
Romance	How old is your boyfriend (girlfriend)?
	When did you last have sex?

From Brown RT, Henderson PB. Treating the adolescent: the initial meeting. *Semin Adolesc Med* 1987;3:79.

rather than another. Hence, if a nurse and a physician, for example, can each interview the teenager, more information may be obtained.

Interviewing the parents is also an essential part of the initial visit. Although it is good practice for those working in adolescent medicine to see the teenager alone, so as to allow him or her the opportunity to discuss private concerns and to develop medical self-responsibility, the practitioner should not ignore the parents. Parents frequently know much more about the family's medical history and about the adolescent's early history. In addition, the parents' perspective on the real problems of their teenager is frequently different from that expressed by the adolescent. Therefore, it is beneficial to interview the parents, using their written form for cues, while the teenager is undressing for the physical examination. After getting the parents' story, the physical examination is performed on the adolescent, and then the parents and their child are brought together for explanation of findings and home-going instructions. The visit could begin by interviewing the parent and child together and then interviewing them individually. If there is confidential material that needs to be discussed with the adolescent, that is done before the joint meeting with the parents. Home-going instructions should be written as well as verbal to allow no room for misinterpretation.

Finally, it is worth mentioning a few words about interview style. The best technique to interview adolescents is the mutual participation style [10]. The interviewer, in this format, invites the teen to participate in a discussion instead of being a passive receiver of another lecture by an adult. For example, when discussing a behavior of the adolescent that may be risky, the clinician could ask the adolescent to relate how he or she would handle such behavior in a child of their own. One could also ask the adolescent to rate the good points and bad points of certain behaviors and then add them up to see if the risk is significant. Medical interviews are said to obtain the necessary information if the questions are asked in an open-ended fashion. Such a question might be, "How are you?" An adolescent, uncomfortable and scared about what may happen in the encounter, even if sick, probably will answer, "Fine," even if there are considerable problems that need to be discussed. A better method is to ask directed questions such as, "Do you have a health problem you'd like me to help you with today?"

THE PHYSICAL EXAMINATION

The physical examination can be a very trying experience for the adolescent, and it occasionally can be wearing on the physician as well. Certain procedures can assist in making it a more bearable experience for all involved.

The first fact that needs to be recognized by the physician is that the teenager will be embarrassed. Most adolescents live in a constant state of embarrassment, so this is not surprising; however, the embarrassment engendered by being naked in front of a stranger is especially disconcerting. Occasionally, the physician's impression of the degree of embarrassment can be skewed by the physician's own discomfort in examining a near-adult when he or she is used to seeing prepubertal children primarily. The physician must recognize this and learn to cope if he or she is to be effective with adolescents.

There are several ways of helping to diminish the level of discomfort for the adolescent being examined. After having the teenager disrobe to his or her underpants, have her or him put on a gown. A small item that can save a lot of discomfort is whether the gown opens in the front or the back. For a general examination in which the most attention will be paid to the front of the chest (heart and breasts), having the gown open in the front saves a lot of awkward manipulation. Having the gown open in the back does the same when the primary concern is looking at the back or listening to the lungs. In addition to the gown, we routinely use a sheet with girls and offer its use to boys. We have the adolescent wrap the sheet around the waist and, when the patient lies down, we move the sheet and gown in tandem so as to expose as little skin as possible.

Discussing the adolescent's own embarrassment is a good way to defuse the anxiety it generates. By telling the patient it is okay to be embarrassed and that adults feel the same way when they have a physical examination, the burden of hiding the embarrassment and trying to act adult is relieved. Using the physical examination as an educational experience helps alleviate anxiety as well. While the examiner is explaining what the various findings are (e.g., "Did you know you had a pulse here in your groin?" or "This graininess in your breast is normal. Why don't you feel it so you'll be sure of what I mean?"), the teenager has moved out of the patient mode and into the student mode, one with which she or he is intimately familiar and, therefore, with which he or she is much more comfortable. While being a student, the patient feels much less stress, and so the anxiety of the examination experience is lessened. The educational aspect of the examination is especially helpful when examining the breasts and the genitalia.

Other than making the adolescent as comfortable as possible, there is little that is different about the examination of the adolescent and that of the adult or child. One's emphasis may differ, however. Pay close attention to the adolescent's face, particularly the skin. Acne is practically a physiologic (rather than pathologic) part of adolescence. It is so common that the physician can forget to note the presence of a few comedones unless a mental note is made to remember. Also, the teenager may never mention concerns about his or her skin unless the physician brings it up. Another area that needs a little extra attention is the thyroid. Thyroid disease can become evident in adolescence, so particular attention to the thyroid gland on physical examination is indicated. An easy way to detect an enlarged thyroid gland is to have the adolescent extend his or her neck fully while the physician views the area from the side. An enlarged gland will be evident in this way. Of course, palpation is also done.

When the parts of the examination that are done in the sitting position are completed, have the teenager lie down. Beginning this part of the examination at the feet and working up the body is effective. When the tops of the thighs are reached in girls, an opportunity arises to look at the crotch of the underpants. This can be an easy way to see if stains from any discharge are present. Examination of the abdomen leads naturally to palpation of the femoral pulses, at which time the physician can look at the pubic hair to rate its Tanner stage.

Breast examination should be performed on every girl and boy. Gynecomastia in a boy who is in early puberty can be entirely normal, whereas its presence in a more developed (stage 4 or 5) boy can be of concern. Either way, the opportunity should be taken to remark on it, either as a normal finding or as something that needs further attention. For girls, breast examination can be extremely embarrassing. However, as mentioned earlier, teaching while you are examining can alleviate much anxiety. Breasts should be examined not only for masses and for Tanner stage but also for disparity in size. Many girls do not know that one breast may be slightly larger than the other one and still be perfectly normal. A more noticeable difference should be noted to the patient and, even if she says it does not bother her, the possibility of correction should be mentioned for future reference. Whether breast self-examination should be taught to adolescents is an issue of some controversy [11,12]. It has been standard for years to teach this technique for early cancer detection to all postpubertal women. However, the value of such instruction in early and middle adolescents has been questioned because of the near-nonexistence of breast cancer in this age group as well as in young adult women. Both authors teach breast self-examination to all girls who are at Tanner stage 5 breast development, primarily to prepare the girls for its later use and to ensure that they will know proper technique when they need to use it.

Examination of the genitalia in boys is important for several reasons. First, it is the only way to check pubertal development. Second, lesions, including those suggestive of a sexually transmitted disease, can be detected. Third, palpation of the scrotum for a varicocele needs to be done. Fourth, testicular self-examination needs to be taught. The incidence of testicular cancer peaks in the young adult years, so all young men should be taught how to palpate their testes and should be instructed on why it is important to do so [13]. Teenage boys take this instruction very seriously because there is little more valuable to them than their testicles. Fifth, every boy wants to hear that he is normal. If the boy gets an erection while having his genitalia examined, do not ignore it. Instead make a comment to the effect that, "This kind of thing can happen to anyone while they are undergoing a physical examination, so don't worry about it." This reassures the boy that he is not unusual. The fact that the erection is totally involuntary does not make it any less embarrassing for him.

TABLE 2. *Screening tests and procedures*

Mandatory	May be advisable
Diphtheria and tetanus (dt) booster (at 15 years of age)	Purified protein derivative of tuberculin (PPD)
Measles, mumps, and rubella (MMR) booster (if not given previously)	Varicella vaccine
	Urinalysis
Hepatitis B immunization	Hearing
Vision	Breast self-examination instruction
Teeth (caries and malocclusion)	Sickle cell screening
Testicular self-examination instruction	Glucose-6-phosphate dehydrogenase (G6PD) screening
Complete blood cell count (CBC)	Cholesterol

The last area usually checked is the back for scoliosis. Idiopathic scoliosis most commonly begins in early adolescence and in girls. Ideally, all girls should be checked early in puberty, because the time to detect significant scoliosis is while it is progressing rapidly, which is during the girl's growth spurt at pubic hair stage 2 and before menarche occurs. The examination is done from the rear with the patient bending over at the waist parallel to the floor with head and arms dangling down loosely. A prominence of one rib hump over the other and a traceable curve are reason for a radiographic examination to measure the degree of the curve, and may warrant referral to an orthopedist (see Chapter 3, under Common Musculoskeletal Problems).

A pelvic examination is routine only for girls who are sexually active. For virgins, when no symptoms are present, the first pelvic examination need not be done until the young woman is about to leave high school. This is as good a time as any for her to begin having routine examinations with Pap smears. A detailed description of the proper approach to this most sensitive examination is presented in Chapter 5.

The physical examination does not have to be a terribly traumatic event for the adolescent. Proper attention to the teenager's delicate feelings and awareness of problems that can be of particular concern to adolescents make it a positive and productive experience for both the adolescent and the physician.

Laboratory tests to look for various conditions and certain screening procedures should be performed at the initial visit. Mandatory tests and those that may be advisable are listed in Table 2.

IMMUNIZATIONS

Adolescence is a time in which many of the childhood immunization sequences come to a conclusion, or at least are finished for several years. Adolescents should have a second tetanus/diphtheria immunization between 12 and 15 years of age. If the second measles–mumps–rubella immunization has not been administered before adolescence, it too should be given. Hepatitis B immunization should be recommended to all adolescents until such time as the infants who are receiving it now reach their adolescence [14]. Varicella vaccine is now available, and it should be offered to all adolescents who do not have a history of natural infection [15]. Currently, it is not known if a second varicella immunization is needed for teenagers who receive their first one as infants. Tuberculosis is very uncommon in children in the United States; therefore, routine purified protein derivative testing should be given only to adolescents who have direct contact with someone with active tuberculosis or to adolescents who have lived in endemic areas, such as some foreign countries [16].

THE SETTING

The physical setting in which the adolescent is seen is somewhat important, although not nearly as important as the personnel. All personnel who come in contact with adolescent patients should, first and foremost, enjoy people in this age group. Many adolescents will tolerate Disney characters on the walls, but they will not take kindly to judgmental, demeaning, intolerant people. One of the key people in the office in this regard is the receptionist. The receptionist who genuinely enjoys teenagers and conveys an interest in them will increase the chances that the whole visit will be perceived positively. A receptionist who is abrupt, cold, or condescending can put a damper on the whole visit.

Although the people who interact with the adolescent are of paramount importance, a physical setting with nondemeaning decor also lends a positive tone to the visit. This does not mean one must display posters of rock groups or use black lights, but subdued, conservative decor with no cartoon characters, in at least part of the office suite, is helpful. Tables in examination rooms used for seeing teenagers should be of adult size, as should chairs both in these rooms and in the waiting area. Another nice touch that appeals to teenagers and to their parents is the ready availability of pertinent health literature in the waiting area and in the rooms. There are many pamphlets, available either free of charge or for a nominal fee, that the physician can obtain and have on hand for the adolescents and their parents to read and take home with them.

SCHOOL-BASED HEALTH CARE

School-based health centers (SBHCs) are becoming increasingly common sites for delivery of ambulatory health services to adolescents. Schools have been the site of delivery of certain services such as vision, hearing, and scoliosis screening for a long time, and schools traditionally have been major sites for health education [17]. More recently, increased efforts have been made to make schools a major loci for integration of social, educational, and health services with a community focus. The Centers for Disease Control and Prevention have been promoting a concept of comprehensive school health programming that does not necessarily include on-site provision of health care. A third effort has been the establishment of many school bases or linked health clinics in middle and high schools for direct provision of health services to underserved adolescents [17]. SBHCs have generated some controversy because of community resistance to provision of sexuality-related services in publicly funded schools, but, in general, these clinics have been successful in bringing services to previously underserved youth. Issues for SBHCs in the coming years, in addition to provision of sexuality-related services, include provision of services when schools are closed and the relationships of SBHCs and third-party payors in a managed care environment [18].

CONSENT AND CONFIDENTIALITY

Two topics that should be broached at the initial visit are consent and confidentiality. It is generally agreed by physicians who specialize in adolescent medicine that each adolescent, and his or her parents, should be informed at the first visit that care will be given confidentially and on the adolescent's own consent when, in the judgment of the physician, the adolescent is deemed capable of understanding that to which he or she is being asked to consent and its implications [19,20]. What should be explicitly stated to both the parents and the patient is that if, in the judgment of the physician, the parents need to know something or if adult judgment is needed for true informed consent, then the physician will so inform the parents. This issue is discussed further in Chapter 9.

REFERENCES

1. American Medical Association. *Guidelines for adolescent preventive services (GAPS)*. Chicago: American Medical Association; 1992.
2. *Adolescent health. Vol. I: Summary and policy options*. Document OTA-H-468. Washington, DC: U.S. Congress, Office of Technology Assessment; April, 1991.
3. Newacheck PW, McManus MA, Gephart J. Health insurance coverage of adolescents: a current profile and assessment of trends. *Pediatrics* 1992;90:589.
4. Lieu TA, Newacheck PW, McManus MA. Race, ethnicity, and access to ambulatory care among US adolescents. *Am J Public Health* 1993;83:960.
5. Ryan SA, Millstein SG, Greene B, et al. Utilization of ambulatory health services by urban adolescents. *J Adolesc Health* 1996;18:192.
6. Ginsburg KR, Slap GB, Cnaan A, et al. Adolescents' perceptions of factors affecting their decisions to seek health care. *JAMA* 1995;273:1913.
7. Society for Adolescent Medicine. Access to health care for adolescents: a position paper of the Society for Adolescent Medicine. *J Adolesc Health* 1992;13:162.

8. Haggerty RJ. The changing role of the physician in child health care. *American Journal of Diseases of Children* 1974;127:545.

9. Brown RT, Henderson PB. Treating the adolescent: the initial meeting. *Seminars in Adolescent Medicine* 1987;3:79.

10. Rosenthal SL, Biro FM. Communication with adolescents and their families. *Adolescent and Pediatric Gynecology* 1991;4:57.

11. Goldbloom RB. Self-examination by adolescents [letter]. *Pediatrics* 1985;76:126.

12. O'Malley MS, Fletcher SW. Screening for breast cancer with breast self-examination: a critical review. *JAMA* 1987;251:2196.

13. Goldenrigh JM. Equal time for men: teaching testicular self-examination. *Journal of Adolescent Health Care* 1986;9:38.

14. The Medical Letter, Inc. New recommendations for immunization against pertussis and hepatitis B. *The Medical Letter* 1992;34:69.

15. The Medical Letter, Inc. Varicella vaccine. *The Medical Letter* 1995;37:55.

16. Doerr CA, Starke JR. Tuberculosis: when to test. *Contemp Pediatr* 1996;13:82.

17. Lear JG. School-based services and adolescent health: past, present, and future. *Adolescent Medicine: State of the Art Reviews* 1996;7:163.

18. Brellochs C, Zimmerman D, Zink T, et al. School-based primary care in a managed care environment: options and issues. *Adolescent Medicine: State of the Art Reviews* 1996;7:197.

19. Smith J, Felice M. Interviewing adolescent patients: some guidelines for the clinician. *Pediatr Ann* 1980;1:38.

20. Johnson RL, Tanner NM. Approaching the adolescent patient. In: Hofmann AD, Greydanus DE, eds. *Adolescent medicine*. 2nd ed. Norwalk, CT: Appleton & Lange; 1989:18.

SUGGESTED READING

Beach RK. Priority behaviors in adolescents: health promotion in the clinical setting. *Adolescent Health Update* 1991;3:1.

Committee on Bioethics. Informed consent, parental permission, and assent in pediatric practice. *Pediatrics* 1995;95:314.

Jenkins RR, Saxena SB. Keeping adolescents healthy. *Contemp Pediatr* 1995;12:75.

Long WA. Practice management and the teenage patient: a practical approach to adolescent care in the clinical setting. *Adolescent Health Update* 1990;2:1.

Litt IF. *Evaluation of the adolescent patient*. Philadelphia: Hanley & Belfus; 1990.

Murray-Garcia J. African-american youth: essential prevention strategies for every pediatrician. *Pediatrics* 1995;96:132.

Orr DP. Charting the journey through adolescence: the role of anticipatory guidance. *Adolescent Health Update* 1989;1:1.

Smith J, Felice M. Interviewing adolescent patients: some guidelines for the clinician. *Pediatr Ann* 1980;1:38.

Society for Adolescent Medicine. Access to health care for adolescents: a position paper of the Society for Adolescent Medicine. *J Adolesc Health* 1992;13:162.

3

Common Medical Problems

ACNE

Acne is a nearly universal disease of adolescents, with an incidence approaching 80% to 90% [1,2]. Unfortunately, acne is so well associated with adolescence that some clinicians overlook or dismiss it. Once acne reaches the inflammatory stage, it can scar the face, back, or chest for life. Not only can early intervention help to prevent this complication, but it can also prevent the psychological scars of acne as well. Given adolescents' normal self-consciousness about themselves and their appearance, helping them to deal with this disorder is extremely important. In one study, 58% of adolescent patients were upset with their appearance, 75% felt embarrassed, and over half were socially inhibited because of their acne [3]. Psychological factors may play an important role in several different ways [4,5]:

- Stress can exacerbate acne.
- Acne patients may suffer from lower self-esteem, social withdrawal, or depression, compared with their clear-complexioned peers.
- Primary psychiatric disease may present with patients focusing on their lesions (e.g., obsessive–compulsive disorder).

Few teenagers actually seek help in treating their acne, particularly from nondermatologists. Teenagers spend over $100 million per year on over-the-counter acne medicines that are not as effective as prescription drugs [6]. Primary care physicians probably can treat 90% of teenagers with the disorder—all but those with severe nodular or cystic acne who require Accutane or acne surgery [7,8]. In addition, offering help to teenagers with blemishes can establish an immediate rapport with them: they are coming to the doctor's office for some other problem or examination, and yet the physician takes the time to talk to them about their appearance.

Etiology

Acne is a disorder of adolescence because of the role that androgens play in stimulating sebaceous glands in the skin [9,10]. Although the exact pathogenesis of acne remains unclear, much is already known (Table 1, Fig. 1). The action takes place in the pilosebaceous units, which consist of the sebaceous glands, ducts, and rudimentary hair follicles that are found on the face, upper chest, and upper back. Follicles are lined by epidermal cells that, in acne patients, are abnormally sticky, because of faulty keratinization. This makes the follicle more likely to plug. Under androgenic stimulation, sebaceous glands empty sebum into the follicle as well. Sebum is a viscous, complex mixture of triglycerides, waxy esters, and other lipids. Although the sebum excretion rate is elevated in patients with acne, it is not completely predictive of who will have lesions and who will be spared [11]. Finally, the follicle is colonized by normal skin bacteria, including *Propionibacterium acnes*, a gram-positive anaerobe. These bacteria contain lipases that can break down triglycerides into free fatty acids and incite a strong inflammatory reaction—hence the need for antibiotics.

This basic unit of trouble—keratin, sebum, and bacteria—is called a *comedo*. If the follicle's opening to the surface is tight, the lesion is a closed comedo or "whitehead"; if the pore is open, it is an open comedo or "blackhead." Although blackheads are unsightly, they are relatively inert and can simply be expressed by an eyedropper or comedo extractor. The blackness of blackheads probably comes from melanin, not dirt or surface oxidation [1]. On the other hand, closed comedones are little

TABLE 1. *Acne myths*

1. Acne is caused or exacerbated by:
   • Chocolate
   • Fried foods
   • Too much or too little sex
2. Only dermatologists should treat acne.
3. Blackheads are caused by dirt.
4. Scrubbing blackheads will get rid of them.
5. Long-term use of tetracycline is harmful.
6. Acne is a part of adolescence and will go away on its own.
7. All teenagers with acne need to take Accutane.

Adapted from Strasburger VC. Acne: what every pediatrician should know about how to treat it. *Pediatr Clin North Am* 1977 (in press).

time bombs, waiting for the follicular wall to rupture and set in motion a potentially devastating inflammatory process. When a follicle ruptures, sebum and free fatty acids (from hydrolysis of triglycerides) infiltrate the surrounding dermis, activating complement and attracting polymorphonuclear leukocytes [10,12,13]. Inflammatory acne elicits a repair response in which dermal collagen is laid down, producing the pitting scars typical of this disorder. If the inflammation extends beyond single pilosebaceous units, then nodulocystic acne is produced, which usually requires referral to a dermatologist.

Acne is classified according to whether it is comedonal or inflammatory (Table 2). It is absolutely essential to begin treatment as early as possible during the comedonal stage to prevent subsequent inflammation and scarring.

Contributing Factors

Because acne presumably has a multifactorial etiology, many factors either contribute to or exacerbate it. Acne, especially severe acne, tends to have a genetic predisposition. Any androgenic stimulation worsens acne, hence the typical premenstrual "flare" when cycles are progestin dominant, or the worsening of acne when androgenic oral contraceptives (OCs) are used (e.g., Lo-Ovral, Ovral, Loestrin

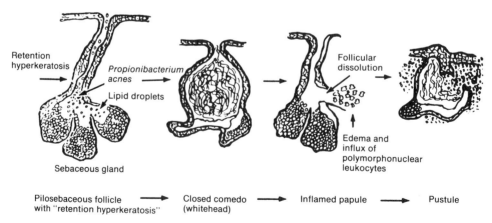

FIG. 1. Pathogenesis of acne. Although blackheads are unsightly, whiteheads (closed comedones) are responsible for the sequence of events leading to follicular rupture, inflammation, and scarring. (Reprinted with permission from Hurwitz S. Acne vulgaris: pathogenesis and management. *Pediatr Rev* 1994;15:47, as adapted from *American Journal of Diseases of Children* 1979;133:536. Copyright 1979, American Medical Association.)

TABLE 2. *Classification and treatment of acne*

Grade I (comedones)
 Benzoyl peroxide 2.5–5% gel at bedtime *or*
 Retin-A 0.025–0.05% cream at bedtime
Grade II (comedones and papules)
 Benzoyl peroxide 2.5–5% gel at bedtime *or*
 Retin-A 0.025–0.05% cream at bedtime
 Topical antibiotics once or twice a day if any inflammation is present
Grade III (pustules)
 Benzoyl peroxide 2.5–5% gel in the morning *and*
 Retin-A 0.025–0.05% cream or 0.025% gel at bedtime
 Topical antibiotics twice a day
 Systemic antibiotics, 500–750 mg twice a day, if necessary
 Consider trying Azelex 20% cream, twice a day, if pustules or scars are hyperpigmented (use instead
  of Benzoyl peroxide and Retin-A)
Grade IV (nodulocystic acne)
 Benzoyl peroxide 2.5–5% gel in the morning *and*
 Retin-A 0.025–0.05% cream or 0.025% gel at bedtime
 Topical antibiotics twice a day
 Systemic antibiotics, 500–1000 mg twice a day
 Referral to a dermatologist—candidate for Accutane

1.5/30). Also, acne may be a marker for such hormonal disorders as polycystic ovarian disease or adrenal disorders [14]. Female teenagers who present with severe acne and others signs of androgen excess such as hirsutism, virilization, or irregular menses should be screened appropriately (e.g., a free testosterone level, a dehydroepiandrosterone sulfate (DHEAS) level, and a determination of follicle-stimulating hormone/luteinizing hormone ratio) [14,15]. Menstrual factors also play a role in worsening of acne just before onset of menses owing to a decrease in the actual size of follicles [16].

Immunologic mechanisms can be extremely important: the host response may make the difference between mild and severe acne. For example, tetracycline has been shown to decrease neutrophil chemotaxis, which may help to explain its usefulness in treatment [17]. Any agent that adds to the plugging of follicles will also worsen acne. This means that oil-based cosmetics must be avoided at all costs (Table 3). Likewise, hair that is worn over the forehead is not helpful.

In hot, dry climates, acne patients often improve, particularly during the summer months. Whether this is due to ultraviolet light or diminished stress is unclear. However, a few patients experience worsening of acne in summertime, especially if they sweat excessively. Other factors that are known to exacerbate acne include stress, drugs (e.g., steroids, lithium), and an XYY genotype [1,7].

One factor that has never been *scientifically* implicated in acne is diet. There is no evidence that chocolate, fatty or greasy foods, nuts, or junk food make acne worse. Excellent, controlled, double-blinded trials demonstrated that large doses of chocolate had no effect on acne [18]. Likewise, trials with other suspect foods have not shown any harmful effect [19]. Yet, it is probably still prudent to recommend avoidance of certain foods if patients are convinced that they "break out" in response to them, and to counsel families about good nutrition in general [20].

Classification

Treatment of acne depends on proper classification of the lesions, because different medications have differing modes of action. Acne is broadly classified into noninflammatory and inflammatory categories, and then further subdivided as follows:

Noninflammatory
- Comedonal acne
- Papular acne
Inflammatory
- Papulopustular acne
- Pustular acne
- Nodulocystic acne

TABLE 3. *Cosmetics: acceptable vs. comedogenic choices*

	Comedogenic	Noncomedogenic
Allercreme	Satin Finish Matte Finish Velvet Finish	Oil Free, Matte Finish
Almay		Fresh Look Oil Free Oil Free Foundation
Elizabeth Arden	Ardena Moisture Oil	Extra Control Oil Free Visible Difference
Clinique	Continuous Coverage Cover Rub	Pore Minimizer Stay-True
Max Factor	Pure Magic	Maxi-Unshine Oil Free
Mary Kay	Day Radiance	
Merle Norman	Aqua Base Warm Blusher	
Revlon	Natural Wonder Acne Spot Cover Ultimate II Formula 2 Highlighter	Fresh All Day Medicated Make-up
Moisturizers		
	Cocoa Butter Soft Sense Skin Lotion Vaseline Intensive Care	Keri Lyt Moisturel Neutrogena Purpose

Treatment

Early treatment of acne is essential and requires a coordinated plan of attack, including prescribing the correct medications, counseling, and guidance about contributory factors. Because acne is initially stimulated by the increase in androgen hormones, which is the earliest endocrinologic change in puberty, it is not uncommon to see 8- to 10-year-old girls with a few comedonal or papular lesions [21]. Early comedonal acne seems to correlate with more severe involvement later on, and is associated with higher levels of testosterone and DHEAS [21]. *Treating noninflammatory acne early, before inflammation and scarring can occur, is essential and represents one of the most important aspects of preventative health care in adolescent medicine.* Experience with a few drugs is all that is necessary (Tables 2, 4), and the physician's arsenal is far more effective than what is available over-the-counter.

Benzoyl Peroxide

Benzoyl peroxide—available in cream, lotion, or gel form—is the mainstay of acne treatment for most patients. It is an irritant and keratolytic agent that causes follicular desquamation, lowers free fatty acids in the epidermis, and helps to disrupt the compaction within the follicle. In addition, it functions as a topical antiseptic by suppressing the growth of *P. acnes*. Available in concentrations of 2.5%, 5%, and 10%, benzoyl peroxide's efficacy depends on its vehicle and solvent. Over-the-counter preparations in-

TABLE 4. *Potency of Retin-A preparations*

Degree of irritation	Vehicle	Concentration
Low	Cream	0.025% (new)
	Cream	0.05%
	Cream	0.1%
	Gel	0.01%
	Gel	0.025%
High	Solution	0.05%

clude lotions, creams, soaps, and washes, all of which may be less effective than gels, which are available by prescription only. A variety of 2.5%, 5%, and 10% gels are available, either in an alcohol or acetone base (both of which can be drying) or an aqueous base. The 2.5% gel is as effective against *P. acnes* as the 10% gel, but has considerably fewer side effects [22]. Common preparations include:

Alcohol or Acetone Base	Water Base
Benzagel	—
Benzac	Benzac-W
Desquam-X	Desquam-E
PanOxyl	PanOxyl Aq
Persa-Gel	Persa-Gel W
—	Xerac

Benzoyl peroxide is synergistic with tretinoin, and the two used together create an ideal treatment regimen for many patients. Also available is Benzamycin, which combines 5% benzoyl peroxide with 3% erythromycin in a water-based gel form.

Using benzoyl peroxide successfully requires adequate instruction. As a bleaching agent, benzoyl peroxide can be toxic to T-shirts, blouses, and sheets. Patients with oily, dark skin can tolerate the alcohol or acetone-based preparations better than fairer patients, who should use the water-based products. Its use should be initiated in gradual, step-wise fashion: after an initial test application on the forearm for a few hours (rarely, patients may have an allergic contact dermatitis), a low concentration is applied as a thin film to all acne-prone areas, initially every other day, gradually increasing within 2 to 3 weeks to twice daily-use of a 2.5% to 5% preparation. Because absorption is increased by moisture, *benzoyl peroxide preparations should never be applied immediately after washing the face.* Acne lesions on the chest and back can usually be treated with a 5% to 10% gel. Patients should be counseled that they may experience a little dryness or tingling, but persistent irritation warrants less frequent use.

Tretinoin (Retin-A)

Tretinoin (Retin-A) is a powerhouse of a drug, superior in many ways to benzoyl peroxide, but its use requires good compliance, counseling, and patient selection (not dry-skinned or poorly compliant patients). Topical vitamin A acid has a variety of actions: 1) increased cell turnover in the pilosebaceous ducts, 2) decreased stickiness of epidermal cells, and 3) expulsion of existing comedones. As such, it may take 2 to 3 months for a clinical effect to be seen, except that many patients may initially experience a *worsening* of their acne as microcomedones are expelled in the first 2 weeks. Therefore, patients must be counseled accordingly. For patients looking for immediate improvement, this is not the ideal drug.

Retin-A is available as a cream (0.025%, 0.05%, and 0.1%), gel (0.01% or 0.025%), or liquid (0.05%). Erythema, peeling, and dryness are frequent side effects, especially if the medication is not used properly. Retin-A is the drug of choice in pure comedonal acne. For patients with inflammatory acne, it can be used along with benzoyl peroxide and a topical antibiotic. Patients should be instructed *never to apply Retin-A to wet skin* and to wait at least 20 to 30 minutes after washing their faces before using it. Again, a very small amount of drug is all that is necessary. Treatment should begin with one of the lowest-strength preparations (0.025% or 0.05% cream, or 0.01% gel) two or three times weekly, gradually increasing to every other night, then nightly, and eventually twice a day. Because Retin-A thins the epidermis, liberal use of a noncomedogenic sunscreen with a sun-protective factor of 15 or greater should be prescribed during the summer and in sunny climates. Although skin cancers have developed in mice treated with Retin-A and ultraviolet light, there is no evidence of this effect in humans [23].

Topical Antibiotics

Since the early 1980s, topical antibiotics have been developed that are equivalent in effect to approximately 500-mg doses of oral tetracycline [24]. The following topical preparations are currently available:

Clindamycin	Cleocin-T 1% solution, gel, lotion (Upjohn)
Erythromycin	A/T/S 2% solution (Hoechst-Roussel)
	Benzamycin 3% gel with 5% benzoyl peroxide (Dermik)
	Erygel 2% gel (Allergan)

	Erycette 2% solution (Ortho)
	Eryderm 2% solution (Abbott)
	Erymax 2% solution (Allergan)
	T-Stat 2.0% solution, pads (Westwood)
Tetracycline	A/T/S 2% solution (Hoechst-Roussel)
	Meclan 1% cream (Ortho)

All of these medications have a drying effect, the gel being most drying, followed by the solutions, creams, and, finally, the ointments.

Of these preparations, topical clindamycin and erythromycin are most frequently used. All inhibit the growth of *P. acnes*. Although a few cases of pseudomembranous colitis have been reported with Cleocin, the risk appears to be extremely small because less than 5% of the drug is absorbed systemically [25]. However, the drug should be discontinued if significant diarrhea occurs. Topical tetracycline preparations can stain and also fluoresce under black light, as used in nightclubs and discotheques. But they do have the advantage of being contained in a moisturizing base, which is less drying.

Systemic Antibiotics

Although topical antibiotics get the drug immediately where it needs to go and are used frequently as initial agents, they have not completely replaced systemic antibiotics. If topical formulations are unable sufficiently to disrupt the inflammatory process within a few weeks, a course of systemic therapy is indicated in conjunction with the topical regimen. Again, tetracycline and erythromycin are the mainstays of systemic treatment. Tetracycline is one of the safest drugs in the formulary when used in long-term situations [1,26]. Side effects include candidal vaginitis, gastrointestinal irritation, and, rarely, pseudotumor cerebri and erythema multiforme [24,27]. Tetracycline is usually used in a dosage of 500 to 750 mg twice a day for 6 months, which is then gradually decreased to the lowest possible dose, often 250 to 500 mg once daily. It must be taken on an empty stomach because it is bound by milk or milk products.

Alternatively, similar doses of erythromycin can be used and are equally effective, but not as well tolerated. Doxycycline and minocycline are now available generically and are less expensive than previously, but have potentially greater side effects and should be reserved for patients with tetracycline-resistant acne [1,6,24]. Some dermatologists prefer minocycline because it is easy to use (100–200 mg/day), penetrates the sebaceous follicle better, and does not need to be taken on an empty stomach [28]. In rare cases, it has been associated with autoimmune hepatitis and a systemic lupus erythematosus-like syndrome, however [29].

Some concern exists about the development of antibiotic-resistant *P. acnes* [30], but the exact incidence of such strains and clinical implications remain unclear.

Oral Isotretinoin (Accutane)

In 1982, the U.S. Food and Drug Administration (FDA) approved the use of 13-*cis*-retinoic acid for treatment of acne. As a vitamin A derivative, Accutane has definite toxicity. On the other hand, it provides an impressive "knock-out punch" to sebaceous glands, totally abolishing sebum production during therapy [31]. *Use of Accutane is best left to dermatologists and should be confined to patients with severe cystic acne that is unresponsive to conventional therapy.*

Accutane is prescribed for a 16- to 20-week course of treatment, costing approximately $500 to $700 for the drug. Frequently, a second 20-week course is needed. Remarkably, acne remains quiescent even after therapy has been discontinued and the sebum excretion rate returns to normal [32]. Virtually all patients experience significant dryness of the face, lips, nasal mucosa, and conjunctivae. Bone pain is also a common side effect (15% of patients). Complete blood count, liver function tests, cholesterol, and triglycerides should be monitored. The drug can cause extremely high levels of serum lipids, although no liver damage occurs and the levels revert to normal once Accutane is discontinued [33].

By far the most dangerous and controversial side effect of Accutane is its teratogenicity, which affects 60% or more of exposed fetuses [34,35]. It should never be administered to a pregnant patient, and adequate birth control measures should be used. Unfortunately, much of the controversy surrounding Accutane derives from physicians either using the drug inappropriately or failing to monitor their patients for the possibility of pregnancy [36–38]. When used appropriately, Accutane is an important and necessary drug in the physician's armamentarium against severe cystic acne. It represents the only drug with proven efficacy in this otherwise dismal and scarring disorder.

Other Treatments

Patients with unsightly comedonal acne benefit from use of a comedone extractor (or eyedropper) to remove the blackheads. Careless "picking" or "popping" pimples, on the other hand, may exacerbate inflammation and lead to further scarring. Topical steroids are not generally useful and may worsen acne, but intralesional injection of triamcinolone into nodules or cysts can be helpful at times. Such patients warrant referral to a dermatologist unless the physician is experienced in such techniques.

New Treatments

In 1996, the FDA approved azelaic acid 20% cream (Azelex) for topical treatment of acne [39–41]. Azelaic acid is a "natural" product derived from wheat. It is comedolytic, can have fewer side effects than other topical medications, and may be particularly useful in causing the violaceous hue of pustules and scars to fade [41]. However, several months of treatment are required to produce this effect. The cream is used twice a day and comes in 30-g tubes.

Also recently approved is adapalene gel 0.1% (Differin), which is the first new topical retinoid in more than 25 years [42]. Although it is as effective as Retin-A gel 0.025%, it is less irritating, but few dermatologists have extensive experience with it.

Other products being investigated include topical antiandrogens, naphthoic acid, and tea-tree oil [42–44].

Treatment Tips

Primary care practitioners should remember that most teenagers will not ask to have their acne treated; instead, they will be using over-the-counter products and will think that only a dermatologist can treat their skin. However, teens appreciate any help once it is offered. Differentiating between noninflammatory and inflammatory acne is crucial: *significant pustular acne necessitates the immediate and vigorous use of oral antibiotics in addition to topical therapy* (the former may then be tapered or eliminated as the lesions are brought under control topically) [26,43,45]. Unfortunately, scarring is not predictable.

Some female teens will inevitably be taking OCs for birth control, dysfunctional uterine bleeding, or severe dysmenorrhea. Careful selection of OCs that contain the newer progestins (e.g., norgestimate, desogestrel) improve acne, whereas pills with androgenic progestins (e.g., norgestrel, levonorgestrel) may worsen acne. For this reason, acne can actually develop in 5% to 20% of patients using Norplant (it contains levonorgestrel) [14].

TABLE 5. *Common therapeutic mistakes in treating acne*

1. Too little explanation and counseling
2. Too little concern
3. Too complex a medication regimen
4. Inappropriate use of:
Estrogens
X-ray treatment
Vaccines
Dietary manipulation

TABLE 6. *Cost of common acne drugs*

Drug	Formulation	Cost[a]
Oral antibiotics		
Tetracycline	500 mg po bid	$ 2.25
Doxycycline	100 mg po bid	$ 2.90
Minocycline	100 mg po bid	$36.90
Topical antibiotics		
Clindamycin		
Cleocin T (Upjohn)	1% gel (solution, lotion)	30 g = $22.04
Erythromycin		
Emgel (Glaxo)	2% gel	27 g = $18.97
Erycette (Ortho)	2% solution	60 swabs = $21.24
T-Stat (Westwood)	2% solution	60 ml = $17.21
Erythromycin + Benzoyl peroxide		
Benzamycin (Dermik)	3%/5% gel	23.3 g = $29.99
Adapalene		
Differin (Galderma)	0.1% gel	15 gm = $22.08
Azelaic acid		
Azelex (Allergan)	20% cream	30 g = $28.88
Benzoyl peroxide (generic)	5% gel	45 g = $1.99
Tretinoin		
Retin-A (Ortho)	0.025% cream	20 g = $28.20
Isotretinoin (Accutane)	400 mg po qid	$163.31

[a]Wholesale cost to the pharmacist; 1-month supply.
Data from Adapalene for acne. *The Medical Letter* 1997;39(995):19; and Webster GF. Is it reasonable for a dermatologist to treat acne? *Arch Dermatol* 1996;132:819.

Teenagers are not always the most compliant of patients, but practitioners can adhere to several principles to try to maximize compliance [46] (Table 5):

- Reassure the teenager that acne is both common and treatable.
- Explain that acne cannot be scrubbed away.
- Do not overload teens with data. A few "take-home" messages are optimal.
- Allow teenagers time to ask questions.
- Remember to treat the teenager's back and chest if they are involved, not just the face.
- Give the teenager choices whenever possible (e.g., Retin-A vs. benzoyl peroxide).
- Be aware of the cost of medications (Table 6).
- Do not take noncompliance personally.

Acne is one of the most common and easily treated diseases of adolescents. Scarring can be prevented in most cases, with early and vigorous treatment. But such treatment requires patience, skill, and a commitment to good counseling.

REFERENCES

1. Hurwitz S. Acne vulgaris: pathogenesis and management. *Pediatr Rev* 1994;15:47.
2. Thiboutot DM, Lookingbill DP. Acne: acute or chronic disease? *J Am Acad Dermatol* 1995;32(Suppl):S2.
3. Krowchuck D, Stancin T, Keskinen R, et al. Does acne affect adolescents' self-concept? *American Journal of Diseases of Children* 1990;144:417.
4. Krowchuck DP, Stancin T, Keskinen R, et al. The psycho-social effects of acne on adolescents. *Pediatr Dermatol* 1991;8:332.
5. Koo J. The psychosocial impact of acne: patients' perceptions. *J Am Acad Dermatol* 1995;32(Suppl):S26.
6. Bergfeld WF. The evaluation and management of acne: economic considerations. *J Am Acad Dermatol* 1995;32(Suppl):S52.
7. Hurwitz S. *Clinical Pediatric Dermatology.* 2nd ed. Philadelphia: WB Saunders; 1993.

8. Strasburger VC. Acne: what every pediatrician should know about how to treat it. *Pediatr Clin North Am* 1997 (in press).
9. Goos SD, Pochi P. Endocrine aspects of adolescent acne. *Adolescent Medicine: State of the Art Reviews* 1990;1:289.
10. Leyden JJ. New understandings of the pathogenesis of acne. *J Am Acad Dermatol* 1995;32(Suppl):S15.
11. Kumasaka BH, Odland PB. Acne vulgaris: topical and systemic therapies. *Postgrad Med* 1992;92:181.
12. Dahl MGC, McGibbon DH. Complement C3 and immunoglobulin in inflammatory acne vulgaris. *Br J Dermatol* 1979;101:633.
13. Tucker SB, Rogers RS, Winkelmann RK, et al. Inflammation in acne vulgaris: leukocyte attraction and cytotoxicity by comedonal material. *J Invest Dermatol* 1980;74:21.
14. Lucky AW. Hormonal correlates of acne and hirsutism. Am J Med 1995;98(Suppl):1A.
15. Winston MH, Shalita AR. Acne vulgaris: pathogenesis and treatment. *Pediatr Clin North Am* 1991;38:889.
16. Williams M, Cunliffe WJ. Explanation for premenstrual acne. *Lancet* 1973;2:1055.
17. Kraus SJ. Stress, acne, and skin surface free fatty acids. *Psychosom Med* 1970;32:503.
18. Fulton JE, Plewig G, Kligman AM. Effect of chocolate on acne vulgaris. *JAMA* 1969;210:2071.
19. Anderson PC. Foods as the cause of acne. *Am Fam Physician* 3:102, 1971;.
20. Rosenberg EW, Kirk BS. Acne diet reconsidered. *Arch Dermatol* 1981;117:193.
21. Lucky AW, Biro FM, Simbartl LA, et al. Predictors of severity of acne vulgaris in young adolescent girls: results of a five-year longitudinal study. *J Pediatr* 1997;130:30.
22. Kligman AM. Acne vulgaris: tricks and treatments: II. the benzoyl peroxide saga. *Cutis* 1995;56:260.
23. Matsuoko LY. Acne and related disorders. *Clin Plast Surg* 1993;20:35.
24. Berson DS, Shalita AR. The treatment of acne: the role of combination therapies. *J Am Acad Dermatol* 1995;32(Suppl):S31.
25. Barza M, Goldstein JA, Kane A, et al. Systemic absorption of clindamycin hydrochloride after topical application. *J Am Acad Dermatol* 1982;7:208.
26. Leyden JJ. Therapy for acne vulgaris. *N Engl J Med* 1997;336:1156
27. Stuart BH, Litt IR. Tetracycline-associated intracranial hypertension in an adolescent: a complication of systemic acne therapy. *J Pediatr* 1978;92:679.
28. Rabinowitz L. Acne vulgaris. *Adolescent Medicine: State of the Art Reviews* 1997;8:77.
29. Ferner R, Moss C. Minocycline for acne. *Br Med J* 1996;312:138.
30. Wright M. Expert forecasts antibiotic-resistant *P. acnes* to be even bigger problem for patients. *Dermatology Times* September, 1996;S13;.
31. Peck GL, Olsen TG, Yoder FW, et al. Prolonged remissions of cystic and conglobate acne with 13-*cis*-retinoic acid. *N Engl J Med* 1979;300:329.
32. Abel E. Isotretinoin (Accutane) therapy for acne. *Adolescent Medicine: State of the Art Reviews* 1990;1:315.
33. Bershad S, Rubinstein A, Paterniti JR Jr, et al. Changes in plasma lipids and lipoproteins during isotretinoin therapy for acne. *N Engl J Med* 1985;313:981.
34. Beuke PJ. The isotretinoin teratogen syndrome. *JAMA* 1984;251:3267.
35. Lammer EJ, Chen DT, Hoar RM, et al. Retinoic acid embryopathy. *N Engl J Med* 1985;313:837.
36. Stern RS. When a uniquely effective drug is teratogenic: the case of isotretinoin. *N Engl J Med* 1989;320:1007.
37. Committee on Drugs, American Academy of Pediatrics. Retinoid therapy for severe dermatological disorders. *Pediatrics* 1992;90:119.
38. Mitchell AA, Van Bennekom CM, Louik C. A pregnancy-prevention program in women of childbearing age receiving isotretinoin. *N Engl J Med* 1995;333:101.
39. Fitton A, Goa KL. Azelaic acid: a review of its pharmacological properties and therapeutic efficacy in acne and hyperpigmentary skin disorders. *Drugs* 1991;41:780.
40. Mackrides PS, Shaughnessy AF. Azelaic acid therapy for acne. *Am Fam Physician* 1996;54:2457.
41. Medical Letter. Azelaic acid: a new topical drug for acne. *The Medical Letter* 1996;38(976):52.
42. Shalita A, Weiss JS, Chalker DK, et al. A comparison of the efficacy and safety of adapalene gel 0.1% and tretinoin gel 0.025% in the treatment of acne vulgaris: a multicenter trial. *J Am Acad Dermatol* 1996;34:482.
43. Sykes NL Jr, Webster GF. Acne: a review of optimum treatment. *Drugs* 1994;48:59.
44. Gibson J. Rationale for the development of new topical treatments for acne vulgaris. *Cutis* 1996;57(Suppl):13.
45. Nuguyen QH, Kim YA, Schwartz RA. Management of acne vulgaris. *Am Fam Physician* 1994;50:89.
46. Draelos ZK. Patient compliance: enhancing clinician abilities and strategies. *J Am Acad Dermatol* 1995;32(Suppl):S42.

SUGGESTED READING

Abel E. Isotretinoin (Accutane) therapy for acne. *Adolescent Medicine: State of the Art Reviews* 1990;1:315.
Bergfeld WF, Odom RB. New perspectives on acne. *J Am Acad Dermatol* 1995;32(Suppl):S1.
Cargnello JA. Acne: what's new? *Med J Aust* 1996;165:153.

Goos SD, Pochi P. Endocrine aspects of adolescent acne. *Adolescent Medicine: State of the Art Reviews* 1990;1:289.

Hurwitz S. *Clinical pediatric dermatology.* 2nd ed. Philadelphia: WB Saunders; 1993;.

Hurwitz S. Acne vulgaris: pathogenesis and management. *Pediatr Rev* 1994;15:47.

Kligman AM. Acne vulgaris: I. Tricks and treatments. II. The benzoyl peroxide saga. III. Antibacterials. IV. Treating severe inflammatory acne: the last word. *Cutis* 1995;56:141, 260, and 315; and 1996;57:26.

Leyden JJ. New understandings of the pathogenesis of acne. *J Am Acad Dermatol* 1995;32(Suppl):S15.

Mackrides PS, Shaughnessy AF. Azelaic acid therapy for acne. *Am Fam Physician* 1996;54:2457.

Medical Letter. Adapalene for acne. *The Medical Letter* 1997;39(995):19.

Nuguyen QH, Kim YA, Schwartz RA. Management of acne vulgaris. *Am Fam Physician* 1994;50:89.

Rabinowitz L. Acne vulgaris. *Adolescent Medicine: State of the Art Reviews* 1997;8:77.

Strasburger VC. Acne: What every pediatrician should know about how to treat it. *Pediatr Clin North Am* 1997 (in press).

Sykes NL Jr, Webster GF. Acne: a review of optimum treatment. *Drugs* 1994;48:59.

INFECTIOUS MONONUCLEOSIS

Case Example

A 15-year-old girl is admitted to the hospital for evaluation of her persistent fevers and lymphadenopathy [1]. She has been completely well until 2 weeks ago, when myalgias, arthralgias, and headaches developed. Four days later, she noted enlarged lymph nodes in her neck. A week ago, she consulted her physician, who ordered a complete blood count (normal), chest radiograph (normal), and a Monospot test (negative). During the ensuing week, she began having fevers up to 102°F and night sweats.

On physical examination, the patient is an attractive, healthy-looking, Tanner 5 teenager. She has a temperature of 101.1°F, many soft palate petechiae, large anterior and posterior cervical nodes and a few small axillary nodes, and a palpable spleen tip.

Laboratory data: white blood cell count (WBC) 11,100/mm^3, with 30% neutrophils and 52% lymphocytes (75% atypical); erythrocyte sedimentation rate 6 mm/hr; and platelet count 337,000/mm. A repeat Monospot is positive, and heterophil agglutination is positive at a 1:112 dilution. A repeat chest radiograph shows hilar adenopathy.

An internal medicine specialist reviews the chart, examines the patient, and informs the patient and her family that she has an acute lymphoma and will need a bone marrow aspiration and lymph node biopsy. But, he tries to reassure them, her prognosis for long-term survival after chemotherapy should be excellent.

Comments. Infectious mononucleosis (IM) is one of the most common infectious diseases seen during adolescence, with an attack rate as high as 1% to 5% of adolescents [2,3]. Because "common diseases occur commonly"—although sometimes, atypically—physicians who treat adolescents *must* become familiar with the spectrum of disease indigenous to this age group or risk misdiagnosing their patients, as the physician in the Case Example did. Had this physician appreciated the clinical picture [4], recognized the significance of the laboratory data [5], and understood the fact that hilar adenopathy can be seen in IM [6], he would have avoided making a serious error. All of these topics are discussed in some detail later. The physician in practice can expect to see several cases of IM per year, and the adolescent medicine specialist or college health physician can probably expect to see 10 to 50 cases per year. (By contrast, the incidence of lymphoma in adolescence is approximately 1.3 cases per 100,000 [7].) Among college-age students and military recruits, IM causes more missed days than any other infectious disease [2].

Mononucleosis Syndromes

Although Epstein-Barr virus (EBV) is most commonly associated with IM, it is not the only known cause. Cytomegalovirus (CMV), *Toxoplasma gondii*, rubella, hepatitis A, adenoviruses, and others can all cause a similar clinical picture (Table 7). The easiest differentiation is that all of these agents, with the exception of adenoviruses and occasionally rubella, are not typically associated with an acute pharyngitis [8]. Nor would any of them result in positive heterophil antibody titers. In addition, CMV is more commonly seen in young and middle-aged adults, although it is probably responsible for most cases of non–EBV-related IM during adolescence [3,9]. The subsequent discussion is confined to EBV because it remains the most significant etiologic agent in IM.

TABLE 7. *Differential diagnosis: heterophil-negative mononucleosis syndromes*

Etiology	Age group	Features
Epstein-Barr virus (EBV)	Mostly <25 y	Typical except for negative heterophil; Do EBV-IgM antibody test, if necessary
Cytomegalovirus	Mostly >25 y	Sore throat rare; minimal adenopathy; hepato-splenomegaly common
Toxoplasmosis	Any age	Sore throat rare; some lymphocytosis; cat or raw meat exposure
Hepatitis A	Young adult	Sore throat, adenopathy, splenomegaly rare; fever before jaundice
Herpesvirus-6	Any age	EBV-like illness with atypical lymphs
Adenovirus	Childhood and young adult	Respiratory symptoms usually prominent
Rubella	Childhood	With or without rash

The knowledge of the relationship between EBV and IM is a surprisingly recent one: it was not until 1920 that IM as we know it was described and named [10]. The etiologic importance of EBV was not clarified until the late 1960s [11–13]. Denis Burkitt had hypothesized that a lymphoma that was confined to tropical Africa was caused by a biologic factor transported by an insect vector [14]. Researchers began looking for viral particles in Burkitt's lymphoma tissue; in 1964, Epstein, Achong, and Barr isolated a herpes-like virus [11]. Soon after, the Henles, in Philadelphia [13], developed an assay for serum antibody directed against EBV-infected cell lines. Fortuitously, one of their technicians developed clinical IM. Her preillness serum was negative for the antibody, but her peripheral leukocytes were cultured after the illness and established a continuous line that harbored EBV antigen and a chromosomal marker previously seen only in Burkitt's tumor cell lines [13].

As a member of the family of human herpesviruses, EBV is a first cousin to herpes simplex 1 and 2, varicella-zoster virus, and CMV. Human herpesvirus-6 has been found to mimic acute EBV infection as well [15]. EBV is harbored in the saliva and nasopharyngeal washings of infected patients [16]. Infection requires transmission of infected saliva in substantial quantities—hence its reputation as "the kissing disease"—but it is not otherwise very contagious under normal conditions. One study indicates the possibility of sexual transmission as well, because EBV can be found in the genital tracts of both men and women [17]. EBV also has been associated with nasopharyngeal carcinoma, posttransplant lymphoma, and other rare immunoproliferative syndromes [18–20].

Epidemiology

Epstein-Barr virus is ubiquitous and causes disease in early infancy as well as adolescence [21]. By adulthood, virtually 100% of adults possess antibodies to EBV [20]. In underdeveloped countries, EBV infection is common in childhood, but in the United States, many middle-class adolescents and college-aged young adults have not yet encountered the virus [21]. Therefore, the attack rate is highest among 15- to 19-year-olds, approaching 3 to 4 cases per 100,000 [22]. Studies of entering college freshmen demonstrate that adolescents previously unexposed to EBV have a seroconversion rate of approximately 12% to 15% per year [23–25].

Pathogenesis

EBV infects B lymphocytes contained in lymphoid tissue of the oropharynx. Normally, infection triggers a self-limited (but excessive) immune response: B cells are transformed by the virus into plasmacytoid cells, capable of producing a wide variety of immunoglobulins, including rheumatoid factor, increased levels of IgG and IgM, cold agglutinins, antinuclear antibodies, and heterophil antibodies (Table 8). Within a few days, the T-cell response becomes dominant, with production of "atypical" lymphocytes that are mostly of the T-suppressor/cytotoxic type [21]. These cells search out and destroy the infected B cells [21]. Enlarged lymph nodes, liver, and spleen are the result of increased numbers of both infected B cells and reactive T cells [16]. Infection of B cells and immune surveil-

TABLE 8. *Humoral antibody responses in patients with mononucleosis*

Major antibodies
  Heterophil (Paul-Bunnel-Davidsohn)
  Specific anti-EBV antibodies
  Cold agglutinins (anti-i)
  Smooth muscle antibodies
Minor antibodies
  Rheumatoid factor
  Antinuclear antibodies
  Wasserman reagin (i.e., biologic false-positive VDRL)

EBV, Epstein-Barr virus; VDRL, Venereal Disease Research Laboratory.
  Adapted from Pearson GR. Infectious mononucleosis: the humoral response. In: Schlossberg D, ed. *Infectious mononucleosis.* 2nd ed. New York: Springer-Verlag; 1989:89–99.

lance of them is probably lifelong, which produces continuous levels of specific anti-EBV antibodies and may have important implications in neoplastic disease [2,18].

Clinical Picture

Infectious mononucleosis is the protean adolescent disease and can present in a variety of ways. The "classic" triad of sore throat, fever, and cervical lymphadenopathy is said to occur in 80% of patients, but this figure may be overly optimistic (Table 9, Fig. 2). Certainly, the teenager with a persistent pharyngitis, despite having been given penicillin for a presumed streptococcal infection, warrants screening. Because the incubation period is 30 to 50 days, contacts may be unknown or forgotten. Three separate clinical presentations have been described, but they are not always as well defined as in the textbooks [21,22]:

- *"Angiose syndrome":* the classic triad
- *Glandular form:* cervical lymphadenopathy out of proportion to the pharyngitis
- *Typhoidal or systemic form:* fever predominates, with little or no lymphadenopathy or pharyngitis

Typically, a viral prodrome occurs, with gradual onset of headache, chills, sweating malaise, anorexia, and inability to concentrate. Fever is often present for the first week or two but may remain up to 5 weeks, with afternoon or evening peaks to 100° to 103°F. A sore throat and severe dysphagia are the most troublesome symptoms, and about one third of patients have whitish exudates or grayish membranes on their tonsils. The exact incidence of group A streptococcal coincident infection is controversial: figures as high as 25% to 33% are frequently cited [21], but some researchers believe that

TABLE 9. *Symptoms and signs of infectious mononucleosis*

Symptoms	Frequency (%)	Signs	Frequency (%)
Sore throat	70–90	Adenopathy	95–100
Malaise/fatigue	45–77	Pharyngitis	70–90
Headache	35–55	Pharyngeal exudate	40–60
Anorexia	10–25	Fever	65–100
Myalgias	10–20	Splenomegaly	50–65
Nausea	2–15	Hepatomegaly	5–15
Abdominal pain	2–15	Palatal petechiae	5–15
Cough	5	Rash	0–15
Vomiting	5	Jaundice	5

Adapted from Radetsky M, Overturf GD. Epstein-Barr infections in adolescents and young adults. *Adolescent Medicine: State of the Art Reviews* 1995;6:91.

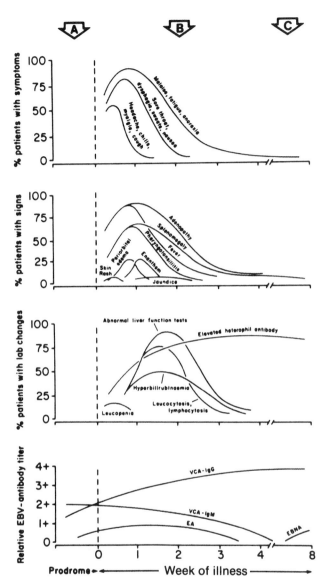

FIG. 2. Typical clinical and laboratory manifestations of infectious mononucleosis. Arrow A indicates asymptomatic prodrome, arrow B indicates the peak of clinical illness, and arrow C indicates early convalescence. (Grose C. The many faces of infectious mononucleosis. *Pediatr Rev* 1985;7:35. Copyright 1985. Reproduced by permission of *Pediatrics.*)

5% is a more accurate figure [3,26]. Adenopathy is uniformly present, but should involve posterior cervical as well as anterior cervical nodes [4].

Unusual presentations can occur. Mesenteric adenopathy can cause acute abdominal pain; axillary adenopathy can cause acute shoulder pain. Complications of IM can result in jaundice [27,28]; various neurologic presentations including coma, encephalitis, seizures, Guillain-Barré syndrome, or acute hallucinations ("Alice in Wonderland" syndrome) [29–32]; and, rarely, severe thrombocytopenia or hemolytic or aplastic anemia [5,33].

Diagnosis

Physicians who treat adolescent patients should always maintain a high index of suspicion about the occurrence of IM. The disease is somewhat milder in younger patients and in those with negative heterophil titers.

Ideally, the following criteria should be met to make a diagnosis of IM (Table 10):

- *Clinical:* Common symptoms: sore throat, posterior cervical lymphadenopathy, fever; other important features include periorbital edema, splenomegaly, palatal petechiae
- *Laboratory:* At least 50% lymphocytes and monocytes, including at least 10% atypical cells; abnormal liver function tests in 80% to 90% of cases
- *Serologic:* Positive monospot, heterophil, or specific EBV antibody tests

As demonstrated in the Case Example, the most common errors in diagnosis are a failure to appreciate IM as a dynamic disease, with a changing clinical and laboratory pattern, and a misunderstanding of its clinical serology. Initially, the WBC is low, but it may rise to 20,000/mm or more by the end of the first week. Mild thrombocytopenia is common. Inexperienced laboratory technicians may have a difficult time differentiating atypical lymphocytes from lymphoblasts, but the former are much more pleomorphic. One frequently overlooked diagnostic test is assessment of serum levels of liver enzymes (lactate dehydrogenase and serum glutamic transaminases), which are mildly elevated in 80% to 90% of patients and usually return to normal within 3 to 5 weeks [34]. Elevations in bilirubin occur less commonly.

One of the most worrisome aspects of IM is splenic enlargement and the risk of rupture. Splenic rupture and neurologic involvement represent the two leading causes of death in IM. Clinically, splenomegaly is found only about 50% of the time [21]; however, in one study of 37 patients with IM, followed with weekly ultrasound studies, *all* had splenomegaly [35]. Its duration could not be reliably predicted based on physical examination alone [35]. However, splenic rupture is exceedingly rare—less than 0.2% of all cases [36]. In many cases, it is the ruptured spleen that brings the patient to medical attention, not the underlying IM [21]. Rupture occurs most often during the second or third week of the illness, although it can occur as early as the first week [36,37]. Half of splenic ruptures occur spontaneously, and another 30% follow minimal exertion [21,38]. Therefore, palpation of the spleen should be done gently, and any complaints of left upper quadrant, shoulder, or chest pain should be thoroughly investigated.

Heterophil antibody is not specifically targeted against EBV but rather is one of the many by-products of EBV infection. It is an IgM-class antibody that the body can manufacture against a variety of antigens in nature. In this case, it is capable of agglutinating red blood cells from other species—hence the name, "heterophil." A number of variations in the test exist to increase accuracy, including

TABLE 10. *Infectious mononucleosis: making the diagnosis*

Clinical:
Maintain high index of
suspicion in teenagers
	Fever, sore throat, malaise ⎫
	Tonsillopharyngitis ⎬ 80%
	Lymphadenopathy, ⎭
	  especially postcervical
	Other findings
	  Splenomegaly
	  Periorbital edema
	  Soft palate petechiae

Laboratory:	Lymphocytosis
	  >50% in differential
	  >4,500/mm³ total
	Atypical lymphocytes:
	  ≥10% total white blood cell count
	  >1,000/mm³ total
	Mildly elevated liver function tests (80–90% of patients)

Serologic:	Positive monospot or heterophil antibody Positive Epstein-Barr virus antibody test

preabsorbing test serum with different factors (e.g., guinea pig kidney cells) or using red blood cells from different species (e.g., sheep, horse). The basic difference between the Monospot and the heterophil antibody test is that the former is qualitative and the latter is quantitative. The Monospot is a rapid slide test that reacts to the presence of heterophil antibody. It requires only 120 seconds and is 96% to 99% accurate, assuming that it is performed properly [3,39,40]. The heterophil antibody test requires 24 hours to measure.

Because heterophil antibody is not specific for EBV, it is unpredictable. For example, children younger than 3 years of age do not ordinarily mount any heterophil response to EBV infection [41]. In teenagers, the heterophil response may be absent entirely, or may rise and fall precipitously (Fig. 3). Usually, a Monospot test is sufficient, but occasionally the clinician may want to follow antibody titers or try to make a retrospective diagnosis. In such cases, measurements of heterophil antibody levels can be performed; and a titer greater than 1:40 is considered positive. Although a variety of diseases can produce heterophil antibody as well (e.g., mumps, malaria, rubella, lymphoma), the levels generated are invariably less than 1 : 40 [3,21,42]. Heterophil antibody can remain elevated for up to a year in 75% of patients, or an anamnestic response can be generated by subsequent infections [3].

Perhaps the most frequent misuse of the Monospot test is the failure to repeat it in the second week of the illness, when it is most likely to be positive. If patients are seen within a few days of the onset of their illness, it is unlikely that they will have had time to mount a heterophil antibody response, although the WBC may still be suggestive of IM.

The most common cause of heterophil-negative IM is still EBV infection. Should a precise diagnosis be required (e.g., a patient with significant weight loss and adenopathy, with a WBC and liver enzyme profile that are not suggestive of IM), a number of specific anti-EBV antibodies can be mea-

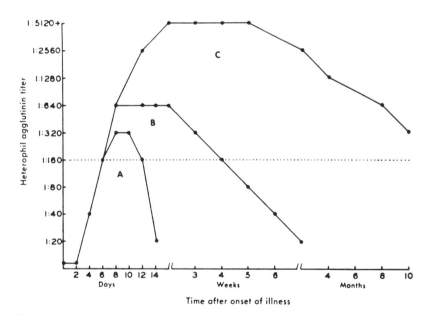

FIG. 3. The rise and fall of heterophil titers in infectious mononucleosis: three possible patterns. Titers above the horizontal dotted line are considered significant. Because of these varying patterns, physicians should not be misled by one negative value. Heterophil antibodies are more likely to be present in adolescents, rather than younger children, and usually peak beginning *after* the first week of the illness. If an absolute serologic diagnosis must be reached and the heterophil titer remains negative, then specific anti-Epstein-Barr virus IgG and IgM titers should be obtained. (Krugman S, Katz SL, Gerson AA, Wilfert CM. *Infectious diseases of children*. 8th ed. St. Louis: CV Mosby; 1985. Copyright 1985. Reproduced by permission.)

TABLE 11. *Interpretation of Epstein-Barr virus serology*

	IgM capsid antigen	IgG capsid antigen	Early antigen (IgG)		Antinuclear antigen
			D	R	
Susceptible	−	−	−	−	−
Acute primary infection (IM)	+	+	+	−	−
Acute infection, asymptomatic	+	+	−	+	−
Old, quiescent infection	−	+	−	−	+
Reactivated infection	±	+	+ or +		+

IM, infectious mononucleosis.
From Sumaya CV. Epstein-Barr virus infections in children. *Curr Probl Pediatr* 1987;17:1. With permission.

sured (Table 11, Fig. 4). Specific IgM and IgG antibodies directed against the viral capsid antigen (VCA) of EBV can be measured and cost $50 to $75 [43]. An elevated IgM but negative IgG indicates acute infection; a negative IgM but elevated IgG indicates past infection. Anti-VCA IgM antibodies are detectable in 97% of patients during the acute phase of their illness [44]. Other antibody determinations (e.g., to the *d* component of early antigen, to nuclear antigen) have been used in the diagnosis of chronic mononucleosis syndrome (see later).

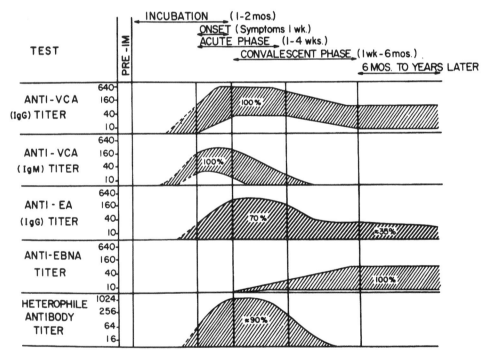

FIG. 4. Pattern of specific Epstein-Barr virus antibodies in infectious mononucleosis (IM) compared with heterophile response. Anti-VCA, viral capsid antigen; anti-EA, early antigens; anti-EBNA, Epstein-Barr nuclear antigens. Percentage in shaded area indicates frequency of detection in acute IM. (Reprinted with permission from Durbin WA, Sullivan JL. Epstein-Barr virus infection. *Pediatr Rev* 1994;15:63. Reproduced by permission of *Pediatrics*.)

Clinical Caveats

Several features of IM in teenagers are worth reemphasizing:

- Splenomegaly occurs in only 50% to 60% of IM patients, usually in the second or third week of their illness. Enlargement is usually pear shaped and *subtle,* and may only be appreciated on deep inspiration. Gross splenomegaly warrants a reconsideration of the diagnosis.
- Periorbital edema is nearly as common as splenomegaly and is a frequently neglected sign of IM [45].
- Petechiae on the soft palate are also frequently overlooked as a sign of IM.
- Anterior cervical lymphadenopathy is unreliable as an indicator of IM. It can be associated with any infection of the upper respiratory system. *Posterior cervical nodes* are more suggestive of the diagnosis, and frequently axillary, inguinal, mesenteric, or postoccipital nodes are involved as well. IM rarely, if ever, involves supraclavicular nodes—a diagnosis of Hodgkin's or non-Hodgkin's lymphoma should be considered in such patients [46,47].
- Most patients demonstrate a mild, chemical hepatitis (80–90%). Therefore, liver function tests may be as useful as serologic tests in the diagnosis of IM.
- In 10% of patients, a variety of rashes have been described: macular, maculopapular, scarlatiniform, petechial, urticarial, or erythema multiforme. Most often, the rash of IM is faint and best seen on the neck and upper chest, similar in quality to the rash of rubella.
- Nearly 100% of IM patients will develop a dramatic maculopapular rash, resembling measles, if given ampicillin or amoxicillin. This does *not* represent a true allergy, and it is safe to continue the drug if necessary. The rash is not IgE-mediated, but probably represents some interaction between a breakdown product of the drug and the virus. Onset is usually 5 to 9 days after administration of the drug, whereas an acute allergic reaction is more likely to occur within 24 to 48 hours and to be urticarial in nature [48].

Complications

A wide variety of complications in IM have been described, involving virtually every organ system (Table 12), and an estimated 20% of patients have some type of complication [8,49]. Fortunately, the disease is rarely fatal, with an estimated case fatality rate of no higher than 1 in 3,000 [50]. In fact, in the medical literature, only a few hundred well documented cases exist [36,50]. The three most important complications are splenic rupture, central nervous system (CNS) involvement, and airway obstruction. In addition, increasing numbers of rare immunoproliferative disorders are being described in predisposed individuals [18,19,51].

Splenic rupture represents the single most common cause of death in IM and is certainly the best known and most feared complication [36,52]. Sudden weakness or fainting can be harbingers of impending shock in IM patients. Spontaneous rupture is common, and often only minor trauma is reported [21,38]. About 20% of patients with splenic rupture present with this as their initial symptom of IM. Conservative, nonsurgical management is increasingly being used, with intensive observation and support [37,53,54], although it is not always successful [55]. Acute abdominal pain can also be caused by pancreatitis or mesenteric adenitis.

The incidence of CNS involvement in IM ranges from 1% to 8% [29,30]. Of these patients, over half present with encephalitis or meningoencephalitis. Approximately 20% of patients with CNS complications demonstrate an acute transverse myelitis or Guillain-Barré syndrome [56].

Tonsillar enlargement is a hallmark of IM, but, rarely, massive enlargement or severe glottic edema can jeopardize the upper airway and become life threatening [57,58]. Such patients deserve hospitalization and intensive observation and benefit from a short course of high-dose glucocorticoids. Peritonsillar abscess is also a well known complication [59,60].

Chronic Mononucleosis

Although EBV is probably not the primary etiologic agent in chronic fatigue syndrome, it is a cause of two related chronic syndromes. The first, a rare, X-linked recessive lymphoproliferative disorder, presents after acute IM with rapid infiltration of the liver, bone marrow, and other organs. It is frequently fatal, as a result of hepatic failure, bleeding, and infection. Kindred studies sometimes reveal

TABLE 12. *Complications of infectious mononucleosis*

Organ system	Specific complications
Respiratory	Acute airway obstruction
	Peritonsillar abscess
	Interstitial pneumonitis
	Hilar lymphadenopathy
	Pleuritis
Neurologic	Encephalitis
	Meningoencephalitis
	Seizures
	Guillain-Barré syndrome
	Bell's palsy
	Transverse myelitis
	Alice in Wonderland syndrome
Psychiatric	Psychosis
Immunologic	Fatal X-linked immunoproliferative disorder
	Hodgkin's disease, B-cell and T-cell lymphoma
	Burkitt's lymphoma
	Nasopharyngeal carcinoma
Hematologic	Hemolytic anemia
	Thrombocytopenia
	Neutropenia (with septicemia)
	Aplastic anemia
Gastrointestinal/abdominal	Pancreatitis
	Hepatitis/hepatic necrosis
	Jaundice
	Reye's syndrome
	Malabsorption
	Splenic rupture
Cardiovascular	Myocarditis
	Pericarditis
Dermatologic	Rash
	Gianotti-Crosti syndrome
Renal	Interstitial nephritis
	Glomerulonephritis
Genital	Orchitis

Adapted from Bartley DC, Del Rio C, Shulman JA. Clinical complications. In: Schlossberg D, ed. *Infectious mononucleosis,* 2nd ed. New York: Springer-Verlag; 1989:35–48; and from Radetsky M, Overturf GD. Epstein-Barr infections in adolescents and young adults. *Adolescent Medicine: State of the Art Reviews* 1995;6:91.

other male relatives who suffered from other immunologic disorders. Affected patients do not always produce anti-EBV antibodies [18,61,62].

The second occurs sporadically and involves a severe and prolonged clinical course, marked by severe pancytopenia, interstitial pneumonitis, hepatitis, malabsorption, wasting, lymphoma, and CNS involvement. These patients demonstrate high levels of antibodies to VCA and early antigen and may respond to acyclovir [21,63]. A similar EBV-related interstitial pneumonitis in children with acquired immunodeficiency syndrome has also been described, but here the virus may have been an incidental finding [64].

For the present, the terms *chronic EBV* and *chronic mononucleosis* should be confined to these two extremely rare disorders rather than used to describe what is properly called the *chronic fatigue syndrome* [21].

Treatment

There is no specific therapy indicated for the treatment of IM. Antibiotics are indicated only if a throat culture or rapid group A streptococcal test is positive. Likewise, steroids are indicated if there is impending airway obstruction. Such patients can be treated with 2 to 4 mg/kg/day of steroids for 5 to

7 days, without a need to taper off the drug. Although steroids are often used for other complications of IM (e.g., persistent high fevers, severe systemic symptoms, hemolytic anemia), they have no scientifically proven efficacy.

Use of steroids in the uncomplicated patient is probably unwise because there are significant theoretical contraindications. Glucocorticoids are immunosuppressive, specifically diminishing the effectiveness of T-cell–mediated immunity [65]. Because IM represents an infection of B cells, and T cells are mobilized to help clear the infection, suppressing them may be unwise. Indeed, studies have shown diminished levels of T-helper and T-suppressor cells in IM patients treated with steroids [21]. Although many uncontrolled trials document that students with IM routinely treated with steroids show decreased duration of fever and length of infirmary stay by a few days, and increased well-being [66,67], such symptomatic relief still does not justify their routine use [3,8,9,68].

Antiviral agents like acyclovir and interferon have been tried; such agents can suppress viral shedding but seem to lack clinical benefit and cannot be recommended at present [69–71]. Intravenous gamma-globulin may be effective in severe thrombocytopenia, however [72].

Aside from making an accurate diagnosis, providing good counseling is probably the most important contribution a physician can make. The following items should be stressed:

- IM is nearly always a self-limited disease that teenagers recover from without difficulty. Often, they feel ill for a week or two, then gradually attain their former level of activity over the next 2 to 4 weeks. Emphasizing the complications or the possibility of chronic mononucleosis only results in a self-fulfilling prophecy.
- Bed rest is indicated only during the febrile period. Thereafter, patients should seek their own individual level of activity.
- If the spleen is palpable, patients should be cautioned against any activity that could result in blunt trauma or increased intraabdominal pressure. This includes such activities as jogging, swimming, rough-housing with friends, contact sports, or straining to pass stool. Patients should be reexamined after 4 to 6 weeks to be "cleared" for physical activities [73].
- Appropriate analgesia is important: liquid codeine preparations may help to ease dysphagia, and saline irrigants may help to relieve pain from membranous tonsillitis.
- Teenagers should never be told that they have "hepatitis." Invariably, they misunderstand and think that they have both IM and hepatitis A or B. Rather, abnormalities in liver function tests can be discussed, if necessary.
- Although physicians have routinely told patients with IM not to consume alcoholic beverages (presumably because of the chemical hepatitis), there is no scientific evidence to support this recommendation.

Infectious mononucleosis can best be explained as being a viral disease, like the common cold. As such, it is self-limited. Patients with splenomegaly can be told that the spleen functions the way an oil filter does in a car, and that it is filtering out the infected white blood cells. Patients can be told that they may have symptoms for a week or two, including fever, but that they should recover without any problems whatsoever. Once they are afebrile, teenagers with IM should be counseled to establish their own level of activity and rest.

REFERENCES

1. Strasburger VC. Why adolescent medicine? Four illustrative cases. *Clin Pediatr* 1984;23:12.
2. Straus SE, Fleisher GR. Infectious mononucleosis: epidemiology and pathogenesis. In: Schlossberg D, ed. *Infectious mononucleosis*. 2nd ed. New York: Springer-Verlag; 1989:8.
3. Radetsky M, Overturf GD. Epstein-Barr infections in adolescents and young adults. *Adolescent Medicine: State of the Art Reviews* 1995;6:91.
4. Chervenick PA. Infectious mononucleosis: the classic clinical syndrome. In: Schlossberg D, ed. *Infectious mononucleosis*. 2nd ed. New York: Springer-Verlag; 1989:29.
5. Mahoney DH Jr, Fernbach DJ. The hematologic response. In: Schlossberg D, ed. *Infectious mononucleosis*. 2nd ed. New York: Springer-Verlag; 1989:80.
6. Rosenthal T, Hertz M. Mediastinal lymphadenopathy in infectious mononucleosis. *JAMA* 1975;233:1300.
7. Young JL, Miller RW. Incidence of malignant tumors in U.S. children. *J Pediatr* 1975;86:254.
8. Sumaya CV. Epstein-Barr virus. In: Feigin RD, Cherry JD, eds. *Textbook of pediatric infectious diseases*. 3rd ed. Philadelphia: WB Saunders; 1992:1547.
9. Bailey RE. Diagnosis and treatment of infectious mononucleosis. *Am Fam Physician* 1994;49:879.

10. Sprunt TP, Evans FA. Mononuclear leukocytosis in reaction to acute infections (infectious mononucleosis). *Bulletin of the Johns Hopkins Hospital* 1920;31:410.
11. Epstein MA, Achong BG, Barr YM. Virus particles in cultured lymphoblasts from Burkitt's lymphoma. *Lancet* 1964;1:702.
12. Evans AS, Niederman JC, McCollum RW. Seroepidemiologic studies of infectious mononucleosis with EB virus. *N Engl J Med* 1968;279:1121.
13. Henle G, Henle W, Diehl V. Relation of Burkitt's tumor-associated herpes-type virus to infectious mononucleosis. *Proc Natl Acad Sci USA* 1968;59:94.
14. Burkitt DP. A sarcoma involving the jaws in African children. *Br J Surg* 1958;46:218.
15. Steeper TA, Horwitz CA, Ablashi DV, et al. The spectrum of clinical and laboratory findings resulting from human herpesvirus-6 (HHV-6) in patients with mononucleosis-like illnesses not resulting from Epstein-Barr virus or cytomegalovirus. *Am J Clin Pathol* 1990;93:776.
16. Straus SE, Cohen JI, Gosato G, et al. Epstein-Barr virus infections: biology, pathogenesis, and management. *Ann Intern Med* 1993;118:45.
17. Naher H, Gissman L, Freese UK, et al. Subclinical Epstein-Barr virus infection of both the male and female genital tract: indication for sexual transmission. *J Invest Dermatol* 1992;98:791.
18. Purtilo DT, Strobach RS, Okano M, et al. Epstein-Barr virus-associated lymphoproliferative disorders. *Lab Invest* 1992;67:5.
19. Kieff E. Epstein-Barr virus: increasing evidence of a link to carcinoma. *N Engl J Med* 1995;333:724.
20. Liebowitz D. Epstein-Barr virus: an old dog with new tricks. *N Engl J Med* 1995;332:55.
21. Durbin WA, Sullivan JL. Epstein-Barr virus infection. *Pediatr Rev* 1994;15:63.
22. Chetham MM, Roberts KB. Infectious mononucleosis in adolescents. *Pediatr Ann* 1991;20:206.
23. Niederman JC, Evans AS, Subrahmanyan L, et al. Prevalence, incidence, and persistence of EB virus antibody in young adults. *N Engl J Med* 1970;282:361.
24. Sawyer RN, Evans AS, Niederman JC, et al. Prospective studies of a group of Yale University freshmen: I. occurrence of infectious mononucleosis. *J Infect Dis* 1971;123:263.
25. Halle TJ, Evans AS, Niederman JC, et al. Infectious mononucleosis at the United States Military Academy: a prospective study of a single class over four years. *Yale J Biol Med* 1974;47:182.
26. Collins M, Fleisher GR, Fager SS. Incidence of beta-hemolytic streptococcal pharyngitis in adolescents with infectious mononucleosis. *Journal of Adolescent Health Care* 1984;5:96.
27. Madigan NP, Newcomer AD, Campbell DC, et al. Intense jaundice in infectious mononucleosis. *Mayo Clin Proc* 1973;48:857.
28. Schaechter J, Tunnessen WW Jr. Diagnosis via a jaundiced "I." *Contemp Pediatr* 1996;13:113.
29. Grose C. Neurologic complications of infectious mononucleosis. In: Schlossberg D, ed. *Infectious mononucleosis.* 2nd ed. New York: Springer-Verlag; 1989:49.
30. Connelly KP, DeWitt LD. Neurologic complications of infectious mononucleosis. *Pediatr Neurol* 1994; 10:181.
31. Copperman SM. "Alice in Wonderland" syndrome as a presenting symptom of infectious mononucleosis in children. *Clin Pediatr* 1977;16:143.
32. Eschel GM, Eyov A, Lahat E, et al. Alice in Wonderland syndrome, a manifestation of acute Epstein-Barr virus infection. *Pediatr Infect Dis* 1987;6:68.
33. Lazarus KH, Baehner RL. Aplastic anemia complicating infectious mononucleosis: a case report and review of the literature. *Pediatrics* 1981;67:907.
34. White N, Juel-Jensen BE. Infectious mononucleosis hepatitis. *Semin Liver Dis* 1984;4:301.
35. Primos WA, Landry GL, Scanlan KA. The course of splenomegaly in infectious mononucleosis. *American Journal of Diseases of Children* 1990;144:438.
36. Bartley DC, Del Rio C, Shulman JA. Clinical complications. In: Schlossberg D, ed. *Infectious mononucleosis.* 2nd ed. New York: Springer-Verlag; 1989:35.
37. Ali J. Spontaneous rupture of the spleen in patients with infectious mononucleosis. *Can J Surg* 1993;36:49.
38. Rutkow IM. Rupture of the spleen in infectious mononucleosis: a critical review. *Arch Surg* 1978;113:718.
39. Basson V, Sharp AA. Monospot: a differential slide test for infectious mononucleosis. *J Clin Pathol* 1969; 22:324.
40. Pochedly C. Laboratory testing for infectious mononucleosis. *Postgrad Med* 1987;81:335.
41. Andiman WA. The Epstein-Barr virus and EB virus infections in childhood. *J Pediatr* 1979;95:171.
42. Horwitz CA., Henle W, Henle G, et al. Persistent falsely positive rapid tests for infectious mononucleosis. *Am J Clin Pathol* 1979;72:807.
43. Henle W, Henle GE, Horwitz C.A. Epstein-Barr virus specific diagnostic tests in infectious mononucleosis. *Hum Pathol* 1974;5:551.
44. Evans AS, Niederman JC, Cenabre LC, et al. A prospective evaluation of heterophile and Epstein-Barr virus-specific IgM antibody tests in clinical and subclinical infectious mononucleosis: specificity and sensitivity of the tests and persistence of antibody. *J Infect Dis* 1975;132:546.
45. Decker MR, Berberian BJ, Sulica VI. Periorbital and eyelid edema: the initial manifestation of acute infectious mononucleosis. *Cutis* 1991;47:323.

46. Lake A, Oski FA. Peripheral lymphadenopathy in childhood: ten-year experience with excisional biopsy. *American Journal of Diseases of Children* 1978;132:357.
47. Knight PJ, Mulne AR, Vassy LE. When is lymph node biopsy indicated in children with enlarged peripheral nodes? *Pediatrics* 1982;69:391.
48. Kraemer MJ, Smith AL. Rashes with ampicillin. *Pediatr Rev* 1980;1:197.
49. Sumaya CV. New perspectives on infectious mononucleosis. *Contemp Pediatr* 1989;6:58.
50. Penman HG. Fatal infectious mononucleosis: a critical review. *J Clin Pathol* 1970;23:765.
51. Sullivan JL. Epstein-Barr virus and the X-linked lymphoproliferative syndrome. *Adv Pediatr* 1983;30:365.
52. Lukes RJ, Cox FH. Clinical and morphologic findings in 30 fatal cases of infectious mononucleosis. *Am J Pathol* 1958;34:586.
53. Wesson DE, Filler RM, Ein SH, et al. Ruptured spleen: when to operate? *J Pediatr Surg* 1980;16:324.
54. Linne T, Eriksson M, Lannergren K, et al. Splenic function after nonsurgical management of splenic rupture. *J Pediatr* 1984;105:263.
55. Vitello J. Spontaneous rupture of the spleen in infectious mononucleosis: a failed attempt at nonoperative therapy. *J Pediatr Surg* 1988;23:1043.
56. Peters CH, Widerman A, Blumberg A, et al. Neurologic manifestations of infectious mononucleosis, with special reference to the Guillain-Barre syndrome. *Arch Intern Med* 1974;80:366.
57. Snyderman NL. Otorhinolaryngologic presentations of infectious mononucleosis. *Pediatr Clin North Am* 1981;28:1011.
58. Kaplan JM, Keller MS, Troy S. Nasopharyngeal obstruction in infectious mononucleosis. *Am Fam Physician* 1987;35:205.
59. Handler SD, Warren WS. Peritonsillar abscess: a complication of corticosteroid treatment in infectious mononucleosis. *Int J Pediatr Otorhinolaryngol* 1979;1:265.
60. Epperly TD, Wood TC. New trends in the management of peritonsillar abscess. *Am Fam Physician* 1990; 42:102.
61. Purtilo DT. X-linked lymphoproliferative syndrome. *JAMA* 1981;105:119.
62. Straus SE. The chronic mononucleosis syndrome. *J Infect Dis* 1988;157:405.
63. Schooley RT, Carey RW, Miller G, et al. Chronic Epstein-Barr virus infection associated with fever and interstitial pneumonitis: clinical and serological features and response to antiviral chemotherapy. *Ann Intern Med* 1986;104:636.
64. Andiman WA, Eastman R, Martin K, et al. Opportunistic lymphoproliferations associated with Epstein-Barr viral DNA in infants and children with AIDS. *Lancet* 1985;2:1390.
65. Mangi RJ, Niederman JC, Kelleher JE Jr, et al. Depression of cell-mediated immunity during acute infectious mononucleosis. *N Engl J Med* 1974;291:1149.
66. Bender CE. The value of corticosteroids in the treatment of infectious mononucleosis. *JAMA* 1967;199:529.
67. Brandfonbrener A, Epstein A, Wu S, et al. Corticosteroid therapy in Epstein-Barr virus infection: effect on lymphocyte class, subset, and response to early antigen. *Arch Intern Med* 1986;146:337.
68. Hickey S, Strasburger VC. Infectious mononucleosis and chronic fatigue syndrome in adolescents. *Pediatr Clin North Am* 1997 (in press).
69. Sullivan JL, Bryon KS, Brewster FE, et al. Treatment of life-threatening Epstein-Barr virus infections with acyclovir. *Am J Med* 1982;73:262.
70. Andersson J, Britton S, Ernberg I. Effect of acyclovir on infectious mononucleosis: a double-blind, placebo-controlled study. *J Infect Dis* 1986;153:183.
71. Van der Horst C, Joncas J, Ahronheim G, et al. Lack of effect of peroral acyclovir for the treatment of acute infectious mononucleosis. *J Infect Dis* 1991;164:788.
72. Cyran EM, Rowe JM, Bloom RE. Intravenous gammaglobulin treatment for immune thrombocytopenia associated with infectious mononucleosis. *Am J Hematol* 1991;38:124.
73. Haines JD. When to resume sports after infectious mononucleosis. *Postgrad Med* 1987;87:331.

SUGGESTED READING

Bailey RE. Diagnosis and treatment of infectious mononucleosis. *Am Fam Physician* 1994;49:879.

Chetham MM, Roberts KB. Infectious mononucleosis in adolescents. *Pediatr Ann* 1991;20:206.

Connelly KP, DeWitt LD. Neurologic complications of infectious mononucleosis. *Pediatr Neurol* 1994;10:181.

Durbin WA, Sullivan JL. Epstein-Barr virus infection. *Pediatr Rev* 1994;15:63.

Epperly TD, Wood TC. New trends in the management of peritonsillar abscess. *Am Fam Physician* 1990;42:102.

Hickey S, Strasburger VC. Infectious mononucleosis and chronic fatigue syndrome in adolescents. *Pediatr Clin North Am* 1997 (in press).

Radetsky M, Overturf GD. Epstein-Barr infections in adolescents and young adults. *Adolescent Medicine: State of the Art Reviews* 1995;6:91.

Reich RM, Mak DG. Infectious mononucleosis in the athlete: diagnosis, complications, and management. *Am J Sports Med* 1982;10:162.

Schlossberg D, ed. *Infectious mononucleosis.* 2nd ed. New York: Springer-Verlag; 1989;.

Straus SE, Cohen JI, Gosato G, et al. Epstein-Barr virus infections: biology, pathogenesis, and management. *Ann Intern Med* 1993;118:45.

Sumaya CV. Epstein-Barr virus. In: Feigin RD, Cherry JD, eds. *Textbook of pediatric infectious diseases.* 3rd ed., Philadelphia: WB Saunders; 1992:1547.

CHRONIC FATIGUE SYNDROME

Fatigue is a puzzling symptom for primary care practitioners to deal with [1], and, although rare, chronic fatigue syndrome (CFS) is now increasingly on the minds of patients and their parents. It may be responsible for up to 15% of patient visits to pediatric infectious disease clinics [2]. In the mid-1980s, the media christened CFS as *chronic mono*, or the *yuppy flu*. Patients were described who had profound and debilitating fatigue and a variety of other symptoms, including sleep disturbances, myalgias, inability to concentrate, and sore throat. A number of early reports implicated Epstein-Barr virus (EBV) as the cause [3,4]. Most of the patients were white women, aged 30 to 50 years [5], and all had elevations in various anti-EBV antibodies.

In fact, the search for a cause of CFS antedates the 1985 publications by half a century. Since 1934, over 30 epidemics of CFS have been reported and been variously ascribed to chronic brucellosis, mass hysteria, postinfluenzal neurasthenia, epidemic myalgic encephalomyelitis, Royal Free disease, and others [6,7]. More recently, human herpesvirus type 6, *Candida* species, enteroviruses, and human retroviruses have all been suggested as possible etiologic agents [7–14]. Increasing numbers of reports are also suggesting either an immunologic basis for the syndrome, on the one hand, or a primary psychological basis on the other [15,16]. This is still a syndrome in search of both an etiology and an adequate definition in adolescents.

Clinical Presentation

Chronic fatigue syndrome was originally described and defined in adults [17]. A number of cases in children and adolescents have now been reported [2,18–24]. Prevalence rates range from 6 cases per 100,000 children younger than 10 years of age, to 48 cases per 100,000 during adolescence, to 110 cases per 100,000 in 30- to 49-year-olds [25]. The initial definition, requiring a 50% reduction in physical activity, has since been revised, but the criteria still remain subjective and poorly defined for children or adolescents [26] (Table 13). In particular, the requirement that symptoms be present for at least 6 months means that many patients experience chronic fatigue without necessarily having CFS.

TABLE 13. *Diagnosis of chronic fatigue syndrome*

1. Unexplained, persistent fatigue for 6 months or more that:
   Is new
   Is not the result of exertion
   Is not relieved by rest
   Results in a substantial reduction in activity level
AND

2. Four or more of the following signs or symptoms:
   Sore throat
   Tender cervical or axillary lymph nodes
   Impaired memory or concentration
   New onset of headaches
   Joint pain
   Sleep difficulty
   Postexertion malaise
   Muscle pain

Adapted from Fukuda K, Straus SE, Hickle I, et al. The chronic fatigue syndrome: a comprehensive approach to its definition and study. *Ann Intern Med* 1994;121:953.

TABLE 14. *Incidence of symptoms reported in children and adolescents with chronic fatigue syndrome*

Symptom	Incidence range (%)
Fatigue/weakness	100
Headaches	75–85
Pharyngitis	50–90
Difficulty concentrating	65
Myalgias/arthralgias	40–90
Fever	35–70
Depression	50–60
Sleeping difficulties	20–55
Weight loss	20–40

Adapted from Glover DM. Chronic fatigue syndrome. *Adolescent Medicine: State of the Art Reviews* 1995;6:101, and from Carter BD, Marshall GS. New developments: diagnosis and management of chronic fatigue in children and adolescents. *Curr Probl Pediatr* 1995;25:281.

Fatigue is the hallmark of CFS and often begins after a flulike illness that fails to clear [15]. The type of fatigue described by such patients is so debilitating that they struggle to get out of bed or to make visits to their physicians. A typical adolescent will be a previously active, athletic, high-achieving girl with an intact, middle-class family. Someone else in the family may have had CFS. By the time medical attention is sought, she will have had symptoms for several weeks or months. School and social activities will have been sharply curtailed, and sleep disturbances, decreased appetite, and a feeling of social isolation are all common. Myriad other symptoms have been described (Table 14).

What Causes Chronic Fatigue Syndrome?

Although a search for a single cause of CFS continues [27], a multifactorial explanation is more likely [16,26] (Fig. 5). Thus, a variety of initiating factors such as viral infection or stress could initiate a complex sequence of immunologic events leading to fatigue and other symptoms [15,16,28]. Research interest has focused on the following broad areas.

Infectious Causes

No one infectious agent has been proven to cause CFS [14,28]. Initially, EBV was thought the most likely culprit. Although it is still possible that some reactivation of the virus occurs in patients with

Chronic Fatigue Syndrome

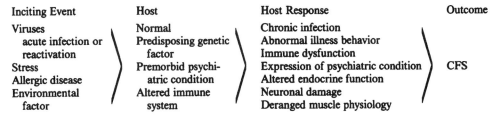

FIG. 5. A multifactorial model for the pathogenesis of chronic fatigue syndrome (CFS). It is unlikely that any one virus, immunologic event, or psychiatric disturbance will ever account entirely for CFS. (Reprinted with permission from Glover DM. Chronic fatigue syndrome. *Adolescent Medicine: State of the Art Reviews* 1995;6:101.)

CFS [15,16], or that some patients thought to have CFS simply have a prolonged case of infectious mononucleosis, considerable evidence exonerates EBV from being the prime etiologic agent [6,14, 16,19,29,30]:

- After their initial infection, many infectious mononucleosis patients display periodic rises in EBV antibody titers [31,32].
- Other herpesviruses may also cause periodic increases in anti-EBV IgM antibody levels [15].
- EBV serology results are notoriously difficult to reproduce and confirm.
- Although EBV infection confers immortality on B cells in vitro, no increase in such cells can be demonstrated in patients with CFS.
- In a double-blinded, placebo-controlled trial of acyclovir in patients with CFS for an average of 7 years, most of the patients improved, whether they received acyclovir or placebo. In addition, those who responded showed no changes in their EBV serologic profiles [33].

Research has focused on human retroviruses, enteroviruses, and human herpesvirus type 6, among others, all without success [19,29,34–37].

Immunologic Causes

A variety of abnormalities in CD4 cells, in vitro lymphocyte stimulation responses, natural killer cells, and cytokine levels have been described [28,38–43], but none is consistently reproducible [28,42]. In general, there seems to be an activation of the immune system, which could reflect viral infection or reactivation, or perhaps psychoimmunologic phenomena [44]. Despite conflicting data, many researchers believe that patients with CFS do have significant disturbances in their cellular immunity, but whether these are primary or secondary is unclear.

Neurally Mediated Hypotension

One of the most exciting recent findings has been that adolescents with chronic fatigue (including some who fulfill the adult criteria) [45] and adults with CFS [46] have positive tilt-table tests, consistent with neurally mediated hypotension and responsive to treatment with a beta-blocker such as atenolol [45,46]. Whether neurally mediated hypotension can be implicated as a cause of CFS or is merely a treatable by-product remains to be seen, but physicians may want to add tilt-table testing to their diagnostic armamentarium.

Psychological Causes

Most series of adolescent CFS patients describe some who have either premorbid or coexisting depression [2,18,20,24,47]. Which comes first, the debilitating fatigue or the depression? Clearly, in a certain percentage of patients, depression and other psychiatric disorders predominate, hence the need for an aggressive psychological evaluation from the outset. But most patients are not depressed in the conventional sense [2]. Their activities may be severely restricted, but they do not have many other affective features of classic depression (Table 15). Conceptually, CFS may be analogous to a conversion reaction in which an infection or other stressor catalyzes certain symptoms to remain in play that give the patient secondary

TABLE 15. *Chronic fatigue syndrome versus depression: clinical features*

Feature	Chronic fatigue syndrome	Depression
Postexercise fatigue	+++	+
Good days/bad days	++	+
Social isolation	+	++
Self-criticism	+	+++
Sense of failure	+	+++
Suicidal ideation	+	+++
Psychomotor retardation	−	+

Adapted from Calabrese L, Danao T, Camara E, et al. Chronic fatigue syndrome. *Am Fam Physician* 1992;45:1205.

TABLE 16. *Chronic fatigue in adolescents: differential diagnosis*

Extremely common	Depression
	Pregnancy
	Stress-related disorders
	Anxiety
	Hyperventilation syndrome
	School avoidance
	Psychosomatic disorder
	Substance abuse
Common	Fibromyalgia
	Eating disorders
	Rapid or excessive change in weight
	Excessive physical activity
	Anemia
	Dysfunctional uterine bleeding
	Nutritional
Uncommon	Cardiomyopathy or congestive failure
	Asthma
	Hyperthyroidism or hypothyroidism
	Connective tissue disease
	Inflammatory bowel disease
	Leukemia/lymphoma
	Acquired immunodeficiency syndrome
	Hepatitis
	Myasthenia gravis
	Obstructive sleep apnea

Adapted from Cavanaugh RM. Evaluating adolescents with fatigue. *Am Fam Physician* 1987;35:163.

gain (e.g., not going to school, diminishing activities) [28]. Some investigators believe that when patients suffer from viral illnesses, their parents' style [15] or their own beliefs about their vulnerability to illness may be a better predictor of their developing CFS than other biologic factors [48]. It is safe to say that CFS patients probably have a psychological vulnerability that normal individuals lack [6,20].

Diagnosis

Chronic fatigue syndrome is as much a diagnosis of exclusion as inclusion (Table 16). Physical examination and laboratory tests in CFS are usually normal. As mentioned, children and adolescents often do not meet the classic criteria, and no specific criteria have been developed exclusively for them. In general, adolescents are far more likely to be suffering from endogenous or situational depression or psychosomatic disorders than from full-blown CFS. Some teens may be experiencing a prolonged convalescence from acute EBV infection (therefore, EBV serologic testing is still indicated), cytomegalovirus infection, or toxoplasmosis [16,48]. Others may be suffering from primary sleep disorders [49]. Unless they fit the clinical picture described previously, most teenagers would be better

TABLE 17. *Basic workup for chronic fatigue syndrome*

Complete blood count	Beck's Depression Inventory
Erythrocyte sedimentation rate	Projective tests
Antinuclear antibody	Psychometric tests
Thyroid function and autoantibody tests	?Tilt-table test
Serology: Epstein-Barr virus	
Sequential multiple analysis,	
20 chemical constituents (SMA-20)	
Urinalysis	

?: Up to physician's discretion.

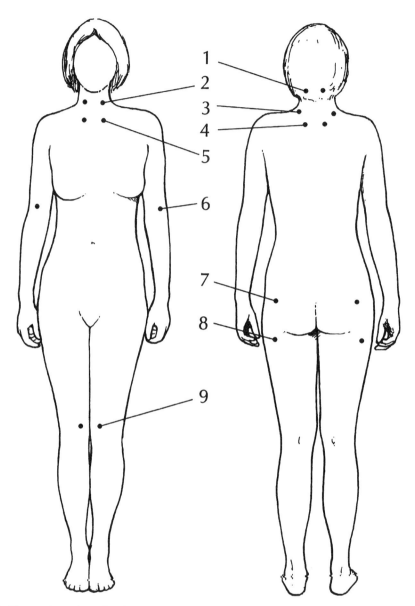

FIG. 6. Diagnostic tender points in patients with fibromyalgia. Tender point locations are paired, 18 in all, with 11 tender points or more required to make the diagnosis according to the 1990 criteria. (Reprinted with permission from Reiffenberger DH, Amundson LH. Fibromyalgia syndrome: a review. *Am Fam Physician* 1996;53:1698.)

served by careful physical examinations, limited laboratory testing, in-depth psychological interviews, and even projective testing rather than extensive viral serologies (Table 17).

One confusing and overlapping syndrome is fibromyalgia, characterized by pain involving both sides of the body in at least 11 of 18 tender-point sites [16,50,51] (Fig. 6). Such patients frequently suffer from fatigue, pharyngitis, sleep disorders, anxiety, and depression (Table 18). In one series of 27 adolescents diagnosed with CFS, 30% also fulfilled the criteria for fibromyalgia [52]. The diag-

TABLE 18. *Chronic fatigue syndrome versus fibromyalgia*

Feature	Chronic fatigue syndrome	Fibromyalgia
Sudden onset	+++	+
Headache	+++	++
Tender lymph nodes	++	−
Fever	++	−
Morning stiffness	++	+++
Sleep disturbance	++	+++
>11 tender points	+	++
Pharyngitis	+	++

Adapted from Calabrese L, Danao T, Camara E, et al. Chronic fatigue syndrome. *Am Fam Physician* 1992;45:1205.

noses of fibromyalgia and CFS may coexist in the same patient; however, whether the two are the *same* is unknown [52,53].

Management of Adolescents with CFS

Teenagers with chronic fatigue and their families may be extremely difficult to treat. Like patients with psychosomatic disorders, these patients and their families may be quite resistant to the notion of psychological assessment and intervention, but that should not deter the practitioner from seeking such input [30]. A multidisciplinary approach is ideal, with the pediatrician or family practitioner at the center. The following principles may be useful [15,16]:

- *Acknowledgment of the disease.* A pattern of normal physical examination findings and laboratory results is absolutely typical of CFS and should not lead the physician to discount the patient's symptoms.
- *Flexibility in definition.* Adolescents who present with chronic fatigue need a similar workup and approach, regardless of whether they fit criteria that were originally established for adults.
- *Thorough medical evaluation.* This helps the patient understand that his or her illness is being taken seriously and allows for exclusion of other diagnoses. Documentation of symptoms and their impact on everyday functioning enables accurate assessment, follow-up, and response to treatment.
- *Comprehensive psychological evaluation and intervention.* Just as in dealing with psychosomatic disorders, physicians working with CFS patients usually need to confront the resistance to psychological input and treatment. The need to rule out psychiatric disease is crucial, but patients can also be reassured that they and their families will need emotional support in dealing with this extremely difficult disease.
- *Reassurance and optimism.* Most children and adolescents with CFS have an excellent prognosis and regain full function within many months [2,18–20,23,24].
- *School and other activities.* A graduated return to normal activities is crucial in CFS patients and does not put them at risk for any untoward medical events. Obviously, this requires commitment from both the teenager and the family.

No medical therapy has proven useful for patients with CFS. Occasional successful trials of therapy (e.g., intravenous immunoglobulin therapy [54]) often do not pan out when repeated [55,56]. Placebo effects are rampant. Of course, specific treatment may be indicated and helpful for depression or sleep disturbance, and physical therapy for prolonged inactivity is recommended. But unconventional or unproven therapies are both unwise and potentially counterproductive [57].

Many experts recommend a cognitive–behavioral psychological regimen, and there is evidence in the literature of the wisdom of this approach [16,23,26,58]. Through cognitive therapy, patients are taught that they are caught in a cycle of increasing activity, isolation, and depression, which only heightens their fatigue. To break the cycle requires positive reinforcement for a gradual progression to increasing levels of activity. Supportive psychotherapy and family counseling may be useful as well.

Most patients with CFS improve with time. In one series, half the teenagers were improved on follow-up 1 to 3 years later [18]. In another pediatric series, 94% of patients improved and 65% were completely recovered [16]. Therefore, despite the seriousness of the illness, physicians can be optimistic with patients and their families.

REFERENCES

1. Cavanaugh R.M. Evaluating adolescents with fatigue. *Am Fam Physician* 1987;35:163.
2. Carter BD, Edwards JF, Kronenberger WG, et al. Case control study of chronic fatigue in pediatric patients. *Pediatrics* 1995;95:179.
3. Jones JF, Ray G, Minnich LL, et al. Evidence for active Epstein-Barr virus infection in patients with persistent, unexplained illnesses: elevated anti-early antigen antibodies. *Ann Intern Med* 1985;102:1.
4. Straus SE, Tosato G, Armstrong G, et al. Persisting illness and fatigue in adults with evidence of Epstein-Barr virus infection. *Ann Intern Med* 1985;102:7.
5. Centers for Disease Control and Prevention. *The chronic fatigue syndrome.* Atlanta: Centers for Disease Control and Prevention; 1990.
6. Katz BZ, Andiman WA. Chronic fatigue syndrome. *J Pediatr* 1988;113:944.
7. Anderson JA, Chai H, Claman HV. Candidiasis hypersensitivity syndrome. *J Allergy Clin Immunol* 1986;78:271.
8. Straus SE. The chronic mononucleosis syndrome. *J Infect Dis* 1988;157:405.
9. Yousef GE, Bell EJ, Mann GF, et al. Chronic enterovirus infection in patients with post-viral fatigue syndrome. *Lancet* 1988;1:146.
10. Renfro L. Yeast connection among 100 patients with chronic fatigue. *Am J Med* 1989;86:165.
11. Dale JK, Straus SE, Ablashi DV, et al. The Inoue-Melnick virus, human herpesvirus type 6, and the chronic fatigue syndrome. *Ann Intern Med* 1989;110:92.
12. Levy JA, Ferro F, Greenspan D, et al. Frequent isolation of HHV-6 from saliva and high seroprevalence of the virus in the population. *Lancet* 1990;335:1047.
13. DeFreitas E, Hilliard B, Cheney PR, et al. Retroviral sequences related to human T-lymphotropic virus type II in patients with chronic fatigue immune dysfunction syndrome. *Proc Natl Acad Sci USA* 1991;88:2922.
14. Ablashi D. Summary: viral studies of chronic fatigue syndrome. *Clin Infect Dis* 1994;18(Suppl):S130.
15. Carter BD, Marshall GS. New developments: diagnosis and management of chronic fatigue in children and adolescents. *Curr Probl Pediatr* 1995;25:281.
16. Glover DM. Chronic fatigue syndrome. *Adolescent Medicine: State of the Art Reviews* 1995;6:101.
17. Holmes GP, Kaplan JE, Gantz NM, et al. Chronic fatigue syndrome: a working case definition. *Ann Intern Med* 1988;108:387.
18. Smith MS, Mitchell J, Corey L, et al. Chronic fatigue in adolescents. *Pediatrics* 1991;88:195.
19. Marshall GS, Gesser RM, Yamanishi K, et al. Chronic fatigue in children: clinical features, Epstein-Barr virus and human herpesvirus 6 serology and long term follow-up. *Pediatr Infect Dis J* 1991;10:287.
20. Walford GA, McC Nelson W, McCluskey DR. Fatigue, depression, and social adjustment in chronic fatigue syndrome. *Arch Dis Child* 1993;68:384.
21. Sidebotham PD, Skeldon I, Chambers TL. Refractory chronic fatigue syndrome in adolescence. *Br J Hosp Med* 1994;51:110.
22. Bell KM, Cookfair D, Bell DS, et al. Risk factors associated with chronic fatigue syndrome in a cluster of pediatric cases. *Rev Infect Dis* 1991;13(Suppl):S32.
23. Vereker MI. Chronic fatigue syndrome: a joint paediatric–psychiatric approach. *Arch Dis Child* 1992;67:550.
24. Pelcovitz D, Septimus A, Friedman SB, et al. Psychosocial correlates of chronic fatigue syndrome in adolescent girls. *Dev Behav Pediatr* 1995;16:333.
25. Lloyd AR, Hickie I, Boughton CR, et al. Prevalence of chronic fatigue syndrome in an Australian population. *Med J Aust* 1990;153:522.
26. Carter BD, Edwards JR, Marshall GS. Chronic fatigue in children: Illness or disease? [letter]. *Pediatrics* 1993;91:163.
27. Levine PH, ed. Chronic fatigue syndrome. *Clin Infect Dis* 1994;18:S1.
28. Krilov LR. Chronic fatigue syndrome. *Pediatr Ann* 1995;24:290.
29. Manian FA. Simultaneous measurement of antibodies to Epstein-Barr virus, human herpesvirus 6, herpes simplex virus types 1 and 2, and 14 enteroviruses in chronic fatigue syndrome: is there evidence of activation of a nonspecific polyclonal immune response? *Clin Infect Dis* 1994;19:448.
30. Fark AR. Infectious mononucleosis, Epstein-Barr virus, and chronic fatigue syndrome: a prospective case series. *J Fam Pract* 1991;32:202.
31. Horwitz CA, Henle W, Henle G, et al. Long-term serological follow-up of patients for Epstein-Barr virus after recovery from IM. *J Infect Dis* 1985;151:1150.
32. Sumaya CV. Endogenous reactivation of Epstein-Barr virus infections. *J Infect Dis* 1977;135:374.
33. Straus SE, Dale JK, Tobi M, et al. Acyclovir treatment of the chronic fatigue syndrome: lack of efficacy in a placebo-controlled trial. *N Engl J Med* 1988;319:1692.
34. Heneine W, Woods TC, Sinha SD, et al. Lack of evidence for infection with known human and animal retroviruses in patients with chronic fatigue syndrome. *Clin Infect Dis* 1994;18(Suppl):S121.

35. Gow JW, Behan WMH, Simpson K, et al. Studies on enterovirus in patients with chronic fatigue syndrome. *Clin Infect Dis* 1994;18(Suppl):S126.

36. Gunn WJ, Komaroff AL, Bell DS, et al. Inability of retroviral tests to identify persons with chronic fatigue syndrome, 1992. *MMWR Morb Mortal Wkly Rep* 1993;42:183.

37. Cavanagh HMA, Gow JW, Simpson K, et al. Special aspects of virology. In: Dawson DM, Sabin TD, eds. *Chronic fatigue syndrome.* Boston: Little, Brown; 1993:91.

38. Barker E, Fujimura SF, Fadem MB, et al. Immunologic abnormalities associated with chronic fatigue syndrome. *Clin Infect Dis* 1994;18(Suppl):S136.

39. Lloyd A, Gandevia S, Brockman A, et al. Cytokine production and fatigue in patients with chronic fatigue syndrome and health control subjects in response to exercise. *Clin Infect Dis* 1994;18(Suppl):S142.

40. Patarca R, Klimas NG, Lugtendorf S, et al. Dysregulated expression of tumor necrosis factor in chronic fatigue syndrome: interrelations with cellular sources and patterns of soluble immune mediator expression. *Clin Infect Dis* 1994;18(Suppl):S147.

41. Ojo-Amaize EA, Conley EJ, Peter JB. Decreased natural killer cell activity is associated with severity of fatigue immune dysfunction syndrome. *Clin Infect Dis* 1994;18(Suppl):S157.

42. Lloyd AR, Klimas N. Summary: immunologic studies of chronic fatigue syndrome. *Clin Infect Dis* 1994;18(Suppl):S160.

43. Bates DW, Buchwald D, Lee J, et al. Clinical laboratory test findings in patients with chronic fatigue syndrome. *Arch Intern Med* 1995;155:97.

44. Ader R, Felten DL, Cohen N, eds. *Psychoneuroimmunology.* 2nd ed. San Diego: Academic Press; 1991.

45. Rowe PC, Bou-Holaigah I, Kan JS, et al. Is neurally mediated hypotension an unrecognised cause of chronic fatigue? *Lancet* 1995;345:623.

46. Bou-Holaigah I, Rowe PC, Kan JS, et al. The relationship between neurally mediated hypotension and the chronic fatigue syndrome. *JAMA* 1995;274:961.

47. Strickland MC. Depression, chronic fatigue syndrome, and the adolescent. *Prim Care* 1991;18:259.

48. Cope H, David A, Pelosi A, et al. Predictors of chronic "postviral" fatigue. *Lancet* 1994;344:864.

49. Sadeh A, Carskadon MA, Acebo C, et al. Chronic fatigue immune dysfunction syndrome: an epidemic [letter]? *Pediatrics* 1992;89:802.

50. Wolfe F, Smythe HA, Yunus MB, et al. The American College of Rheumatology 1990 criteria for the classification of fibromyalgia. *Arthritis Rheum* 1990;33:160.

51. Goldenberg DL. Fibromyalgia syndrome and its overlap with chronic fatigue syndrome. In: Dawson DM, Sabin TD, eds. *Chronic fatigue syndrome.* Boston: Little, Brown; 1993:75.

52. Bell DS, Bell KM, Cheney PR. Primary juvenile fibromyalgia syndrome and chronic fatigue syndrome in adolescents. *Clin Infect Dis* 1994;18(Suppl):S21.

53. Goldenberg DL, Simms RW, Geiger A, et al. High frequency of fibromyalgia in patients with chronic fatigue seen in a primary care practice. *Arthritis Rheum* 1990;33:381.

54. Lloyd A, Hickie I, Wakefield D, et al. A double-blind, placebo-controlled trial of intravenous immunoglobulin therapy in patients with chronic fatigue syndrome. *Am J Med* 1990;89:561.

55. Peterson PK, Shepard J, Macres M, et al. A controlled trial of intravenous immunoglobulin G in chronic fatigue syndrome. *Am J Med* 1990;89:554.

56. Straus SE. Intravenous immunoglobulin treatment for the chronic fatigue syndrome. *Am J Med* 1990;89:551.

57. Gantz N. Management of a patient with chronic fatigue syndrome. In: Dawson DM, Sabin TD, eds. *Chronic fatigue syndrome.* Boston: Little, Brown; 1993:185.

58. Wachsmuth JR, MacMillan HL. Effective treatment for an adolescent with chronic fatigue syndrome. *Clin Pediatr* 1991;30:488.

SUGGESTED READING

Calabrese L, Danao T, Camara E, et al. Chronic fatigue syndrome. *Am Fam Physician* 1992;45:1205.

Carter BD, Marshall GS. New developments: diagnosis and management of chronic fatigue in children and adolescents. *Curr Probl Pediatr* 1995;25:281.

Cavanaugh RM. Evaluating adolescents with fatigue. *Am Fam Physician* 1987;35:163.

Clauw DJ. Fibromyalgia: more than just a musculoskeletal disease. *Am Fam Physician* 1995;52:843.

Dawson DM, Sabin TD, eds. *Chronic fatigue syndrome.* Boston: Little, Brown; 1993.

Demitrack MA, Abbey SE, eds. *Chronic fatigue syndrome: an integrative approach to evaluation and treatment.* New York: Guilford Press; 1996.

Glover DM. Chronic fatigue syndrome. *Adolescent Medicine: State of the Art Reviews* 1995;6:101.

Krilov LR. Chronic fatigue syndrome. *Pediatr Ann* 1995;24:290.

Levine PH, ed. Chronic fatigue syndrome. *Clin Infect Dis* 1994;18:S1.

McGregor RS. Chronic complaints in adolescence: chest pain, chronic fatigue, headaches, abdominal pain. *Adolescent Medicine: State of the Art Reviews* 1997;8:15.

Moder KG. Use and interpretation of rheumatologic tests: a guide for clinicians. *Mayo Clin Proc* 1996;71:391.

Reiffenberger DH, Amundson LH. Fibromyalgia syndrome: a review. *Am Fam Physician* 1996;53:1698.

SYNCOPE

Syncopal spells are surprisingly common, yet not much is written about the subject in the conventional textbooks. As many as half of all teenagers may have at least one syncopal episode during their lifetimes [1]. The workup and treatment can vary considerably, however. In studies of adults, the average cost per workup was $2,463 in 1982, with a definitive cause found in only 13 of 121 patients. To reach those 13 diagnoses, the cost per patient was $22,925 [2]. However, since the early 1990s, major advances have been made in understanding the nature of syncopal spells in children and adolescents, so that a rational approach is now possible.

Etiology

Vasodepressor Syncope

Vasodepressor syncope is a new classification that may be unfamiliar to many practicing physicians. However, it is the most common cause of syncope in the adolescent population and includes simple fainting spells (vasovagal syncope). It is also referred to as neurocardiogenic syncope, neurally mediated syncope, or neuroautonomic syncope [3].

The pathophysiology for vasodepressor syncope is complex: ordinarily, when a patient goes from supine or prone to upright, venous pooling occurs, which leads to decreased venous return. The change in position usually triggers tachycardia and vasoconstriction to compensate for the decreased ventricular output. However, in vasodepressor syncope, ventricular C-fiber mechanoreceptors are thought to misfire, resulting in decreased sympathetic activity (vasodilation) and increased parasympathetic activity (bradycardia)—both of which are inappropriate and lead to inadequate cardiac output and syncope [1].

Cardiac Causes

Syncope can be caused by a number of cardiac abnormalities, including supraventricular tachycardia (SVT), ventricular tachycardia (VT), congenital long QT syndrome, bradyarrhythmias, and structural lesions. SVT is the most commonly found tachycardia in adolescents and is frequently associated with Wolff-Parkinson-White (WPW) syndrome with short PR intervals on electrocardiogram (ECG). However, WPW syndrome alone can cause syncope or even sudden death [1]. VT is relatively uncommon in structurally normal hearts and should raise the question of cocaine or crack use. Congenital long QT syndrome is a rare but significant cause of sudden death in adolescents and is the reason why a screening ECG is always useful in evaluating recurrent or significant syncopal episodes [4].

Structural lesions that may cause syncope include hypertrophic cardiomyopathy, dilated cardiomyopathy, and aortic or pulmonic stenosis. With such lesions, a family history is sometimes positive. Syncope that occurs during exercise is particularly worrisome and can portend sudden death in competitive athletes [5].

Noncardiac Causes

Although a variety of etiologies can lead to syncopal spells, perhaps the largest category of noncardiac causes is idiopathic or unknown [3]. Often, despite intensive workups, patients remain undiagnosed. In such situations, however, it may still be reassuring to the teenager and his or her family that certain life-threatening disorders have been ruled out. Obviously, close follow-up is mandatory.

Seizures and vasodepressor spells can be difficult to distinguish (the latter is sometimes termed "convulsive syncope" when seizure activity occurs) [3]. Both can involve loss of consciousness, tonic–clonic activity, and a postictal phase; however, all of these manifestations usually last longer than a few minutes if seizures are the cause. Atypical migraines, drugs (cocaine, crack, alcohol), diuretic abuse in patients with eating disorders, and conversion reactions can also cause syncopal episodes.

Diagnosis

A careful history is extremely important (Table 19). In one study of adults, the history and physical examination resulted in a diagnosis for 25% of the patients [6]. In particular, a careful history of re-

TABLE 19. *Taking a good syncope history*

Before the event
Recent fluid intake (quantify)
Preceding aura, nausea, sweating?
Presence of headache, palpitations, or lightheadedness?

During the event
Did the patient actually lose consciousness?
Duration of the event
Witnesses
Tonic–clonic activity
Injuries sustained
Loss of continence

Other important questions
Previous spells
Medications
Drug abuse
Past psychiatric symptoms
Precipitating factors
Family history: syncope, arrhythmias, sudden death

Adapted from Schutte DA, Franklin WH. Adolescent syncope: faint or feigned? *Adolescent Medicine: State of the Art Reviews* 1997;8:111.

cent fluid intake often shows that teenagers take inadequate fluids (2,100 ml/24 hours is recommended for a 50-kg teen) [1]. Patients with true syncope often sustain injuries during the episode (more than one third in one series) [3].

Laboratory Evaluation

Although the history and physical examination will greatly determine the extent of the laboratory workup, an ECG should probably be obtained on any patient with true syncope [1]. If the history is consistent with a vasodepressor episode, no further diagnostic testing is necessary. Other tests (e.g., electroencephalography, electrolytes, toxicology screen, computed tomography, or magnetic resonance imaging) may be indicated, depending on the clinical situation.

Tilt-Table Testing

Tilt-table testing [3,7,8] is indicated if a patient has recurrent syncope or even a single syncopal episode that is particularly severe or worrisome (Fig. 7). Patients with vasodepressor syncope or single uncomplicated episodes of syncope do not require such testing [9].

Use of the tilt-table enables clinicians to evaluate a patient's response to orthostatic changes in position. Usually, a patient has fasted overnight, is placed on the table with blood pressure and heart rate monitoring, and is tilted upright 60° to 80° for 45 minutes. The test is 90% specific and 65% to 85% reproducible [1]. In a positive test, the patient's symptoms reoccur, along with either bradycardia or hypotension. Isoproterenol, a sympathomimetic agent, is sometimes used to provoke syncopal spells.

In one study of 54 pediatric and adolescent patients [10], only 5 of 298 studies (excluding tilt-table testing) were abnormal. Of the 27 patients who underwent tilt-table testing, 100% were diagnosed; of the other 27 patients, only 18.5% were given a definitive diagnosis.

Ambulatory Monitoring

Clinicians often order Holter monitoring for their patients with syncope, yet the likelihood that a syncopal event will occur during a given 24-hour period is quite low. However, event recorders exist that can be worn for months if necessary and can record ECG rhythms at the press of a button. At the first sign of difficulty, either the patient or a witness can press the button to start the recording.

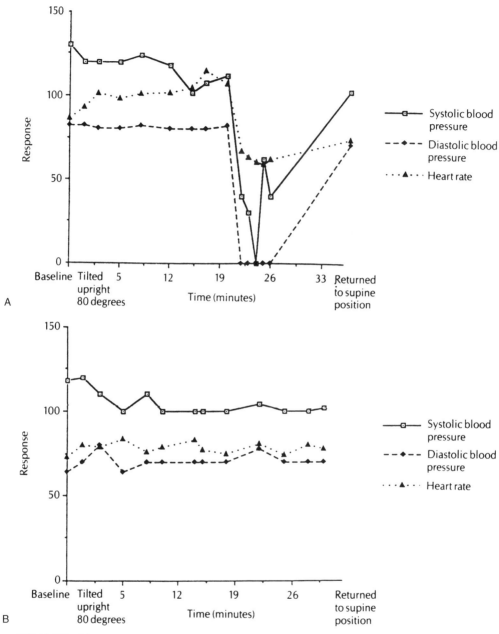

FIG. 7. Tilt-table testing for syncope. Patient is a 15-year-old female athlete with a history of syncope after exercise. **A:** Positive tilt-table test. **B:** After 10 mg of intravenous metoprolol was administered, a repeat test is negative. (Wolfe DA, Grubb BP, Kimmel SR. Head-upright tilt test: a new method of evaluating syncope. *Am Fam Physician* 1993;47:149. Used with permission.)

Exercise Testing

If patients are found to have long QT intervals on ECG, exercise testing can be useful. Similarly, patients with syncope during exercise may require such testing.

Treatment

Vasodepressor Syncope

Fluids are the mainstay of therapy for teenagers with vasodepressor episodes. Patients should drink at least 64 ounces of noncaffeinated fluids a day. Occasionally, urine dipsticks can be prescribed so that teens can maintain their urine specific gravity above 1.010.

For patients who fail fluid therapy, drug therapy can be helpful. In a randomized trial of either atenolol or fludrocortisone acetate for 59 patients with positive tilt-table tests, 83% were cured or improved [11]. Another study of 27 consecutive pediatric patients found an 89% response rate to metoprolol [12]. Sertraline, a selective serotonin reuptake inhibitor commonly used to treat depression, also has been found to be effective when other therapies fail [13]. Also, oral theophylline has been used [3].

Other Causes

Cardiac causes of syncope require consultation with a cardiologist. SVT can be managed with beta blockers, verapamil, or digoxin (but the latter two should not be used in patients with WPW syndrome because activation of alternative conduction pathways may lead to ventricular fibrillation or VT.) Beta blockers are also the drug of choice for treating prolonged QT syndrome. For noncardiac causes, consultation with a neurologist or adolescent psychiatrist or psychologist is useful, depending on the suspected etiology.

REFERENCES

1. Schutte DA, Franklin WH. Adolescent syncope: faint or feigned? *Adolescent Medicine: State of the Art Reviews* 1997;8:111.
2. Kapoor WN, Karpf M, Maher Y, et al. Syncope of unknown origin: the need for a more cost-effective approach to its diagnostic evaluation. *JAMA* 1982;247:2687.
3. Wolfe DA, Grubb BP, Kimmel SR. Head-upright tilt test: a new method of evaluating syncope. *Am Fam Physician* 1993;47:149.
4. Wogciech Z. Risk of cardiac events in family members of patients with long QT syndrome. *J Am Coll Cardiol* 1995;26:1685.
5. Maron BJ, Epstein SE, Roberts WC. Causes of sudden death in competitive athletes. *J Am Coll Cardiol* 1986;7:204.
6. Kapoor WN, Karpf M, Wieand S, et al. A prospective evaluation and follow-up of patients with syncope. *N Engl J Med* 1983;309:197.
7. Thilenius OG, Quinones JA, Husayni TS, et al. Tilt test for diagnosis of unexplained syncope in pediatric patients. *Pediatrics* 1991;87:334.
8. Samoil D, Grubb BP, Kip K, et al. Head-upright tilt table testing in children with unexplained syncope. *Pediatrics* 1993;92:426.
9. Benditt DG, Furguson DW, Grubb BP, et al. Tilt table testing for assessing syncope. *J Am Coll Cardiol* 1996;28:263.
10. Streiper MJ, Auld DO, Hulse JE, et al. Evaluation of recurrent pediatric syncope: role of tilt table testing. *Pediatrics* 1994;93:660.
11. Scott WA, Pongiglione G, Bromberg BI, et al. Randomized comparison of atenolol and fludrocortisone acetate in the treatment of pediatric neurally mediated syncope. *Am J Cardiol* 1995;76:400.
12. O'Marcaigh AS, MacLellan-Tobert SG, Porter CJ. Tilt-table testing and oral metoprolol therapy in young patients with unexplained syncope. *Pediatrics* 1994;93:278.
13. Grubb BP, Samoil D, Kosiniski D, et al. Use of sertraline hydrochloride in the treatment of refractory neurocardiogenic syncope in children and adolescents. *J Am Coll Cardiol* 1994;24:490.

SUGGESTED READING

Hannon DW, and Knilans TK. Syncope in children and adolescents. *Curr Probl Pediatr* 1993;23:358.

Hart GT. Evaluation of syncope. *Am Fam Physician* 1995;51:1941.

O'Marcaigh AS, MacLellan-Tobert SG, Porter CJ. Tilt-table testing and oral metoprolol therapy in young patients with unexplained syncope. *Pediatrics* 1994;93:278.

Samoil D, Grubb BP, Kip K, et al. Head-upright tilt table testing in children with unexplained syncope. *Pediatrics* 1993;92:426.

Schutte DA, and Franklin WH. Adolescent syncope: faint or feigned? *Adolescent Medicine: State of the Art Reviews* 1997;8:111.

Streiper MJ, Auld DO, Hulse JE, et al. Evaluation of recurrent pediatric syncope: role of tilt table testing. *Pediatrics* 1994;93:660.

Wolfe DA, Grubb BP, Kimmel SR. Head-upright tilt test: a new method of evaluating syncope. *Am Fam Physician* 1993;47:149.

COMMON UPPER RESPIRATORY PROBLEMS IN ADOLESCENTS

Pharyngitis

All clinicians are familiar, of course, with the vagaries of trying to diagnose group A streptococcal infection of the tonsillopharynx. What they may not be as familiar with are the many other causes of pharyngitis in adolescents, particularly those that might require antimicrobial treatment.

Viral infection is, by far, the most common etiology of pharyngitis. A variety of organisms are known to involve both the pharynx and the upper respiratory tract, including rhinoviruses, coronaviruses, influenza A and B, and the parainfluenza viruses [1]. Other organisms are more limited to the pharynx and cause distinctive disease, such as Epstein-Barr virus, herpes simplex virus, and coxsackie A.

Group A Streptococcus

Although less common, bacterial pharyngitis is more worrisome because of the risks of complications and epidemiologic considerations. Group A streptococcal infection is the most common bacterial form of acute pharyngitis and, if untreated, can lead to acute rheumatic fever, poststreptococcal glomerulonephritis, streptococcal toxic shock syndrome, and other invasive infections [2,3]. Occurring primarily among school-age children, group A streptococcal infections account for 15% to 20% of all cases of pharyngitis among 5- to 15-year-olds [1].

A number of clinical signs (exudate, tender anterior cervical adenopathy, scarlatiniform rash) and epidemiologic considerations (outbreaks, fall or winter season) may be suggestive of group A streptococcal infection, but there is no sure way of making a diagnosis without an appropriate rapid test or throat culture. Alternatively, symptoms such as rhinitis, conjunctivitis, and cough point to a viral etiology and thus a very low risk of bacterial infection [4]. However, most authorities recommend using an appropriate microbiologic test, no matter how good one's "batting average" supposedly is. Rapid detection tests are highly specific but, unfortunately, not as sensitive. Therefore, a positive test can reliably be used alone to treat a patient for group A streptococcal pharyngitis, but a negative test does not rule out the disease and should be followed with a throat culture [4,5]. Clinicians should also be aware that a single throat culture detects only 88% to 99% of infections [4]. If patients are taking oral tetracyeline or erythromycin for treatment of acne, throat cultures are still useful and should be obtained [6].

Group C and Group G Streptococci

Both group C and group G streptococci are beta-hemolytic and have been associated with epidemics of acute pharyngitis [7,8]. More than half of streptococci isolated in 18-year-olds may be non-group A [8]. Although neither infection leads to acute rheumatic fever, acute glomerulonephritis after group C [9] and group G [10] infection is well described. A 1990 study of college students demonstrated that group C streptococci were associated with endemic pharyngitis with fever, exudative tonsillitis, and anterior cervical adenopathy [11]. They have also been found in milk-borne outbreaks of

TABLE 20. *Prevalence of pharyngeal gonorrhea in adolescents*

Clinic site	No. (%) with genital gonorrhea	No. (%) with pharyngeal gonorrhea
Adolescent clinic (*N* = 240)	6 (2.5)	0 (0.0)
Sexually transmitted diseases clinic (*N* = 594)	196 (33)	20 (3.4)

Brown RT, Lossick JG, Mosure DJ, et al. Pharyngeal gonorrhea screening in adolescents: is it necessary? *Pediatrics* 1989;84:623, with permission.

acute pharyngitis, but there is increasing evidence that both groups C and G are responsible for sporadic cases of pharyngitis as well [1].

Group G streptococci have also been found in food-borne outbreaks due to contaminated egg salad and chicken salad [1]. In 1991, a community outbreak of group G infection was documented, with clinical, serologic, and treatment responses similar to group A outbreaks. However, the group G patients tended to be significantly older (mean age, 11.5 years) [12].

Rapid tests for group A organisms do not detect group C or G infection. However, if asked, laboratories can provide typing of beta-hemolytic colonies that are not group A.

Neisseria gonorrhoeae, Mycoplasma pneumoniae, and Chlamydia pneumoniae

Pharyngeal gonorrhea usually occurs in the context of concurrent genital gonorrhea. In a prospective study of 240 teens in a general adolescent clinic, none had a positive throat culture for *N. gonorrhoeae*; of 594 teens at a sexually transmitted disease clinic, 3.4% had positive throat cultures, but in only 2 of 20 patients was the pharynx the only infected site [13] (Table 20). Therefore, routinely culturing teenagers' throats for gonorrhea is not productive except in the clinical setting of suspected sexually transmitted disease [13].

Mycoplasma pneumoniae and *C. pneumoniae* both cause tonsillopharyngitis in the clinical context of lower respiratory tract infection [4,14]. Once thought to cause pharyngitis in adults, *Chlamydia trachomatis* has been exonerated [1,4].

Treatment

Oral penicillin V for 10 days remains the drug of choice for group A (as well as groups C and G) infections [15–17]. Erythromycin has been the drug of choice for patients with penicillin allergy. Other macrolides, clindamycin, and various cephalosporins are also effective (Table 21). Clindamycin may be particularly effective in eliminating the chronic carrier state [18]. A full 24 hours' worth of antibiotics should be administered before teenagers return to school [19].

Sinusitis

Trying to distinguish between acute sinusitis and a simple upper respiratory infection (URI) is enough to give any clinician a headache. Americans spend an estimated $5 billion annually for medications to treat rhinitis and sinusitis and another $60 billion for surgical interventions [20]. During the past decade, annual outpatient visit rates for sinusitis have tripled from 30 to 90 per 1,000 people aged 15 years and older [21]. Are there good data to suggest that we know what we are doing when we diagnose acute sinusitis?

Diagnosis

Experts have wrestled with how to diagnose acute sinusitis for the past several decades (Fig. 8). Numerous problems exist:

- Simple URIs can be complicated, perhaps 5% to 10% of the time, by acute sinusitis [22]. In one of the few double-blinded, placebo-controlled trials of treating adult patients with antibiotics for their

TABLE 21. *Cost of some commonly used oral antibiotics*

Drug	Adult dosage	Cost[a]
Amoxicillin (generic)	250 mg tid	$ 2.41
Augmentin	500 mg bid	$57.63
Azithromycin	250 mg qd	$36.23
Cefixime	400 mg qd	$67.33
Cefuroxime axetil	250 mg bid	$64.17
Clarithromycin	250 mg bid	$61.75
Dirithromycin	500 mg qd	$26.25
Erythromycin (generic)	250 mg qid	$ 7.53
Ery-tab		$ 6.65
Eryc		$12.00
Penicillin V (generic)	250 mg tid	$ 1.73
Trimethoprim–sulfamethoxasole (generic)	160 mg bid	$ 1.79
	160 mg bid[b]	$ 1.79
Septra	160 mg bid[b]	$24.10

[a]Cost to the pharmacist, average wholesale price.
[b]Of trimethoprim.
Adapted from Dirithromycin. *The Medical Letter* 1995;37(962):109, and Ceftibuten: a new oral cephalosporin. *The Medical Letter* 1996;38(970):23.

URIs, it was found that of 314 adults, the 20% who harbored *Hemophilus influenzae*, *Moraxella catarrhalis*, or *Streptococcus pneumoniae* (by nasopharyngeal aspiration) responded better to a 5-day course of amoxicillin/clavulanate [23].

• The true gold standard for diagnosing acute sinusitis is sinus aspiration and culture, not a very practical test in pediatric or adult medicine [24].
• Signs and symptoms can overlap greatly among acute sinusitis, URI, and allergic rhinitis.
• Patients with acute sinusitis have a spontaneous clinical cure rate as high as 40% to 50% [22].
• Imaging only complicates the picture [25]: plain sinus films are abnormal in a sizable number of healthy children [26–28] (Table 22); 5% of teenagers may have abnormal computed tomography (CT) scans of their sinuses in the absence of suspected sinus disease [29]; and plain films and CT scans do not always agree [30] (Table 23). In one study of children with chronic sinusitis, 74% had plain films and CT scans that did not correlate. If plain films were negative, 45% had abnormal CT scans; if plain films were positive, 34% had no abnormal findings on CT scan [31].
• In adults with common colds, 87% of maxillary sinuses and 65% of ethmoid sinuses are abnormal on CT scan [32].

How, then, should the problem be approached?

Nearly every expert would agree with clinicians who treat the triad of high fever, copious and purulent nasal discharge, and facial pain [25]. Others report that certain clusters of symptoms (e.g., purulent nasal discharge, cough, and sneezing) can be sensitive but not specific, or specific (maxillary toothache) but not sensitive [24]. Other experts suggest that the 10-day mark can be used to separate a simple viral URI from acute sinusitis, whereas 30 days separates acute from chronic sinusitis [33]. One complicating factor is that the paranasal sinuses are lined with respiratory epithelium that is contiguous with the rest of the respiratory tree; therefore, a low degree of sinusitis is inevitable with any cold [32].

In a typical URI, the patient may not be completely free of symptoms by day 10, but the symptoms should have peaked before then and the patient's condition begun to improve. The quality of the nasal discharge may have changed during the course of the URI from clear to purulent and back to clear or mucoid before resolving. By contrast, patients with acute sinusitis seem to have persistent symptoms, which may include nasal discharge (of any quality), cough (often worse at night), headache, facial pain, fever, and malaise [33]. In chronic sinusitis, nasal discharge can be present or absent; cough or persistent throat clearing may be present; mouth breathing is common; and chronic, headache, sore throat, and halitosis are common.

Sinusitis must be differentiated from allergic rhinitis, the most common allergic disorder in the United States, affecting more than 20 million people [20]. Here, again, there is significant overlap: al-

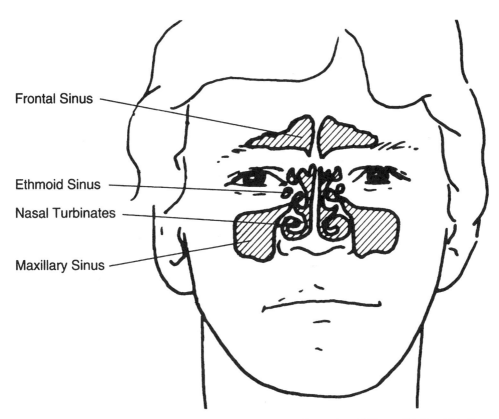

FIG. 8. Coronal view of paranasal sinuses. (Adapted with permission from Williams JW, Simel DL. Does this patient have sinusitis? Diagnosing acute sinusitis by history and physical examination. *JAMA* 1993;270:1242.)

TABLE 22. *Abnormal sinus radiographs in children without clinical symptoms of sinusitis*

Age	Healthy children	Children without URI	With URI
Study 1			
6–9 y	27–30%	—	—
9–12 y	14–17%	—	—
Study 2			
6–14 y	—	27%	57%
Study 3			
1–16 y	—	10%	52%

Study 1: Maresh MM, Washburn AH. Paranasal sinuses from birth to late adolescence. *Am J Dis Child* 1940;60:841.

Study 2: Shopfner CE, Rossi JO. Roentgen evaluation of the paranasal sinuses in children. *AJR Am J Roentgenol* 1973;118:176.

Study 3: Kovatch AL, Wald ER, Ledesma-Medina J, et al. Maxillary sinus radiographs in children with nonrespiratory complaints. *Pediatrics* 1984;73:306.

URI, upper respiratory infection.

Adapted from Abbasi S, Cunningham AS. Are we overtreating sinusitis? *Contemp Pediatr* 1996;13:49.

TABLE 23. *Comparison of plain films with computed tomography (CT) scans for diagnosing sinusitis*

Sinus	Full CT scan (gold standard)	Plain films	Limited CT scan
Frontal	100%	20%	100%
Ethmoid	100%	54%	73%
Maxillary	100%	75%	97%
Sphenoid	100%	0%	82%

Adapted from Garcia DP, Corbett ML, Eberly SM, et al. Radiographic imaging studies in pediatric chronic sinusitis. *J Allergy Clin Immunol* 1994;94:523.

lergic rhinitis can lead to or be confused with acute or recurrent episodes of sinusitis [22]. A thorough history may help to distinguish patients with seasonal symptoms (e.g., due to grass or pollen) or perennial symptoms (e.g., due to dust or animal dander). Patients often have conjunctivitis, itching, and tearing, in addition to sneezing and nasal pruritus. Control of environmental allergens when possible [34], judicious use of antihistamines [35,36], and corticosteroid nasal sprays [37] (Table 24) help control most symptoms. Numerous nonsedating oral antihistamines are available (e.g., Hismanal, Allegra, Claritin), but they are all expensive (average wholesale cost to pharmacist, $50–$60 for 30 days' treatment) [38].

Imaging remains controversial. Some experts believe that a single Waters view of the sinuses is an easy and cost-effective alternative to a limited CT scan [30], some think that a plain sinus series should be obtained [22], some foresee a limited or complete CT scan becoming the new gold standard [24], and others believe that imaging of any kind can be flawed and therefore clinicians should rely more on clinical findings [25].

Treatment

Antimicrobial therapy should be targeted at the organisms most frequently responsible for infection: *H. influenzae*, *M. catarrhalis*, *S. pneumoniae*, group A streptococci, and alpha-hemolytic streptococci [39,40]. In chronic sinusitis, these organisms can be found along with others, including *Staphylococcus aureus* and various anaerobes (*Prevotella*, *Fusobacterium*, and *Peptostreptococcus* species) [20,40]. Some experts prefer to start treatment with amoxicillin, despite the possibility of beta-lactamase–producing *H. influenzae*, *M. catarrhalis*, or *S. aureus* organisms, because it is inexpensive (see Table 21), well tolerated, and seems to be as efficacious as other antibiotics [39,41]. Others prefer

TABLE 24. *Some steroid nasal sprays for allergic rhinitis*

Drug	Initial dosage	Wholesale cost[a]
Beclomethasone Beconase Vancenase	1 spray in each nostril bid or qid	$18.01
Beconase AQ Vancenase AQ	1–2 sprays in each nostril bid	$19.44
Budesonide Rhinocort	2 sprays in each nostril bid or 4 sprays qd	$32.40
Flunisolide Nasalide	2 sprays in each nostril bid	$31.82
Fluticasone propionate Flonase	2 sprays in each nostril qd or 1 spray bid	$38.88
Triamcinolone acetonide Nasacort	2 sprays in each nostril qd	$45.19

[a]Cost to pharmacist for 30 days' treatment.
Fluticasone propionate nasal spray for allergic rhinitis. *The Medical Letter* 1995;37(940):5.

amoxicillin–potassium clavulanate (Augmentin) because of its activity against nearly all suspected pathogens [33]. Most experts would also choose this drug to treat patients with chronic sinusitis. In adults with maxillary sinusitis, trimethoprim–sulfamethoxazole has been found to be effective [39] for as short as a 3-day course [42], although a 7- to 10-day course for acute sinusitis is more typical. In addition, treatment with corticosteroid sprays may be useful, although no controlled clinical trials have yet been performed. On the other hand, the most recent randomized trial of decongestant–antihistamine combinations failed to demonstrate the usefulness of these agents in treating acute maxillary sinusitis [43].

REFERENCES

1. Bisno AL. Acute pharyngitis: etiology and diagnosis. *Pediatrics* 1995;97(Suppl):949.
2. Denny FW Jr, Henderson FW. Group A invaders. *Contemp Pediatr* 1996;13:104.
3. Holm SE. Invasive group A streptococcal infections. *N Engl J Med* 1996;335:590.
4. Denny FW Jr. Tonsillopharyngitis 1994. *Pediatr Rev* 1994;15:185.
5. Pichichero ME, Disney FA, Green JL, et al. Comparative reliability of clinical, culture, and antigen detection methods for diagnosis of group A beta-hemolytic streptococcal tonsillopharyngitis. *Pediatr Ann* 1992;21:798.
6. Dajani AS. Value of throat cultures in adolescents taking daily antibiotics for acne. *Pediatr Infect Dis J* 1994;13:842.
7. Hayden GF, Murphy TF, Hendley JO. Non-group A streptococci in the pharynx: pathogens or innocent bystanders? *American Journal of Diseases of Children* 1989;143:794.
8. Denny FW Jr. Group A Streptococcal infections: 1993. *Curr Probl Pediatr* 1993;23:179.
9. Duca E, Teodorovici GR, Radu C, et al. A new nephritogenic streptococcus. *Journal of Hygiene* 1969;67:691.
10. Gnann JW Jr, Gray BM, Griffin FM Jr, et al. Acute glomerulonephritis following group G streptococcal infection. *J Infect Dis* 1987;156:411.
11. Turner JC, Hayden GF, Kiselica D, et al. Association of group C β-hemolytic streptococci with endemic pharyngitis among college students. *JAMA* 1990;264:2644.
12. Gerber MA, Randolph MF, Martin NJ, et al. Community-wide outbreak of group G streptococcal pharyngitis. *Pediatrics* 1991;87:598.
13. Brown RT, Lossick JG, Mosure DJ, et al. Pharyngeal gonorrhea screening in adolescents: is it necessary? *Pediatrics* 1989;84:623.
14. Williams WC, Williamson HA Jr, LeFevre ML. The prevalence of *Mycoplasma pneumoniae* in ambulatory patients with nonstreptococcal sore throat. *Fam Med* 1991;23:117.
15. Shulman ST, Gerber MA, Tanz RR, et al. Streptococcal pharyngitis: The case for penicillin therapy. *Pediatr Infect Dis J* 1994;13:1.
16. Shulman ST. Evaluation of penicillins, cephalosporins, and macrolides for therapy of streptococcal pharyngitis. *Pediatrics* 1996;97(Suppl):955.
17. Medical Letter. The choice of antibacterial drugs. *The Medical Letter* 1996;38(971):25.
18. Tanz RR, Poncher JR, Corydon KE, et al. Clindamycin treatment of chronic pharyngeal carriage of group A streptococci. *J Pediatr* 1991;119:123.
19. Snellman LW, Stang HJ, Stang JM, et al. Duration of positive throat cultures for group A streptococci after initiation of antibiotic therapy. *Pediatrics* 1993;91:1166.
20. Guarderas JC. Rhinitis and sinusitis: office management. *Mayo Clin Proc* 1996;71:882.
21. McCaig LF, Hughes JM. Trends in antimicrobial drug prescribing among office-based physicians in the United States. *JAMA* 1995;273:214.
22. Wald ER. Sinusitis. *Pediatr Rev* 1993;14:345.
23. Kaiser L, Hueston WJ, Clark JR. Effects of antibiotic treatment in the subset of common-cold: patients who have bacteria in nasopharyngeal secretions. *Lancet* 1996;347:1507.
24. Williams JW, Simel DL. Does this patient have sinusitis? Diagnosing acute sinusitis by history and physical examination. *JAMA* 1993;270:1242.
25. Abbasi S, Cunningham AS. Are we overtreating sinusitis? *Contemp Pediatr* 1996;13:49.
26. Maresh MM, Washburn AH. Paranasal sinuses from birth to late adolescence. *American Journal of Diseases of Children* 1940;60:841.
27. Shopfner CE, Rossi JO. Roentgen evaluation of the paranasal sinuses in children. *AJR Am J Roentgenol* 1973;118:176.
28. Kovatch AL, Wald ER, Ledesma-Medina J, et al. Maxillary sinus radiographs in children with nonrespiratory complaints. *Pediatrics* 1984;73:306.
29. Diament MJ, Senac MO Jr, Gilsanz V, et al. Prevalence of incidental paranasal sinuses opacification in pediatric patients: a CT study. *J Comput Assist Tomogr* 1987;11:426.
30. Garcia DP, Corbett ML, Eberly SM, et al. Radiographic imaging studies in pediatric chronic sinusitis. *J Allergy Clin Immunol* 1994;94:523.

31. Lusk RP, Lazar RH, Muntz HR. The diagnosis and treatment of recurrent and chronic sinusitis in children. *Pediatr Clin North Am* 1989;36:13.
32. Gwaltney JM Jr, Phillips CD, Miller RD, et al. Computed tomographic study of the common cold. *N Engl J Med* 1994;330:25.
33. Wald ER. Chronic sinusitis in children. *J Pediatr* 1995;127:339.
34. Fireman P. Diagnosis of allergic disorders. *Pediatr Rev* 1995;16:178.
35. Peggs JF, Shimp LA, Opdycke RAC. Antihistamines: the old and the new. *Am Fam Physician* 1995;52:593.
36. Kemp JP. Special considerations in the treatment of seasonal allergic rhinitis in adolescents: the role of antihistamine therapy. *Clin Pediatr* 1996;35:383.
37. Medical Letter. Fluticasone propionate nasal spray for allergic rhinitis. *The Medical Letter* 1995;37(940):5.
38. Medical Letter. Fexofenadine. *The Medical Letter* 1996;38(986):95.
39. Giebink GS. Criteria for evaluation of antimicrobial agents and current therapies for acute sinusitis in children. *Clin Infect Dis* 1992;14(Suppl):S212.
40. Brook I, Yocum P, Frazier EH. Bacteriology and β-lactamase activity in acute and chronic maxillary sinusitis. *Arch Otolaryngol* 1996;122:418.
41. Lindbaek M, Hjortdahl P, Johnsen UL-H. Randomised, double blind, placebo controlled trial of penicillin V and amoxycillin in treatment of acute sinus infection in adults. *Br Med J* 1996;313:325.
42. Williams JW Jr, Hollerman DR Jr, Samsa GP, et al. Randomized controlled trial of 3 vs 1 days of trimethoprim/sulfamethoxazole for acute maxillary sinusitis. *JAMA* 1995;273:1015.
43. McCormick DP, John SD, Swischuk LE, et al. A double-blind, placebo-controlled trial of decongestant–antihistamine for the treatment of sinusitis in children. *Clin Pediatr* 1996;35:457.

SUGGESTED READING

Abbasi S, Cunningham AS. Are we overtreating sinusitis? *Contemp Pediatr* 1996;13:49.
Bisno AL. Acute pharyngitis: etiology and diagnosis. *Pediatrics* 1995;97(Suppl):949.
Denny FW Jr. Tonsillopharyngitis 1994. *Pediatr Rev* 1994;15:185.
Denny FW Jr, Henderson FW. Group A invaders. *Contemp Pediatr* 1996;13:104.
Fireman P. Diagnosis of allergic disorders. *Pediatr Rev* 1995;16:178.
Guarderas JC. Rhinitis and sinusitis: office management. *Mayo Clin Proc* 1996;71:882.
Kaplan EL, ed. Group A streptococcal infections. *Pediatrics* 1995;97(Suppl):945.
Kemp JP. Special considerations in the treatment of seasonal allergic rhinitis in adolescents: the role of antihistamine therapy. *Clin Pediatr* 1996;35:383.
Peggs JF, Shimp LA, Opdycke RAC. Antihistamines: the old and the new. *Am Fam Physician* 1995;52:593.
Perkins A. An approach to diagnosing the acute sore throat. *Am Fam Physician* 1997;55:131.
Pichichero ME. Group A streptococcal tonsillopharyngitis: cost-effective diagnosis and treatment. *Ann Emerg Med* 1995;25:390.
Pichichero ME, ed. Streptococcal infections. *Pediatr Ann* 1992;21:795.
Rosendaal FR. Invasive group A streptococcal infections. *N Engl J Med* 1996;335:590.
Shulman ST. Streptococcal pharyngitis: diagnostic considerations. *Pediatr Infect Dis J* 1994;13:567.
Wald ER. Sinusitis in children. *N Engl J Med* 1992;326:319.
Wald ER. Sinusitis. *Pediatr Rev* 1993;14:345.
Wald ER. Chronic sinusitis in children. *J Pediatr* 1995;127:339.
Williams JW, Simel DL. Does this patient have sinusitis? Diagnosing acute sinusitis by history and physical examination. *JAMA* 1993;270:1242.
Wood RA. Asthma, allergies, and sinusitis in adolescence. *Adolescent Medicine: State of the Art Reviews* 1997;8:125.

ASTHMA

Asthma is the most common chronic illness in childhood [1,2]. It occurs in 8% to 9% of white children and 11% to 12% of African-American children at some time during their lives. The ratio of asthma in boys versus girls is 1.4 : 1 [3]. In all, asthma affects nearly 2.5 million youngsters younger than 18 years of age. African-American children have 2.5 times the prevalence of asthma in whites, and inner-city children have a prevalence 1.5 times greater than other children [4]. In 1990, children between the ages of 5 and 17 years had 160,000 hospitalizations, 860,000 emergency room visits, and over 1.25 million physician visits due to asthma [5]. Linkages to the following have been established [6]:

- Roach antigens in inner-city housing
- Maternal history of asthma

- Lack of prenatal care
- Low maternal weight gain during pregnancy
- History of bronchiolitis
- Positive-pressure ventilation at birth
- Maternal smoking during pregnancy

Asthma is a syndrome characterized by increased tracheobronchial reactivity to various stimuli. This results in widespread, reversible airway narrowing that changes in severity either as a result of therapy or spontaneously. Persistent or chronic airway inflammation may also be present and may be the primary problem in many patients. This is characterized by the presence of inflammatory mediators, inflammatory cells (especially eosinophils), bronchial wall edema, and epithelial cell changes. Asthma is almost always associated with some kind of IgE-related reaction and therefore has an allergic basis. Asthma has been characterized, in the past, as being either extrinsic (caused by factors external to the patient) or intrinsic (caused by factors within the patient's body). It might be more accurate to say that asthma attacks can be triggered by external or internal factors, but that IgE-mediated (i.e., allergic) and inflammatory-mediated processes cause them [7].

Asthma almost always begins in the early childhood years. By 5 years of age, asthma is present in more than 80% of those in whom it will develop [8]. Although asthma is twice as common among boys in childhood, the rates begin to even out during adolescence and, by the fourth and fifth decades of life, it is twice as common among women [9]. One of the prime morbidities of asthma is school absenteeism. In 1 year, more than 10 million days of school were missed because of asthma [5]. Asthma accounts for one fourth of the days lost from school due to chronic illness. Children younger than 17 years with asthma are reported to have absentee rates 24% higher than the general absentee rate, as indicated for one school district where this was studied [9]. Asthma also is responsible for more days of activity restriction than any other chronic illness in children aged 17 years and younger [9]. School absenteeism from asthma accounts for loss of parental income at the rate of almost a billion dollars per year [4].

Although asthma usually is not thought of as fatal, it can be. The increase in asthma deaths has not spared adolescents [10]. These deaths often appear to be due to sudden, severe attacks that prove irreversible. A review of asthma deaths in England, New Zealand, and Sweden revealed the following reasons for such deaths: patient and family members did not recognize the severity of the illness in some cases; in others, the physician failed to recognize the severity of the illness; sometimes there was delay in getting emergency care; the patient was noncompliant; home monitoring was poor; beta-adrenergic drugs were used improperly; or, there was delay in and improper use of corticosteroid drugs [9,11–13]. Many of these problems are common in adolescents with any chronic illness, including asthma. Another factor may be overuse of bronchodilators without use of antiinflammatory drugs [14]. Beta-adrenergic drugs themselves have not been found to be related to deaths from asthma [15]. Goldenhersh and Rachelefsky [9] list the following risk factors for life-threatening asthma:

- Early onset of severe asthma, particularly before 1 year of age
- Frequent need for hospitalization to control asthma
- Dependence on corticosteroids, either oral or inhaled
- Noncompliance or abuse of medication
- Labile asthma with pronounced "morning dipping," diurnal obstruction
- *Brittle* asthma with unexpected rapid deterioration of pulmonary function
- Teenager with long-standing asthma of early onset
- Depressive symptoms with chronic asthma

The risk of a severe or fatal attack is compounded in adolescents by several factors. These include the normal adolescent rebellion against parental authority, the need in some adolescents, particularly those with low self-esteem, for risk-taking behaviors, and the belief among early and middle adolescents that "it can't happen to me." All of these factors can result in poor compliance with medication regimens and, therefore, an increased risk of exacerbation of asthma. An additional factor is the lack of awareness by some teenagers with asthma that their disease is poorly controlled. The lungs of these patients are in a state of chronic hyperinflation with consequent loss of elastic recoil, and have airways that are narrowed by chronic inflammatory changes [16]. Feeling tight and occasionally wheezing can become second nature to an adolescent with poorly controlled asthma. In a sense, he or she forgets what it feels like to be totally free of symptoms, so nothing is done to alleviate them [17]. The feeling of respiratory normality, then, is actually one of respiratory compromise. The patient then is at a significantly increased risk for rapid escalation of symptoms to a critical level. When airways are chronically edematous and inflamed, it takes little bronchospasm to close them completely, and relieving that small bit of bronchospasm does little to open airways that now have a greater degree of edema and inflammation. This situation can lead rapidly to a severe attack that takes days to correct, if it can be corrected at all.

Presentation

Most teenagers with asthma have been wheezing for years. Many are well known to practitioners. However, several have symptoms that have never been diagnosed as asthma. They have variably been said to be suffering from a chronic cough, recurrent bouts of "bronchitis," and the like. Some, particularly those who have a heart murmur or who have mitral valve prolapse, may have been mislabeled and followed inappropriately for years when what they really may have is exercise-induced asthma (EIA).

Teenagers with EIA may present during adolescence when they first try out for a scholastic sports team, or they may never try out for sports because they know that they get short of breath whenever they exercise [18]. A specific syndrome that frequently affects adolescents, EIA occurs in 80% of those people with asthma and in 40% with allergic rhinitis [19]. Typically, bronchospasm occurs 5 to 10 minutes after beginning strenuous exercise when the heart rate is in the range of 170 beats per minute [20]. Mild EIA is associated with approximately a 15% decrease in lung function; a drop of 20% is considered moderately severe; a drop of 40% is very severe. These drops in lung function are as measured on a Wright peak flow meter. Symptoms are usually more severe and more frequent in cold, dry air as opposed to warm, moist air. Therefore, people with EIA typically have more problems in the winter when exercising outdoors. Whether a specific patient will have exercise-induced symptoms at any one particular time depends on the degree of exercise, the ambient conditions in which the patient exercises (e.g., temperature, humidity, pollutants, pollen), and intrinsic factors such as coexisting upper respiratory infections, active hay fever, and the like (Table 25).

An interesting facet of EIA is the refractory period. This is a period of up to an hour after resolution of exercise-induced bronchospasm in which a person can begin to exercise without further wheezing. Many people with EIA have learned that if they rest until the tightness goes away, they will get a "second wind" and be able to resume exercise without the recurrence of symptoms [21].

Some people with asthma appear to have another asthma attack several hours after the immediate EIA attack without any further provocation. This has been called the *late-phase attack*. It does not occur in all patients with EIA, and even its existence has been questioned by some authorities [19].

Treatment of EIA must be individualized. If a patient is already on asthma medication, that may be enough to prevent an attack of EIA. However, such a patient may be similar to those on no chronic medication; he or she may need treatment before each period of exercise (Table 26). The most efficacious treatment is inhalation of a beta$_2$-adrenergic agonist within a half hour of beginning exercise. Alternatively, inhaled cromolyn sodium can be used 30 to 60 minutes before exercise [4]. Some oral medications, such as beta$_2$-adrenergic agonist tablets or theophylline tablets, can be effective if taken

TABLE 25. *Exercise-induced asthma contributing factors*

Air conditions: low humidity, pollutants, cold air
Exposure to allergens in sensitive people
Overall asthma control
Poor physical conditioning
Respiratory infections
Time since last episode
Type, intensity, and duration of exercise
Underlying bronchial hyperreactivity

Adapted from Rupp NT. Diagnosis and management of exercise-induced asthma. *Phys Sports Med* 1996;24:77.

TABLE 26. *Historical factors in the patient suggesting exercise-induced asthma*

Altered, decreased, or discontinued exercise program
Chest discomfort, coughing, dyspnea, or wheezing during exercise
Complaints of decreased or limited endurance
Out-of-shape label used to describe a well conditioned athlete
No problems in warm, humid environments or with swimming
Variation in symptoms according to outdoor temperature or season

Adapted from Rupp NT. Diagnosis and management of exercise-induced asthma. *Phys Sports Med* 1996;24:77.

1 to 2 hours before activity, but the inhalers are without systemic side effects and most teenagers consider them more convenient.

One condition that can rebuff all efforts to control asthma is chronic sinus infection. Many people with asthma find no relief from their symptoms until their sinus problems are successfully addressed. This condition is particularly common in teenagers with allergies [16].

Another group of adolescents with difficult-to-control asthma is those who do not regularly visit a physician for maintenance control of their disease. Instead, they rely on the local emergency room for treatment of exacerbations. It is incumbent on emergency room physicians to check the records of any child presenting with asthma to see whether frequent visits have been made and to then refer that child to a source of continuing care, with social worker intervention if it appears that the parents will not follow through with recommendations. Establishment of case management teams in health care systems to which the clinician belongs enables tracking of asthma patients and more effective care.

Children and teenagers with chronic cough frequently baffle physicians. If problems (e.g., foreign bodies, chronic lung disease, vocal cord lesions) can be ruled out, a trial of asthma therapy is indicated. Many improve dramatically. If this does not work, pulmonary function tests with pharmacologic challenge and bronchodilators are indicated [22]. An additional factor that can exacerbate asthma is gastroesophageal reflux. The physician should ask for a history of heartburn in teenagers with asthma. Consider gastroesophageal reflux as a possibility in asthma that is very difficult to control, especially when the patient is on theophylline, which can aggravate the problem.

Management

The goal of asthma management is to keep every patient free of symptoms and totally participating in all desired activities. The first step to achieve that goal is to define the degree of the patient's problem. This can be done in several ways. The number of emergency visits and hospitalizations for acute attacks can be tallied. Pulmonary function tests can be performed at various times to objectify the level of the patient's disease. An increased frequency of use of inhaled $beta_2$-adrenergic drugs is also a marker of more severe disease. The use of peak flow meters increasingly has become the gold standard in the management of asthma. As is outlined in Figure 9, peak expiratory flow rate (PEF) can be used effectively to monitor severity of asthma and to dictate treatment intensity. This method has been promulgated by both national and international panels on the management of asthma [23]. Finally, the psychosocial situation can be assessed. Adolescents with moderate to severe asthma have been shown to have a higher degree of irrational thinking and emotionality compared to those with mild asthma and to adolescents without asthma. If the patient with asthma has evidence of depression, excessive anxiety surrounding the disease, or family dysfunction, psychosocial intervention is indicated [24,25].

The next step is to design a treatment protocol to fit each patient's unique situation. The patient should be given a peak flow meter and instructed on its proper use. Then the patient should be sent home to monitor PEF for a week, with instructions to call or go to the emergency room if function falls below preset limits. The PEF diary then should be reviewed, and rates for green zone, yellow zone, and red zone should be set. The concept of the colored zones uses PEF rates as shown in Figure 9.

The total medication regimen should be reviewed to determine whether it is well fitted to the patient's particular symptoms and, equally important, to each patient's life-style. The patient's desired

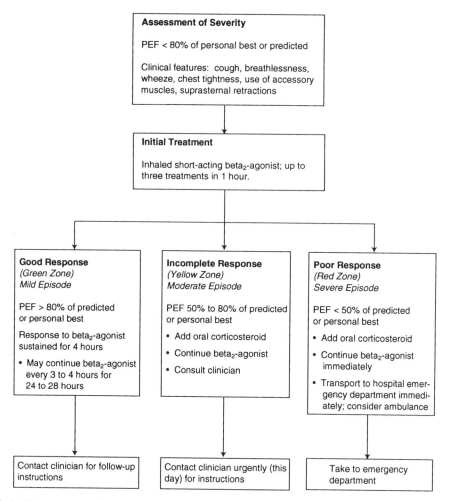

Assessment of Severity

PEF < 80% of personal best or predicted

Clinical features: cough, breathlessness, wheeze, chest tightness, use of accessory muscles, suprasternal retractions

Initial Treatment

Inhaled short-acting beta₂-agonist; up to three treatments in 1 hour.

Good Response
(Green Zone)
Mild Episode

PEF > 80% of predicted or personal best

Response to beta₂-agonist sustained for 4 hours

• May continue beta₂-agonist every 3 to 4 hours for 24 to 28 hours

Incomplete Response
(Yellow Zone)
Moderate Episode

PEF 50% to 80% of predicted or personal best

• Add oral corticosteroid
• Continue beta₂-agonist
• Consult clinician

Poor Response
(Red Zone)
Severe Episode

PEF < 50% of predicted or personal best

• Add oral corticosteroid
• Continue beta₂-agonist immediately
• Transport to hospital emergency department immediately; consider ambulance

Contact clinician for follow-up instructions

Contact clinician urgently (this day) for instructions

Take to emergency department

FIG. 9. Management of an acute asthma attack at home. (Adapted from the *International Consensus Report on Diagnosis and Management of Asthma.* Public Health Service publication No. 92-3091, 1992.)

and current activities should be reviewed, and efforts should be made to make those two pictures congruent. A very important component of the whole management package should be an assessment of the patient's home situation. If family life and, consequently, supervision of this adolescent is not optimal, all the medical regimens in the world will not control this teenager's asthma. Be sure to check whether there are smokers or pets in the patient's house. Little can be done by the physician to counteract a continuing supply of antigen such as a dog or cat, or continuing supplies of pollutants as from a family member who smokes cigarettes in the house. With the increasing attention to the need to decrease medical costs and with the recognition of the contribution of asthma to those costs, efforts to manage more closely patients with asthma have been instituted. As mentioned earlier, case management services, especially for those patients with moderate to severe asthma, have been shown to decrease use of emergency services and inpatient hospital care. Clear instructions about how to monitor asthma using a peak flow meter and clear instructions on when to seek emergency care (using the colored zone approach), along with detailed and repetitive instruction about use of inhalers, can help patients to improve their asthma management significantly.

Medical Therapy

Maintenance Therapy

The mainstay of maintenance therapy has increasingly become inhaled drugs (Table 27). One of the drugs of choice for the child or early adolescent who needs daily medication is cromolyn sodium [26]. Cromolyn sodium is primarily a preventive drug, not a therapeutic one. The drug decreases bronchial hyperreactivity through inhibiting degranulation of mast cells and decreases inflammation in general by inhibiting secretory properties of neutrophils, eosinophils, and monocytes. Two puffs (1 mg/puff) from a metered-dose inhaler two to four times daily are sufficient to keep many patients wheeze free. Cromolyn also may have a place in the treatment of asthma in the hospital [27]. Nedocromil, a drug similar to cromolyn, can be used in its stead.

In many adolescents, inhaled steroids should be the first choice in treating chronic asthma [16,26]. Inhaled corticosteroids prevent bronchospasm and inflammation and, as such, are key factors in long-term control. Although oral corticosteroids certainly treat and prevent bronchial edema and inflammation, there are problems associated with long-term use of these drugs. Therefore, they are reserved for treatment of patients just coming off of intravenous steroid therapy and for short bursts of treatment in patients with exacerbations of their disease [4,28]. There are a few patients who require long-term treatment with oral corticosteroids, but these patients should be managed by a pulmonologist or an allergist, not a primary care physician. Instead of the oral forms, many teenagers with asthma can be maintained on inhaled steroids. These include triamcinolone, beclomethasone, fluticasone, and flunisolide. These drugs are given by a metered-dose inhaler, two to four puffs two to four times daily. Twice-daily dosage can be as effective as more frequent use, a boon in poorly compliant teenagers. The inhaled steroids produce very low serum levels of steroids and, therefore, have no effect on the adrenal glands in mature adolescents and adults. They also have no effect on growth [29,30]. The only major side effect is oral *Candida* infection, which can be prevented by the use of a spacing chamber between the inhaler and the patient's mouth or by rinsing out the mouth with water after inhaler use.

If cromolyn and steroids are not sufficient, many experts add theophylline in a sustained-release form. Given that compliance is a problem in many adolescents with asthma, the short-acting forms of theophylline are not really an option. The theophylline capsules or tablets (e.g., Slo-bid, Theo-Dur) are usually taken two times daily. One dose at bedtime may be useful in suppressing nocturnal symptoms. Although clinical improvement and maintenance has been demonstrated with serum levels of 5 to 20 μg/ml, there is no specific level that should be sought [27]. Each adolescent finds relief at his or her own optimum level. Ultra–sustained-release preparations are available that allow once-daily dosing, but these present increased problems if ingested in an overdose. Theophylline is a xanthine similar to caffeine, and it carries the same side effects. These include jitteriness, insomnia, and bed-wetting. The side effects can be present even at therapeutic doses [31].

The next category of asthma drugs is the beta$_2$-adrenergic stimulators. These include albuterol, metaproterenol, bitolterol, terbutaline, and salmeterol. All of these medications are bronchodilators and have little, if any, effect on bronchial edema or inflammation. It is best, therefore, to save the beta$_2$-adrenergic agonists for treatment of exacerbations and for prevention of wheezing from prospective exposures to known stimulants and for EIA [14,27]. In the adolescent, either tablets or inhalers may be used. Inhalers have a quicker onset of action and fewer side effects. They have a thera-

TABLE 27. *Inhalant medications for treating asthma*

Acute treatment
  Albuterol
  Metaproterenol
  Terbutaline
  Isoetharine
  Ipratroprium bromide

Maintenance
  Cromolyn sodium, nedocromil
  Steroids: triamcinolone, beclomethasone, flunisolide, fluticasone
  Salmeterol

TABLE 28. *Key activities in the management of status asthmaticus*

Obtain patient history.
Perform physical examination.
Obtain arterial blood gases.
Carry out periodic monitoring on peak flow meter.
Establish intravenous line.
Administer oxygen.
Administer aerosolized β_2-adrenergic agonists.
Administer aerosolized cromolyn sodium.
Give intravenous steroids early in course.
Administer intravenous aminophylline.

peutic duration of 4 to 6 hours. In patients who are using beta$_2$-adrenergic agonists in this fashion, an increased frequency of use is a signal that the asthma is not being well controlled. Nonselective beta-adrenergic agonists such as isoproterenol have little place in modern asthma therapy, because all sites of actions in the lungs are beta$_2$-responsive [27]. The long-acting beta agonist, salmeterol, can be helpful in the patient who needs additional long-term bronchodilation, but it is not effective for immediate, short-term use. Excessive use of salmeterol may lead to tolerance [14].

Troleandomycin, anticholinergics, calcium channel-blocking agents, and other treatments, including gold, inhaled heparin, and methotrexate, are not used very often in children and adolescents and should be reserved for use by an allergist or pulmonologist.

Therapy of Acute Attacks

Treatment of acute attacks (Table 28) usually begins with inhaled beta agonists such as albuterol, terbutaline, or isoetharine. Inhaled beta$_2$-adrenergic agonists are preferred both for efficacy and patient comfort, including lack of systemic side effects [27,32]. Inhaled ipratropium bromide can be added to the beta agonists if the symptoms persist [33]. If relief is not obtained, intravenous therapy with corticosteroids is needed. Intravenous corticosteroids should be initiated early in the emergency room treatment of asthma because even one intravenous dose may prevent hospitalization. The use of intravenous aminophylline is no longer indicated in the management of an acute asthma attack [34]. Figure 10 demonstrates a nomogram for management of asthma in an emergency department.

The decision to hospitalize should be made if there are signs of respiratory failure such as severe respiratory distress, exhaustion, alteration in consciousness, pulsus paradoxus, severe retractions, hypoxia, hypotension, hypercapnia (carbon dioxide tension [PCO_2] in excess of 40 mm Hg), and electro-cardiographic abnormalities, or if there is extrapleural air. The patient also should be hospitalized if there is vomiting or refusal to take medications at home, if there is no one reliable to care for the adolescent at home, or if there are two or more visits to the emergency room in less than 48 hours [18]. Patients with severe bronchoconstriction have decreased intensity and duration of response to beta$_2$-adrenergic agonists. Therefore, these drugs can be given as often as needed, even continuously [28]. Treatment failure is signaled by a PCO_2 of 55 mm Hg or greater after 1 or 2 hours of intensive therapy or by a rise of 5 to 10 mm Hg of PCO_2 per hour during aggressive therapy in a patient who is becoming fatigued. In these situations, ventilation should be considered, and the patient should be managed in an intensive care unit with the assistance of a pulmonologist or an intensivist. Blood gases should be followed in the acute phase, and coexisting infections should be treated appropriately. During recovery, pulmonary function tests are an accurate method of gauging resolution of the attack. While the adolescent is hospitalized, the home situation should be reevaluated to assess whether adequate supervision is available and to determine whether there are excessive stresses that may have led to the exacerbation of the disease. If not already in place, case management services should be initiated.

Asthma and Sinusitis

Patients with asthma and allergies should have their allergies attended to appropriately. If allergies are neglected, asthma management will be difficult at best. In addition, frequent exacerbations of

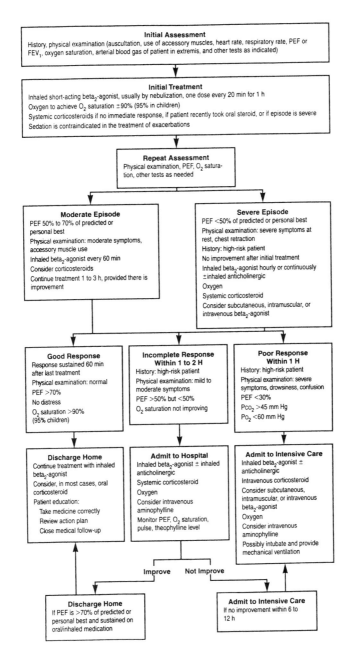

FIG. 10. Management of an acute asthma attack in the emergency department and hospital. (Adapted from the *International Consensus Report on Diagnosis and Management of Asthma.* Public Health Service publication No. 92-3091, 1992.)

asthma should lead the physician to investigate the possibility of chronic sinusitis. A history of chronic postnasal drip, of coughing when recumbent, and of chronic productive cough should be sought.

Sinus radiographs should be obtained, and careful examination of the nose and percussion of the sinuses should be performed. If sinusitis is found, antibiotic therapy should be initiated and continued for at least 3 weeks. Amoxicillin is usually adequate, but trimethoprim–sulfamethoxazole or another antibiotic may be used. In addition to antibiotics, medications to shrink the nasal and sinus membranes are needed. Oral antihistamine–decongestants are helpful in the allergic patient, and decongestants alone can be used in the nonallergic patient. Topical decongestants (nose drops or sprays) can be used acutely for a few days, and acute and long-term treatment with nasally inhaled corticosteroids is frequently beneficial. Nasally inhaled corticosteroids, used on a long-term basis, may prevent recurrence of the sinusitis and of the wheezing that frequently accompanies it.

Finally, a critical component of management of any chronic illness such as asthma is assisting the adolescent in learning constructive ways with which to cope with life stresses. This is necessary because maladaptive coping mechanisms can include psychologically induced worsening of asthma. First, adolescents must learn to recognize the internal signals that stress is building. Then, they must learn to recognize how they unconsciously cope. Once that is done, positive coping skills such as self-relaxation, self-talk, imaging, and so forth, can be learned and put to use. Asthma is a very common, and potentially severe, disease. However, it should not prevent full activity by any adolescent who suffers from it. The management of asthma can be a very rewarding experience, and most issues can be managed by the primary care physician.

REFERENCES

1. Stiles GL, Caron MG, Lefkowitz RJ. β-Adrenergic receptors: biochemical mechanisms of physiological regulation. *Physiol Rev* 1984;64:661.
2. McFadden ER Jr. Beta receptor agonists: metabolism and pharmacology. *J Allergy Clin Immunol* 1981;68:91.
3. Gergen PJ, Mullally KE, Evans RE III. National survey of prevalence of asthma among children in the United States, 1976—1980. *Pediatrics* 1988;81:1—7.
4. Murphy SJ, Kelly HW. Advances in the management of acute asthma in children. *Pediatr Rev* 1996;17:227.
5. Reed CE. Adrenergic bronchodilators: pharmacology and toxicology. *J Allergy Clin Immunol* 1985;76:335.
6. Oliveti JF, Kercsmar CM, Redline S. Pre- and perinatal risk factors for asthma in inner city African-American children. *Am J Epidemiol* 1996;143:570.
7. Burrows B, Martinez FD, Halonea M, et al. Association of asthma with serum IgE levels and skin-test reactivity to allergens. *N Engl J Med* 1989;320:271.
8. Blair H. Natural history of childhood asthma. *Arch Dis Child* 1977;52:613.
9. Goldenhersh MJ, Rachelefsky GS. Childhood asthma: overview. *Pediatr Rev* 1989;10:227.
10. Sly RM. Increases in deaths from asthma. *Ann Allergy* 1984;53:20.
11. Johnson AJ, Nunn AJ, Somner AR, et al. Circumstances of death from asthma. *Br Med J* 1984;288:1870.
12. Sears MR, Rea HH, Beaglehole R, et al. Asthma mortality in New Zealand: a two year national study. *New Zealand Medical Journal* 1985;98:271.
13. Foucard T, Graff-Lonnevig V. Asthma mortality rate in Swedish children and young adults 1973:88. *Allergy* 1994;49:616.
14. Nelson HS. β-Adrenergic bronchodilators. *N Engl J Med* 1995;333:499.
15. Mullen M, Mullen B, Carey M. The association between β-agonist use and death from asthma. *JAMA* 1993;270:1842.
16. Barnes PJ. A new approach to the treatment of asthma. *N Engl J Med* 1989;321:1517.
17. Rubinfeld AR, Pain MCF. Perception of asthma. *Lancet* 1976;1:882.
18. Rachelefsky GS, Katz RM, Seigel SC. Chronic sinus disease with associated reactive airway disease in children. *Pediatrics* 1984;73:526.
19. McCarthy P. Wheezing or breezing through exercise-induced asthma. *Phys Sports Med* 1989;17:125.
20. Exercise and asthma: a roundtable. *Phys Sports Med* 1984;12:58.
21. Rupp NT. Diagnosis and management of exercise-induced asthma. *Phys Sports Med* 1996;24:77.
22. Cloutier MM, Loughlin GM. Chronic cough in children: a manifestation of airway hyperreactivity. *Pediatrics* 1981;67:6.
23. National Institutes of Health. *Global initiative for asthma: global strategy for asthma management and prevention.* NHLBI/WHO workshop report, March, 1993. Publication No. 95-3659.Bethesda, MD: National Institutes of Health; January, 1995.
24. Silverglade L, Tosi DJ, Wise PS, et al. Irrational beliefs and emotionality in adolescents with and without bronchial asthma. *J Gen Psychol* 1994;121:199.
25. Bussing R, Halfon N, Benjamin B, et al. Prevalence of behavior problems in US children with asthma. *Arch Pediatr Adolesc Med* 1995;149:565.
26. Spector SL, Nicklas RA, eds. Practice parameters for the diagnosis and treatment of asthma. *J Allergy Clin Immunol* 1995;96(Suppl 5, pt. 2):858, .
27. Goldenhersh MJ, Rachelefsky GS. Childhood asthma: management. *Pediatr Rev* 1989;10:259.
28. McWilliams B, Kelly HW, Murphy S. Management of acute severe asthma. *Pediatr Ann* 1989;18:774
29. Merkus PJFM, van Essen Zandvliet EEM, Duiverman EF, et al. Long-term effect of inhaled corticosteroids on growth rate in adolescents with asthma. *Pediatrics* 1993;91:1121.

30. Barnes PJ. Inhaled glucocorticoids for asthma. *N Engl J Med* 1995;332:868.
31. Szefler SJ, Bender BG, Jusko WJ, et al. Evolving role of the theophylline for treatment of chronic childhood asthma. *J Pediatr* 1995;127:176.
32. Becker AB, Nelson NA, Simons FER. Inhaled salbutamol (albuterol) vs. injected epinephrine in the treatment of acute asthma in children. *J Pediatr* 1983;102:465.
33. Schuh SS, Johnson DW, Callahan S, et al. Efficacy of frequent nebulized ipratropium bromide added to frequent high-dose albuterol therapy in severe childhood asthma. *J Pediatr* 1995;126:639; .
34. Strauss RE, Wertheim DL, Bonagura VR, et al. Aminophylline therapy does not improve outcome and increases adverse effects in children hospitalized with acute asthmatic exacerbations. *Pediatrics* 1994;93: 205.

SUGGESTED READING

Barnes PJ. A new approach to the treatment of asthma. *N Engl J Med* 1989;321:1517.
Burrows B, Martinez FD, Halonea M, et al. Association of asthma with serum IgE levels and skin-test reactivity to allergens. *N Engl J Med* 1989;320:271.
Eggleston PA. Are β-adrenergic bronchodilators safe? *Pediatrics* 1997;99:729.
Goldenhersh MJ, Rachelefsky GS. Childhood asthma: management. *Pediatr Rev* 1989;10:259.
Goldenhersh MJ, Rachelefsky GS. Childhood asthma: overview. *Pediatr Rev* 1989;10:227.
McCarthy P. Wheezing or breezing through exercise-induced asthma. *Phys Sports Med* 1989;17:125.
McWilliams B, Kelly HW, Murphy S. Management of acute severe asthma. *Pediatr Ann* 1989;18:774.
Murphy SJ, Kelly HW. Advances in the management of acute asthma in children. *Pediatr Rev* 1996;17:227.
National Institutes of Health. Global initiative for asthma: global strategy for asthma management and prevention. NHLBI/WHO workshop report, March, 1993. Publication No. 95-3659. Bethesda, MD: National Institutes of Health; January, 1995;.
O'Hollaren MT, Yunginger JW, Offord KP, et al. Exposure to an aeroallergen as a possible precipitating factor in respiratory arrest in young patients with asthma. *N Engl J Med* 1991;324:359.
Oren J, Hemady Z. Asthma and adolescence. *Adolescent Medicine: State of the Art Reviews* 1991;2:617.
Rosenstreich DL, Eggleston P, Kattan M, et al. The role of the cockroach allergy and exposure to cockroach allergen in causing morbidity among inner-city children with asthma. *N Engl J Med* 1997;336:1356.
Spector SL, Nicklas RA. Practice parameters for the diagnosis and treatment of asthma. *J Allergy Clin Immunol* 1995;96:858.

HEADACHES

Headache is an extremely common complaint in adolescents. It would be difficult to find an adolescent who never had a headache, but the number who find it necessary to seek medical care for this condition is considerably smaller. In one large epidemiologic study, 15.7% of 15-year-olds had experienced frequent nonmigrainous headaches, 5.3% had migrainous headaches, and 54% had infrequent nonmigrainous headaches [1,2]. Other studies show different rates, but the fact remains that headaches are a common problem in adolescents (Table 29). For the most part, these are amenable to evaluation and treatment by the primary care physician and rarely require referral to a neurologist or neurosurgeon. In fact, referral to a social worker, psychologist, or psychiatrist is more frequently needed. The most important part of the evaluation of headache in an adolescent is obtaining a complete and detailed history. The history should be much more than just a cataloging of symptoms. A thorough review of the other boxes (see Chapter 2) of the patient's life often reveals factors that are responsible for the patient's organic symptoms or that contribute significantly to them. Even with headaches of organic origin, such as migraines, a review of the other four areas of the patient's life can be very helpful in determining exacerbating factors. For instance, family pressures such as divorce can cause so-called tension headaches or can exacerbate headaches of organic origin such as migraines. Drug misuse can cause headaches, and headaches from environmental factors such as dry heat in the winter or indoor pollution such as from carbon monoxide must be ruled out.

One authority [3] has classified headaches in children and adolescents into four categories: acute, acute recurrent, chronic progressive, and chronic nonprogressive.

Acute Headaches

An acute headache is one that occurs as a single event that the patient has never before experienced. A diagnosis must be made quickly if the headache is associated with other rapidly progressing organic

TABLE 29. *Selected studies on the prevalence of headache in childhood, including age and sex incidence of migraine[a]*

Author	No. of patients	Survey method[b]	Headache of all types	Childhood migraine	Adolescent migraine
Bille [1]	8,993	Patient questionnaire Ascertainment: all past years	58.7% (age 7–14 y)	Male 2.5% Female 2.4% (age 7–9 y)	Male 4.0% Female 6.4% (age 13–15 y)
Dalsgaard-Neilsen et al. [2]	2,027	Patient and parent interview by author Ascertainment: all past years	—	Male 3.1% Female 2.8% (age 7–9 y)	Male 8.4% Female 9.5% (age 15–17 y)
Deubner [3]	600	Patient and parent interview Ascertainment: previous year	Male 74% Female 85% (age 10–20 y)	Male 14% Female 20% (age 10–12 y)	Male 18% Female 23% (age 13–15 y)
Sillanpää [4]	2,921	Student questionnaire Ascertainment: previous year	37.0% (age 7 y) 69% (age 14 y)	Male 2.9% Female 2.5% (age 7 y)	Male 6.4% Female 14.8% (age 14 y)

[a]See table 3-31 for criteria of migraine used by the study authors.
[b]Note that Bille and Dalsgaard-Neilsen et al. recorded headache experience during the lifetime of the patient, whereas Deubner and Sillanpää data relate to prevalence in the 1 year before assessment.
Adapted from Barlow CF. *Headaches and migraine in childhood. Clinics in Developmental Medicine* 1984;91.

signs such as neck stiffness, vomiting, or obtundation. The possible causes can include recent trauma, systemic illness, acute sinusitis, and central nervous system (CNS) infections.

Acute Recurrent Headaches

Acute recurrent headaches occur periodically and are separated by pain-free periods. The most common headache that presents this way is migraine. Another possibility in this group is sinus headache, although sinus headache frequently presents more similarly to chronic nonprogressive headaches. Another acute recurrent headache is that caused by vasomotor rhinitis.

Chronic Progressive Headaches

Chronic progressive headaches are those indicative of serious organic pathologic processes, such as those symptomatic of increased intracranial pressure. A history of progressive and worsening symptoms is found in these cases, and neurologic deficits may be present.

Chronic Nonprogressive Headaches

Chronic nonprogressive headaches do not seem to change over time, although they may occur daily or weekly. Neither are they accompanied by symptoms suggestive of CNS disease. The physical examination is frequently normal, but occasionally it may reveal findings indicative of allergies or sinus congestion. Probably the most common diagnosis in this group is headache of nonorganic origin.

Evaluation

History

As stated earlier, the first and most important part of the diagnostic process is a complete, accurate, and detailed history. The authors find that categorizing factors by the five boxes system (see Chapter 2) makes this process easier.

Factors to consider in the organic area include all the standard questions the physician asks when presented with any patient with a complaint of pain: intensity, character, frequency, location, alleviating and exacerbating factors, and the normal activities that are limited by the pain. Whether the symptoms are progressive is a key factor. A history of systemic symptoms should be sought, as well as a history of recent head trauma and information about sleeping patterns. A history of similar symptoms in close family members is frequently helpful, as when, for example, a sibling, parent, or grandparent had headaches and then developed a brain tumor, or when a parent has had migraines. A careful history of current or recent medications should be taken. Birth control pills should be asked about specifically, because many teenagers do not consider them in the category of "medicines." Also, the clinician should not forget to ask about vitamin and mineral supplements. Adolescents are very concerned about their bodies and are susceptible to inducements, self-generated or otherwise, to take substances that are purported to enhance strength and endurance. Excessive amounts of vitamin A in these products can cause pseudotumor cerebri. Table 30 shows a series of questions to help elucidate the cause of headaches.

In questioning about the home box, the physician should seek information about the actual house environment, such as the form of heating system in the patient's house and the presence of pets. This is also the area in which a history of recent life change, such as a move, or a history of parental discord should be sought. Relationship to meals should be ascertained. This becomes important in the rare adolescent with "Chinese restaurant syndrome," that is, a sensitivity to monosodium glutamate [4].

Questions in the school and work area should delve into issues such as school attendance patterns, recent school changes, number of hours spent at work, and the work environment. Headaches can be associated with working in environments with too little ventilation or with a lot of noise, for example. If the patient plays in a rock band, the exposure to excessive noise can be considerable. Lack of sleep from trying to work at a full-time job while going to school and keeping up a social life is a common pattern in adolescents; headaches are often associated with this life-style. A drop in school grades that persists for more than one grading period is often the earliest objective sign of depression or substance abuse in this age group, two problems that can easily generate headaches. As in all the other areas of history, corroboration by parents of information given by the adolescent often is very helpful.

The topic of peers must also be assessed thoroughly. The lack of an identifiable best friend can be a sign of depression. Having friends who use a lot of drugs or alcohol is a red flag as well. Out of school, nonwork activities should be explored. For instance, leisure time spent with friends in an activity such as boxing can be a significant historic factor in a teenager complaining of headaches. This is an area in which parents can be most helpful. They should be asked whether the teenager spends excessive time alone and whether their child's friends are new and display worrisome behaviors.

Finally, the romance box should be explored. The whole area of sexuality is rife with factors that can contribute to the complaint of headaches. A recent failed romance, concerns about homosexuality, worries about acquired immunodeficiency syndrome (most often unrealistic), and worry about

TABLE 30. *Evaluating adolescents who complain of headaches*

1. How long have you had headaches?
2. How did the headaches begin?
3. Do you have single or multiple types of headache?
4. Do you have a chronic medical condition?
5. Are you on any medication? Which types? How often do you take it/them?
6. Do you take anything that makes the headache better or go away?
7. Have you noticed any activity that makes the headache begin or get worse?
8. When you have a headache, do you stop what you are doing?
9. Does anyone else in your family have headaches? How often?
10. Have the headaches stayed the same or become worse?
11. About how often do you get a headache?
12. About how long do they last?
13. Are there any warning signs before you get a headache?
14. Is there a special time or circumstance when the headaches are more likely to begin?
15. Where exactly is the pain located?
16. What is the pain like?
17. Are there any other symptoms you notice when you have a headache?

Adapted from Rothner AD. A practical approach to headaches in adolescents. *Pediatr Ann* 1991;20:201.

being pregnant are some items from this area that can contribute to the development of headaches in an adolescent.

Physical Examination

The physical examination is the next evaluative tool. Signs that may be particularly pertinent include those of increased intracranial pressure, elevated blood pressure, severely congested nasal mucosa, the presence of allergic shiners, tenderness on percussion of the sinuses, severe dental caries, immobile tympanic membranes, adenopathy, and skin lesions (such as café au lait spots, possibly indicative of neurofibromatosis, and those that could indicate possible intravenous drug use). A thorough neurologic examination is indicated, although most frequently all findings are normal. The head should be auscultated for bruits, which could indicate arteriovenous malformations. Among the ocular problems of refractive error, strabismus, and astigmatism, only the latter problem has been associated with headaches to any significant degree [5]. In any case, a thorough eye examination is indicated.

Laboratory and Other Evaluations

As with all diagnostic endeavors, the choice of laboratory and other tests and evaluations depends on the direction in which the history and physical examination have led the physician. For adolescents in whom there is no evidence of organic derangement or in whom the diagnosis of migraine headache is highly likely, frequently no additional workup is needed. These patients' headaches usually fall into the acute recurrent or chronic nonprogressive categories. On the other hand, for the patient who presents with concrete organic findings, such as engorged optic discs or significant weight loss and adenopathy, the diagnostic path to follow is clear and includes appropriate imaging studies for possible CNS lesions and laboratory studies for any suspected systemic disorders. For patients with upper respiratory findings, imaging studies of the sinuses can be helpful although not totally diagnostic. Dental evaluation is indicated when significant oral abnormalities are found or when temporomandibular joint dysfunction is suspected. Ophthalmologic evaluation is indicated when eye problems are present.

Blood tests are not helpful very often, except when other findings indicate possible benefit. This may happen with a girl with headaches, pallor, and fatigue. She may have anemia, so a complete blood cell count is indicated. Imaging techniques such as computed tomography scans and magnetic resonance imaging are not very helpful except when the physical examination indicates the possibility of an organic lesion [6]. Electroencephalography should be reserved for teenagers who have either a history compatible with the diagnosis of seizure disorder or findings that suggest the possibility of a focal CNS lesion. Without ample cause, a lumbar puncture is not indicated.

A most helpful evaluation can be that performed by a social worker, a psychologist, or a psychiatrist. Which of these should be consulted depends in part on the nature of the problem discovered and also on the availability of a particular mental health professional in the clinician's area. It should be noted, however, that the necessary psychosocial evaluation and intervention can often be performed by the adolescent's primary care physician without resorting to outside help.

Specific Syndromes

Acute Headaches

Acute headaches may be caused by life-threatening and other serious problems such as those leading to increased intracranial pressure (e.g., mass lesions and pseudotumor cerebri). Pseudotumor can occur in teenagers who ingest excessive quantities of vitamin A and in those who use outdated tetracycline (see Acne section). Accutane treatment for acne can also precipitate this condition. Among the mass lesions that may be encountered are brain tumors and lesions such as subarachnoid and subdural hematomas. Other causes of acute headaches include upper respiratory conditions such as sinusitis and dental conditions such as severe caries, malocclusion, and temporomandibular joint dysfunction. All of these are readily diagnosable by the primary care physician, although referral may be needed for treatment. Localized acute headache may follow head trauma, so a history of trauma should be sought assiduously. Ocular abnormalities such as refractive errors and astigmatism are rare causes of acute headaches, as previously stated.

Acute Recurrent Headaches

The prototypical syndrome in the category of acute recurrent headaches is migraine. The primary neuronal hypothesis is thought to explain the cause of migraine. This hypothesis considers migraine to be an inherited sensitivity of the trigeminal vascular system. Internal or external stimuli cause cortical, thalamic, or hypothalamic mechanisms to initiate the headache. These structures stimulate the locus ceruleus and nucleus raphe dorsalis in the brain stem, which, in turn, move through the cortex to produce the spreading wave of neuronal depression and then to the cranial vasculature to produce a cascade of neurogenic inflammation and secondary vascular reactivity. Vasoactive peptides stimulate immune-sensitive cells such as mast cells and platelets, resulting in inflammation of dural and pial blood vessels from which pain sensation is transmitted by the trigeminal nerve [7–9]. Spreading cortical depression also has been associated with onset of migraine with aura [10]. Serotonin has been implicated in migraines, and this has led to the use of serotonin antagonists as treatment for migraines.

Various surveys have shown that migraine headaches occur in many children. In one of the better surveys, approximately 11% of children suffered from migraines by the age of 14 years. Approximately 6% of boys and 15% of girls of that age suffer from this phenomenon [11]. Table 29 shows more epidemiologic data. Criteria from various authors for diagnosis of migraine appear in Table 31. From these, it can be seen that the periodicity of the syndrome is a key diagnostic element. Table 32 shows the frequency of symptom occurrence in a population of 300 patients. The main factors that suggest this diagnosis to the physician appear to be 1) periodicity, 2) positive family history, 3) throbbing quality of the pain, and 4) gastrointestinal symptoms. Relief brought by lying down in a quiet,

TABLE 31. *Criteria for the diagnosis of migraine*

Author	Essential criteria		Necessary symptoms
Vahlquist [8], Bille [1], and Sillanpää [4]	Periodic	*plus*	Three of the following: Aura Nausea Vomiting Family history
Prensky [9]and Jay and Tomasi [10]	Recurrent with symptom-free intervals	*plus*	Three of the following: Abdominal pain or nausea or vomiting Unilateral Throbbing Relief after sleep Aura (visual, sensory, motor) Family history
Deubner [3]	Periodic	*plus*	Three of the following: Unilateral Nausea with or without vomiting Neurologic symptoms (scotomas, scintillations, paresthesias)
Congdon and Forsythe [11]	Periodic	*plus*	Three of the following: Aura Nausea Vomiting Family history
Kurtz et al. [12]	Recurrent with anorexia or nausea	*plus*	One of the following: Vomiting Specific visual disturbance

Adapted from Barlow CF. *Headaches and migraine in childhood. Clinics in Developmental Medicine* 1984;91.

TABLE 32. *Characteristics of juvenile migraine (personal series of 300 patients)*

Characteristic	Percentage of cases
Family history of migraines	89.7
Headache	
Throbbing quality	66.0
Hemicranial distribution	22.0
Associated gastrointestinal symptoms	
Nausea or vomiting	62.0
Anorexia alone	12.0
Total	74.0
Aura	
Visual (teichopsia, scotomas)	5.0
Numbness (face, hands, usually bilateral)	0.5
Other factors	
Associated vertigo or light-headedness[a]	19.0
Nocturnal occurrence (occasional)[b]	9.0
Morning awakening (occasional)[b]	4.0

[a]During aura or headache.

[b]Most headaches in these patients occurred during the daytime hours, in contrast to some patients with mass lesions or hydrocephalus, in whom headaches customarily occurred at night or on awakening.

From Barlow CF. *Headaches and migraine in childhood. Clinics in Developmental Medicine* 1984;91.

dark place and going to sleep is also a very frequent finding in adolescents with migraine. The presence of an aura is not a consistent finding, although personal experience would suggest that patient awareness of an impending headache (a symptom more vague than a specific aura) is more frequent than the 5.5% listed in Table 32.

A frequently misunderstood factor is the presence of two relatively distinct types of migraine headache patterns—migraine with aura, and migraine without aura. The aura ranges from a vague feeling of malaise to scintillating scotomas to a full-blown seizure, and the headache tends to be unilateral. Migraine without aura is usually bilateral. No other major differences occur. With no aura and with no specific part of the head involved, migraine without aura is the more difficult to diagnose and is more difficult to treat episodically, because acute therapy depends in large part on initiation of therapy before the onset of pain. Frequency of attacks varies from once every few years to few to several times per week. Migraines almost never occur daily.

Precipitating factors for migraines are many, but all seem to have in common the increase of stress on the patient, either psychological or physical or both. In patients who have yet to be diagnosed, the fear of the headache itself may be a precipitating factor in the generation of an ever-increasing frequency of headaches. Being informed of the diagnosis and of its essentially benign nature lessens anxiety, and frequency of headaches decreases. Migraine sufferers have an increased frequency of attacks with increased psychological stress [12–14]. Physical stress such as upper respiratory infections and other illnesses can also increase the frequency of attacks [12]. Interestingly, a propensity for motion sickness is common in migraine victims [15]. Hormonal changes of the menstrual cycle have been associated with migraines, as have hormonal manipulations such as taking oral contraceptive pills [16]. Foods rich in tyramine [17] and foods high in nitrates such as hot dogs, chocolate, and bacon have been implicated in some people as well [12].

Treatment for migraines is directed at stopping the attacks before they begin or at their onset (Table 33). In adolescents, episodic treatment is the most desirable because of the teenager's tendency to deal with things on an immediate basis. Prophylactic therapy is less desirable because of adolescents' typically poor compliance with long-term treatment regimens and because of the side effects of drugs used for prophylaxis. Acute treatment, with the medication being taken at the first sign of an aura or, if lacking an aura, at the first hint of head pain, is tried first with nonsteroidal antiinflammatory drugs

TABLE 33. *Diagnosing migraine*

Sudden onset	Preceded by symptoms
Five attacks, lasting from 4 to 72 hours Characteristics (2 of 4) 　1. Worsened by physical activity 　2. Unilateral 　3. Moderate or severe 　4. Pulsating Concomitant features (1 or 2) 　1. Fear of light or sound 　2. Vomiting/nausea	Two attacks Characteristics (3 of 4) 　1. Aura lasting more than 1 hour 　2. Aura developing slowly over 4 minutes or several 　　in succession 　3. Aura indicating focal cerebral or brain stem 　　dysfunction 　4. Headache before, with, or within 1 hour of aura

Adapted from Singer HS. Migraine headaches in children. *Pediatr Rev* 1994;15:94.

[18]. Drug compounds containing vasoconstrictors such as isometheptane (Midrin) are listed as only possibly effective by the U.S. Food and Drug Administration [18]. More recently, sumatriptin, a 5-hydroxytryptamine$_{1D}$ agonist and potent vasoconstrictor, has become available for treatment of acute attacks unresponsive to other therapies. Sumatriptin can be given either by subcutaneous injection or orally. Relief can be expected for more than two thirds of the drug's users. Side effects are mostly limited to feelings of flushing and hot/cold flashes [19,20]. If the attacks come too frequently for these acute treatments or if the lack of an aura precludes the effectiveness of acute therapy, then prophylactic medication, such as propranolol or cyproheptadine, may be useful. Once the headaches are controlled with chronic prophylaxis, another try at acute therapy is advisable. Self-hypnosis and self-relaxation may be helpful in the prevention and treatment of migraines as well [21]. Another, more recent approach to therapy is intranasal lidocaine nose drops. Lidocaine nose drops stopped migraines in 55% of patients in one study, but the headaches commonly recurred early after treatment [22].

Other acute recurrent headache syndromes include vasomotor or allergic-type sinus headaches. These are usually frontal in location, can be throbbing or constant, change intensity with change in the position of the head, and frequently are precipitated by a change in the weather, particularly when a low-pressure front moves in. If the patient is allergic, antihistamine medications can prevent or treat these headaches. For these (as well as for nonallergic) patients, steroid nasal inhalers can be effective treatment and prophylaxis. These vasomotor headaches can be viewed as a migraine variant. Medications helpful in treating migraines, such as cyproheptadine and Midrin, may be useful.

Chronic Progressive Headaches

Headaches that are increasingly severe and recurrent most commonly signal an organic condition such as pseudotumor cerebri or benign intracranial hypertension. They also can be signs of subdural hematomas or intracranial abscesses. Other symptoms such as nausea, morning vomiting, ataxia, weakness, seizures, lethargy, or personality changes are present with these conditions, and neurologic findings on physical examination are common. An enhanced computed tomography scan is usually the best diagnostic tool in these situations [23].

Pseudotumor cerebri is most commonly found without a clear etiology [5,23]. It usually presents with headache, papilledema, and sixth cranial nerve palsy. Some specific associated conditions include obesity, menstrual disorders, vitamin A intoxication, use of 13-*cis*-retinoic acid, pregnancy, systemic lupus erythematosus, infectious mononucleosis, and administration of thyroid medications, nalidixic acid, steroids, or contraceptives; steroid withdrawal may also precipitate pseudotumor cerebri. Even with removal of the apparent causative factor, the disorder may persist. Treatment includes serial lumbar punctures to remove cerebrospinal fluid, oral dexamethasone, oral acetazolamide, and glycerol. It may take up to 3 months for symptoms to begin to resolve and as long as 12 months for headaches to disappear. Few patients suffer a recurrence.

TABLE 34. *Diagnosing tension headaches*

Episodic	Chronic

Ten episodes, less than 15 per month
Lasting from 30 minutes to 7 days
Characteristics (at least 2 of the following)
  1. Pressing/tightening
  2. Mild or moderate
  3. Bilateral
  4. Not aggravated by physical activity
Both of the following
  1. No vomiting or nausea
  2. Either fear of light or sound but not both
	More than 15 per month for longer than 6 months
	
	Characteristics (at least 2 of the following)
	  1. Pressing/tightening
	  2. Mild or moderate
	  3. Bilateral
	  4. Not aggravated by physical activity
	Both of the following
	  1. No vomiting
	  2. Only one of the following:
	    a. Fear of light
	    b. Fear of sound
	    c. Nausea

Adapted from Singer HS. Migraine headaches in children. *Pediatr Rev* 1994;15:94.

Chronic Nonprogressive Headaches

What are commonly called *tension headaches* are among the chronic nonprogressive type. This group includes headaches that are a sign of depression, headaches that signal a somatiform disorder, and headaches that may be a result of previous trauma. The cause of tension, or muscle contraction, headaches is unknown. Actually, this type of headache may not be related directly to contraction of the frontalis or temporalis muscles at all [24]. It is the most common headache in adolescents, occurring in 16% of patients in one study by 15 years of age [1]. It is most common in girls [23]. Other somatiform symptoms are frequent in patients with this problem. The pain is nonprogressive and is rarely associated with other symptoms except for fatigue. Such headaches can be present all day long and can recur for days at a time. The pain is usually not incapacitating, is described as dull in character, and is not specifically located, and mild analgesics such as acetaminophen usually are helpful to some degree. These headaches do not wake patients from a sound sleep. Factors that are related to the headaches frequently can be elicited in the history, possibly including family conflicts, school problems, and peer problems (Table 34). The only diagnosis that must be included seriously in the differential diagnosis is chronic sinus or vasomotor headaches. Laboratory tests and imaging procedures are not helpful except as they may reassure doubting parents that no significant organic lesion is present.

Psychosocial evaluation of these patients is mandatory. With sufficient time, the primary care physician can readily elicit causative or contributing factors and, frequently, minimal and basic counseling can bring relief. An example is a 17-year-old young man seen by one of the authors. This youth had been suffering from moderately severe, dull, frontoparietal headaches and fatigue for several weeks since he had the flu at Thanksgiving. Because he had been ill at the time, he had been relieved of the burden of his full-time, 40-hour-per-week job, which he had been performing as well as going to school. Both his social life and his studies had been suffering because of his work schedule, but he felt that he had to work those hours or he would be fired. He had never discussed this fear with his parents or with his supervisor at work. After this fear had been elicited by the physician, his mother and he negotiated with his boss and found that it was fine with his employer if he worked fewer hours. With that information, the headaches rapidly disappeared. At other times, more intensive psychosocial evaluation and intervention is needed, and the patient must be referred to a psychosocial consultant.

REFERENCES

1. Bille BS. Migraine in school children. *Acta Paediatrica Scandinavica Supplement* 1962;136:1.
2. Linet MS, Stewart WF, Celentano DD, et al. An epidemiologic study of headache among adolescents and young adults. *JAMA* 1989;261:2211.
3. Rothner AD. Pathophysiology of recurrent headaches in children and adolescents. *Pediatr Ann* 1995;24:458.
4. Schaumberg HH, Byck R, Gerstl R. Monosodium L-glutamate: its pharmacologic role in Chinese restaurant syndrome. *Science* 1969;163:825.

5. Prensky AL. Differentiating and treating pediatric headaches. *Contemp Pediatr* 1984;1:12.
6. Maytal J, Bienkowski RS, Patel M, et al. The value of brain imaging in children with headaches. *Pediatrics* 1995;96:413.
7. Moskowitz M. The visceral organ brain: implications for the pathophysiology of vascular head pain. *Neurology* 1991;41:182.
8. Welch KMA, Barkley GL, Tepley N, et al. Central neurogenic mechanisms of migraine. *Neurology* 1993;43:51.
9. Solomon GD. The pharmacology of medicines used in treating headaches. *Seminars in Pediatric Neurology* 1995;2:165.
10. Olesen J. Understanding the biologic basis of migraine [editorial]. *N Engl J Med* 1994;331:1713.
11. Sillanpää M. Changes in the prevalence of migraine and other headaches during the first seven school years. *Headache* 1983;23:15.
12. Barlow CF. *Headaches in childhood.* London: Spastics International Medical Publishers; 1984.
13. Leviton A, Slack WV, Mosek B, et al. A computerized behavioral assessment of children with headaches. *Headache* 1984;24:182.
14. Maratos J, Wilkinson M. Migraine in children: a medical and psychiatric study. *Cephalalgia* 1982;2:179.
15. Barabas G, Matthews WS, Ferrari M. Childhood migraine and motion sickness. *Pediatrics* 1983;72:188.
16. Silberstein SD, Merriam GR. Sex hormones and headache. *J Pain Symptom Manage* 1993;8:98.
17. Olness KN, MacDonald JT. Recurrent headaches in children: diagnosis and treatment. *Pediatr Rev* 1987; 8:307.
18. Welch KMA. Drug therapy of migraine. *N Engl J Med* 1993;329:1476.
19. The Subcutaneous Sumatriptan International Study Group. Treatment of migraine attacks with sumatriptan. *N Engl J Med* 1991;325:316.
20. Cady RK, Wendt JK, Kirchner, et al. Treatment of acute migraine with subcutaneous sumatriptan. *JAMA* 1991;265:2831.
21. Olness K, MacDonald JT, Uden DL. Comparison of self-hypnosis and propranolol in the treatment of juvenile classic migraine. *Pediatrics* 1987;79:593.
22. Maizels M, Scott B, Cohen W, et al. Intranasal lidocaine for treatment of migraine. *JAMA* 1996;276:319.
23. Rothner AD. Headaches in children and adolescents. *Postgrad Med* 1987;81:223.
24. Philips HC, Hunder MS. A psychophysiological investigation of tension headache. *Headache* 1982;22:173.

SUGGESTED READING

Barlow CF. *Headaches in childhood.* London: Spastics International Medical Publishers; 1984.
Dunn DW, Purvin VA. Headaches in adolescents: practical management strategies for the pediatrician. *Adolescent Health Update* 1990;3:1.
McCrory P. Recognizing exercise-related headache. *Phys Sports Med* 1997;25:33.
Olness KN, MacDonald JT. Recurrent headaches in children: diagnosis and treatment. *Pediatr Rev* 1987;8:307.
Rothner AD. A practical approach to headaches in adolescents. *Pediatr Ann* 1991;20:200.
Rothner AD. Headaches in children and adolescents. *Postgrad Med* 1987;81:223,.
Singer HS. Migraine headaches in children. *Pediatr Rev* 1994;15:94.
Smith MS. Comprehensive evaluation and treatment of recurrent pediatric headache. *Pediatr Ann* 1995;24:450.
Strasburger VC, Reeve A. Chronic pains in adolescence: basic principles of psychosomatic medicine. *Adolescent Medicine: State of the Art Reviews* 1991;2:677.

COMMON MUSCULOSKELETAL PROBLEMS

Musculoskeletal aches and pains are extremely common in adolescents. Considering all that is happening to their bodies, this is not surprising. Although very few of these symptoms reflect any significant pathologic process, those symptoms that bring the adolescent to the clinician require serious consideration because of the *possibility* of a serious problem. Despite this caution, it is safe to say that most of these investigations will bear little fruit. Adolescents are active, healthy people who, when they have musculoskeletal complaints, usually have simple problems with no major implications.

The musculoskeletal problems that are most common in adolescents are discussed. Mention is made of less common, but serious, problems. Nonetheless, this review is not intended to be exhaustive.

Scoliosis

Scoliosis is a lateral deviation, either postural or structural, from the vertical course of the spine of at least 10° [1]. *Postural scoliosis* may be due to several causes, including leg length discrepancy,

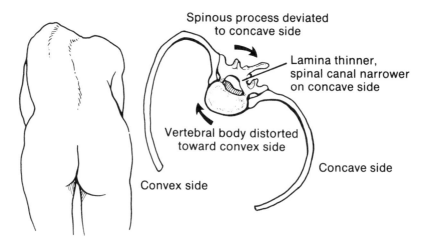

FIG. 11. Rib deformity in scoliosis.

muscular weakness, or tightness on one side of the back. Characteristic of this type of curve is a pelvic tilt when the patient is standing upright. The primary problem is not the spine, and diagnosis and treatment are directed elsewhere.

This discussion focuses on *structural curves* of idiopathic origin, the most common type. Idiopathic scoliosis has a genetic component in its etiology; it seems to follow an autosomal dominant pattern with variable penetrance. Adolescents with scoliosis may have a defect in the elastic fiber, fibrillin, similar to that in the fibrillin of patients with Marfan's syndrome [2]. Structural curves have a rotatory component. The spinous processes of the affected vertebrae rotate toward the concave side, whereas the vertebral bodies are distorted toward the convexity, and a rib prominence develops on the convex side (Fig. 11).

Prevalence

Studies differ on the prevalence of scoliosis in various populations of children and adolescents because of differing criteria used for diagnosis and different populations screened. In school screenings, prevalence has been reported to range from 0.3% to 15.3% [3–9]. For larger curves only, the prevalence has been reported to be 1% to 3% [3,7,8]. In other words, detectable scoliosis can be found in 10% or more of 13- to 14-year-olds [10], and up to two thirds are found to have no detectable curve [11,12]. Of every 1,000 children screened, only 1 to 3 require bracing, and only 1 in 2,000 to 3,000 require surgical correction [10].

Curve Significance

The significance of a detected curve in a latency-age child, or in an adolescent, depends on several factors. First, the degree of the curve is significant. The degree of curve is commonly accepted to be the Cobb angle as measured on a standing posteroanterior radiograph of the spine. This angle is defined by the following technique: parallel lines are drawn to the articular surfaces of the last superior and inferior vertebrae involved in the curve; the perpendicular is then drawn to each of these lines, and the angle of intersection of each of these lines is measured (Fig. 12). This is done for each curve present. Curves of 20° to 29° have much more chance of progression than do curves of less than 20°, and there is a direct correlation between the magnitude of the original curve and the incidence of progression [13].

The sex of the child or adolescent with the curve has implications for prognosis. Equal proportions of boys and girls are referred from school screening examinations [3,9,13], but curves in girls have a much greater chance of progressing to clinical significance [14,15]. There is a 1 : 1 ratio of girls to

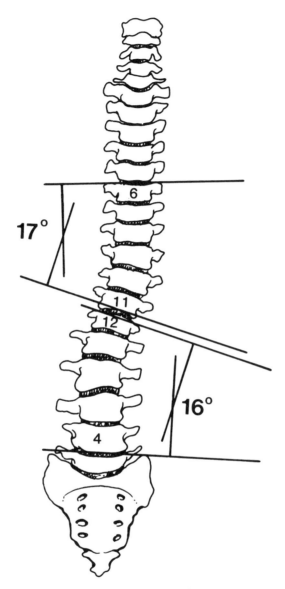

FIG. 12. Cobb angle.

boys with curves of 6° to 10°, 1.4 : 1 for curves of 11° to 20°, 5.4 : 1 for curves exceeding 21°, and 7.2 : 1 for those cases under treatment [9].

Age and maturity are other factors important in curve progression. The time of peak progression of a curve occurs at the time of peak height velocity in adolescents (i.e., the adolescent growth spurt) [15]. The actual beginning of this increase in curve angle occurs at the beginning of puberty with the appearance of secondary sex characteristics (i.e., Tanner rating 2) [16–18]. The older an adolescent becomes (i.e., the more mature), the less a curve progresses [13,15]. Likewise, progression is less likely after menarche [13], by which time most of a girl's height has been achieved.

Finally, the pattern of the curve has been related to risk of progression [13,17]. The rule is that double curves progress more frequently than single curves, and a single thoracic curve progresses more frequently than a single lumbar curve.

These factors must be considered together when evaluating any one adolescent. Therefore, a curve of more than 20° found in a young girl who has not yet reached menarche and who has not completed her period of peak height velocity is much more likely to increase than the same curve found in a girl who has been regularly menstruating and, consequently, has completed most of her growth. The chance of significant progression of a curve of less than 20° in a boy who is at Tanner stage 4 or 5 is much less than either of the preceding examples. One of the problems with these kinds of statements, however, is that they are based on statistical analyses, and for any given patient they may be meaningless. Still, they do allow for a reasonable assessment of risk of curve progression and, therefore, of the need for treatment.

Screening for Scoliosis

A screening program should be designed to detect in people a condition of which they would otherwise be unaware and in whom detection and treatment will cure, slow, or stop the progression of the condition. The screening procedure should be relatively inexpensive and easily applied to a large percentage of the population in question. In addition, the follow-up needed for those detected in the screening program should be effective and worth the effort in cost and results.

Scoliosis screening programs are currently mandated in more than 15 U.S. states and in some foreign countries [17]. These programs are in schools because that is where large numbers of children can be reached in an organized fashion and where, usually, there are health personnel who can provide the expertise necessary to implement such a program. The children screened are typically in grades 5 through 9 (ages 11–14 years), although, because puberty begins before age 11 in many girls, an argument could be made for starting these programs earlier.

Screening tests have certain characteristics that must be measured before they are blindly accepted. These are sensitivity (will the test identify all possible patients?), specificity (will the test accurately identify those who do not have the condition for which it is being used?), and positive predictive value (PPV), that is, predictive value of a positive test, the probability that a person with a positive test actually has the condition for which he or she is being tested. The PPV varies with the prevalence of the condition in the population being tested. If a condition is prevalent, the PPV may be high even if the test is not that sensitive; if the condition is rare, many detected on screening with a sensitive test may not actually have the condition.

Sensitivity of scoliosis screening is considered high; almost all people with the condition are detected. Specificity is also considered to be high because almost all of those children without scoliosis are accurately identified. If children identified on scoliosis screening are divided into two populations—a population with detectable scoliosis and another population with treatable scoliosis—one finds PPVs of widely differing significance [10]. In the detectable population, PPV is high; 60% to 70% of those identified on screening do have a radiologically detectable curve. For the treatable population, however, the PPV is low because fewer than 5% of those detected on screening actually turn out to have scoliosis that requires treatment [18]. Although there is much enthusiasm for screening programs because of the high detection rate, possibly more attention should be paid to the PPV for the treatable population [18–20].

Nevertheless, screening is a fact of life in most communities; it should be a procedure that is performed routinely in the clinician's office as well because it is so easy to do. The child is examined in her underwear or with no clothes on from the waist up. She is instructed to bend over from the waist and to hang her hands and head down loosely. The examiner sights along her spine from the rear and from the head and looks for a rib hump on one side or the other. Detection of such a hump is the positive sign and is due to the rotatory phenomenon mentioned earlier. While the child is in this position, it is prudent also to view her from the side to detect any exaggerated kyphosis. Other signs for which the clinician can search are elevation of one shoulder, asymmetry or prominence of the scapulae, tilting of the hips or differing hip levels, increased space between one arm and the waist, failure of the occiput of the head to align directly over the crease of the buttocks, and, of course, a noticeable curve of the spine (Fig. 13).

Once a sign of scoliosis is detected, the clinician must decide whether to pursue further evaluation. Knowledge of risk of progression is essential to help the primary physician or other clinician make an intelligent decision at this point. Children or adolescents who are female, are relatively immature, and who have curves of from 20° to 29° are at highest risk for progression [1]. Therefore, a girl who has any curve and is at Tanner stage 1 through 3 should have a low-dose, standing posteroanterior radiograph of the spine. If the curve is less than 20°, the primary clinician should follow with another examination

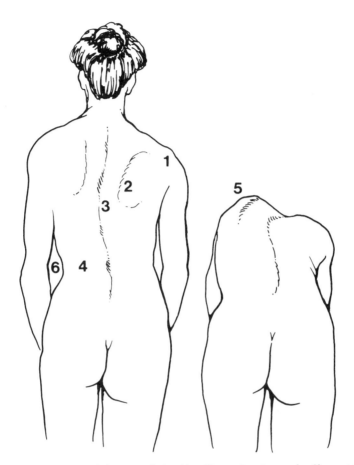

FIG. 13. Six signs of scoliosis: 1) depressed shoulder, 2) prominent scapula, 3) curved spine, 4) hip asymmetry, 5) rib hump, and 6) increased elbow–hip space.

and film in 6 months. If the curve has progressed significantly (i.e., 3–5° or more), referral to an orthopedist experienced in treatment of these children and adolescents should be made. If the curve is more than 20° on this first film, then referral should be made immediately [21]. In the adolescent who is relatively mature (i.e., Tanner stage 4 or 5), curves up to 30° have relatively little risk of significant progression [22]. Still, with curves of large magnitude, it is prudent to refer to an orthopedist.

Treatment

There are three useful methods of treating scoliosis: 1) bracing, 2) surgery with instrumentation and fusion, and 3) benign neglect. Exercise never has been shown to have any effect on the progression or outcome of a structural curve. For most children detected in a screening program, no treatment is needed.

Bracing

The actively growing child with a progressing curve of 20° to 40° should be treated with nonsurgical methods (i.e., bracing) [23], and *only* with documented progression should a curve of less than 29° be treated [17]. The patient with the best chance of responding to the bracing is a relatively immature patient (Tanner stage 2 or 3) with a single right thoracic curve of 25° to 40° that is progressive. A curve greater than 40° stands little chance of improving with this type of brace regardless of whether the child is immature [24]. Wearing a thoracolumbosacral orthosis for 23 hours daily for up to 4 years can be a trying experience for even the most dedicated and motivated patient. Excellent patient education and a high degree of rapport between the patient, her family, and the treatment team (which always should include the primary care clinician) is essential if any success is to be obtained. The best sign of success of brace treatment is the initial response [25]. Those patients obtaining a 50% reduction in the curve while in the brace for the first 6 months of treatment are most likely to have a good end result. Because the goal of treatment is to keep the curve at less than 40°, reduction in the curve is not mandatory for success; it is lack of progression that marks successful treatment [26]. Underarm bracing is not the preferred treatment with single thoracic curves, but it is preferred when bracing is indicated in lumbar and thoracolumbar curves [25].

Who, then, is the patient with a good prognosis with bracing? It is the relatively immature patient who is flexible, has a smaller rotational prominence, and has a normal lateral radiograph. The patient who is more likely not to respond to treatment is the one who has a highly structural curve with poor flexibility and who has a large rotational prominence and a thoracic lordosis. True double thoracic curves are notoriously resistant to brace treatment [25].

Surgery

The primary goal of surgery is stabilization of the curve so that there will be no further progression, which is the same goal as nonsurgical treatment. Surgery also presents the possibility of some correction of preexisting curvature, with concomitant cosmetic improvement. Modern techniques consistently yield a 50% reduction in deformity without excessive risk [23,27]. The two components of any surgical correction are fusion of the spine and stabilization by instrumentation (i.e., with metal stabilizing devices such as bars, struts, and internal braces). The best known of these instruments is the Harrington rod, the type most indicated for correction of a single thoracic curve. Fusion must be extensive enough for permanent stabilization of the curve but not so extensive that it compromises function and creates a new set of problems.

Surgery is indicated for curves that are progressing rapidly past 40° or for curves that already exceed 50° [28]. Surgery is also needed for patients whose curves continue to worsen while undergoing bracing or electrical stimulation treatment. Surgery done properly has fairly good results, but it has risks, as do all major operations, and should be done only when specifically indicated [27,29].

Other Back Problems

Curvatures of the spine other than scoliosis can also cause problems in adolescents. One of these is *kyphosis*. A gradual posterior curve of the thoracic spine is normal. When the adolescent is viewed from the side while he or she is bending over from the waist with hands and head hanging down, a gradual curve from the neck to the buttocks should be seen. The normal lumbar lordosis can be seen to have flattened out as well, producing a smooth line. When the curve is more sharply angled in the thoracic area, excessive kyphosis can be present. To confirm this impression, a standing lateral radiograph of the spine should be obtained. The curve should not measure more than 40°. If it does, pathologic kyphosis is present. With a curve of 40° to 60° in a relatively immature adolescent (Tanner stage 1–3), bracing may be successful in halting progression of the curve. With a progressive curve of more than 40° that does not respond to bracing or with a curve of greater than 60°, surgical fusion with instrumentation is indicated [30].

It is well to remember that at least 95% of the teens with apparent kyphosis have a postural and not a structural problem. Counseling and attention to posture should alleviate the problem in these adolescents. A condition that can lead to structural kyphosis is Scheuermann's disease. On spinal radiographs, irregularity of the apophyseal growing areas of the thoracic vertebrae may be apparent [30]. This condition accounts for a large number of young kyphosis patients who will need bracing or surgery.

A relatively common problem in adolescents is *back pain*. Although most frequently it is the low back that hurts, thoracic back pain can be a problem. Often, this is caused by muscle strain, especially in students who carry extremely heavy book bags or purses slung over the same shoulder all the time. Low back pain in the adolescent is usually not due to muscle spasm or degenerative disease, the most frequent causes in adults [31]. The comparison of causes in youths versus adults is seen in Table 35. The most common cause, spondylolysis/spondylolisthesis, is more fully discussed in Chapter 6. When

TABLE 35. *Low back pain comparison between adults and children participating in sports*

Lesion	Adult	Child	P
Ankylosing spondylitis	1	0	—
Discogenic	48	11	0.05
Degenerated	22	1	—
Herniated	24	9	—
Both	2	1	—
Hamstring strain	0	1	—
Hyperlordotic mechanical back pain	0	26	—
Lumbosacral strain	27	6	0.05
Neoplasm	2	0	—
Osteoarthritis	4	0	—
Scoliosis	7	8	—
Spinal stenosis	6	0	—
Spondylolysis/-isthesis	5	47	0.05
Trochanteric bursitis	0	1	—
Total	100	100	

Adapted from Micheli LJ, Wood R. Back pain in young athletes. *Arch Pediatr Adolesc Med* 1995; 149:15.

low back paraspinal muscle strain is suspected, then rest and nonsteroidal antiinflammatory drugs are indicated. Muscle relaxants can be of value. Small doses of diazepam also are helpful in the early stages of treatment. Once pain is gone, patients should be instructed on proper lifting technique (i.e., bend at the knees and use the legs to lift) and on daily use of flexion exercises for the back.

Getting an adolescent to comply with this full treatment regimen can be difficult, and one or two repeat courses may be necessary. However, if a reasonable course of therapy is not successful, other diagnoses should be sought. Radiologic examination should be sufficient to diagnose spondylolysis and spondylolisthesis. Other imaging studies such as bone scans, computed tomography scans, and magnetic resonance imaging should be helpful with the others. Laboratory tests should include a complete blood cell count and a differential count, an erythrocyte sedimentation rate, rheumatoid factor, and a human leukocyte antigen (HLA)-B27 if ankylosing spondylitis is suspected [32].

Slipped Capital Femoral Epiphysis

The most significant hip problem in adolescents is slipped capital femoral epiphysis (SCFE). The pathologic lesion is actually a fracture through the growth plate of the femoral head, with slippage of the femoral head downward and medial to the femoral neck.

The most common form of SCFE is the gradual one, which occurs most often in adolescents who are obese and who are about to enter, or are in, their pubertal growth spurt [33,34]. The acute form occurs after sudden and severe trauma and is not considered further here. The gradual form occurs in 2.8 to 10 per 100,000 pubertal adolescents, is more prevalent in boys than in girls (between 2 and 4 to 1), seems to occur more frequently in blacks than in whites, and is unilateral three times more frequently than bilateral. Approximately 25% of teens with SCFE will have the problem on the other side within 2 years [33].

History reveals a complaint of pain that usually is in or around the hip but may be confined to the lower thigh or even the knee. A limp is frequently reported as well. Physical examination reveals a limp with a characteristic gait wherein the leg is externally rotated at the hip. There is limited passive hip motion, especially with internal rotation, flexion, and abduction. Fever and other systemic signs are absent. Diagnosis is confirmed by anteroposterior and frogleg hip radiographs, which show increased epiphyseal width and displacement of the femoral head posteriorly and inferiorly. Sometimes this is apparent only on the front leg view [35]. Differential diagnosis includes late-onset Legg-Calvé-Perthes disease, monoarticular juvenile rheumatoid arthritis (JRA), idiopathic chondrolysis, osteochondrosis dissecans, and a low-grade septic joint. The latter is most commonly caused by gonorrhea (see Chapter 5). All these can be ruled out relatively easily by a thorough history, physical examination, and selected laboratory tests and imaging studies.

Treatment is surgical, with earlier diagnosis producing better results. There is some urgency to stabilize the problem surgically because of the risk of avascular necrosis [33]. The procedure most often involves insertion of bone pegs across the slipping epiphysis. If not treated optimally or early, chronic hip problems may develop.

Chest Problems and Costochondritis

Most chest pain in adolescents is of musculoskeletal origin. There have been several studies of the causes of chest pain in adolescents [36–38] (Table 36). Musculoskeletal causes have been noted as the most frequent organic causes of pain, with costochondritis the most common of these. The other major causes have been called variously psychogenic, functional, or idiopathic. Another cause can be hyperventilation [37]. Most of what is called *chest pain of nonorganic origin* in adolescents is actually pain of organic origin, and most of that is costochondritis. The problems lie in the examination technique and in ascribing the cause of the pain to psychological factors when, actually, these factors often exacerbate or make a patient more aware of pain that is from an organic source.

Compared with adults and even with children, adolescents have little organic heart disease, but what adolescents *do* have in abundance is a preoccupation with their bodies and a blossoming awareness of their own mortality. This combination makes teenagers acutely aware of persistent chest pains, especially when they are on the left side of the chest [36]. With persistent left-sided chest pain, it is the rare adolescent (and his or her parents) who does not worry just a little that he or she might be having a heart attack and might die. When these teens are seen by the physician, it is natural that they appear psychologically distressed. This distress can easily be mistaken as the cause of the pain when a meticulous examination of the chest wall is not performed. However, when a meticulous, firm, one-finger palpation of each sternocostal cartilage is performed, most often the cause is found to be costochondritis [39].

Costochondritis is defined as pain that is reproducible by palpation of the affected chest cartilage when no signs or symptoms of other abnormalities are present [40]. The pain is usually sharp and may radiate laterally from the sternal area or down into the upper abdomen. It is frequently associated with a particular movement or position, and the patients often report a history of upper respiratory infection or of heavy exercise in the 3 months preceding the visit to the physician [36]. When the pain is unilateral, it more frequently emanates from the left side [36]. This may be due to the fact that teenagers are aware that the heart is on the left side of the chest, and so right-sided chest pain is more often ignored. More women than men are seen by physicians for this condition [36,41,42]. It is important to emphasize that this diagnosis can be made only after history and physical examination have excluded other chest or upper abdominal pathologic processes. When there is a hint of other pathologic findings, further testing, such as imaging and laboratory studies, is indicated.

TABLE 36. *Causes of chest pain in adolescents*

Musculoskeletal
Costochondritis
Traumatic injury
Muscle strain
Rib cage anomaly
Infectious or inflammatory
Pleurisy
Pneumonitis
Bronchitis
Herpes zoster
Esophagitis or esophageal reflux
Pericarditis
Mitral valve prolapse
Arrhythmia
Hyperventilation
Psychosomatic
Idiopathic

Management of costochondritis is fairly simple. After other causes of the pain are ruled out, and the clinician has demonstrated that the pain can be reproduced by palpation of the affected cartilage, a simple explanation and education in very concrete terms usually suffice. It is very important to be explicit in this counseling. Phrases such as, "The pain is not coming from your heart," "This is not a heart attack," and "You're not going to die from this" should be used. It is also important to tell the adolescent and parents that this pain may not resolve very rapidly because the ribs move all the time with each breath. They should expect recurrence of the pain for up to several months. However, because they now know what is causing the pain and, more important, what is not causing the pain, they can ignore it or use mild analgesics.

A mention of hyperventilation as a cause of chest pain is necessary. Hyperventilation syndrome is relatively common as a manifestation of anxiety in adolescents. The symptoms produced by chronic hyperventilation can be very worrisome and can focus the adolescent's attention on his or her body. Although chronic hyperventilation may cause chest pain [43–45], it is more likely that the acute awareness of somatic problems in the anxious, hyperventilating adolescent makes him or her more concerned about a chest pain of organic origin, and when that pain is left sided, the youngster worries all the more [37].

Mitral valve prolapse (MVP) is another condition in which chest pain may be a symptom. Chest pain is said to occur in approximately 60% of patients with MVP and is more common in men [46,47]. A study of 9- to 14-year-olds, however, showed no increase in chest symptoms in MVP patients compared with control subjects [48]. Several causes have been postulated for this pain, including stretching of the chordae tendineae, myocardial ischemia, excessive myocardial oxygen consumption, coronary artery vasoregulatory abnormalities, and, possibly, arrhythmias [49]. Therefore, careful auscultation of the heart is essential in any adolescent with chest pain. If a characteristic diastolic click is heard, an echocardiogram and cardiology consultation should be obtained. Although chest pain is frequently associated with MVP, most adolescents with chest pain do not have this condition.

Pectus Excavatum

The major chest deformity encountered in childhood and adolescence is pectus excavatum. Other defects such as pectus carinatum (pigeon chest), Poland's syndrome, and minor rib abnormalities occur.

Pectus excavatum was first described in 1590 [50], and surgical correction was first described in 1911 [51] and again in 1920 [52]. Modern treatment was begun in 1931 [53]. Pectus excavatum occurs in 1 in 300 births, is rare in blacks, and occurs in boys five times more often than in girls [50]. Its cause is unknown. Often visible at birth, pectus excavatum becomes more apparent as the child grows older. It is frequently seen in Marfan's syndrome and is also associated with Hurler's syndrome [54]. The major reason for concern is cosmetic. Severe deformities can compromise cardiac and pulmonary function by the severe anteroposterior compression of the heart and lungs, which can be alleviated by surgical correction of the defect [55–58]. The most devastating effects are psychological. These children are typically described as shy and retiring and frequently will not participate in physical and social activities with their peers owing to their embarrassment about their deformities.

Treatment, which helps the cosmetic problem but which may not help the functional deficits [59], consists of surgical correction. The surgery is most easily performed and requires the shortest recovery time when the child is younger than 5 years [50]. Unfortunately, some children are missed and do not present until they are adolescents. One method of selecting children and adolescents for surgical treatment is use of the *pectus index* [60]. This is calculated by using the transverse diameter of the chest as the numerator and the sternal-to-vertebral distance as the denominator. If the index is greater than 3.25, surgery is believed to be justified. Surgery consists of removing the defective cartilages, elevating the sternum to the normal position, and fixing it in place with or without an internal splint. If a splint is used, it can be removed under general anesthesia a year later [59]. The results of surgical treatment are generally good. One series of 161 patients showed excellent results in 84% of the repairs and good results in 15% [50].

Arthritis

The differential diagnosis of arthritis in adolescents is extensive (Table 37). The primary categories include collagen vascular disorders and infectious arthritides.

TABLE 37. *Differential diagnosis of arthritis
in adolescents*

Collagen vascular disorder
Juvenile rheumatoid arthritis
Ankylosing spondylitis
Systemic lupus erythematosus
Dermatomyositis
Scleroderma
Polyarteritis nodosa
Psoriasis
Sjögren's syndrome
Henoch-Schönlein syndrome

Infectious or parainfectious process
Gonococcal disease
Reiter's syndrome
Rheumatic fever
Lyme arthritis

Traumatic injury
Slipped capital femoral epiphysis
Legg-Calvé-Perthe disease
Chondromalacia patellae

Other conditions with arthritis as a feature
Hemophilia
Sickle cell disease
Serum sickness
Inflammatory bowel disease
Sarcoidosis

Collagen vascular disorders that have arthritis as a major component include JRA, systemic lupus erythematosus (SLE), and spondyloarthropathies [61]. Reiter's syndrome can be included here; it is discussed in Chapter 5. Gonorrhea is the leading cause of septic arthritis in adolescents by far (see Chapter 5). The organisms that cause commonly cause arthritis in children are rarely do so in adolescents.

Juvenile rheumatoid arthritis can present during adolescence in any of its forms: systemic, monoarticular, pauciarticular (four or fewer joints involved) types 1 and 2, and rheumatoid factor-positive or -negative polyarticular (five or more joints involved). Pauciarticular type 2 and rheumatoid factor-positive or -negative polyarticular JRA appear more often in late childhood and adolescence than do the other forms [61,62]. As opposed to pauciarticular type 1, which occurs predominantly in younger girls, type 2 occurs more often in boys older than 8 years.

Type 2 pauciarticular JRA is not associated with iridocyclitis or with antinuclear antibodies. It affects the major joints of the lower extremity most often, and patients frequently have a family history of spondyloarthropathies such as ankylosing spondylitis, Reiter's syndrome, psoriatic arthritis, or inflammatory bowel disease. More than half of these patients are positive for HLA-B27 [63]. Patients in this group also may have episodes of enthesitis (inflammation at the sites of attachment of ligaments, tendons, and fasciae to bone) [64–67]. As time goes on, patients with this form of JRA are increasingly found to have other spondyloarthropathies and not JRA [68–71].

Although rheumatoid factor-negative polyarticular JRA without prominent systemic manifestations has a relatively good prognosis, many patients with the rheumatoid factor-positive variety are not so fortunate [61]. This latter form often is severe, involves highly destructive disease, positive antinuclear antibodies, and rheumatoid nodules, and may rarely be complicated by rheumatoid vasculitis. It is associated with a genetic marker, HLA-DR4 [72,73].

Clinically, most patients with JRA have morning stiffness and swollen, painful joints. Symptoms must be present for at least 6 weeks and usually are present for months or years [74]. Onset of arthritis often is gradual and insidious. Fever may be present, usually in the systemic type. Laboratory tests are helpful in some types, but not diagnostic. The clinical picture over time is what makes the diagnosis of JRA.

TABLE 38. *Classification of systemic lupus erythematosus (SLE), revised*

Four or more of the following criteria are adequate for a diagnosis of SLE:
Antinuclear antibody
Arthritis
Discoid rash
Hematologic disorder: hemolytic anemia, leukopenia (less than 4,000/μL), or thrombocytopenia (less than 100,000/μL)
Immunologic disorder: positive LE cell preparation, abnormal titer of anti-DNA antibody, anti-Sm antibody, or false-positive Venereal Disease Research Laboratory test
Malar rash
Neurologic disorder
Oral ulcers
Photosensitivity
Renal disorder: persistent proteinuria or cellular casts
Serositis: pleuritis or pericarditis

Adapted from Lindsley CB. The adolescent with arthritis. *Compr Ther* 1996;22:48.

Systemic lupus erythematosus is a serious, multisystem disease that occurs with some frequency in adolescents. Although joint problems are not the symptoms of primary concern in SLE, they are frequent. Arthritis occurs in 60% to 85% of cases, and intermittent arthralgia is even more common. The arthritis tends to be episodic, nonerosive, and polyarticular [74]. Myalgia is also common, occurring in 50% of cases [75]. The revised criteria for classification of SLE are presented in Table 38.

Another unusual condition with arthritis as a prime component is *Reiter's syndrome,* which is diagnosed by recognition of the triad of symptoms of arthritis, conjunctivitis or uveitis, and urethritis or cervicitis. It usually follows dysentery or can be acquired by sexual transmission of a chlamydial or, possibly, a mycoplasmal infection. Enthesopathy can also be a feature of this condition (see Chapter 5) [72].

A more recent addition to the list of possible causes of arthritis in adolescents is *Lyme disease.* Because of this disease's protean symptoms and increasing geographic occurrence, all physicians should be aware of it as a possible cause of indolent arthritis. Lyme disease is caused by the spirochete *Borrelia burgdorferi* and is transmitted by various ticks, especially *Ixodes dammini* [64]. The physician could be consulted at any time during the three distinct phases of this illness (Table 39). The joint manifestations of this condition range from recurring arthralgias in the early phase to migratory symp-

TABLE 39. *Symptoms of Lyme disease*

Acute phase
Rash at bite site (erythema chronicum migrans)
Fever
Chills
Headaches
Stiff neck
Fatigue
Arthralgias
Myalgias
Sore throat
Lymphadenopathy
Abdominal pain
Malaise

Subacute phase
Arthropathy
Neurologic problems
Cardiac problems

Chronic phase
Chronic arthritis (5–10%)
Chronic neurologic problems

toms, usually without swelling, in the second stage, to a pauciarticular chronic arthritis in the chronic or late stage [76]. Children and younger adolescents seem to have joint pains and frank arthritis less frequently than do adults [77]. There is some evidence that some patients with Lyme disease may be predisposed, genetically, to development of chronic arthritis [65].

Other Common Joint Problems

Blount's disease, or tibia vara, is a disorder of the knee that can produce bowed legs and tibial torsion. There is a severe form in early childhood and a milder juvenile form that occurs in early adolescence, most often unilaterally [78]. On radiography, the affected extremity shows enlargement or a beaklike projection at the medial aspect of the proximal tibial metaphysis. There is medial angulation of the tibia at the knee. Without correction, there can be permanent bowlegging and shortening of the affected limb.

Another condition that may affect the knee of an adolescent is *osteochondritis dissecans*, which consists of separation of a portion of bone and overlying articular cartilage, most commonly from the medial femoral condyle and occasionally from the lateral aspect [80]. It is most common in boys and is unilateral 90% of the time [79,80]. Adolescents with open physes are considered a different population from those with closed epiphyses. Adults with the problem usually have the onset while still adolescents [81]. The femoral head, the capitellum, and the talus may also be affected. Early on, the cartilage is intact, with only the bone being separated. Symptoms at this stage are nonspecific, with a vague aching sensation after exercise. Later, when the fragment separates from its condyle and moves in its bed, limping, swelling, and limited range of motion occur. Examination reveals tenderness over the affected area, especially with the knee flexed. Radiographs reveal the separation. Treatment involves early immobilization for 6 to 10 weeks in a long leg cast. This is successful for most adolescents with open physes. Surgical correction using arthroscopic fixation with pins or screws is needed in those whose epiphyses have closed [81].

Popliteal cyst, or *Baker's cyst*, is a painless cyst of variable size that arises from the gastrocnemius bursa and communicates with the knee joint, or arises from the knee joint itself. It is similar to a ganglion cyst of the wrist. Treatment is required only if the cyst is large enough to cause pain or to limit motion. Spontaneous resolution is common [79,80].

Finally, the primary care clinician may be confronted with a condition known as *fibromyalgia*. This condition has been defined as a nonarticular rheumatism characterized by aching and stiffness in the presence of focal tender points [82]. The name is descriptive without implying pathogenesis. The pain of this condition is primarily proximal and often difficult to localize. Although some patients complain of pain in specific joint regions (neck, shoulders, back, knees, hands), many vaguely refer to generalized musculoskeletal discomfort. Apparent muscle weakness may represent a guarding against pain. Morning stiffness and easy fatigability are frequently reported. Emotional distress, excessive fatigue, and unresolved conflicts or decisions can exacerbate the symptoms. Physical examination reveals no significant pathologic findings in the joints, bones, or muscle strength or integrity. The patient may seem tense and uncomfortable during the musculoskeletal examination. The clinician should check for tenderness at specific "tender points." Firm palpation of these sites usually elicits verbal expressions of pain and withdrawal from the examiner's probing finger. However, these "points" also can be tender in people who do not have symptoms of fibromyalgia. Laboratory testing should reveal no abnormalities. Treatment consists primarily of thoroughly explaining to the patient what he or she does not have (i.e., any disease with serious prognostic implications). Taking the patient's complaints seriously and offering symptomatic treatment while urging a return to full activity are critical components of therapy. Underlying causes of depression and conflict in a patient's life should be sought assiduously and, if found, treated with counseling or psychotherapy. A key component of treatment is to have the patient enter a graded exercise program. This can help considerably. Fibromyalgia is part of a spectrum of conditions, including chronic fatigue syndrome and irritable bowel syndrome, in which physical symptoms result from nonorganic causes.

REFERENCES

1. Skaggs DL, Bassett GS. Adolescent idiopathic scoliosis: an update. *Am Fam Physician* 1996;53:2327.
2. Hadley-Miller N, Mims B, Milewicz DM. The potential role of the elastic fiber system in adolescent idiopathic scoliosis. *J Bone Joint Surg [Am]* 1994;76:1193.

3. Asher M, Greene P, Orrick J. A six year report: spinal deformity screening in Kansas school children. *Journal of the Kansas Medical Society* 1980;81:968.
4. Brooks HL, Azen SP, Gerberg E, et al. Scoliosis: a prospective epidemiological study. *J Bone Joint Surg [Am]* 1975;57:968.
5. Dickson RA, Stamper P, Sharp AM, et al. School screening for scoliosis: cohort study of clinical course. *Br Med J* 1980;73:265.
6. Leaver JM, Alvik A, Warren MD. Prescriptive screening for adolescent scoliosis: a review of the incidence. *Int J Epidemiol* 1982;11:101.
7. Lonstein JE. Screening for spinal deformities in Minnesota schools. *Clin Orthop* 1972;126:33.
8. Lonstein JE, Bjorklund S, Wanninger MH, et al. Voluntary school screening for scoliosis in Minnesota. *J Bone Joint Surg [Am]* 1982;64:481.
9. Rogala EJ, Drummond DS, Gurr J. Scoliosis: incidence and natural history. A prospective epidemiological study. *J Bone Joint Surg [Am]* 1978;60:173.
10. Berwick DM. Scoliosis screening. *Pediatr Rev* 1984;5:238.
11. Lonstein JE, Bjorklund S, Wanninger MH, et al. Voluntary school screening for scoliosis in Minnesota. *J Bone Joint Surg [Am]* 1982;64:481.
12. Morais T, Bernier M, Turcotte F. Age- and sex-specific prevalence of scoliosis and the value of school screening programs. *Am J Public Health* 1985;75:1377.
13. Lonstein JE, Carlson MJ. The prediction of curve progression in untreated idiopathic scoliosis during growth. *J Bone Joint Surg [Am]* 1984;66:1061.
14. Bunnell WP. The natural history of idiopathic scoliosis before skeletal maturity. *Spine* 1986;11:773.
15. Duval-Beaupre G. Pathogenic relationship between scoliosis and growth. In: Zorab PA, ed. *Scoliosis and growth.* Edinburgh: Churchill Livingstone; 1971:58.
16. Marshall WA, Tanner JM. Variations in patterns of pubertal changes in girls. *Arch Dis Child* 1969;44:291.
17. Pedriolle R, Vidal J. Thoracic idiopathic curve evolution and prognosis. *Spine* 1985;10:785.
18. Lonstein JE. Natural history and school screening for scoliosis. *Orthop Clin North Am* 1988;19:227.
19. Goldberg CJ, Dowling FE, Fogarty EE, et al. School scoliosis screening and the United States Preventive Services Task Force: an examination of long-term results. *Spine* 1995;20:1368.
20. United States Preventive Services Task Force. Screening for adolescent idiopathic scoliosis: policy statement. *JAMA* 1993;269:2664.
21. Berwixck DM. Scoliosis screening: a pause in the chase [editorial]. *Am J Public Health* 1985;75:1373.
22. Lonstein JE, Winter RB. The Milwaukee brace for the treatment of adolescent idiopathic scoliosis: a review of one thousand and twenty patients. *J Bone Joint Surg [Am]* 1994;76:1207.
23. Weinstein SL, Ponseti IV. Curve progression in idiopathic scoliosis. *J Bone Joint Surg [Am]* 1983;65:447.
24. Winter RB, ed. Adolescent idiopathic scoliosis. *N Engl J Med* 1986;314:1379.
25. Lonstein JE, Winter RB. Adolescent idiopathic scoliosis: nonoperative treatment. *Orthop Clin North Am* 1988;19:239.
26. Carr WA, Moe JH, Winter RB, et al. Treatment of idiopathic scoliosis in the Milwaukee brace, long term results. *J Bone Joint Surg [Am]* 1980;62:599.
27. Nachemson AL, Peterson LE. Effectiveness of treatment with a brace in girls who have adolescent idiopathic scoliosis: a prospective, controlled study based on data from the Brace Study of the Scoliosis Research Society. *J Bone Joint Surg [Am]* 1995;77:815.
28. Boachie-Adjei O, Lonner B. Spinal deformity. *Pediatr Clin North Am* 1996;43:883.
29. Bunnell WP. Spinal deformity. *Pediatr Clin North Am* 1986;33:1475.
30. Connolly PJ, von Schroeder HP, Johnson GE, et al. Adolescent idiopathic scoliosis: long-term effect of instrumentation extending to the lumbar spine. *J Bone Joint Surg [Am]* 1995;77:1210.
31. Watts HG. The spine. In: Behrman RE, Vaughan VC, eds. *Nelson textbook of pediatrics.* 13th ed. Philadelphia: WB Saunders; 1987:1352.
32. Micheli LJ, Wood R. Back pain in young athletes. *Arch Pediatr Adolesc Med* 1995;149:15.
33. Greydanus DE, Hofmann AD. Spine and joint disorders. In: Hofmann AD, Greydanus DE, eds. *Adolescent medicine.* 2nd ed. Norwalk, CT: Appleton & Lange; 1989:204.
34. Brown RT. Costochondritis in adolescents. *Journal of Adolescent Health Care* 1981;1:198.
35. Pantell RH, Goodman BW Jr. Adolescent chest pain: a prospective study. *Pediatrics* 1983;71:881.
36. Selbst SM. Chest pain in children. *Pediatrics* 1985;75:1068.
37. Brown RT. Adolescent chest pain [letter]. *Pediatrics* 1983;72:914.
38. Colabro JJ. Costochondritis [letter]. *N Engl J Med* 1977;296:947.
39. Walsh TD. Costochondritis [letter]. *N Engl J Med* 1977;297:1071.
40. Scobie BA. Costochondral pain in gastroenterologic practice. *N Engl J Med* 1976;295:1261.
41. Wheatley CE. Hyperventilation syndrome: a frequent cause of chest pain. *Chest* 1975;68:195.
42. Missri JC, Alexander S. Hyperventilation syndrome: a brief review. *JAMA* 1978;240:2093.
43. Evans DW, Lum LC. Hyperventilation: an important cause of pseudoangina. *Lancet* 1977;1:155.
44. Boudoulas H, King BD, Fontana ME, et al. Mitral valve prolapse syndrome: clinical presentation and diagnostic evaluation. In: Boudoulas H, Wooley CF, eds. *Mitral valve prolapse and the mitral valve prolapse syndrome.* Mount Kisco, NY: Futura; 1988:525.
45. Boudoulas H, Wooley CF. Chest pain in patients with mitral valve prolapse. *Primary Cardiology* 1985;11:16.

46. Arfken CL, Lachman AS, McLaren MJ, et al. Mitral valve prolapse: associations with symptoms and anxiety. *Pediatrics* 1990;85:311.
47. Boudoulas H, Kolibash AJ Jr, Baker P, et al. Mitral valve prolapse and the mitral valve prolapse syndrome: a diagnostic classification and pathogenesis of symptoms. *Am Heart J* 1989;118:796.
48. Ellis DG. Chest wall deformities. *Pediatr Rev* 1989;11:147.
49. Meyer L. Zur chirurgischen Behandlung der angeborenen Trichterbrust. *Verhandlungen der Berliner Medicin-ishen Gesellschfaft* 1911;42:364.
50. Sauerbruch F. *Die Chirugie der Brustorgane.* Berlin: Verlag von Julius Springer; 1940:440.
51. Ravitch MM. *Congenital deformities of the chest wall and their surgical correction.* Philadelphia: WB Saunders; 1977:78–81.
52. Smith DW. *Recognizable patterns of human malformation.* Philadelphia: WB Saunders; 1982.
53. Welch KJ. Chest wall deformities. In: Holder TM, Ashcraft KW, eds. *Pediatric surgery.* Philadelphia: WB Saunders; 1980:162.
54. Howard R. Funnel chest: its effect on cardiac function. *Arch Dis Child* 1959;34:5.
55. Beiser GD, Epstein SE. Impairment of cardiac functions in patients with pectus excavatum, with improvement after operation. *N Engl J Med* 1972;287:267.
56. Cahill JM, Lees GM, Robertson HT. A summary of preoperative and postoperative cardiorespiratory performance in patients undergoing pectus excavatum and carinatum repair. *J Pediatr Surg* 1984;19:430.
57. Shamberger RC. Congenital chest wall deformities. *Curr Probl Surg* 1996;33:478.
58. Haller JA, Kramer SS, Leitman SA. Use of CT scans in selection of patients for pectus excavatum surgery: a preliminary report. *J Pediatr Surg* 1987;22:904.
59. Stephens RB. Slipped capital femoral epiphysis. *Pediatr Rev* 1996;17:69.
60. Gerberg LF, Micheli LJ. Nontraumatic hip pain in active children: a critical differential. *Phys Sports Med* 1996;24:69.
61. Greydanus DE, Hofmann AD. The hip. In: Hofmann AD, Greydanus DE, eds. *Adolescent medicine.* 2nd ed. Norwalk, CT: Appleton & Lange; 1989:208.
62. Lindsley CB. The adolescent with arthritis. *Compr Ther* 1996;22:48.
63. Schaller JG. Arthritis in children. *Pediatr Clin North Am* 1986;33:1565.
64. Schaller JG, Ochs HD, Thomas ED, et al. Histocompatibility antigens in childhood onset arthritis. *J Pediatr* 1976;88:926.
65. Rennebohm RM. Rheumatic diseases of childhood. *Pediatr Rev* 1988;10:183.
66. Steere AC, Dwyer E, Winchester R. Association of chronic Lyme arthritis with HLA-DR4 and HLA-DR2 alleles. *N Engl J Med* 1990;323:219.
67. Jacobs JC, Berdon WE, Johnston AD. HLAB27 associated spondyloarthritis and enthesopathy in childhood: clinical, pathologic, and radiographic observations in 58 patients. *J Pediatr* 1982;100:521.
68. Rosenberg AM, Petty RE. A syndrome of seronegative enthesopathy and arthropathy in children. *Arthritis Rheum* 1982;25:1041.
69. Lindley CB, Schaller JG. Arthritis associated with inflammatory bowel disease in children. *J Pediatr* 1974;84:16.
70. Rosenberg AM, Petty RE. Reiter's disease in children. *American Journal of Diseases of Children* 1979; 133:394.
71. Schaller JG, Bitnum S, Wedgwood RJ. Ankylosing spondylitis with childhood onset. *J Pediatr* 1969;74:505.
72. Shore A, Ansell BM. Juvenile psoriatic arthritis: an analysis of 60 cases. *J Pediatr* 1982;100:529.
73. Nepom BS, Nepom GT, Mickelson E, et al. Specific HLA-DR4-associated histocompatibility molecules characterize patients with seropositive juvenile rheumatoid arthritis. *J Clin Invest* 1984;74:287.
74. Schaller JG, Hansen J. Rheumatoid factor-positive juvenile rheumatoid arthritis: the childhood equivalent of classic adult rheumatoid arthritis. *Arthritis Rheum* 1982;25:S18.
75. Labowitz R, Schumacher HR. Articular manifestations of systemic lupus erythematosus. *Ann Intern Med* 1971;74:911.
76. Isenberg DA, Snaith ML. Muscle disease in systemic lupus erythematosus. *J Rheumatol* 1981;8:917.
77. Steere AC. Musculoskeletal manifestations of Lyme disease. *Am J Med* 1995;98:4A.
78. Dietz WH Jr, Gross WL, Kirkpatrick JA Jr. Blount disease (tibia vara): another skeletal disorder associated with childhood obesity. *Pediatrics* 1982;101:735.
79. Greydanus DE, Hofmann AD. Leg aches. In: Hofman AD, Greydanus DE, eds. *Adolescent medicine.* 2nd ed. Norwalk, CT: Appleton & Lange; 1989:211.
80. Smith JB. Knee problems in children. *Pediatr Clin North Am* 1986;33:1439.
81. Schenck RC, Goodnight J. Osteochondritis dissecans. *J Bone Joint Surg [Am]* 1996;78:439.
82. Bennett RM. Fibrositis: misnomer for a common rheumatic disorder. *West J Med* 1981;134:405.

SUGGESTED READING

Boachie-Adjei O, Lonner B. Spinal deformity. *Pediatr Clin North Am* 1996;43:883.
Boudoulas H, Kolibash AJ Jr, Baker P, et al. Mitral valve prolapse and the mitral valve prolapse syndrome: a diagnostic classification and pathogenesis of symptoms. *Am Heart J* 1989;118:796.

Brown RT. Recurrent chest pain in adolescents. *Pediatr Ann* 1991;20:194.

Bunnell WP. The natural history of idiopathic scoliosis before skeletal maturity. *Spine* 1986;11:773.

Lonstein JE. Natural history and school screening for scoliosis. *Orthop Clin North Am* 1988;19:227.

Lonstein JE, Winter RB. Adolescent idiopathic scoliosis: nonoperative treatment. *Orthop Clin North Am* 1988;19:239.

Micheli LJ, Wood R. Back pain in young athletes: significant differences from adults in causes and patterns. *Arch Pediatr Adolesc Med* 1995;149:15.

Peterson H. Growing pains. *Pediatr Clin North Am* 1986;33:1365.

Rennebohm RM. Rheumatic diseases of childhood. *Pediatr Rev* 1988;10:183.

Richards BS. Slipped capital femoral epiphysis. *Pediatr Rev* 1996;17:69.

Schaller JG. Arthritis in children. *Pediatr Clin North Am* 1986;33:1565.

Shamerger RC. Congenital chest wall deformities. *Curr Probl Surg* 1996;33:478.

Sherry DD. Limb pain in childhood. *Pediatr Rev* 1990;12:39.

Skaggs DL, Bassett GS. Adolescent idiopathic scoliosis: an update. *Am Fam Physician* 1996;53:2327.

Szer I. Arthritis. *Adolescent Medicine: State of the Art Reviews* 1991;2:539.

Szer IS. Musculoskeletal pain syndromes that affect adolescents. *Arch Pediatr Adolesc Med* 1996;150:740.

URINARY SYSTEM PROBLEMS

Urinary Tract Infections

Adolescents, particularly girls, frequently present to practitioners with complaints of burning or pain when urinating. Occasionally, the clinician will see a teenager with the full-blown picture of pyelonephritis (i.e., dysuria, flank pain, fever, and possibly vomiting). Although urinary tract infections (UTIs) are not as common in adolescents as they are in younger children [1], they are common enough to warrant discussion. What is seen more frequently, however, is a symptom complex that may be caused by a UTI but that has other possible causes as well. This is the real challenge in adolescents—ferreting out the UTIs from other pathologic processes.

Epidemiology

In early infancy, UTIs occur more frequently in boys than in girls. As children age, the proportions reverse, and in school-aged children the rates of asymptomatic bacteriuria have been reported to be 0.3% in boys and 1% to 2% in girls. In adolescents, the risk of acquiring significant bacteriuria is greater than 2%, primarily among girls [1]. Therefore, the following discussion centers on female adolescents.

Urinary symptoms suggestive of UTI in patients younger than 15 years of age were found to be associated with positive cultures for a urinary pathogen in only 18% of cases [2]. In another study in adolescents, isolated bacterial UTI was diagnosed, using bacterial counts of 10^4 to 10^5 organisms per milliliter in only 17% of girls presenting with dysuria [3]. Up to one fourth of adult women may experience an episode of acute dysuria each year [4]. Dysuria accounts for more than 3 million office visits annually in the United States [5].

Urinary symptoms in adolescent girls can be caused by many other factors (Table 40). These include local irritants such as chemically treated feminine hygiene products and sexually transmitted

TABLE 40. *Causes of acute dysuria in adolescent women without evidence of pyelonephritis*

Lower urinary tract infection, bacterial
Lower urinary tract infection, viral
Chlamydial urethritis
Vaginitis
Subclinical pyelonephritis
No recognized pathogen
Local irritants

agents such as *Chlamydia trachomatis* [6,7], *Trichomonas vaginalis* [8], *Neisseria gonorrhoeae* [9], herpes simplex, *Ureaplasma* and *Mycoplasma* species, and *Candida* species [8]. Urinary symptoms in teenaged boys are almost always due to sexually transmitted pathogens, particularly *C. trachomatis* and, possibly, *Ureaplasma* species.

There is an association of UTI with recent sexual intercourse in young women (so-called "honeymoon cystitis") [10,11]. This association seems to decrease if the women void immediately after intercourse [12]. In addition, self-administered, one-dose antibiotic therapy may be helpful in these women. Recurrence of UTI within 6 months of the first episode, which occurred in 26% of women in one college study, was correlated with symptoms of hematuria and urgency with the first infection but not with frequency of intercourse, method of contraception, or voiding after intercourse [13].

Clinical Assessment

The most important single point to remember about UTI in adolescents is that the symptoms may be due to another cause, so a thorough assessment is warranted. The usual presentation of a teenaged girl with a UTI is dysuria. Occasionally, back pain, fever, and vomiting are present. If they are, pyelonephritis should be suspected. Some authors have discussed the difference between the perception of "internal" versus "external" dysuria as a distinguishing factor between an actual UTI and a vaginitis or vulvitis picture [3]. We have not found this to be a helpful item in distinguishing between the two conditions.

A previously documented UTI is helpful because it may indicate a recurrence. A history of recent sexual intercourse preceding the onset of symptoms is also helpful because it can suggest to the practitioner the diagnosis of honeymoon cystitis [14]. The presence of a vaginal discharge or of lesions on the vulva can also indicate the possibility that a sexually transmitted disease is the cause of the symptoms. When the symptoms indicate pyelonephritis, especially with a urinalysis showing white blood cells with white cell casts, red blood cells, and bacteria, hospitalization and intravenous administration of antibiotics are prudent measures.

The usual picture, however, is one of a young woman who complains of lower urinary tract symptoms but little else. This patient has cystitis, urethritis, or vaginitis. One of the problems in diagnosing UTIs in adolescents is that the age group includes prepubertal, early pubertal, and physically mature girls. Therefore, the causes of UTI-type symptoms encompass those common in children and those common in adults. If the girl is prepubertal or in early puberty, then the symptoms of urgency, frequency, and dysuria are most likely due to either a UTI or local irritating factors. If the girl is more mature, then the symptoms are most likely indicative of vulvovaginal infection or of a urethritis or cystitis. Because most girls in this age group are pubertal or postpubertal, we concentrate on the causes of the symptoms in this group (see Table 40).

The physical examination should include palpation of the abdomen and the costovertebral angles. Tenderness with palpation over the bladder is relatively common with a UTI but is not diagnostic. However, a culture should always be taken before starting treatment, and a follow-up culture after treatment should be performed. In general, a pelvic examination is appropriate if the patient is sexually active and should include all the usual cultures, a Pap smear, and a wet mount to look for trichomonads or evidence of bacterial vaginosis. Vulvar and vaginal lesions indicative of either herpetic infection or of human papillomavirus infection should be sought assiduously during the examination.

Laboratory assessment should include a urinalysis, most usually a dipstick assay for blood, protein, nitrites, and leukocyte esterase, and a microscopic examination of the urine as well. A simple, first-time cystitis or urethritis may require only dipstick urinalysis, especially if a culture is being performed. As previously stated, many girls do not have a classic infection, with 10^5 organisms per milliliter present. A teenager may have a vaginal infection or sexually transmitted disease, or she may have a UTI with 10^2 to 10^4 organisms per milliliter. If there are mixed flora on the first culture and treatment has not been started, then catheterization of the bladder for culture may be indicated. If a first-time infection has been documented, then a repeat culture a week or two after termination of therapy is indicated. If return of symptoms follows treatment of a presumptive UTI, culture is mandatory. For office use, sending urines out for formal culture at a laboratory usually is not necessary. There are several in-office techniques available, of which the dipslide seems to give the best results [15].

What about imaging studies of the urinary tract in an adolescent patient with UTIs? Such studies are indicated in the authors' opinion after a bout of pyelonephritis and after more than one lower-tract UTI with documented cultures and no history of recent sexual intercourse. Despite the extensive literature, there are no clear-cut recommendations for teenagers [15,16]. The choice of which type of imaging technique to request is clear. The first choice should be renal and bladder ultrasound and, possibly, a voiding urethrogram. Intravenous pyelography should be reserved for instances in which very detailed depiction of the renal anatomy is necessary [16].

Treatment

If there are absolutely no pelvic symptoms, especially if the girl is a virgin, the physician may elect to forego a pelvic examination and treat presumptively given the following conditions: no systemic signs or symptoms, no history of a previous UTI, no history of vaginal symptoms, and presence of pyuria and microscopic hematuria on urinalysis. Occasionally, the practitioner encounters a patient who may have a UTI but also may have *C. trachomatis* infection. In that case, treatment that is appropriate for the latter infection (i.e., doxycycline) almost certainly will treat the UTI as well.

Almost all organisms that cause UTI in adolescents and young adult women are sensitive to most of the commonly used antibiotics. Although there is a large selection of drugs and more are being introduced every year, the practitioner needs to be familiar with only two or three inexpensive antibiotics to treat most UTIs, including sulfa drugs (such as sulfisoxazole [Gantrisin] or trimethoprim–sulfamethoxazole), amoxicillin, and, possibly, a tetracycline such as doxycycline or a quinolone such as ciprofloxacin. Other drugs that may be used include various cephalosporins and nitrofurantoin.

Whether treating presumptively or after documentation with a culture, the length of treatment is uncertain. Although single-dose treatment may be effective for adults with simple UTIs [17–19], it has not proven superior to the usually recommended 10-day course of therapy [15,20]. With adolescents, there are other factors to consider. For example, will the adolescent comply with a long course of therapy or in taking the recommended number of doses each day? These kinds of issues caused the authors of one study to recommend one-dose treatment in simple UTIs in adolescents [21]. Other authors note that there are more recurrences of infection with short-course therapy compared with conventional 10- to 14-day treatment; therefore, they advocate the longer course [10,16]. We agree that a 7- to 10-day course of therapy is advisable in most adolescents with simple, first-time UTI. With recurrences, we also would advise the longer course.

Hematuria and Proteinuria

Hematuria

Hematuria is a very common urine abnormality that, in adolescents, is rarely indicative of serious disease [22]. However, this finding can augur a serious condition on occasion, so it must be investigated to a certain degree before being considered innocuous. Hematuria may be either gross or microscopic.

Incidence

Because there are no good data on the incidence of hematuria in adolescents, we must extrapolate from data on children and adults. The studies in school-aged children indicate that the incidence of new cases of microhematuria is between 0.17% to 0.3%. Prevalence rates may vary between 0.5% to 2.0% [22]. In adults, the prevalence of hematuria has been estimated to be between 4.0% and 13.0% [23,24]. In adolescents, the reported rate is higher than that in children because of contamination with menstrual blood and bleeding from sexually transmitted infections.

Clinical Presentation

Five patterns of hematuria have been defined [22] (Table 41). Types 1 and 2 are microscopic, types 3 and 4 are gross, and type 5 is mixed. Microscopic hematuria detected on routine urine screen is probably the most common presentation of hematuria in adolescents; nevertheless, this presentation is not so common as to warrant routine urinalysis on asymptomatic patients. Microscopic hema-

TABLE 41. *Patterns of hematuria*

Type	Pattern
1	Persistent, microscopic
2	Intermittent, microscopic
3	Persistent, gross
4	Intermittent, gross
5	Intermittent, gross, *and* persistent, microscopic

Adapted from Boineau FG, Lewy JE. Evaluation of hematuria in children and adolescents. *Pediatr Rev* 1989;11:101.

turia can be defined as three or more consecutive urine samples positive for hemoglobin on urine test strips and six or more red blood cells per high-power field in a fresh urine sediment specimen [22]. This latter specimen is obtained by centrifuging 15 ml of fresh urine at 1,500 rpm for 5 to 10 minutes, discarding the supernatant, and resuspending the sediment in 1 to 2 ml of residual urine. A uniform drop of this sediment is then pipetted onto a glass slide and examined with a microscope under high power.

Another common occurrence is hematuria discovered in a patient who has genitourinary symptoms consistent with either a UTI or a vaginal infection. A teenager presenting with asymptomatic gross hematuria is rare. The evaluation of hematuria is outlined in Table 42.

Etiology

Numerous causes of hematuria in adolescents are listed in Table 43. The most important of these for the clinician to consider are UTI, benign familial hematuria, IgA nephropathy, hypercalciuria, and

TABLE 42. *Evaluation of hematuria*

Clinical features
Historic information
   Associated symptoms
   Precipitating events
   Pattern of hematuria
   Familial occurrence
Physical examination
   Edema
   Blood pressure
   Skin lesions
   Joint involvement

Laboratory studies
Quantification of proteinuria
Microscopic examination of sediment
Red blood cell morphology and size
Urine culture
C_3, antinuclear antibody, anti-DNA
Serum creatinine
Urine calcium

Imaging studies
Urinary tract ultrasound
Intravenous pyelogram
Voiding cystourethrogram

Adapted from Boineau FG, Lewy JE. Evaluation of hematuria in children and adolescents. *Pediatr Rev* 1989;11:101.

TABLE 43. *Causes of hematuria*

Renal	Developmental
Glomerular	Simple cysts
Glomerulonephritis: proliferative glomerular lesions	Polycystic kidney disease
Postinfections (poststreptococcal, postviral)	Multicystic disease
Henoch-Schönlein purpura	Medullary sponge kidney
IgA nephropathy	
Mesangiocapillary	*Postrenal*
Systemic lupus erythematosus	Renal pelvic
Mesangial proliferative	Vascular abnormalities
Glomerulopathy: nonproliferative	Malformations
Familial nephritis (Alport's syndrome and variants)	Papillary necrosis
Vasculitis (microangiopathic)	Hydronephrosis
Benign familial hematuria	Nephrolithiasis
Membranous nephropathy	Trauma
Focal and segmental glomerulosclerosis	Ureteral
Nephrosclerosis	Nephrolithiasis
Hypercalciuria	Inflammation
Nonglomerular	Bladder
Interstitial nephropathy	Inflammation
Infections (bacterial pyelonephritis, tuberculosis)	Obstruction
Metabolic (nephrocalcinosis)	Stones
Drug- or poison-induced (analgesics, antimicrobials)	Drugs such as cyclophosphamide
Acute tubular necrosis	Tumors
Vascular	Trauma
Malformations (aneurysms, hemangiomas)	Urethral
Venous or arterial thrombosis	Inflammation
Sickle cell nephropathy	Trauma
Tumor	Prostatic
Wilms' tumor	Inflammation
Others	

From Boineau FG, Lewy JE. Evaluation of hematuria in children and adolescents. *Pediatr Rev* 1989;11:101. Reproduced by permission of *Pediatrics.*

acute postinfectious (usually poststreptococcal) glomerulonephritis. Other causes of hematuria that have less favorable prognoses are decidedly less common. In addition, they usually present with other findings: proteinuria, azotemia, urine-concentrating defects, or a history of other family members with renal disease and hearing loss, as in hereditary nephritis (Alport's disease).

Urinary tract infection and acute glomerulonephritis usually have associated symptoms or signs that make them relatively easy to diagnose. Acute glomerulonephritis presents with gross hematuria in nearly half of those affected, and all victims have microscopic hematuria. Frequently, hypertension is present and, occasionally, malaise, lethargy, and other constitutional symptoms. Laboratory investigation usually reveals elevated antistreptococcal antibodies and a low C3 or CH_50 (or both) [22]. The other, more common causes of hematuria are usually without additional symptoms. One clue as to whether the red blood cells in the urine are from a glomerular source is the finding of distorted, misshapen red blood cells of different sizes on examination of urine with a phase-contrast microscope. This is not an instrument commonly found in clinical laboratories, however, so it is not a commonly available procedure [25].

Benign familial hematuria usually presents with the incidental finding of microscopic hematuria. Red blood cell casts are sometimes present. Benign familial hematuria is more prevalent in women and girls, and laboratory studies are helpful only in that they are normal. If other family members are checked, several other cases usually are found. Inheritance is autosomal dominant [26].

Immunoglobulin A nephropathy (Berger's disease) usually presents with intermittent episodes of gross hematuria followed by spontaneous clearing. It is more common in men and boys, and mild proteinuria is present occasionally. Family members are not affected. IgA is present in the mesangial regions of all glomeruli, and focal nephritis may be present on light microscopy of biopsy specimens [27]. It has been determined that a significant proportion of patients with IgA nephropathy progress to end-stage renal disease. Several factors are predictive of such progression. These include hypertension at biopsy, the presence of glomerular sclerotic changes, especially when this was associated with proliferation or sclerosis in 20% or more of the glomeruli, black race, proteinuria at biopsy, older age at presentation, crescents, and male sex. Of these factors, most important are glomerular sclerosis, proteinuria, and hypertension [28].

Hypercalciuria may be present in up to one third of children with isolated hematuria [29]. Some of these children may go on to form renal calculi [30,31]. Renal excretion of calcium can be quantified by comparing it to creatinine excretion, which is expressed as the calcium–creatinine ratio (Ca/Cr). White female adolescents normally have a higher Ca/Cr than black girls or boys [32]. Mean values and 95th percentile values for Ca/Cr are shown in Table 44.

Another cause of hematuria in adolescents is blunt trauma to the kidneys, especially considering the propensity of adolescents for accidents. If blood pressure is normal and if there are no more than 50 red blood cells per high-power field, there is no serious renal injury. If the injury is serious, there will be significant hematuria and, sometimes, shock [33]. Clinicians should also be aware that patients with sickle cell trait and sickle cell disease can have sporadic gross hematuria [22].

Last, clinicians should be aware that all that looks like hematuria may not be red blood cells. Tables 45 through 48 show causes of red urine, of red urine without hematuria, of hemoglobinuria without hematuria, and of myoglobinuria.

Proteinuria

As with hematuria, isolated proteinuria in adolescents is usually an innocuous finding with no prognostic significance. However, when associated with other factors such as hematuria, hypertension, and edema, it may signify renal disease. Pediatricians and other clinicians who see children should remember that adolescent girls may have protein in their urine owing to menstruation or to a sexually transmitted disease. Protein and blood in the urine may also signal a UTI (Table 49).

In a study of a large population of Finnish school children aged 8 to 15 years, the significance of proteinuria was determined. Protein was found in 10.7% of 8,954 children in at least one of four urine specimens. The key finding was that when not associated with hematuria, proteinuria proved to be transient or intermittent in every child when a large enough number of urine samples was tested [34].

Proteinuria usually is discovered on routine urinalysis when a urine test strip turns positive. These test strips are graded on their color responsiveness to the concentration of protein present in the urine. The color gradations range from trace to +4. Strongly alkaline urine may give a false-positive reaction, and a dilute urine may give a false-negative result. These test strips are very sensitive; therefore, a trace to a +2 reading usually can be ignored. By using the ratio of protein to creatinine (Pr/Cr) in a random urine specimen, the significance of the proteinuria can be determined without having to go through all the uncertainties of a 24-hour urine collection. If the Pr/Cr exceeds

TABLE 44. *Selected percentile values of urinary calcium/creatinine ratios in normal adolescents*

Adolescent group	Percentage of group demonstrating these ratios[a]			
	50%	75%	90%	95%
White girls	0.23 (0.08)	0.34 (0.12)	0.51 (0.18)	0.54 (0.19)
Black girls	0.14 (0.05)	0.25 (0.09)	0.45 (0.16)	0.59 (0.21)
White boys	0.14 (0.05)	0.25 (0.09)	0.42 (0.15)	0.68 (0.24)
Black boys	0.08 (0.03)	0.17 (0.06)	0.31 (0.11)	0.51 (0.18)

[a]Ratios expressed as millimoles per liter per millimoles per liter (milligrams per deciliter per milligrams per deciliter).

Reprinted by permission of Elsevier Science Publishing Co., Inc., from Seifert-McLean CM, et al. Urinary calcium excretion in healthy adolescents. *J Adolesc Health Care* 1989;10:300. Copyright 1989 by the Society for Adolescent Medicine.

TABLE 45. *Common causes of red urine*

Negative dipstick test: dyes, drugs, pigment
No red blood cells on microscopy: free hemoglobin or myoglobin
Red blood cells, no casts: tumor, cysts, stones, obstruction
Red blood cells, casts:
　No proteinuria: IgA, nephropathy, familial nephritis, or benign familial hematuria
　Proteinuria: acute glomerulonephritis, Henoch-Schönlein purpura, systemic lupus erythematosus,
　　chronic glomerulonephritis
　Heavy proteinuria: nephrotic syndrome

From Boineau FG, Lewy JE. Evaluation of hematuria in children and adolescents. *Pediatr Rev* 1989;11:101. Reproduced by permission of *Pediatrics.*

TABLE 46. *Causes of red urine without hematuria*

Pink, red, Coke-colored, burgundy
Drug and food ingestion: aminopyrine, anthocyanin, azo dyes, beets, blackberries, chloroquine,
　deferoxamine mesylate, ibuprofen, methyldopa, nitrofurantoin, phenazopyridine, phenolphthalein,
　rhodamine B, rifampin, sulfasalazine, urates

Dark brown, black
Disease-associated: alkaptonuria, homogentisic aciduria, melanism, methemoglobinemia, tyrosinosis
Drug and food ingestion: alanine, resorcinol, thymol

From Boineau FG, Lewy JE. Evaluation of hematuria in children and adolescents. *Pediatr Rev* 1989;11:101. Reproduced by permission of *Pediatrics.*

TABLE 47. *Causes of hemoglobinuria without hematuria*

Drugs and chemicals: aspidium, betanaphthol, carbolic acid, carbon monoxide, chloroform, fava beans,
　mushrooms, naphthalene, pamaquine, phenylhydrazine, quinine, snake venom, sulfonamides
Other: hemolytic anemias (all types), uremic syndrome, septicemia, paroxysmal nocturnal hemoglobin-
　uria, freshwater drowning, mismatched blood transfusions, cardiopulmonary bypass, severe pro-
　longed exercise

Adapted from Boineau FG, Lewy JE. Evaluation of hematuria in children and adolescents. *Pediatr Rev* 1989;11:101.

TABLE 48. *Causes of myoglobinuria*

Rhabdomyolysis from:
　Extensive burns
　Crush injuries
　Electrical shock
　Severe myositis
　Major, prolonged seizures

TABLE 49. *Causes of asymptomatic proteinuria*

Transient proteinuria
Fever
Emotional stress
Exercise
Extreme cold
Abdominal surgery
Congestive heart failure
Infusion epinephrine

Orthostatic proteinuria
Transient
Fixed and reproducible

Persistent proteinuria
Benign proteinuria (sporadic or familial)
Acute glomerulonephritis, mild
Chronic glomerular diseases that can lead to nephrotic syndrome
   Lupus glomerulonephritis
   Henoch-Schönlein glomerulonephritis
   Glomerulonephritis associated with chronic shunt infections or subacute bacterial endocarditis
Chronic interstitial nephritis
Congenital and acquired structural abnormalities of urinary tract
   Hydronephrosis
   Polycystic disease
   Renal hypoplasia or dysplasia
   Reflux nephropathy

From Feld LG, et al. Evaluation of the child with asymptomatic proteinuria. *Pediatr Rev* 1984;5:248. Reproduced by permission of *Pediatrics.*

3.5, then the proteinuria is in the nephrotic range. A Pr/Cr of 0.2 or less is within normal limits [35] (Table 50).

A common finding in adolescents is orthostatic or postural proteinuria. This occurs in an intermittent pattern in up to 70% of young men with isolated proteinuria. Fixed and reproducible postural proteinuria is found in approximately 20% of patients with isolated proteinuria, occurring about equally in men and women [36]. This pattern of proteinuria has been shown to be indicative of no future pathologic findings [37–39].

TABLE 50. *Definition of significant proteinuria*

Qualitative
Grade +1 (30 mg/dl) on dipstick examination of two of three random specimens collected 1 week apart
   if urine specific gravity ≤1.015
Grade +2 (100 mg/dl) on similarly collected urine specimens if urine specific gravity ≥1.015

Semiquantitative
Urine protein–creatinine ratio (expressed in terms of milligrams per deciliter per milligrams per deciliter)
   of ≥0.2 on an early-morning urine specimen

Quantitative
Normal: ≤4 mg/m²/hr in a timed 12- to 24-hour urine collection
Abnormal: 4–40 mg/m²/hr[a] in a timed 12- to 24-hour urine collection
Nephrotic range: ≥40 mg/m²/hr[a] in a timed 12- to 24-hour urine collection

[a]For example, in a 1-m² child (age 8 years, weight 60 lb), abnormal is from 100 to 1,000 mg; nephrotic range is greater than 1,000 mg.
From Norman ME. An office approach to hematuria and proteinuria. *Pediatr Clin North Am* 1987;3:545.

REFERENCES

1. Feld LG, Greenfield SP, Ogra PL. Urinary tract infections in infants and children. *Pediatr Rev* 1989;11:71.
2. Dickerson JA. Incidence and outcome of symptomatic UTI in children. *Br Med J* 1974;1:1330.
3. Waters WE. Prevalence of symptoms of urinary tract infection in women. *British Journal Preventive and Social Medicine* 1969;23:263.
4. Koch HK. *The National Ambulatory Medical Care Survey: 1975 summary*. Hyattsville, MD: Department of Health, Education, and Welfare; 1978:1–62.
5. Demetriou E, Emans SJ, Masland RP Jr. Dysuria in adolescent girls: Urinary tract infection or vaginitis? *Pediatrics* 1982;70:299.
6. Tait A, Rees E, Jameson RM. Urethral syndrome associated with chlamydial infection of the urethra and cervix. *Br J Urol* 1978;50:425.
7. Stamm WE, Wagner KF, Amsel R, et al. Causes of the acute urethral syndrome in women. *N Engl J Med* 1980;303:409.
8. Ris HW, Dodge RW. *Trichomonas* and yeast vaginitis in institutionalized adolescent girls. *American Journal of Diseases of Children* 1973;125:206.
9. Curran JW. Gonorrhea and the urethral syndrome. *Sex Transm Dis* 1977;4:119.
10. Nicolle L, Harding GKM, Preiksaitis J, et al. The association of urinary tract infection with sexual intercourse. *J Infect Dis* 1982;146:579.
11. Pfan A, Sacks T, Englestein D. Recurrent urinary tract infection in premenopausal women: prophylaxis based on an understanding of the pathogenesis. *J Urol* 1983;129:1152.
12. Adatto K, Doebele KG, Galland L, et al. Behavioral factors and urinary tract infections. *JAMA* 1981;241:2525.
13. Foxman B. Recurring urinary tract infection: incidence and risk factors. *Am J Public Health* 1990;80:331.
14. Strom BL, Collins M, West SL, et al. Sexual activity, contraceptive use, and other risk factors for symptomatic and asymptomatic bacteriuria. *Ann Intern Med* 1987;107:816.
15. Eichenwald HF. Some aspects of the diagnosis and management of urinary tract infection in children and adolescents. *Pediatric Infectious Disease* 1986;5:760.
16. Parrott TS. Cystitis and urethritis. *Pediatr Rev* 1989;10:217.
17. Stamm WE, Turck M. Urinary tract infection. *Adv Intern Med* 1983;28:141.
18. Brenner AE, Simon RR. Cystitis and pyelonephritis. *Ann Emerg Med* 1983;12:228.
19. Farrar WE. Infections of the urinary tract. *Med Clin North Am* 1983;67:187.
20. Shapiro ED. Short course antimicrobial treatment of urinary tract infections in children: a critical analysis. *Pediatric Infectious Disease* 1982;1:294.
21. Fine JS, Jacobson MS. Single-dose versus conventional therapy of urinary tract infections in female adolescents. *Pediatrics* 1985;75:916.
22. Boineau FG, Lewy JE. Evaluation of hematuria in children and adolescents. *Pediatr Rev* 1989;11:101.
23. Mohr DN, Offord KP, Owen RA, et al. Asymptomatic microhematuria and urologic disease: a population-based study. *JAMA* 1986;256:224.
24. Kassirer JP. The wild goose chase and the elephant's relevance. *JAMA* 1986;256:256.
25. Rizzoni G, Braggion F, Zacchelo G. Evaluation of glomerular and nonglomerular hematuria by phase-contrast microscopy. *J Pediatr* 1983;103:370.
26. Blumenthal SS, Fritsche C, Lemann J Jr. Establishing the diagnosis of benign familial hematuria. *JAMA* 1988;259:2263.
27. Hogg RJ. Recent advances in the diagnosis of hematuria in children. *Pediatr Ann* 1988;17:560.
28. Hogg RJ, Silva FG, Wyatt RD, et al. Prognostic indicators in children with IgA nephropathy: report of the Southwest Pediatric Nephrology Study Group. *Pediatr Nephrol* 1994;8:15.
29. Stapleton FB, Roy's III, Noe HN, et al. Hypercalciuria in children with hematuria. *N Engl J Med* 1984;310:1345.
30. Roy's III, Stapleton FB, Noe HN, et al. Hematuria preceding renal calculus formation in children with hypercalciuria. *J Pediatr* 1981;99:712.
31. Kalia A, Travis LB, Brouhard BH. The association of idiopathic hypercalciuria and asymptomatic gross hematuria in children. *J Pediatr* 1981;99:716.
32. Seifert-McLean CM, Cromer BA, Mosher G, et al. Urinary calcium excretion in healthy adolescents. *Journal of Adolescent Health Care* 1989;10:300.
33. Stalker HP, Kaufman RA, Stedje K. The significance of hematuria in children after blunt abdominal trauma. *Am J Radiol* 1990;154:569.
34. Vehaskari VM, Rapola J. Isolated proteinuria: analysis of a school-age population. *J Pediatr* 1982;101:661.
35. Ginsberg JM, Chang BS, Matarese RA, et al. Use of single voided urine samples to estimate quantitative proteinuria. *N Engl J Med* 1983;309:1543.
36. Glassock RJ. Postural (orthostatic) proteinuria: no cause for concern [editorial]. *N Engl J Med* 1981;305:639.
37. Springberg PD, Garrett LE, Thompson AL, et al. Fixed and reproducible orthostatic proteinuria: results of a 20 year follow-up study. *Ann Intern Med* 1982;97:516.

38. Ryland DA, Spreiter S. Prognosis in postural (orthostatic) proteinuria: forty to fifty year follow-up of six patients after diagnosis by Thoma Addis. *N Engl J Med* 1981;305:618.
39. Feld LG, Schoeneman MJ, Kaskel FJ. Evaluation of the child with asymptomatic proteinuria. *Pediatr Rev* 1984;5:248.

SUGGESTED READING

Boineau FG, Lewy JE. Evaluation of hematuria in children and adolescents. *Pediatr Rev* 1989;11:101.
Braverman PK. Urinary tract infection. *Adolescent Medicine: State of the Art Reviews* 1991;2:659.
Daniels S, Loggie J. Essential hypertension. *Adolescent Medicine: State of the Art Reviews* 1991;2:551.
Demetriou E, Emans SJ, Masland RP Jr. Dysuria in adolescent girls: urinary tract infection or vaginitis? *Pediatrics* 1982;70:299.
Feld LG, Greenfield SP, Ogra PL. Urinary tract infections in infants and children. *Pediatr Rev* 1989;11:71.
Feld LG, Schoeneman MJ, Kaskel FJ. Evaluation of the child with asymptomatic proteinuria. *Pediatr Rev* 1984;5:248.
Hogg RJ. Recent advances in the diagnosis of hematuria in children. *Pediatr Ann* 1988;17:560.
Hooton TM, Scholes D, Hughes JP, et al. A prospective study of risk factors for symptomatic urinary tract infection in young women. *N Engl J Med* 1996;335:468.
Kurtin P. Hematuria and proteinuria. *Adolescent Medicine: State of the Art Reviews* 1991;2:649.
Parrott TS. Cystitis and urethritis. *Pediatr Rev* 1989;10:217.
Strom BL, Collins M, West SL, et al. Sexual activity, contraceptive use, and other risk factors for symptomatic and asymptomatic bacteriuria. *Ann Intern Med* 1987;107:816.

DIABETES MELLITUS

Insulin-dependent diabetes mellitus (IDDM), or type 1 diabetes, is the most common endocrine disorder of childhood and adolescence [1]. It affects 1 in 400 people in this age group. The incidence rate is approximately 15 per 100,000 per year at a prevalence of approximately 2 per 1,000 [2]. IDDM is a result of the failure of the pancreas to produce insulin because of beta-cell destruction. The nutritional derangements that result are also accompanied by cardiovascular, renal, neurologic, and ocular complications. Even when treated optimally, IDDM often augurs a shorter-than-expected life span and significant morbidity.

Pathogenesis

Research has deciphered the genetics of IDDM to a great degree. There are correlations of IDDM with human leukocyte antigens (HLA) located on the short arm of chromosome 6 [1]. At least 90% of whites with type 1 diabetes have HLA-DR3 or HLA-DR4, and 1 in 50 people with both of these antigenic markers has IDDM. Genetic susceptibility to the disease is not sufficient to result in clinical disease. This is apparent from studies of identical twins in whom the concordance rate for IDDM is, at best, 50% [3]. If the disease is not due solely to genetics, then an environmental cause must be operative. The most likely candidates for such a cause are viruses.

The best model in humans is the congenital rubella syndrome [4]. In this syndrome, as many as 40% of those affected will have IDDM, and most of those are positive for HLA-DR3 or HLA-DR4 [1]. Moreover, cases of IDDM seem to start most often in a seasonal pattern, reflecting the incidence of certain viruses in a community.

The first event leading to IDDM is damage to the pancreatic beta cells in genetically susceptible people. This damage uncovers new antigenic sites that the body's immune system treats as foreign antigens. The body produces antibodies and sets out to destroy these cells. Immunologically active cells appear and seem to be directed against the pancreatic beta cells. Immunologic markers can detect people in whom diabetes is likely to occur, which could be helpful with siblings of people with IDDM. However, only 12% to 15% of new IDDM cases appear in families that already have a diabetic member [1].

Diagnosis

The diagnosis of IDDM usually presents no problem. The child has poor weight gain and fatigue, and may become dehydrated. However, glucosuria can be present for a long time before the classic symptoms of polyuria and polydipsia occur. In female adolescents, candidal vaginitis may be the presenting complaint, and children may present with a recrudescence of nocturnal enuresis. Changes in vision, behavior problems, and decreasing school performance may also be the first symptoms reported to the physician. When glucosuria is found, blood glucose of more than 200 mg/dl is strongly indicative of IDDM. Checking for fasting glucosuria and the performance of glucose tolerance tests are rarely necessary.

Management

The child or adolescent with newly diagnosed IDDM may be managed on an outpatient basis if mechanisms are available for extensive education. Hospitalization is required if the patient first presents with severe ketoacidosis. The issues of outpatient diabetes management are listed in Table 51. The overriding concern of the physician managing a child or adolescent with IDDM should be the maintenance of normal growth and development, both emotional and physical, while keeping the blood glucose as close to normal as possible. Lack of good glycemic control has been correlated with risk of long-term complications [5].

Education and involvement of the family are crucial for good diabetes control [6–10]. A chronic illness can exacerbate problems in a family system, resulting in family dysfunction and poor care and control of the patient's problem. If the physician identifies or suspects difficulties of this kind, he or she should strongly recommend family counseling to prevent future crises. This counseling may be done by the primary care physician, a social worker, a psychologist, or by a psychiatrist. Education in coping effectively with stress is helpful as well.

Good nutrition is one of the cornerstones of diabetes management. Adolescents and their families should have their diets assessed by a dietitian familiar both with the eating habits of teenagers and with the tenets of nutrition for diabetics. In addition, the dietitian should be familiar with eating patterns of various cultural groups, so that he or she can recommend healthful foods that are culturally acceptable. Often, it is more helpful to try to alter an entire family's eating pattern rather than to concentrate solely on the habits of the patient. The practitioner should also realize that, often, adolescents may not eat with the family. This occurs more frequently as the adolescent gets older. Therefore, allowances must be made for the teenager who is rarely home. For instance, if the adolescent works at a fast-food restaurant, he or she may get one or two meals there each day. The dietitian must be able to help the adolescent choose healthful foods from those that are available in the venue in which the teenager finds himself or herself.

The nutritional requirements of children with IDDM are similar to those of other children of similar age, size, and level of development. While an adolescent is in puberty, particularly during the pubertal growth spurt, more calories are needed. The teenager should be alerted to decrease intake to approximately 35 kcal/kg/day when growth is finished to avoid obesity [1]. The diet should be composed of 15% protein, 55% to 60% carbohydrates, and approximately 30% fats. Nearly 70% of the carbohydrates should be ingested in the form of complex carbohydrates such as starch, and the intake of sucrose or other highly refined sugars should be severely limited. Complex carbohydrates and fiber help to modulate blood glucose levels. The ingestion of large quantities of fructose-containing beverages should be discouraged, because fructose may increase blood glucose levels up to 100 mg/dl or more before it drops rapidly, thereby provoking hypoglycemia [1,2]. The protein should be from lean, relatively fat-free meats and fish, and the fats should be predominantly of the polyunsaturated variety. Three meals per day and snacks at least at mid-afternoon and at bedtime are necessary, with calories proportioned among them.

Two major advances have occurred in the manufacture of insulin, the mainstay of diabetic management. First, the purification of all marketed insulins has improved dramatically, and second, synthetic human insulin is now readily available. The better purification of insulin has led to fewer allergic responses, the virtual elimination of lipodystrophy, and significantly lower anti-insulin antibody titers [11]. There are no advantages to using human insulin compared with pork insulin, nor are there proved disadvantages [1,11], although there is a recent suggestion that human insulin may mask symptoms of hypoglycemia [1,2].

A combination of short-acting and intermediate-acting insulin is given in at least two doses daily. The dosage of intermediate-acting insulin (NPH or Lente) should range from 0.5 to 1.5 units per kilogram of body weight per day. It should be adjusted for each patient by measuring blood glucose before

TABLE 51. *General issues in managing diabetes in adolescents*

Factors
Patient
  Easily understood directions
  Staff understanding of patient–parent relations and interests
Clinical
  Convenient location
  Flexible scheduling
  Consistent appointment reminders
  Staff aware of patient–parent interaction
Regimen
  Simple
  Emphasis on benefits of monitoring
  Well documented negotiations
  Parent understanding of goals
  Short-term compromise for long-term success

Requirements of provider
Understand normal adolescent development
Enjoy working with adolescents
Understand diabetes management
Confidence in skills for managing diabetes
Able to compromise on aspects of care
A physician or a team able to provide consistent care

Alcohol and drugs
  Increased danger of hypoglycemia
  Use may express anger/rebellion
  Treatment: consider counseling
Insulin
  Injections two times per diem
  Daily dosage (total): 1–1.5 U/kg
  Ratio of intermediate- to short-acting insulin: 2 : 1 to 3 : 1
Monitoring
  Glycosylated hemoglobin tests may uncover falsified home records
  Unrealistic demands/expectations may lead to misrepresentation
  Confront the patient and emphasize the importance of accurate reports
Nutrition
  With dietitian, tailor a meal plan to the patient
Parental supervision
  Increase adolescent's responsibility for care
  Tie driving privileges to good control and adherence
  Wear medical ID bracelet
  Irresponsibility can lead to poor control
Recurrent ketoacidosis
  Linked to poor compliance and psychosocial adjustment
  Immediately refer for counseling
Sex and marriage
  Easy access to birth control information
  Before conception, well controlled diabetes
  Couple attends clinic and diabetes education sessions
Sports
  Physician reassurance of school officials
  Adjust regimen for safe participation

Adapted from Sperling MA. Diabetes in adolescence. *Adolescent Medicine: State of the Art Reviews* 1994;5:87.

meals and before the bedtime snack. During puberty, the doses may increase significantly; more frequent injections may be needed because of relative insulin resistance due to hormonal changes. This pubertal insulin resistance may necessitate an increase in insulin dose of 30% to 50% [12–14]. The resistance subsides as puberty ends. Regular insulin can be given on a sliding scale at 0.05 to 0.1 U/kg per dose. Some diabetes experts use a fixed dose of regular insulin based on blood glucose tests; the sliding scale is used only when the patient is ill. Blood glucose levels should be maintained at as close to 100 mg/dl as possible. Consistent levels of 70 mg/dl or lower or 180 mg/dl or higher indicate a need to adjust the dose of insulin.

If the dose of daily insulin reaches 2.0 U/kg/day, then the *Somogyi phenomenon* should be suspected; this is a hyperglycemic surge from counterregulatory hormones that increase glucose production after hypoglycemia [15] (Table 52). Nightmares and severe hypoglycemia may occur often in the early morning hours, whereas some patients may be totally asymptomatic. Clues to the diagnosis are rapid swings of blood glucose levels and prebreakfast ketonuria without glucosuria [11]. After this is diagnosed, the insulin dose should be reduced, and the bedtime blood glucose level should be targeted at 100 mg/dl.

Occasionally, the practitioner encounters the *dawn phenomenon*, which is defined as significant early morning hyperglycemia in the absence of antecedent hypoglycemia. To document this phenomenon, blood glucose determinations need to be done between 2:00 AM and 6:00 AM. Normal blood glucose levels will be seen initially, followed by a significant rise between 4:00 and 6:00 AM. Resolution is achieved by delaying the evening intermediate-acting insulin injection or reducing the bedtime snack (Table 53).

Blood glucose monitoring is an integral part of diabetes management. Using an autolancet, a drop of blood is placed onto a chemical paper strip. The glucose level is read either by a portable glucose-determining machine or by color changes in the strip. Blood glucose measurements should be performed at least three times a day. Blood glucose levels should also be checked at least once weekly before lunch and before bedtime snack to ensure that the morning regular insulin dose is appropriate [1]. Another method of monitoring requires blood glucose determinations three to four times daily on two varying days of the week, with spot checks on the other days. This can be helpful with adolescents who rebel against frequent daily blood glucose checks [12]. Adolescents with IDDM should be encouraged to check their blood glucose at any time they feel that they may be hypoglycemic or hyperglycemic.

Exercise is another significant component of overall care for the adolescent with IDDM. Exercise increases glucose utilization for the same insulin dose; it allows addition of items to the diet that may not be tolerated without the increased caloric utilization. It increases general and cardiovascular fitness. Blood glucose should be checked before and after exercise until a pattern is attained that can

---

TABLE 52. *Somogyi phenomenon: hypoglycemia begets hyperglycemia*

Mechanisms
Counterregulatory hormone surge, increasing glucose production after hypoglycemia

Symptoms
Night sweats
Night terrors
Classic hypoglycemia
Asymptomatic

Clues
Rapid swings in glucose
Prebreakfast ketonuria without glucosuria
Insulin dose greater than 1.5 U/kg/day

Management
Document hypoglycemia, hyperglycemia
Reduce dose of evening insulin
Target blood glucose at bedtime to 80–120 mg/dl
Consider delay in intermediate insulin injection

From Sperling MA. Outpatient management of diabetes mellitus. *Pediatr Clin North Am* 1987;34:919.

TABLE 53. *Dawn phenomenon*

Definition
Marked by early morning hyperglycemia, which occurs in insulin-dependent diabetes mellitus in
  absence of hypoglycemia

Mechanisms
"Normal" early morning increase in insulin requirement unmet
Nocturnal surges in growth hormone

Symptoms
None

Clues
Early morning hyperglycemia and ketonuria

Management
Document blood glucose 2–6 AM
Delay intermediate insulin injection

From Sperling MA. Outpatient management of diabetes mellitus. *Pediatr Clin North Am* 1987;34:919.

predict increased caloric needs or decreased insulin needs. Regular exercise on, at least, an every-other-day basis can significantly reduce hemoglobin A_1c concentrations and help normalize blood lipids [1]. If patients are poorly controlled, exercise does not improve control. Unless pronounced complications exist, diabetes should be no deterrent to participation in competitive sports.

In the effort to control blood glucose as tightly as possible, there is the danger that the patient will experience frequent bouts of hypoglycemia. The best way to avoid this condition is to anticipate it and to deter its occurrence. Snacks containing only short-acting carbohydrates should be avoided. If there is heavy exercise, additional snacks should be provided. All patients and their families should be taught to use glucagon. Hypoglycemia may occur as long as 12 to 18 hours after prolonged exercise.

Diabetic Ketoacidosis

Diabetic ketoacidosis (DKA) is the leading cause of hospitalization among adolescents and children with IDDM [16]. Sixty-five percent of all patients admitted for DKA are younger than 19 years of age. Although the incidence of DKA is believed to be decreasing, the number of patients with IDDM is increasing, so the number of admissions remains unchanging [16]. DKA is the most common cause of death in IDDM patients younger than 24 years.

Pathogenesis and Clinical Features

The triad of symptoms of DKA consists of hyperglycemia, ketosis, and metabolic acidosis. DKA can be viewed as a superfasted state in which the body's tissues are deprived of their normal homeostatic substrate, glucose [17]. Stress is the usual trigger in a person deprived of adequate insulin. Without the insulin to counteract the increased activity of the counterregulatory hormones (such as growth hormone, epinephrine, glucagon, and cortisol), ketosis and metabolic acidosis ensue. Hyperglycemia causes an osmotic diuresis that leads to dehydration, electrolyte depletion, and hypertonicity. Metabolic acidosis, secondary to ketosis, causes compensatory hyperventilation and hypocapnia, which cause changes in renal, central nervous system, cardiovascular, bowel, and blood oxygen transport functions. The stress that precipitates DKA can be anything from an upper respiratory infection to the emotional stress of breaking up with a boyfriend or girlfriend.

Management

Diabetic ketoacidosis can be managed on an outpatient basis if detected early, or on an inpatient basis otherwise. Development of DKA is slow; therefore, assiduous following of blood glucose at home should detect persistent hyperglycemia and allow time for the patient to seek outpatient management of the problem. However, once the process of DKA is well established, hospitalization is necessary. The principles of management are the same either way: give insulin to reduce the hyperglycemia, replace fluid and electrolyte losses, and reverse the process of ketosis (Table 54).

Educating the patient about checking for ketonuria is the key to home management of DKA [16]. If the teenager feels ill or is vomiting, or if the blood glucose exceeds 240 mg/dl, then urine ketones should be measured. If the ketone level is moderate or large, the physician should be called. Supplements of subcutaneous regular insulin are given, approximately 5% to 10% of the total daily dose for moderate ketonuria and 10% to 20% for large ketonuria. The blood sugar checks, urine ketone checks, telephone calls, and regular insulin supplements are repeated every 3 hours until the urine ketone measurement is small or negative. Phone contact with the care team is vital. Liquids are begun slowly in the form of fruit juices, and when the blood glucose is lower than 120 mg/dl, sugar-containing fluids are begun. If the vomiting persists, the parents are instructed to bring the child to the hospital emergency room. If there are deep (Kussmaul) respirations, sunken eyes, and more than mild lethargy, the child must be admitted.

When home management fails or DKA is not detected early enough in adolescents, hospital management is indicated. First, after vital signs are determined, if there is obtundation, a secure airway may have to be established and nasogastric suction begun. The next order of business is to establish an intravenous line both to replace fluids and electrolytes and to provide access for intravenous insulin therapy. Blood for appropriate laboratory tests is obtained, and fluid therapy is begun. The patient can be assumed to be dehydrated. If comparative weights are not available, assume 10% dehydration unless the patient is in shock. Normal saline in the amount of 10 to 20 ml/kg of body weight is given initially, with avoidance of sudden fluid loads in an attempt to prevent cerebral edema. After initial rehydration, 0.45% sodium chloride is given according to the calculated deficit. Urine losses are replaced with the same solution. When vomiting has ceased and the patient is awake, progressive oral fluids may be offered. The remainder of the fluid deficit may be replaced over the next 24 to 36 hours. Blood tests of serum electrolytes, sugar, and venous pH should be obtained hourly for the first 4 hours and then every 2 hours until the serum pH reaches 7.30 [16,17].

Electrolytes need to be replaced as well. Serum sodium is usually measured as low, but this is due primarily to the hyperglycemia (1.6 mmol/L decrease in serum sodium for every 100 mg/dl rise in

TABLE 54. *Treatment plan for diabetic ketoacidosis*

Physiologic principle	Method
Restoration of fluid volume	Physiologic (0.9%) saline, 10–20 ml/kg, during first hour. If indicated, repeat during second hour.
	After initial reexpansion, change to half-physiologic saline (0.45%), usually at one and a half times maintenance. In the first 4 hours, urine loss is also replaced using 0.45% saline. Five percent dextrose is added when the serum glucose reaches 250 mg/dl.
Inhibition of lipolysis and return to the utilization of glucose	As soon as the blood glucose value is known, intravenous insulin is started at 0.1 U/kg/hr. Continue until the venous pH value reaches 7.30 (or the serum ketone levels are small or negative at a 1 : 2 dilution of serum). Five or 10% is added to maintain the blood glucose value at approximately 200 mg/dl.
Replacement of body salts	Sodium as above.
	Potassium is never added to the intravenous fluids until the serum potassium level is known to be in the normal or low range. After the pH exceeds 7.10, 20 mEq/L potassium phosphate and 20 mEq/L potassium acetate are usually added to each liter bottle of intravenous fluids.
Correction of acidosis	If the pH is less than 7.0, sodium bicarbonate, 1–2 mEq/kg (not to exceed one ampule of 44 mEq/hr), is infused for 60/120 min. This is added to 0.45% saline rather than to 0.9% saline.

From Chase HP, et al. Diabetic ketoacidosis in children and the role of outpatient management. *Pediatr Rev* 1990;11:297. Reproduced by permission of *Pediatrics*.

serum glucose above a normal level of 100 mg/dl). Even though the actual sodium level in the serum may be close to normal, the losses of sodium are high, and it must be replaced. This is accomplished in the rehydration fluids.

Potassium is also lost in significant quantities. Because potassium is an intracellular ion, there can be severe losses with normal serum values. It is prudent to obtain an electrocardiogram strip initially to determine whether there are characteristic electrocardiographic changes of low potassium. Potassium should never be replaced initially, especially if the patient is not urinating. Usually, potassium replacement can be started in the second hour of therapy. It is rarely necessary to administer more than 40 mEq/L of potassium, half as the chloride or acetate salt and half as the phosphate. As the DKA is corrected, it is not unusual to see the serum potassium value fall because of the movement into the cells of the ion.

Correction of the acidosis must also be accomplished. Primarily, acidosis is corrected as the fluid losses are replaced and as the glucose reenters the cells with insulin administration. Bicarbonate is rarely needed unless the acidosis is unusually severe. Even then, only enough should be used to raise the pH to 7.10. There are several reasons for not using bicarbonate unless it is absolutely needed: it may precipitate rapid transfer of potassium into cells, thereby lowering serum potassium, with resultant cardiac problems [16], or it may cause a shift of fluids across the blood–brain barrier.

The last cornerstone of DKA treatment is insulin administration. Insulin corrects lipolysis and reduces hyperglycemia. Insulin is given by constant intravenous infusion after the blood glucose level is known, but *always* within the first hour of treatment. If the level is lower than 250 mg/dl, 5% glucose is added to the solution. The insulin solution is made by adding 30 units of regular insulin to 150 ml of 0.9% saline (1 U/5 ml). Fifty milliliters is run through the tubing to cover all binding sites, and then the infusion is piggybacked to the intravenous line and infused using an infusion pump. The rate is 0.1 unit of insulin per kilogram of body weight per hour. In a mature adolescent of adult size, the rate can be set at 7 U/hr [16]. The aim is to decrease the blood glucose by 100 mg/dl/hr. When the blood glucose falls below 250 mg/dl, 5% glucose is added to the infusate and, if the blood glucose falls below 100 mg/dl while there is still acidosis, then 10% glucose is added. One way of switching to subcutaneous insulin is to maintain the blood glucose at 200 mg/dl until the pH exceeds 7.30 and the patient is eating, and then to give the first dose of subcutaneous regular insulin while the intravenous insulin is still running. The infusion is stopped after 30 to 60 minutes. The patient's usual dose is then resumed. If this is a new patient, he or she can be started on 0.5 to 1.0 U/kg/day, with two thirds of the dose given as intermediate-acting insulin and one third as regular insulin. Two thirds of the total dose is given before the morning meal and one third before the evening meal. Individual adjustments then can be made according to home blood glucose monitoring.

TABLE 55. *Checklist for management of diabetic ketoacidosis*

- Weigh the patient and record vital signs and hydration status.
- Start fluids and insulin treatment after blood glucose and urine ketone levels are determined at bedside.
- Know the serum sodium, potassium, bicarbonate, and blood pH levels before initiating therapy with potassium or bicarbonate.
- Determine serum osmolality if blood glucose level is very high (>1,000 mg/dl).
- Run insulin solution through intravenous tubing and buretrol before initiating insulin therapy, using a constant-infusion pump.
- Keep an accurate flowchart of precise intake and output records. Check vital signs, neurologic status, and pupils at regular intervals.
- Add glucose to the intravenous fluids when blood glucose level falls below 250 mg/dl. Do not discontinue intravenous insulin if pH remains lower than 7.30.
- Before discharging the patient, make sure pH exceeds 7.30 (or serum ketone levels are less than moderate).
- Give subcutaneous insulin before discontinuation of intravenous insulin. Make an appointment with patient and diabetes care provider in the near future so that similar episodes may be avoided by proper education, changes in treatment, or psychologic intervention.

From Chase HP, et al. Diabetic ketoacidosis in children and the role of outpatient management. *Pediatr Rev* 1990;11:297. Reproduced by permission of *Pediatrics*.

Cerebral edema is a rare, unpredictable complication of DKA that usually occurs when biochemical values are improving during therapy [18]. Mortality is near 90% [19]. Although the exact cause is unknown, the usual recommendations are to avoid large amounts of hypotonic fluids, to regulate the decline in glucose levels, and to give insulin slowly. These recommendations have not been proved effective, but they are prudent nonetheless. It is critical to recognize the early signs of increased intracranial pressure and to take action promptly. Signs include headaches, lethargy, and, eventually, dilated pupils. Treatment includes decreasing the patient's carbon dioxide by intubation and hyperventilation and the use of mannitol and fluid restriction. Evidence suggests that it is important to follow serum sodium concentrations as serum glucose concentration declines. Serum sodium concentration that fails to rise indicates excessive free water and may increase the risk of brain herniation [20,21]. Tips for managing DKA are given in Table 55.

The Office Visit

Adolescents with IDDM should be seen by the physician frequently in the first few months after diagnosis and then on a regular schedule of three to four times yearly if no problems intervene. At these visits, a thorough physical examination should be done, with attention to blood pressure, growth and development, eyes, skin, and joints. An easy test for joint mobility is to have teenagers put their hands in apposition and see whether the palms and fingers can press fully against one another. If not, then limitation of joint mobility is present. This may be a sign that other microvascular complications of diabetes are present [22] Table 56 lists the minimal components of the annual evaluation. Blood work done should include a hemoglobin A_1c determination (test for glycosylated hemoglobin), which is the best quantifiable method for evidence of long-range control. It reflects the degree of elevated blood glucose for the preceding 6 to 8 weeks [23,24], and it cannot be affected by patient manipulation. The methods for hemoglobin A_1c determination and the normal values may differ by laboratory, so physicians should familiarize themselves with the standard values of the laboratory being used. Given the new information derived from the Diabetes Control and Complications Trial [5], it is clear that the glycosylated hemoglobin should be below 8.1% [25]. The blood glucose levels should be in the 80 to 120 mg/dl range when fasting, and at any other time of day should fall within the 80 to 180 mg/dl range [2,12]. If microalbuminuria does develop, use of angiotensin-converting enzyme inhibitors may be indicated. These substances decrease the risk of progression to nephropathy by more than 60% [26,27].

The adolescent with noninsulin-dependent diabetes mellitus (NIDDM) is unusual, but not as unusual as previously, given the increase in obesity among American adolescents [28]. These patients are usually obese and almost never ketotic. They are usually discovered to have NIDDM because of

TABLE 56. *Elements of minimum annual evaluation of adolescents with insulin-dependent diabetes mellitus*

- Height, weight, growth percentile, and maturation.
- Blood urea nitrogen, creatinine, and microalbumin levels and creatinine clearance. Urine cultures should be considered for all girls.
- Antimicrosomal and antithyroglobulin antibodies at onset. If positive, annual thyroxine, thyroxine-binding globulin, and thyroid-stimulating hormone levels. If initially negative, reevaluate if thyroid is enlarged or growth rate changes. All girls should be reevaluated at puberty.
- Cholesterol and triglyceride levels and high- and low-density lipoprotein fractions.
- Blood pressure.
- Peripheral pulses.
- Deep-tendon reflexes.
- Neurologic examination (sensory nerves, touch and position sense). If abnormal, nerve conduction velocities should be measured.
- Ophthalmologic examination with dilation by certified ophthalmologist every other year for prepubertal children and yearly for postpubertal adolescents.
- Gynecologic and urologic evaluations when indicated.
- Psychosocial assessment of teenager and family.

Adapted from Ginsberg-Fellner F. Insulin-dependent diabetes. *Pediatr Rev* 1990;11:239.

glucosuria on a routine physical examination. They rarely have symptoms and find it exceedingly difficult to believe there is really anything wrong with them. Consequently, they often require insulin for control of their blood sugars because they find it very difficult to control their diets.

The key to prolonged health and the avoidance of complications in patients with IDDM is keeping the blood glucose as close to normal as possible. The stresses of adolescence, both physical and psychosocial, can make such control exceedingly difficult. However, with good communication between the practitioner and his or her staff and the patient and the patient's family, the chances for success rise considerably. Good nutrition, adequate exercise, and early and effective psychosocial intervention and support are also important. The primary care practitioner, with occasional support from the regional or local pediatric diabetologist, can be successful in the care of these patients and can find that care amply rewarding.

REFERENCES

1. Ginsberg-Fellner F. Insulin-dependent diabetes. *Pediatr Rev* 1990;11:239.
2. Arslanian S, Drash AL. Insulin-dependent diabetes mellitus in children and adolescents. *Current Therapy in Endocrinology and Metabolism* 1994;5:380.
3. Tattersall RB, Pike PA. Diabetes in identical twins. *Lancet* 1972;2:1120.
4. Ginsberg-Fellner F, Witt ME, Fedun B, et al. Diabetes mellitus and autoimmunity in patients with the congenital rubella syndrome. *Rev Infect Dis* 1985;70(Suppl 1):S170.
5. Diabetes Control and Complications Trial Research Group. Effect of intensive diabetes treatment on the development and progression of long-term complications in adolescents with insulin-dependent diabetes mellitus: Diabetes Control and Complications Trial. *J Pediatr* 1994;125:177.
6. Wysocki T, Hough BS, Ward KM, et al. Diabetes mellitus in the transition to adulthood: adjustment, self-care, and health status. *Dev Behav Pediatr* 1992;13:194.
7. Wysocki T. Associations among teen-parent relationships, metabolic control, and adjustment to diabetes in adolescents. *J Pediatr Psychol* 1993;18:441.
8. Jacobson AM, Hauser ST, Lavori P, et al. Family environment and glycemic control: a four-year prospective study of children and adolescents with insulin-dependent diabetes mellitus. *Psychosom Med* 1994;56:401.
9. La Greca AM, Auslander WF, Greco P, et al. I get by with a little help from my family and friends: adolescents support for diabetes care. *J Pediatr Psychol* 1995;20:449.
10. Jacobson AM. The psychological care of patients with insulin-dependent diabetes mellitus. *N Engl J Med* 1996;334:1249.
11. Sperling MA. Outpatient management of diabetes mellitus. *Pediatr Clin North Am* 1987;34:919.
12. Sperling MA. Diabetes in adolescence. *Adolescent Medicine: State of the Art Reviews* 1994;5:87.
13. Dunger DB. Diabetes in puberty. *Arch Dis Child* 1992;67:569.
14. Editorial [unsigned]. Insulin resistance in puberty. *Lancet* 1991;337:1259.
15. Bolli G, Gottesman I, Campbell P, et al. Glucose counterregulation and waning of insulin in the Somogyi phenomenon. *N Engl J Med* 1984;311:1214.
16. Chase HP, Garg SK, Jelley DH. Diabetic ketoacidosis in children and the role of outpatient management. *Pediatr Rev* 1990;11:297.
17. Krane EJ. Diabetic ketoacidosis: biochemistry, physiology, treatment, and prevention. *Pediatr Clin North Am* 1987;34:935.
18. Rosenbloom AL, Riley WJ, Weber FT, et al. Cerebral edema complicating diabetic ketoacidosis in childhood. *J Pediatr* 1980;96:357.
19. Scibilia J, Finegold D, Dorman J, et al. Why do children with diabetes die? *Acta Endocrinologica Supplement (Copenhagen)* 1986;113:326.
20. Harris GD, Fiordalisi I, Harris WL. Minimizing the risk of brain herniation during treatment of diabetic ketoacidemia: a retrospective and prospective study. *J Pediatr* 1990;117:22.
21. Finberg L. Fluid management of diabetic ketoacidosis. *Pediatr Rev* 1996;17:46.
22. Rosenbloom AL. Skeletal and joint manifestations of childhood diabetes. *Pediatr Clin North Am* 1984;31:569.
23. Bunn HF. Evaluation of glycosylated hemoglobin in diabetic patients. *Diabetes* 1980;30:613.
24. Kirschenbaum DM. Glycosylation of proteins: its implications in diabetic control and complications. *Pediatr Clin North Am* 1984;31:611.
25. Viberti G. A glycemic threshold for diabetic complications? [editorial] *N Engl J Med* 1995;332:1293.
26. Viberti G, Mogensen CE, Groop LC, et al. Effect of captopril on progression to clinical proteinuria in patients with insulin-dependent diabetes mellitus and microalbuminuria. *JAMA* 1994;271:275.
27. Borch-Johnson K, Wenzel H, Viberti GC, et al. Is screening and intervention for microalbuminuria worthwhile in patients with insulin dependent diabetes? *Br Med J* 1993;306:1722.
28. Pinhas-Hamiel O, Dolan LM, Daniels SR. Increased incidence of non-insulin-dependent diabetes mellitus among adolescents. *J Pediatr* 1996;128:608.

SUGGESTED READING

Anderson B, Ho J, Brackett J, et al. Parental involvement in diabetes management tasks: Relationships to blood glucose monitoring adherence and metabolic control in young adolescents with insulin-dependent diabetes mellitus. *J Pediatr* 1997;130:257.

Chase HP, Garg SK, Jelley DH. Diabetic ketoacidosis in children and the role of outpatient management. *Pediatr Rev* 1990;11:297.

Diabetes Control and Complication Trial Research Group. Effect of intensive diabetes treatment on the development and progression of long-term complications in adolescents with insulin-dependent diabetes mellitus: Diabetes Control and Complications Trial. *J Pediatr* 1994;125:177.

Drush AL, Arslanian SA. Can insulin-dependent diabetes mellitus be cured or prevented? A status report on immunomodulatory strategies and pancreas transplantation. *Pediatr Clin North Am* 1990;37:1467.

Ginsberg-Fellner F. Insulin-dependent diabetes. *Pediatr Rev* 1990;11:239.

Leslie ND, Sperling MA. Relation of metabolic control to complications in diabetes mellitus. *J Pediatr* 1986;108:491.

Spack N. Diabetes mellitus. *Adolescent Medicine: State of the Art Reviews* 1991;2:000.

Sperling MA. Outpatient management of diabetes mellitus. *Pediatr Clin North Am* 1987;34:919.

Weissberg-Benchell J, Glasgo AM, Tynan WD, et al. Adolescent diabetes management and mismanagement. *Diabetes Care* 1995;18:77.

THYROID PROBLEMS

Thyroid problems are among the most common endocrinologic problems in school-aged children and adolescents [1]. Most disorders are heralded or accompanied by an enlargement, either diffuse or nodular, of the thyroid gland. The differential diagnosis of an enlarged thyroid gland, or goiter, is listed in Table 57, and the pathogenesis of an enlarged thyroid is given in Table 58. *Goiter* is defined by the World Health Organization as an enlargement of the lateral lobe of the gland that exceeds the size of the terminal phalanx of the patient's thumb [2].

Basic Physiology

Thyroid hormone production is regulated by a negative feedback system (Fig. 14). The hypothalamus produces thyrotropin-releasing hormone (TRH), which stimulates the production and release of thyroid-stimulating hormone (TSH [thyrotropin]) from the pituitary. TSH acts on the thyroid gland to stimulate the production and release of thyroxine (T_4) and triiodothyronine (T_3). Most T_4 and T_3 circulate bound to thyroid-binding proteins, which render them inactive. It is the small unbound portion of the hormones that is metabolically active. TSH production is affected by the level of T_4. As free T_4 declines, TSH production is stimulated. As T_4 and T_3 levels rise, TSH production and response to TRH decline. In thyroid hormone production, TSH binds to thyroid cell surface receptors, activates adenylate cyclase, and generates adenosine monophosphate, which serves as the intracellular second messenger. Iodine, as the iodide, is attached to thyroglobulin molecules, and monoiodothyronine and diiodothyronine are combined into T_3 and T_4. These are stored in the thyroid colloid until needed, when they are brought back into the cells and reconverted into free T_4 and T_3. Most of the active hormone is released as T_4. Most of the T_3 that is active at the tissue level is converted from T_4 in the peripheral tissues.

Autoimmune Thyroid Disease

Chronic autoimmune thyroiditis is the most common organ-specific autoimmune disorder in humans [3]. Autoimmune thyroid disease can be divided into two broad categories—chronic lymphocytic thyroiditis and autoimmune thyroiditis. Chronic lymphoid thyroiditis, or Hashimoto's disease, is the most common cause of thyroiditis in childhood and adolescence. It is an autoimmune, inflammatory disorder that causes 55% to 65% of all euthyroid goiters [1]. The incidence of Hashimoto's thyroiditis may be increasing [4]. The incidence of this disease peaks in early to middle puberty. Chronic lymphoid thyroiditis seems to cluster in families, and it occurs more frequently in patients with chromosomal syndromes and in children with other autoimmune diseases, such as insulin-dependent diabetes mellitus.

The inflammation and damage in this condition stem from humoral and cell-mediated immune processes (Fig. 15). Either anti-thyroglobulin or anti-microsomal (or anti-thyroperoxidase) antibodies, or both, are present in nearly all patients with chronic lymphoid thyroiditis, but they are not specific for this disease. Most patients with Hashimoto's thyroiditis have anti-microsomal antibodies in the range of 1 : 100 to over 1 : 1,000 [5]. The pathologic features of the gland include diffuse lympho-

TABLE 57. *Classification of adolescent thyromegaly*

A. Diffuse goiter
  1. Autoimmune thyroid disease
    a. CLT
      CLT of childhood and adolescence
      Hashimoto's thyroiditis
      Fibrous variant of CLT
    b. Thyrotoxicosis
      Graves' disease
      Toxic thyroiditis
  2. Endemic goiter: iodine deficiency
  3. Enzymatic deficiencies: familial thyroid dyshormonogenesis
  4. TSH-mediated thyromegaly
    a. TSH-secreting pituitary adenoma
    b. Resistance to thyroid hormone
      1) Generalized (pituitary and peripheral tissues)
      2) Isolated pituitary with hyperthyroidism
  5. a. Antithyroid drugs
    b. Antithyroid agents and foods
  6. Inflammatory: acute and subacute thyroiditis (bacterial or viral)
  7. Idiopathic (simple or colloid goiter)
B. Nodular goiter
  1. Benign tumors or cysts
    a. Hyperfunctioning (hot) adenomas
      1) Hyperthyroid or euthyroid
    b. Nonfunctioning (cold) adenomas
      1) Solitary follicular adenoma
      2) Multinodular goiter: adenomatous hyperplasia
      3) Cyst: solitary or multiple
  2. Malignant thyroid tumors: epithelial cell
    a. Carcinoma
      1) Papillary
      2) Papillary with follicular components
      3) Follicular
      4) Medullary
  3. Malignant thyroid tumors: nonepithelial cell
    a. Lymphoma
    b. Histiocytoma
  4. Autoimmune (Hashimoto's) thyroiditis: lymphoid follicles
  5. Nonthyroidal masses
    a. Lymphadenopathy
    b. Branchial cleft cyst
    c. Thyroglossal duct cyst

CLT, chronic lymphocyte thyroiditis; TSH, thyroid-stimulating hormone.
From Foley TP Jr. Goiter in adolescents. *Endocrinol Metab Clin North Am* 1993;22:593, with permission.

cytic infiltration replacing normal thyroid tissue. Thyroid follicular reactive hyperplasia and fibrosis may follow. Other antibodies may be present, including thyroid-stimulating immunoglobulins, which may be involved in the less common thyrotoxic form of chronic lymphoid thyroiditis [1,6]. There is an increased incidence of subsequent thyroid cancer in patients with this disease [7].

Clinically, the patient is usually asymptomatic and has a diffusely enlarged, nontender thyroid gland. The surface of the gland is usually granular, pebbly, or even nodular. A few patients have laboratory evidence of hypothyroidism. Rarely, they may have transient thyrotoxicosis with suppressed TSH levels and elevated T_4 and T_3. This hyperthyroidism is transient; if it persists, Graves' disease or a functioning thyroid nodule should be considered.

Laboratory evaluation begins with the measurement of TSH and free T_4. If symptoms of hyperthyroidism are present, then a T_3 measurement should be done. Titers of anti-thyroglobulin and anti-

TABLE 58. *Pathogenesis of thyromegaly*

Stimulation
Thyrotropin
    Inhibition of thyroidal hormonogenesis
    Excessive hypothalamic and pituitary secretion
Thyrotropin receptor antibodies
    Thyroid-stimulating antibodies
    Thyroid growth-stimulating antibodies

Inflammation
Noninfection
    Lymphocytic (autoimmune)
Infection
    Bacterial
    Viral
    Other pathogens

Infiltration
Nonneoplasia
    Cysts
Neoplasia
    Adenoma
    Carcinoma
    Lymphoma
    Histiocytosis

From Foley TP Jr. Goiter in adolescents. *Endocrinol Metab Clin North Am* 1993;22:593, with permission.

microsomal antibodies should be performed as well. A patient with a diffusely enlarged thyroid gland, positive anti-thyroglobulin and anti-microsomal antibody titers, and thyroid hormone levels consistent with a euthyroid or hypothyroid picture has chronic lymphoid thyroiditis. No further workup is required [1]. In the thyrotoxic form, radioactive iodine uptake studies may be helpful. The radioactive iodine uptake is normal or decreased in this disease, whereas in Graves' disease, it is elevated.

Long-term follow-up includes both physical assessment and laboratory evaluations every 6 to 12 months. The condition resolves completely in approximately 50% of the patients, but as many as 25% will have transient or permanent hypothyroidism. In these teenagers, thyroid hormone therapy definitely is indicated, using levothyroxine in the smallest dose necessary to decrease the TSH to normal levels. The usual dose in adolescents is 1 to 2 µg/kg of body weight. After growth has ceased, a trial period without the medication is warranted. Normal thyroid hormone levels after 6 to 8 weeks denote complete recovery [8].

Other Causes of Goiter

Colloid goiter, or idiopathic simple goiter, is the second most common cause of euthyroid goiter in childhood [1,9]. This type of goiter is not associated with inflammatory, infectious, or neoplastic processes in a patient with euthyroidism. The cause is unknown. There is a female preponderance and a tendency to family clustering with this type of goiter. No reported association with malignancy exists. The natural history of colloid goiter is resolution, and therefore no treatment is necessary [1].

Graves' disease is the primary cause of hyperthyroidism and goiter in adolescents. Nearly all patients with Graves' disease have a goiter, and approximately half of the patients have exophthalmos [10]. Other signs of hyperthyroidism—nervousness, emotional lability, weight loss, heat intolerance, tachycardia, and a widened pulse pressure—are usually present. The differential diagnosis of Graves' disease includes the occasional transient hyperthyroidism of chronic lymphoid thyroiditis, TSH-secreting pituitary adenomas, and autonomous thyroid nodules. Serum TSH levels are below normal in

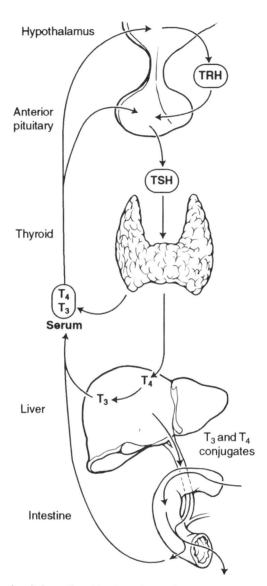

FIG. 14. The hypothalamic–pituitary–thyroid axis and extrathyroidal pathways of thyroid hormone metabolism. Triiodothyronine (T_3) and thyroxine (T_4) inhibit the secretion of thyrotropin (TSH) both directly and indirectly, by inhibiting the secretion of thyrotropin-releasing hormone (TRH). TSH stimulates the synthesis and secretion of T_4 and T_3 by the thyroid gland. T_4 is converted to T_3 in the liver (and many other tissues) by the action of T_4 monodeiodinases. Some of the T_4 and T_3 is conjugated with glucuronide and sulfate in the liver, excreted in the bile, and partially hydrolyzed in the intestine; the T_4 and T_3 formed there may be reabsorbed. Drug interactions can occur at any of these sites. (From Surks MI, Sievert R. Drugs and thyroid function. *N Engl J Med* 1995;333:1688, with permission.)

Graves' disease. The T_4 and T_3 levels are elevated, as is the serum thyroid-stimulating immunoglobulin level.

Thyroid nodules in adolescents warrant a radionuclide scan with I-123. This compound offers a 100-fold dose reduction compared with I-131. "Warm" or "cold" nodules (i.e., ones with either little activity or a moderate amount) should be sampled for biopsy because they may be malignant. A "hot"

Chronic Lymphocytic Thyroiditis

Defect in Cell-Mediated Immunity

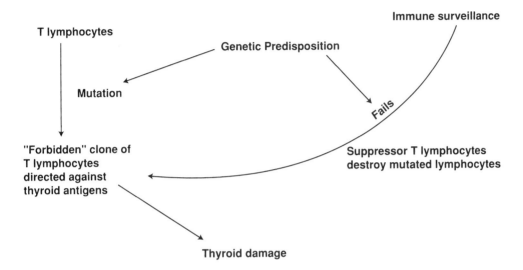

1. Antibody-dependent cell mediated cytotoxicity (ADCC)
2. Complement-dependent antibody mediated cytotoxicity (CDAC)
3. Natural killer cell mediated cytotoxicity (NKCC)

FIG. 15. In adolescents with an inherited genetic predisposition to chronic lymphoid thyroiditis, an apparent failure of suppressor T-cell lymphocyte function results in autoimmune thyroid damage by antibody-mediated, complement-mediated, and natural killer cell-mediated cytotoxicity.

nodule usually signifies an autonomous nodule that is functioning independently of central control, and does not require a thyroid biopsy. This would be reflected by a low TSH level. Ultrasonography also can be used to assess thyroid masses. This technique is most useful when the mass is asymmetric, lateral, or above the usual location for the thyroid. Radionuclide scan is still the primary assessment tool [11,12].

Other causes of an enlarged thyroid gland include acute suppurative thyroiditis, subacute thyroiditis, iodine deficiency (uncommon in the United States), and goitrogens such as iodides (kelp or seaweed, iodide-containing expectorants, amiodarone), ethionamide, and paraaminosalicylic acid.

Many factors other than the thyroid gland, the pituitary, and the hypothalamus can affect the level of the various thyroid hormones. For example, anything that decreases the amount of circulating thyroxine-binding globulin can give an apparent low reading for T_4 if free T_4 is not measured. These factors include testosterone, corticosteroids, severe illness, cirrhosis, nephrotic syndrome, and an inherited condition. Factors that can raise the thyroxine-binding globulin level and give a falsely elevated T_4 level include oral contraceptives, pregnancy, estrogens, hepatitis, acute intermittent porphyria, and some inherited conditions. Measurement of free T_4 is crucial to distinguish between true thyroid problems and these other factors. Lithium is an example of a drug that interferes with thyroid synthesis and decreases thyroid hormone secretion [13].

REFERENCES

1. Bachrach LK, Foley TP Jr. Thyroiditis in children. *Pediatr Rev* 1989;11:184.
2. Delange F, Bastani S, Benmiloud M, et al. Definitions of endemic goiter and cretinism, classification of goiter size and severity of endemieas, and survey techniques. In: Dunn JT, Pretell EA, Daza CH, et al, eds. *Towards the eradication of endemic goiter, cretinism, and iodine deficiency.* PAHOS scientific publication No. 502. Washington, DC: Pan American Health Organization; 1986:373.
3. Dayan CM, Daniels GH. Chronic autoimmune thyroiditis. *N Engl J Med* 1996;335:99.
4. Faber J, Cohn D, Kirkegaard C, et al. Subclinical hypothyroidism in Addison's disease. *Acta Endocrinologica (Copenhagen)* 1979;91:674.
5. Foley TP Jr. Acute, subacute, and chronic thyroiditis. In: Kaplan SA, ed. *Clinical pediatric and adolescent endocrinology.* Philadelphia: WB Saunders; 1982:96.
6. Fisher DA, Pandian MR, Carlton E. Autoimmune thyroid disease: an expanding spectrum. *Pediatr Clin North Am* 1987;34:907.
7. Hamburger JL, Miller JM, Kini SR. Lymphoma of the thyroid. *Ann Intern Med* 1983;99:685.
8. Foley TP Jr. Goiter in adolescents. *Endocrinol Metab Clin North Am* 1993;22:593.
9. Mahoney CP. Differential diagnosis of goiter. *Pediatr Clin North Am* 1987;34:891.
10. Uretsky SH, Kennerdell JS, Gutair JP. Graves' ophthalmopathy in childhood and adolescence. *Arch Ophthalmol* 1980;98:1963.
11. Hopwood NJ, Kelch RP. Thyroid masses: approach to diagnosis and management in childhood and adolescence. *Pediatr Rev* 1993;14:481.
12. LaFranchi S. Adolescent thyroid disorders. *Adolescent Medicine: State of the Art Reviews* 1994;5:65.
13. Surks MI, Sievert R. Drugs and thyroid function. *N Engl J Med* 1995;333:1688.

SUGGESTED READING

Bachrach LK, Foley TP Jr. Thyroiditis in children. *Pediatr Rev* 1989;11:184.
Foley TP Jr. Goiter in adolescents. *Endocrinol Metab Clin North Am* 1993;22:593.
LaFranchi S. Adolescent thyroid disorders. *Adolescent Medicine: State of the Art Reviews* 1994;5:65.
Mahoney CP. Differential diagnosis of goiter. *Pediatr Clin North Am* 1987;34:891.
Sadeghi-Nejat A. Thyroid disorders in adolescents and young adults. *Adolescent Medicine: State of the Art Reviews* 1991;2:509.
Zimmerman D, Gan-Gaisano M. Hyperthyroidism in children and adolescents. *Pediatr Clin North Am* 1990;37:1273.

HYPERTENSION IN ADOLESCENTS

Hypertension, or high blood pressure, is a major contributor to cardiovascular morbidity and mortality in adults. Although the consequences of hypertension are not evident in most affected adolescents, the condition must be detected early so that appropriate steps can be taken to prevent the long-term effects. Moreover, hypertension has a close association with other morbid conditions, including obesity, hyperlipidemia, noninsulin-dependent diabetes mellitus, and, in women, polycystic ovary syndrome [1,2]. Insulin resistance appears to be a root causal factor for all of these conditions (Fig. 16). Remedial steps to address one of these conditions can have beneficial effects for the other components of this complex of symptoms.

Prevalence

The prevalence of hypertension in children and adolescents is estimated to be approximately 2% [3–5]. One screening study, however, found 15% of inner city adolescents to be hypertensive. In children, prolonged elevation of diastolic blood pressure and periodic elevation of systolic pressure are correlated with hypertension [6]. Indeed, periodic elevations of systolic pressure may be more diagnostic of future cardiovascular disease [7,8] (Fig. 17). Most adolescents with hypertension have mild elevations of blood pressure, but about 5% to 10% have higher blood pressures (e.g., greater than 20 mm Hg above the 95th percentile for age). Most of these adolescents have another cause of hypertension, primarily renal or renovascular disease [5]. The primary focus of this discussion is adolescents with primary or essential hypertension.

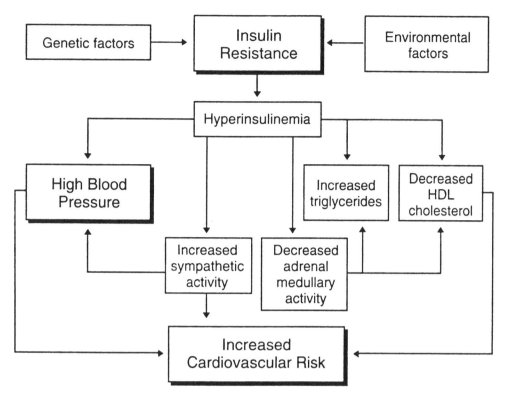

FIG. 16. Postulated relations among insulin resistance, high blood pressure, and increased cardiovascular risk. The sympathetic nervous system and adrenal medulla are the effector links between insulin resistance and hypertension and cardiovascular disease. (Reaven GM, Kithell H, Lansberg L. Hypertension and associated metabolic abnormalities: the role of insulin resistance and the sympathoadrenal system. *N Engl J Med* 1996;334:374. *"Copyright 1996 Massachusetts Medical Society. All rights reserved."* with permission).

Detection

There are no physical findings specific for primary hypertension in the adolescent. Blood pressure rises steadily from the beginning of puberty to physical maturity [4,9]. Hypertension in children and adolescents has been defined as systolic or diastolic pressure above the 95th percentile for age and sex [10,11]. In mature adolescents, the 95th percentile is very close to the accepted cutoff for adults, 140/90. In 1996, an update on blood pressure standards for adolescents was published using height as the major correlate for blood pressure because of the prevalence of obesity in this country [12]. The standards for adolescents 12 to 17 years of age are shown in Table 59. Causes of hypertension are listed in Table 60.

Diagnosing hypertension requires proper technique and proper equipment. The mercury manometer and auscultation are the standards against which other devices and techniques are measured. Aneroid manometers and digital Doppler devices need to be calibrated periodically against a mercury manometer. Taking blood pressure readings properly seems to be a simple task, but there are many ways to obtain inaccurate readings. Proper cuff size, calibration of manometers, and consistent, proper technique of detecting pressures are all necessary. The size of the cuff used is very important. The cuff should span two thirds of the length of the upper arm. A palpatory estimate of the systolic pressure should be performed first. The examiner should palpate disappearance and reappearance of the pulse with inflation and deflation of the cuff. This prevents using an arbitrary pressure goal for inflating the cuff and avoids the misinterpretation of sounds that can occur early in deflation when the

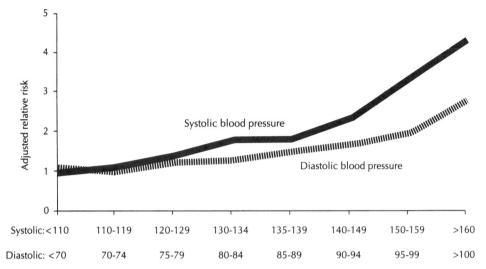

FIG. 17. Relative risk for cardiovascular disease according to systolic and diastolic blood pressures. Risks deriving from increases in systolic blood pressure are greater than the risks of relatively similar increases in diastolic blood pressure (i.e., a blood pressure increase of 140 to 149 mm Hg has a greater risk than a blood pressure increase of 90 to 94 mm Hg). (Moser M. Management of hypertension, part I. *Am Fam Physician* 1996;53:2295, with permission).

TABLE 59. *Blood pressure standards for adolescents*[a]

Age (y)	Percentile	5th	10th	25th	50th	75th	90th	95th
Boys								
12	90th	115/75	116/75	117/76	119/77	121/78	123/78	123/79
	95th	119/79	120/79	121/80	123/81	125/82	126/83	127/83
13	90th	117/75	118/76	120/76	122/77	124/78	125/79	126/80
	95th	121/79	122/80	124/81	126/82	128/83	129/83	130/84
14	90th	120/76	121/76	123/77	125/78	126/79	128/80	128/80
	95th	124/80	125/81	127/81	128/82	130/83	132/84	132/85
15	90th	123/77	124/77	125/78	127/79	129/80	131/81	131/81
	95th	127/81	128/82	129/83	131/83	133/84	134/85	135/86
16	90th	125/79	126/79	128/80	130/81	132/82	133/82	134/83
	95th	129/83	130/83	132/84	134/85	136/86	137/87	138/87
17	90th	128/81	129/81	131/82	133/83	134/84	136/85	134/85
	95th	132/85	133/85	135/86	138/87	136/88	140/89	140/89
Girls								
12	90th	116/75	116/75	118/76	119/76	120/77	121/78	122/78
	95th	120/79	120/79	121/80	123/80	124/81	125/82	126/82
13	90th	118/76	118/76	119/77	121/78	122/78	123/79	124/80
	95th	121/80	122/80	123/81	125/82	126/82	127/83	128/84
14	90th	119/77	120/77	121/78	122/79	124/79	125/80	126/81
	95th	123/81	124/81	125/82	126/83	128/83	129/84	130/85
15	90th	121/78	121/78	122/79	124/79	125/80	126/81	127/82
	95th	124/82	125/82	126/83	128/83	129/84	130/85	131/86
16	90th	122/79	122/79	123/79	125/80	126/81	127/82	128/82
	95th	125/83	126/83	127/83	128/84	130/85	131/86	132/86
17	90th	122/79	123/79	124/79	125/80	126/81	128/82	128/82
	95th	126/83	126/83	127/83	129/84	130/85	131/86	132/86

[a]Systolic/diastolic blood pressure (mm Hg) by percentile of height. Standard growth curves determine height percentile. The disappearance of Korotkoff's sounds (K5) determine diastolic blood pressure.
Adapted from Sardegna K, Loggie JMH. Hypertension in teens. *Contemp Pediatr* 1996;13:96.

TABLE 60. *Causes of hypertension*

Cause	Acute hypertension	Chronic hypertension	
Idiopathic		Primary (essential)	
Renal	Poststreptococcal glomerulonephritis	Focal segmental glomerulosclerosis	Interstitial nephritis Polycystic kidney
	Schönlein-Henoch purpura	Chronic glomerulonephritis	disease
	IgA nephropathy	Crescentic glomeru-	Medullary cystic
	Hemolytic–uremic syndrome	lonephritis	disease
	Acute tubular necrosis	Collagen vascular diseases	Hydronephrosis
		Alport's syndrome	Hypoplastic kidney
		Reflux nephropathy	Hemangiopericytoma
Endocrine		Pheochromocytoma	Hyperthyroidism
		Primary aldosteronism	(systolic)
Vascular	Renal or renovascular trauma	Coarctation of the aorta	Arteriovenous fistula
		Renal artery stenosis[a]	Tuberous sclerosis
		Takayasu's arteritis	
Neurogenic	Increased intracranial pressure	Dysautonomia	
	Guillain-Barré syndrome		
Metabolic	Hypercalcemia		
	Hypernatremia		
Drugs	Cocaine	Nonsteroidal anti-	Anabolic steroids
	Phencyclidine amphetamines	inflammatory drugs	Oral contraceptives
	Jimson weed	Corticosteroids	
		Alcohol	
Miscellaneous	Burns	Heavy metal poisoning	

[a]Including neurofibromatosis, fibromuscular dysplasia, and Williams syndrome.
From Sardegna K, Loggie JMH. Hypertension in teens. *Contemp Pediatr* 1996;13:96. Medical Economics Publishing, Inc., Montvale, NJ: Reprinted by permission.

cuff has been overinflated. Cuff inflation should be rapid, and deflation should occur at a rate of approximately 2 mm Hg per second. If a sound is missed, the cuff should be deflated and the patient should be allowed to rest for 2 to 3 minutes before the reading is attempted again. Never reinflate the cuff while it is deflating [4].

The National Heart, Lung, and Blood Institute recommends using the disappearance of the Korotkoff sounds to determine diastolic blood pressure in adolescents. The patient must be sitting comfortably in a quiet environment with the arm held steadily at heart level, preferably resting on a solid surface. The patient should not have a full bladder and should not have used any form of nicotine or of any other stimulant in the previous 30 minutes. The data on normal blood pressures apply to adolescents who have been sitting quietly for only 5 to 10 minutes, so it is recommended to adhere to that schedule when the reading has to be repeated. The authors do believe, however, that if a noxious procedure, such as taking off clothes for a physical examination or having a pelvic examination performed, is anticipated by the adolescent, another blood pressure determination should be performed after the procedure is finished. When elevated blood pressure is found, blood pressure determinations in the legs should always be performed to detect the rare adolescent with coarctation of the aorta.

To make a firm diagnosis of hypertension in an asymptomatic adolescent, the patient should have elevated blood pressures at three readings per visit for three weekly visits. Corroborating factors include obesity and a family history of essential hypertension. Oligomenorrhea in an overweight girl, with or without hypertension, should suggest insulin resistance and polycystic ovary syndrome. If such a girl is normotensive, she still has a significant chance for development of hypertension, especially if she has a family history of this condition.

Physical examination in the adolescent who has elevated blood pressure should emphasize detection of conditions that cause secondary hypertension. Table 61 lists findings and suggested etiologies. White girls with hypertension always should have abdominal auscultation to detect a renal artery bruit. In addition to the physical findings listed, attention should be paid to the presence of acanthosis nigricans, because this skin condition is correlated with polycystic ovary syndrome and insulin resistance, which, in turn, is correlated with hypertension [2,13].

TABLE 61. *The hypertension-directed physical examination*

Signs and symptoms	Suggestive etiology
Growth failure Enuresis Edema Polydipsia Polyuria Abdominal bruit	Renal
Rash/skin findings Joint symptoms	Collagen vascular
Increased systolic pressure Increased pulse pressure	Hyperthyroidism
Virilization Striae Increased heart rate Abnormal fat distribution Menstrual irregularities Genital abnormalities	Endocrine
Differential blood pressure Claudication Murmur "Notched ribs" on chest Radiograph	Coarctation of the aorta
Episodic headaches Sweating Palpitation Abdominal pain	Pheochromocytoma

From Greydanus DE. Hypertension in adolescence. *Adolescent Health Update* 1993;6:1, with permission.

Based on findings in the individual adolescent, the evaluation of hypertension requires minimal laboratory and imaging studies to help further define possible causes and effects of the condition [4,6]. If the blood pressure is very high, secondary hypertension primarily from renal disease should be suspected. Studies to be performed in all adolescents with hypertension include urinalysis, serum blood urea nitrogen and creatinine, and renal ultrasound. A urine culture, a hemoglobin or hematocrit, and a lipid profile also may be indicated based on the history and physical findings. Although many authors suggest that the renal ultrasound can be omitted in the obese adolescent who has a family history of essential hypertension, such adolescents also can have occult renal disorders such as renal dysplasia that may be detected by ultrasound. Of course, in female adolescents, a pregnancy test is imperative. If the blood pressure is very high or if there is reason to suspect that it is of long standing, then an echocardiogram should be performed for determination of ventricular wall thickness.

Management

In the adolescent with primary hypertension, the first management strategy is to encourage weight loss and an increase in aerobic exercise (Fig. 18). (It should be noted that there is a subset of adolescent boys with primary hypertension who are thin and who have a hyperdynamic precordium.) Although the success of prescribed weight loss regimes is abysmal, an attempt still should be made. A diet with no more than 25% to 30% fat and no more than 10% saturated fat is recommended [14].

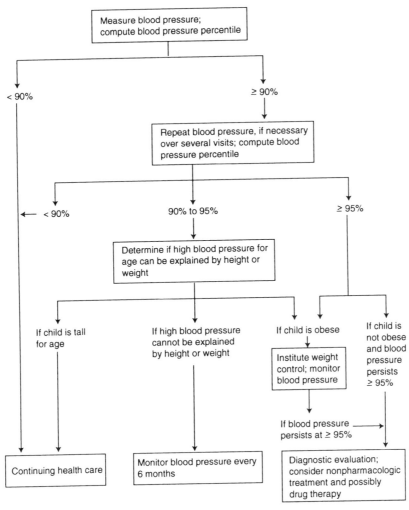

FIG. 18. Algorithm for detecting and treating hypertension in children. (Adapted from the Task Force on Blood Pressure Control in Children. Report of the second Task Force on Blood Pressure Control in Children—1987. Pediatrics 1987;79:1. Reproduced with permission from *Cleveland Clinic Journal of Medicine.*

Sodium restriction to at least 1,500 to 2,000 mg/day is recommended, although that is very difficult to achieve with modern American teenagers [4]. Although growing adolescents need only 500 mg/day sodium, the average American has a daily sodium intake of anywhere from 1,800 to 5,000 mg, with some reporting intakes of as much as 8,000 mg [11]. The chances of significant sodium reduction are slim at best, with one study reporting total failure to get teenage boys to comply with a low-sodium diet for any length of time [15]. Still, adolescents and their families should receive instruction in ways to reduce overall sodium and fat intake. They should be taught to read food labels, and to keep a list of the sodium and fat contents of common foods in their house as a reference. Although there are no official recommendations to increase potassium and calcium intakes, there are studies that correlate increased intakes of these minerals with decreased prevalence of hypertension [16–18]. Aerobic exercise is an important concomitant of hypertension management of weight loss [4–6]. There is even indication that weight training, especially when combined with aerobic exercise, has an added benefi-

TABLE 62. *Recommendations for selection of initial antihypertensive drug for patients with various coexisting conditions[a]*

Coexisting condition	Diuretic	β-Blocker	ACE inhibitor[b]	α₁-Blocker	Nondihydropyridine	Dihydropyridine
Older age	++	+/−	+	+	+	+
Black race	++	+/−	+/−	+	++	++
Angina pectoris	+	++	+	+	++	++
Postmyocardial infarction	+	++	+	+	+	−
Congestive heart failure with systolic dysfunction	++	−	++	+	−	−
Cerebrovascular disease	+	+	+	+/−	+	+
Renal disease						
Serum creatinine <220 μmol/L	++	+/−	++[c]	+	+	+
Serum creatinine ≥220 μmol/L	++[d]	+/−	−	+	+	+
Diabetes mellitus without nephropathy	+[c]	+/−[c]	+	+	+	+
Diabetes mellitus with nephropathy	+[c]	+/−[c]	++	+	+	+
Dyslipidemia	+[c]	+/−[c]	+	++	+	+
Prostatism	+	+	+	++	+	+
Migraine	+	++	+	+	++	+
Atrial fibrillation (with rapid ventricular rate)	+	++	+	+	++	+
Paroxysmal supraventricular tachycardia	+	++	+	+	++	+
Senile tremor	+	++	+	+	+	+

[a]Symbols used indicate the following: ++, preferred; +, suitable; +/−, usually not preferred; −, usually contraindicated.
[b]ACE, angiotensin-converting enzyme.
[c]Requires special monitoring.
[d]Loop diuretic preferred.
From Kaplan NM, Gifford RW Jr. Choice of initial therapy for hypertension. *JAMA* 1996;275:1577 (with permission).

TABLE 63. *Oral drugs for mild to moderate hypertension*

Name	Dose range[a]	Dosage interval	Major adverse effects	Comments
Diuretics				
Chlorothiazide	250–500 mg	Daily	Hypovolemia, electrolyte imbalance, hyperuricemia, hyperlipidemia, hyperglycemia, rash, agranulocytosis, sexual problems	May take 10–14 d for maximum effect.
Hydrochlorothiazide	25–50 mg	Daily	Same as chlorothiazide	May take 10–14 d for maximum effect.
β-Blockers				
Atenolol	25–200 mg	Daily or in divided doses every 12 h	Decreased exercise tolerance, impotence, depression, increased low-density lipoprotein	
ACE inhibitors				
Lisinopril[b]	10–40 mg	Daily	Angioedema (early), chronic cough, rash	Lipid neutral.
Enalapril maleate[b]	5–40 mg	Daily or in divided doses every 12 h	Same as lisinopril	Has to be metabolized to active form; lipid neutral.
Calcium channel blockers				
Verapamil long acting[c]	240–480 mg	Daily or in divided doses every 12 h	Somnolence, reduced heart rate, constipation, gum hyperplasia	Give at bedtime if on daily dosing; lipid neutral; effect usually within 1 week.
Diltiazem long acting[c]	60–180 mg	Twice daily	Same as verapamil	Maximum effect of any dose seen after ±14 d; lipid neutral.
Nifedipine long acting[d]	30–120 mg	Daily	Peripheral edema, flushing, headache, nausea	
Amlodipine[d]	2.5–10 mg	Daily	Peripheral edema, headache, flushing, palpitations	May take 2–6 wk for full effect at any given dose.

ACE, angiotensin-converting enzyme.
[a]First dose given is usual starting dose.
[b]If patient is taking a diuretic, use half the starting dose.
[c]Not usually given with β-blockers.
[d]Use with caution with β-blockers—may produce hypotension.
From Sardegna K, Loggie JMH. Hypertension in teens. *Contemp Pediatr* 1996;13:96. Medical Economics Publishing, Inc., Montvale, NJ: Reprinted by permission.

133

cial effect on elevated blood pressure [19]. Life-styles that are not conducive to good health habits should be discouraged. These would include irregular and inadequate sleep, high-stress situations, and irregular or poor diets with little exercise. Stress must be addressed assiduously with psychosocial intervention and with instruction in stress management techniques.

Although some experts prescribe a trial (6–12 months) of nonpharmacologic therapy for hypertension, the failure rate with this approach is high either because of severity of the condition or, more likely, because of noncompliance with the therapeutic regimen. Drug therapy is the most dependable approach with this population. Some specialists start drug therapy simultaneously with nonpharmacologic methods [Mahan J, personal communication]. Several classes of antihypertensive agents exist today, and the choice of an initial agent can be difficult. The various drugs are listed in Table 62. Typical choices for adolescents are listed in Table 63. Adolescents seem to accept angiotensin-converting enzyme (ACE) inhibitors and calcium channel blockers quite well. Although diuretics or beta-adrenergic receptor blockers are recommended as first choice in adults with hypertension [20], these agents have side effects that make them much less desirable for adolescents. Beta blockers are contraindicated in patients with asthma, and they are not well accepted by active adolescents, in whom they reduce exercise tolerance. However, they may be useful in adolescents with a hyperdynamic precordium. Diuretics can cause electrolyte disorders and lipid elevations, and therefore they are not desirable for adolescents. ACE inhibitors and calcium channel blockers have the advantage for adolescents of once-daily dosing. They do not affect lipid levels. In patients with apparent insulin resistance, alpha$_1$-adrenergic antagonists decrease blood pressure, lower insulin resistance, and help decrease serum lipid levels. Long-acting calcium channel blockers are also appropriate in this type of patient [1]. Compliance with medical therapy is always an issue in adolescents. Proper education, regular office visits, and periodic blood pressure checks at home or at school help the adolescent stay focused on blood pressure control.

Special Conditions

Athletes with hypertension should be encouraged to continue their sport once their blood pressure is well regulated because aerobic conditioning is correlated with improved blood pressure. Weight training can be helpful, but power lifting or competitive weight lifting should be discouraged [14,21].

Contraception should be emphatically encouraged in female adolescents who are hypertensive. The risks of estrogen or progestins as contraceptives are much less than the risk of pregnancy. Neither Depo-Provera nor levonorgestrel (Norplant) implants have been found to raise blood pressure [22,23]. Where possible, abstinence should be actively encouraged.

Length of Therapy

Nonpharmacologic therapy should be lifelong. Pharmacologic therapy should be continued at least for 12 months, and then a trial of reduced therapy should be given. If the pressure returns to high levels, drug therapy should be considered for the long term.

Prematurely labeling an adolescent as a hypertensive can have significant long-term consequences. Health insurance can be hard to find, and, if found, it can be very expensive. Certain career paths can be shut off with this label. Clinicians should do as much as possible to control this condition by the end of adolescence. When drug therapy is required, the results in compliant youths can be rewarding.

REFERENCES

1. Reaven GM, Lithell H, Landsberg L. Hypertension and associated metabolic abnormalities: the role of insulin resistance and the sympathoadrenal system. *N Engl J Med* 1996;334:374.
2. Nestler JE, Jakubowicz DJ. Decreases in ovarian cytochrome P450c17α activity and serum free testosterone after reduction of insulin secretion in polycystic ovary syndrome. *N Engl J Med* 1996;335:617.
3. Sinaiko AR, Gomex-Marin O, Prineas RJ. Prevalence of significant hypertension in junior high school-aged children: the children and adolescent blood pressure program. *J Pediatr* 1989;114:664.
4. Sardegna KM, Loggie JMH. Hypertension in teens. *Contemp Pediatr* 1996;13:96.
5. Jung FF, Ingelfinger JR. Hypertension in children. *Pediatr Rev* 1993;14:169.
6. Greydanus DE, Rowlett JD. Hypertension in adolescence. *Adolescent Health Update* 1993;6:1.

7. Sagie A, Larson MG, Levy D. The natural history of borderline isolate systolic hypertension. *N Engl J Med* 1993;329:1912.
8. Weisman DN. Systolic or diastolic blood pressure significance [commentary]. *Pediatrics* 1988;82:112.
9. Wein MR, Stafford EM, Gregory G, et al. The relationship between sexual maturity rating, age, and increased blood pressure in adolescents. *Journal of Adolescent Health Care* 1988;9:465.
10. National Heart, Lung and Blood Institute. Report of the Task Force on blood pressure control in children. *Pediatrics* 1977;59:797.
11. National Heart, Lung and Blood Institute. Report of the second task force report on blood pressure control in children. *Pediatrics* 1987;79:1.
12. National Heart, Lung and Blood Institute. Update on the 1987 task force report on high blood pressure in children and adolescents. *Pediatrics* 1996;98:649.
13. Arslanian S, Suprasongsin C. Differences in the in vivo insulin secretion and sensitivity of healthy black versus white adolescents. *J Pediatr* 1996;129:440.
14. U.S. Departments of Agriculture and Health and Human Services. *Nutrition and your health: dietary guidelines for Americans*. Washington, DC: U.S. Departments of Agriculture and Health and Human Services;1990.
15. Sinaiko AR, Gomez-Marin O, Prineas RJ. Effect of low sodium diet or potassium supplementation on adolescent blood pressure. *Hypertension* 1993;21:991.
16. McCarron DA, Morris CD, Henry HJ, et al. Blood pressure and nutrient intake in the United States. *Science* 1984;224:1392.
17. Gillman MW, Hood MY, Moore LL, et al. Effect of calcium supplementation on blood pressure in children. *J Pediatr* 1995;127:186.
18. Gillman MW, Oliveria SA, Moore LL, et al. Inverse association of dietary calcium with systolic blood pressure in young children. *JAMA* 1992;267:2340.
19. Hagberg J, Ehsani AA, Goldring D, et al. Effect of weight training on blood pressure and hemodynamics in hypertensive adolescents. *J Pediatr* 1984;104:147.
20. Kaplan NM, Gifford RW Jr. Choice of initial therapy for hypertension. *JAMA* 1996;275:1577.
21. Daniels SR, Meyer RA, Strife CF, et al. Distribution of target-organ abnormalities by race and sex in children with essential hypertension. *J Hum Hypertens* 1990;4:103.
22. Smith RD, Cromer BA, Hayes JR, et al. Medroxyprogesterone acetate (Depo-Provera) use in adolescents: uterine bleeding and blood pressure patterns, patient satisfaction, and continuation rates. *Adolescent and Pediatric Gynecology* 1995;8:24.
23. Cromer BA, Smith RD, Blair JM, et al. A prospective study of adolescents who choose among levonorgestrel implant (Norplant), medroxyprogesterone acetate (Depo-Provera), or the combined oral contraceptive pill as contraception. *Pediatrics* 1994;94:687.

SUGGESTED READINGS

American Academy of Pediatrics Committee on Sports Medicine and Fitness. Athletic participation by children and adolescents who have systemic hypertension. *Pediatrics* 1997;99:637.
Brouhard BH. Hypertension in children and adolescents. *Cleve Clin J Med* 1995;62:21.
Greydanus DE, Rowlett JD. Hypertension in adolescence. *Adolescent Health Update* 1993;6:1.
Jung FF, Ingelfinger JR. Hypertension in childhood and adolescence. *Pediatr Rev* 1993;14:169.
Reaven GM, Lithell H, Landsberg L. Hypertension and associated metabolic abnormalities: the role of insulin resistance and the sympathoadrenal system. *N Engl J Med* 1996;334:374.
Sardegna KM, Loggie JMH. Hypertension in teens. *Contemp Pediatr* 1996;13:96.
Sinaiko AR. Hypertension in children. *N Engl J Med* 1996;335:1968.

ATTENTION DEFICIT/HYPERACTIVITY DISORDER

Any condition that interferes with the successful achievement of an adequate education for an adolescent can be termed a learning disorder. Such a condition can be purely organic, purely psychosocial, or a combination of both. A list of medical conditions that predispose to disorders of attention and learning is given in Table 64. This list does not include the major de novo conditions that interfere with learning—attention deficit/hyperactivity disorder (AD/HD) and learning disabilities. This section is devoted to AD/HD. Mention is made of learning disabilities as well as those conditions that tend to be comorbid with AD/HD.

Although the true prevalence of AD/HD is not known, in 1995 it was estimated that over 2 million school-age children were diagnosed with this problem and were receiving pharmacologic treatment for it [1]. Many older adolescents and adults are being diagnosed with this disorder as well [2]. One of the major problems with counting the numbers of adolescents with AD/HD is the difficulty in making the diagnosis. Many other conditions have symptoms that overlap with AD/HD, and by the time a

TABLE 64. *Predisposing conditions to disorders of learning and attention*

Environmental
Emotional deprivation ("psychosocial malnutrition")
Familial dysfunction
Lead poisoning
Nutritional deprivation
Traumatic brain injury

Infectious/inflammatory
Congenital infection
Human immunodeficiency virus encephalopathy
Meningitis/encephalitis
Sydenham chorea

Malignancy
Brain tumors/noncentral nervous system malignancies
Treatment of malignancies: radiation and chemotherapy effects

Medical
Chronic hypoxia
Chronic illness
Subclinical seizures

Medication effects
Anticonvulsants
Antihistamines
Corticosteroids
Ethanol and recreational drugs
Methylxanthines

Sequelae of prematurity
Hydrocephalus
Hypoxic ischemic encephalopathy
Intraventricular hemorrhage
Periventricular leukomalacia

Teratogenic
Fetal alcohol syndrome and effects

Vascular
Stroke

Adapted from Capin DM. Developmental learning disorders: clues to their diagnosis and management. *Pediatr Rev* 1996;17: 284.

child reaches adolescence, much emotional and psychological overlay can obscure any real deficit in attending to necessary educational tasks.

The *Diagnostic and Statistical Manual* of the American Psychiatric Association, 4th edition (DSM-IV) criteria for the diagnosis of AD/HD are listed in Table 65. A child or adolescent must show at least six symptoms of inattention or hyperactivity as described in the table for a diagnosis to be made. It seems that we have reached the point where the diagnosis of attention deficit disorder can be made without identification of a problem with attention [3]. Some salient points from the DSM-IV include:

- The "slash" in AD/HD indicates that deficits of attention, hyperactivity, and impulsivity can occur separately or concurrently.
- Symptoms must be "maladaptive and inconsistent with developmental level."
- Symptoms must be present across settings at home or at school.
- AD/HD should not be diagnosed if symptoms are better accounted for by other conditions.

The clinician must be aware that all that looks like AD/HD is not AD/HD. A differential diagnosis for AD/HD is listed in Table 66. Several problems also coexist with AD/HD in greater frequency than they do with the normal population. These are listed in Table 67.

TABLE 65. *Diagnosing attention deficit/hyperactivity disorder*

1. Either a or b
   a) Six or more of the following **inattention** symptoms lasting for at least six months which are maladaptive or inconsistent with level of development:
      i) Frequently fails to pay close attention to detail and/or makes careless mistakes in homework, schoolwork, work, or other activities
      ii) Frequently inattentive to tasks or play activities
      iii) Frequently inattentive when spoken to directly
      iv) Frequently does not complete tasks or follow instructions (not due to failure to understand directions)
      v) Frequently has problems in organization of tasks/activities
      vi) Frequently avoids or is reluctant to engage in activities requiring sustained mental effort
      vii) Frequently loses items necessary for task completion (e.g., pencils, tools, toys)
      viii) Frequently distracted by extraneous stimuli
      ix) Frequently forgetful in daily activities
   b) Six or more of the following **hyperactivity/impulsivity** symptoms that have lasted for at least six months which are maladaptive or inconsistent with level of development:
      i) Frequently fidgets (hands/feet) or squirms in chair
      ii) Frequently leaves seat
      iii) Frequently runs around or climbs when inappropriate
      iv) Frequently "chatty" or loud during activities when inappropriate
      v) Frequently "on the go" or acts as if "driven by a motor"
      vi) Frequently talks excessively
      vii) Frequently blurts out the answer to an unfinished question
      viii) Frequently cannot wait a turn
      ix) Frequently interrupts others
2. Impairment from the symptoms is evident in two or more settings, such as home, school, or work.
3. Clinically significant impairment must be evident in school, occupational, or academic functioning.
4. Impulsive or hyperactive symptoms that caused impairment were manifest before 7 years of age.
5. The symptoms are not manifested uniquely during a pervasive developmental disorder, schizophrenia, or other psychotic disorder, and are not better accounted for by another mental disorder, such as dissociative, personality, mood, or anxiety.

Adapted from *Diagnostic and statistical manual.* 4th ed. Washington, DC: American Psychiatric Association; 1994.

TABLE 66. *Differential diagnosis*

General	Neurodevelopmental	Psychosocial
Anemia	"Average" child in "high-achieving" family	Anxiety disorder
Chronic illness causing frequent school absence	Hearing impairment	Chaotic social environment
Hypothyroidism/hyperthyroidism	Increased intelligence (classroom boredom)	Child abuse/neglect
Lead exposure	Language disorders	Conduct disorder
Malnutrition	Learning disabilities	Depression
Side effect of medication	Mental retardation	Dissociative disorder
Antihistamines	Neurodegenerative disorder	Drug abuse syndromes
Anticonvulsants	Normal preschoolers	Inconsistent parenting/understructured family
Bronchodilators	Perceptual disorders	Manic–depressive illness
Sleep disturbance	Pervasive developmental disorder/autism	Mood disorder
	Slower learning	Oppositional defiant disorder
	Tourette's syndrome	Parental psychopathology
	Uncontrolled seizure disorder	Personality disorder
	Visual impairment	Poor limit-setting at home
		Posttraumatic stress disorder
		Reactive emotional states/adjustment disorder
		Schizophrenia/thought disorder

Adapted from Brown FR III, Boigt RG, Elksnin N. AD/HD: a neurodevelopmental perspective. *Contemp Pediatr* 1996;13:25.

TABLE 67. *Comorbid conditions in children with developmental learning disorders*

Anxiety disorders
Bipolar disorder
Depression
Eating disorders
Movement disorders
Sleep disorders
Substance abuse

Adapted from Capin DM. Developmental learning disorders: clues to their diagnosis and management. *Pediatr Rev* 1996;17: 284.

Diagnosing and Managing AD/HD

1. The symptoms of inattention, poor impulse control, and/or hyperactivity are interfering significantly with the adolescent's ability to function appropriately.

☐ Yes; continue. ☐ No; no further intervention is necessary.

2. The symptoms of inattention, poor impulse control, and/or hyperactivity are solely related to some other medical, neurodevelopmental, psychiatric, or psychosocial condition.

☐ No; continue. ☐ Yes; treat the true etiology of symptoms.

3. The symptoms of inattention, poor impulse control, and/or hyperactivity are inappropriate for the adolescent's level of developmental function.

☐ Yes; continue. ☐ No; special education services as needed.

4. Demands and expectations at school and home are congruent with the adolescent's developmental abilities.

☐ Yes; continue ☐ No; adjust demands and expectations.

5. Behavioral/educational interventions are successful in remediating symptoms.

☐ No; continue ☐ Yes; no further intervention necessary.

6. A trial of stimulant medication is successful in resolving symptoms of inattention, poor impulse control, and hyperactivity.

☐ No; continue ☐ Yes; no further intervention necessary. (Continue behavioral/ educational interventions).

7. You are sure that AD/HD is the correct diagnosis and the persisting symptoms are amenable to medication management.

☐ Yes; continue ☐ No; reevaluate patient (return to beginning); increase educational/behavioral intervention.

8. Try a secondary medication, such as imipramine or clonidine.

FIG. 19. Diagnosing and managing attention deficit/hyperactivity disorder. (Adapted from Brown FR III, Voigt RG, Elksnin N. AD/HD: a neurodevelopmental perspective. *Contemp Pediatr* 1996;13:25.)

Diagnosis of AD/HD is best approached using the system in Figure 19. The basic approach is to ascertain whether the problem behaviors are interfering with the adolescent's ability to function in various settings. The clinician must then decide if the symptoms/behaviors can be accounted for by another condition. If not, then an attempt must be made to see whether the demands on the patient are developmentally appropriate for this adolescent. If so, then behavioral and educational efforts should be made to alleviate the symptoms. If these interventions are not helpful, a trial of stimulant medication should be attempted. Behavior checklists and psychological testing are frequently used to help make the diagnosis of AD/HD, but by themselves they are not totally reliable. It is the total picture as filtered through the clinician's perception and experience that makes the final diagnosis.

Stimulant medications do help alleviate the inability to attend to necessary tasks for adolescents with AD/HD. Usually, methylphenidate is the drug of first choice. Amphetamines and pemoline are other stimulants that are used relatively commonly. If these drugs, used in appropriately sufficient doses, do not work, a reassessment of the diagnosis should be made. If the diagnosis seems firm, then other drugs that can be used include tricyclic antidepressants, such as imipramine and desipramine, and the antihypertensive, clonidine. In adolescents with coexistent conditions such as Tourette's syndrome or psychological disorders, the medications used must be balanced; there can be adverse, as well as beneficial, effects. A review of studies of effectiveness of stimulants in adolescents indicates that they do seem to work [4].

Many adolescents with AD/HD do have coexisting psychological problems, many of which may be generated from the problems of the AD/HD with which these adolescents must cope [3,5]. Therefore, frequent counsel is a necessary adjunct to pharmacologic treatment. Families need to be included in this counseling to enable them to help their affected child best.

Mention should be made of the common coexistence of AD/HD with Tourette's syndrome. The comorbidity of these conditions is said to be anywhere from 21% to 54%, with boys more likely to have the motor disturbances than girls, and with AD/HD symptoms more pronounced in those patients with more severe Tourette's syndrome [6,7]. The general approach to treating adolescents with both problems is to use stimulant medication cautiously, if at all. A better medication for those so affected might be clonidine. Whether this drug is treating the problems of attention directly or just affecting the ability to attend by decreasing the motor disturbance and aggression is unknown [3].

Other learning disorders, such as dyslexia, also occur in adolescents, and their diagnosis relies on more specific neuropsychological testing.

REFERENCES

1. Baren M, Swanson J. How *not* to diagnose ADHD. *Contemp Pediatr* 1996;13:53.
2. Biederman J, Faraone S, Keenan K, et al. Further evidence for family-genetic risk factors in ADHD. *Arch Gen Psychiatry* 1992;49:728.
3. Brown FR III, Voight RG, Elksnin N. AD/HD: a neurodevelopmental perspective. *Contemp Pediatr* 1996; 13:25.
4. Wilens TE, Biederman J. The stimulants. *Psychol Clin North Am* 1992;15:191.
5. Huntington DD, Bender WN. Adolescents with learning disabilities at risk? Emotional well-being, depression, and suicide. *Journal of Learning Disorders* 1993;26:159.
6. Biederman J, Newcorn J, Sprich SE. Comorbidity of attention deficit hyperactivity disorder with conduct, depressive, anxiety, and other disorders. *Am J Psychiatry* 1991;148:564.
7. DePaul GJ, Barkley RA. Medication therapy. In: Barkley RA, ed. *Attention-deficit hyperactivity disorder: a handbook for diagnosis and treatment*. New York: The Guilford Press; 1990:573.

SUGGESTED READING

Brown FR III, Voight RG, Elksnin N. AD/HD: a neurodevelopmental perspective. *Contemp Pediatr* 1996;13:25.
Capin DM. Developmental learning disorders: clues to their diagnosis and management. *Pediatr Rev* 1996;17:284.

4

The Adolescent With Chronic Illness Or Disability

Chronic illness or *disability* has been defined as any chronic physical or psychological state creating a permanent condition, with residual disability affecting one or more organ systems [1]. Such a condition can create significant difficulty for a person of any age. When the victim is an adolescent, problems can be compounded considerably.

A large number of adolescents suffer from chronic disorders. According to the 1988 National Health Interview Survey (NHIS) data, an estimated 31.5% of adolescents have at least one chronic (lasting at least 3 months) condition. That extrapolates to about 9 million of a total of about 28 million 10- to 17-year-olds [2]. The prevalence estimates for various disorders are listed in Table 1. The category of chronic disorders includes conditions as innocuous as myopia or seasonal allergies and others as severe as myelomeningocele, cancer, and cystic fibrosis. Chronic disorders may also include conditions such as learning disability or mental retardation, and psychiatric conditions such as schizophrenia or eating disorders. The degree of disability engendered by a chronic condition in an adolescent results from a combination of factors that include the actual degree of dysfunction resulting from the condition, the patient's perceived degree of dysfunction, the association of the condition with the stage of cognitive and of psychosocial development of the adolescent, and the perception of the condition by the patient's family, friends, and society in general. NHIS data revealed that 6.2% of the noninstitutionalized adolescent population had a chronic health condition that caused some limitation in daily activities. Nearly 4% had a major limitation of function, and 0.5% were unable to participate in a major activity such as work or school [3]. Condition categories most likely to be associated with disability included:

- Mental disorders, including mental retardation and substance abuse disorders (32%)
- Respiratory conditions such as asthma and bronchitis (21%)
- Musculoskeletal system or connective tissue diseases, including arthritis and limb deformities (15%)
- Central nervous system deformities, including epilepsy and cerebral palsy (6%)
- Ear and mastoid process conditions, predominantly hearing loss and deafness (4%)

These data also give us a picture of who has these problems. This is listed in Table 2. In this chapter, we attempt to convey an overall picture of the impact of chronic disorders on adolescents. Because teenagers with chronic disorders have more in common with each other than the differences they have due to their specific conditions [4], details of specific diseases are left to those chapters that deal with each disorder separately.

CHRONIC DISORDERS AND GROWTH AND DEVELOPMENT

To comprehend the impact of chronic illness or disability on an adolescent, an understanding of adolescent growth and development is mandatory (see Chapter 1). With such an understanding, the multiple impact of a chronic disorder becomes evident [5]. An adolescent is changing rapidly in all areas of life. The major physical changes of size increase and secondary sex characteristic differentiation occur primarily in early and middle adolescence. The significant cognitive changes (i.e., the transition into effective use of abstract thought) occur throughout adolescence. Changes in the way

TABLE 1. *Estimates of adolescents' chronic conditions*

General condition	Cases/1,000 adolescents (U.S.)
Respiratory allergies	130.3
Asthma	46.8
Frequent/severe headache	45.8
Eczema/skin allergies	35.2
Frequent/repeated ear infections	33.6
Other	30.0
Digestive allergies	21.1
Musculoskeletal impairments	20.9
Speech defects	18.9
Heart disease	17.4
Deafness and hearing loss	17.0
Blindness and visual impairments	16.0
Frequent diarrhea/bowel trouble	9.6
Arthritis	8.7
Anemia	5.8
Diabetes	1.5[a]
Cerebral palsy	1.2[a]
Sickle cell disease	0.9[a]

[a]Relative standard error exceeds 30% of estimate value.

Adapted from Newacheck PW, McManus MA, Fox HB. Prevalence and impact of chronic illness among adolescents. *American Journal of Diseases of Children* 1991;145:1367.

TABLE 2. *Sociodemographics of two groups suffering from chronic conditions*

	Physical conditions (per 100 cases)	Activity-limiting conditions (per 100 cases)
Source	NHIS, CHS, 1988	NHIS, 1984
Age		
Combined ages	31.5	6.2
10–13/10–14 y	31.0	6.6
14–17/15–18 y	31.9	5.7
Gender		
Male	32.1	7.2
Female	30.9	5.2
Race and ethnicity		
White	34.8	6.2
Black	23.7	6.2
Hispanic	24.0	6.7
Other	25.5	5.5
Poverty status		
Above poverty level	32.4	5.9
Below poverty level	30.1	8.6
Region		
Northeast	31.5	6.0
Midwest	33.0	6.3
South	28.0	6.5
West	35.5	6.0
Residence		
Metropolitan	28.8	6.3
Other	32.8	6.0

NHIS, National Health Interview Survey; CHS, Child Health Survey.

Adapted from Westbrook LE, Stein REK. Epidemiology of chronic health conditions in adolescents. *Adolescent Medicine: State of the Art Reviews* 1994;5:197.

adolescents view themselves and in the way they relate to others (i.e., psychosocial changes) are also occurring throughout adolescence. An adolescent without any significant health problems can have a difficult enough time coping with all these changes, which occur more or less concurrently. Consider the impact of a chronic health disorder on one or more of these components of development; the effect can be devastating, but with positive support from family, friends, and health professionals, adolescents with chronic conditions can do very well.

First, consider the effects of a chronic ailment on physical growth and development. During no other time in life does a person's body habitus grow and change faster than during puberty. These rapid changes depend on optimal health. Any compromise of the organism's ability to supply energy for these changes can delay them or compromise the final outcome. The conditions in which this delay and compromise of growth are most obvious are those such as sickle cell disease and cystic fibrosis. A lack of normal genetic programming can also compromise growth and development, as can be seen in Turner's syndrome. Although outcome may be normal, certain conditions can delay onset and progression of puberty. An example of such a condition is anorexia nervosa. Conversely, a chronic condition such as diabetes mellitus can be exacerbated by puberty. The hormonal flux of puberty decreases insulin sensitivity [6] and can, therefore, increase insulin requirements and decrease an adolescent's ability to control the disease.

The effects of chronic disorders on cognitive development usually are not as overt as in other areas of development. That may be due, in part, to our inability to measure changes in this area with as much sensitivity as in other areas of development. Some obvious conditions in which cognitive delays or deficiencies can be seen include learning disabilities, malnutrition, lead poisoning, untreated hypothyroidism, and conditions with increased intracranial pressure. Also, children who have intellectual deficiencies not very evident during latency may witness the emergence of those deficiencies when their peers are advancing into formal operational thought and they lag behind. More obvious lack of cognitive development may be evident in victims of head trauma. In addition, medications used to treat some conditions may cause learning difficulties [7].

The most sensitive sign of a problem in cognitive development usually is trouble in maintaining good grades in school. This difficulty frequently occurs when the adolescent is confronted with subjects that have a significant amount of abstract or conceptual content, such as geometry or literature. Neuropsychological testing can be very helpful in elucidating the specific disabilities and in suggesting methods of coping with or overcoming them [8,9].

The most pervasive effects of a chronic disorder usually are felt in the area of psychosocial development [10–15]. As the reader may recall from Chapter 1, the adolescent must be well on the road to achieving mastery of four tasks in order to enter adulthood in a fully functional state. These tasks are 1) effective separation from parents and achievement of the capability to function independently; 2) development of a realistic vocational goal; 3) development of a mature level of sexuality, both as one views oneself and as one relates to others; and 4) development of a realistic and positive self-image. Each adolescent's journey to adulthood can be divided into an early, a middle, and a late stage.

ISSUES THAT AFFECT ADOLESCENTS AND THEIR DISORDER

The impact of the adolescent's specific problem on psychosocial development depends on a number of factors:

- When in the patient's life the problem was acquired
- Whether the problem is progressive or static
- Whether the problem is constantly present or is episodic in occurrence and, if episodic, whether the occurrences are predictable
- The degree of difficulty imposed on daily life by the actual mechanics of coping with the chronic problem
- Whether the problem is visible and, if it is visible, to what degree the problem is disfiguring
- The attitudes of parents, siblings, and peers
- The way in which society views this particular type of problem
- The mechanisms used by the adolescent to cope with his or her problem
- The degree of medical care needed to deal with the problem

We review each of these factors and the way in which it affects psychosocial development.

Timing

The impact of a chronic disorder on an adolescent can vary significantly based on when the problem was acquired. For example, an adolescent may find it easier to cope with a problem that has been present since birth or early childhood than with a problem that has its onset in late childhood or during adolescence. Such an early start gives the teenager time to master the difficulties presented by the condition so that, on reaching adolescence, more effort can be expended on the usual problems that all youngsters encounter. Similarly, a problem that begins in late adolescence is easier to cope with than one that starts earlier in adolescence, because the teenager is well on the way to mastery of the four psychosocial tasks and because cognitive and physical development are nearing adult levels. More psychosocial resources, therefore, can be devoted to coping with the new problem, and those resources can be used in a more adult fashion.

Separation from Parents and Achieving Independence

A disorder that begins in early or middle adolescence, on the other hand, can have a major negative impact on the achievement of effective psychosocial development. The early adolescent is struggling ineffectively to achieve independence from his parents, but he works toward it nonetheless. As the child enters middle adolescence, he refines this effort into more intellectual areas and gravitates toward the peer group. A chronic disorder that begins at these times can severely retard the middle adolescent's efforts, making him more dependent on his parents and other adults. This is also true for the adolescent having a preexisting condition. For example, the adolescent with myelodysplasia probably is wheelchair bound and needs assistance in many activities of daily living. Through diligent effort, she can master some of these by herself, but many still require parental assistance. Her mobility is severely limited compared with her normal peers, and, therefore, her association with the peer group is severely compromised outside of school. Add to that her probable inability to control defecation, or the presence of an ostomy appliance with its unavoidable odors, and this adolescent's ability to spend time with peers is even more severely compromised [10–15].

Setting a Vocational Goal

In trying to achieve a realistic vocational goal, the adolescent with a chronic disorder is again at a significant disadvantage. If she has a seizure disorder, the jobs for which she can prepare may be severely limited. With a well controlled disorder, an adolescent may fantasize about a career as a pilot, for example, and, indeed, she may have all the skills and attributes necessary for such a career. However, her disability would make it impossible to achieve. She may choose to lie about having a disorder, but is she going to find a physician who will be a party to her deception when she fills out medical forms for her employment application? The time of onset of a disorder is significant in this area, although perhaps in a different manner than for achieving independence. Here it may be more advantageous to acquire a problem earlier in adolescence than later. This would give the youth more time to come to grips with the limitations placed on her by the disorder, whereas acquiring the problem later in adolescence could abort a whole career plan. For example, consider the 17-year-old who was a sure bet for a track or football scholarship until he contracted osteosarcoma and required an amputation. Adjusting to his new limitations will take a major effort.

Sexual Maturation

The adolescent with a chronic disorder faces problems in the area of sexuality as well. The early adolescent spends much of the energy in this area in fantasizing about ideal partners. For the normal adolescent, there is always the possibility that these dreams could come true, but what about the teenager with an ostomy? How compromised is his fantasy life because of his defect? When other middle adolescents are entering into the dating game, will this adolescent feel as if he can venture forth with the same vigor as his buddies? Usually not. As we discuss later, the visibility of the problem can have a significant impact on how the adolescent feels he can approach the area of intimacy, but, visible or not, he cannot help feeling that his capabilities in this area are compromised. If these problems are generated by a chronic disorder in early or middle adolescence, they do not fade away in late adolescence. This is the time when an adolescent should be entering into more intimate relationships in an adult fashion. A disorder that retards development in sexuality during early or middle adolescence has a profound impact on his ability to enter into relationships at this time. Similarly, a problem that has its onset in late adolescence can bring sexuality development to an abrupt halt, from which it will be extremely difficult to recover.

Forming a Healthy Self-Image

The task of developing a realistic and positive self-image is one that we pursue all our lives. During adolescence, however, a major portion of the effort is expended. The completion of puberty allows a realistic assessment of one's physical characteristics and, ideally, acceptance of one's perceived physical imperfections. In the same way, the maturation of one's ability to use formal operational thought in late adolescence allows the realistic appraisal of one's personality characteristics and, ideally, acceptance thereof. At each subsequent stage of life development, we reintegrate these impressions and come up with an adjusted self-appraisal, but our basic impression of ourselves occurs in adolescence, and it is at this time that we should begin to like what we see.

Consider the difficulties in achieving these goals for an adolescent with a chronic disorder. The key to acceptance of a defect or disease and subsequent achievement of a positive and realistic self-image may be the manner in which the patient is treated by those close to him or her. This is more fully discussed later in this chapter. Studies do show, however, that the self-concept of adolescents with chronic illness is not significantly different from that of normal adolescents [16–19].

The timing of the onset of a chronic disorder can markedly affect a person's ability to form a realistic and positive self-image. A disorder that predates adolescence can be incorporated into one's self-image before the upheavals of adolescence. One that begins early in adolescence can make the achievement of a realistic and positive self-appraisal of physical characteristics even more difficult than it normally is. Consequently, the usual fine tuning of the physical self-image during middle adolescence may be delayed or prevented. A disorder that occurs during middle adolescence can abort this whole process and push its resolution into a much later period of life. When a disorder has its onset in late adolescence, self-image can be destroyed and must be rebuilt, but at least cognitive maturity allows for easier acceptance and reintegration.

Progression of the Disorder

A known quantity is always easier to accept than one that is unknown. In the same way, a problem that occurs with predictability is easier to accept than one that catches its victim unaware. Thus, an adolescent who has a chronic problem such as a missing limb finds acceptance of the defect easier than one who has a problem such as a seizure disorder, which can emerge at any time. Similarly, an adolescent with asthma who knows what triggers her attacks and who is used to the severity of her condition finds acceptance of her condition easier than one who has cystic fibrosis, with its sporadic exacerbations and downhill course.

A static condition such as a missing limb enables the adolescent to master the skills needed to deal with the problem and then go on with development without having continually to learn new ways of coping, except those dictated by changing developmental needs. This allows quicker separation from dependence on parents, more ease in realistic self-appraisal and, therefore, realistic vocational choices, more ease in learning to enter intimate relations, and earlier development of a realistic and positive self-image. For an adolescent who has a condition that is nonprogressive but sporadic in occurrence, successful coping is more difficult. The fear generated by never knowing when the problem will surface makes development in all four task areas more difficult. Similarly, a condition with a progressive, downhill course requires considerable coping skills just to exist from day to day, let alone making significant progress in the four developmental tasks.

Visibility of the Disorder

It might be believed that coping with a visible defect is more difficult than coping with a condition that is not readily apparent to others. After all, being seen as obviously abnormal makes almost all daily encounters potentially difficult. However, children and adolescents with inapparent problems have just as much, if not more, difficulty coping than do those with more obvious disabilities.

Certainly, a visible disorder requires an initial effort on the patient's part to get used to facing the world successfully. Once that skill is mastered, however, the patient with a visible disorder can go on with the rest of development relatively unhindered. There is no question that such a patient will always have problems because of the visible defect—a port wine stain, for example. However, he or she knows how people will react and, one would hope, has developed the necessary skills to deal with such reactions. Adolescents in the early and middle stages of development have special difficulty with a visible defect because of their emerging awareness of their physical selves. Problems that were present before adolescence are usually less troublesome, but, regardless of when the disorder began, the teenager must cope if he or she wants to proceed with life.

This is not so for the adolescent with an inapparent problem. With a problem that no one can see, there is always the temptation to try to hide it, even to the point of denying that the problem exists. Adolescents with noninsulin-dependent diabetes mellitus have a particular problem in this area because they rarely, if ever, feel ill from their disease. They do not suffer from bouts of ketoacidosis, and they frequently question whether there is really anything wrong. Hypertension is a condition with similar dynamics. These invisible problems allow the adolescent to fantasize that he or she is absolutely normal, thereby compromising treatment compliance and also preventing the patient from successfully integrating the fact of his or her condition into his or her development. Dire consequences can result.

Degree of Disability

An obvious factor with considerable impact on the adolescent with a chronic disorder is the actual degree of disability engendered by his or her condition. An adolescent with an ostomy, for example, has much less difficulty proceeding with development than a peer with myelodysplasia. The sheer mechanics of everyday life dictate that the myelodysplasia patient will find existence, and therefore normal development, more difficult. Even so simple a difference as having to take an insulin injection once versus twice daily can have a major impact on an adolescent's life. The once-daily injection can be given in the morning so that the rest of the day is free for normal activities. The adolescent who must have a second shot, however, always has to adjust plans and activities to allow for that second injection. This can have myriad effects, including disruption of peer relationships and lack of compliance with therapy.

Youngsters who are wheelchair bound constantly face such difficulties. Public access laws have helped considerably, but many school buildings, for example, were constructed before public access for the handicapped was mandated. Therefore, adolescents who are wheelchair bound frequently can be with their peers only if their peers happen to have classes on the first floor of such buildings.

Attitudes of Others

The attitudes of significant others in an adolescent's life can have a major impact on that teenager's ability to cope successfully with his or her chronic disorder. Obviously, the greatest impact is from the attitudes of the parents. A possibly oversimplified way of stating the magnitude of the impact of parental attitudes is to say that if the parents treat the child as a child with a problem, he or she will have a much greater chance of achieving normality than if the parents treat him or her as a problem who happens to be a child. In other words, the more parents are able to allow their child to be normal and are able to facilitate their child's normal activities, the more normal that child will be.

Parental responses to their child's disorder can manifest in several ways. All of these responses are to be expected from any parent at one time or another. It is when responses that are detrimental to the child's development persist that the physician should become concerned and should contemplate intervention beyond simple education and reassurance. There is no doubt that parents are under considerable stresses in many ways when their child is chronically ill or disabled [5].

One response that all parents feel, especially when the child is first diagnosed with his or her disorder and when there are exacerbations, is *anxiety*. Anxiety manifests itself in several ways. An obvious one is simply excessive worrying by the parents. Another manifestation that can annoy health workers and detract from their effectiveness is overprotectiveness, with its attendant excessive contacts with the health care staff. This can generate hostility in the staff's attitude toward that parent and, possibly, toward the child as well. *Anger* in the parents that lingers longer than expected can also generate hostility among the staff unless the physician and others realize what is generating the anger—usually fear—and can help the parents deal with it. *Depression*, again an expected response at appropriate times, can cause parents to distance themselves from the care of their child. Parents may feel overwhelmed and ineffective. Noncompliance with care plans can result, so the physician and his or her staff must be ready to intervene when this response becomes evident.

Denial is necessary, to a degree, in both parents and the affected child. Frequently, use of denial is the only way that parents can make it from day to day and continue to function. It is when denial becomes pervasive and interferes with the care of their child that it becomes harmful, necessitating professional intervention. For example, one of the authors cared for a young man of 13 years who had a seizure disorder and who alternated living with his divorced parents. When he lived with his mother, his seizures were under excellent control. However, when he returned to his mother after a typical weekend stay with his father, he frequently would have seizures. It became apparent that his father could not cope with the idea of his son having epilepsy. He therefore directed his son to stop taking his medication when he arrived for the weekend because he really did not need the medicine. This caused the blood level of the medications to drop below the therapeutic level at approximately the time the boy arrived back at his mother's house on Sunday night.

The last aberrant response of parents to their chronically ill child is *guilt*. Feelings of guilt are almost universal among parents when they first confront the fact that their child has an unresolvable problem. With appropriate assurances by the physician and staff, these feelings resolve into a more realistic and functional state. When guilt persists, however, the parent can become ineffective or even detrimental to the child's welfare. Parents who have excessive guilt feelings can demonstrate them either by distancing from the patient or by becoming overprotective in an attempt to compensate for how they feel.

Many of these aberrant feelings can be prevented before they intrude on the parents' ability to care for their child, if the physician and staff initiate preventive counseling shortly after the diagnosis is made. By teaching parents to expect these emotions and by giving tips on how to live with and eventually overcome them, their excessive expression can be prevented.

Parents can also aid in the adolescent's achievement of appropriate independence by allowing the teenager the degree of independence commensurate with his or her ability to be independent. However, giving total control for the care of a chronic problem to an early adolescent (13- or 14-year-old) can be too much of a burden. It may be more appropriate for the parents to continue to aid their teenager in the care of the chronic problem until formal operational thought is somewhat more established, say at 16 or 17 years of age. That support during early adolescence may be crucial to later successful management of a chronic problem by an adolescent.

Coping Mechanisms

Adolescents use a variety of coping mechanisms to handle the stress of chronic illness (Table 3). *Denial* is one of the primary coping mechanisms used by adolescents who have a chronic disorder. This mechanism can be either harmful or helpful. It is helpful when it enables a teenager with cystic fibrosis, for example, to continue with as normal a life as possible in the face of almost certain early

TABLE 3. *Coping mechanisms of adolescents with chronic illness or disability*

Denial
Intellectualization
Regression
Depression, suicide
Acting out
Acceptance
Adjustment

demise. It becomes harmful when it allows an adolescent with diabetes to feel relatively invulnerable, thereby decreasing compliance with therapeutic diet, for instance.

Intellectualization is a defense mechanism by which emotionally troubling material is blocked from emotional consideration and is only dealt with intellectually. This method of coping with the stress of chronic illness or disability is most commonly found in early adolescents. As with some other coping mechanisms, intellectualization can be helpful in assisting teenagers to come to grips with their problems and eventually cope with them emotionally. In the extreme, it allows the adolescent to block out any negative emotions and, therefore, not overcome and effectively cope with them. A good example was a 13-year-old boy who had hydrocephalus with an effectively functioning shunt but also incapacitating headaches that prevented him from going to school. On questioning, it was found that he knew everything there was to know about hydrocephalus and shunts, and yet he was at a loss to explain the cause of his headaches. When asked about any ridicule he might have suffered at school because of his obviously larger-than-normal head, he acknowledged that that had indeed been a problem. Although he could readily state that the ridicule was a problem, he showed no emotion when discussing the issue and could not relate his headaches and subsequent school avoidance to the ridicule. A few sessions of counseling alleviated the immediate problem and helped prepare him for a successful return to school.

Regression is a common coping mechanism in patients of any age. It is particularly troublesome in adolescents who have yet to achieve feelings of mastery and control, and therefore are more prone to revert to childlike behaviors when under stress. The younger the adolescent, the more likely resorting to this mechanism will cause problems for the adults charged with his or her care. Helping an adolescent scale the heights of maturity so as to cope more effectively with a problem is best accomplished with patience, support, and firm limits, just as one would approach a younger child exhibiting similar behavior. In the long run, regression is best countered by assisting affected adolescents to achieve competence in everyday activities to the highest degree allowed by their disability and level of maturity.

Depression occurs with some consistency in adolescents with chronic illnesses or disabilities, but it is most often situational, as opposed to chronic. Effective coping with life's daily activities and successful interaction with peers help to avoid depression. Examples of factors that may predispose to chronic depression, expressed either by classic signs or by acting-out behaviors, include a visible deformity: a condition whose manifestations are sporadic and unpredictable (such as seizures); difficulty obtaining employment; difficulty interacting with the opposite sex; and difficulty obtaining a driver's license and insurance. Clinicians can assist in preventing or limiting such depression by aiding such youths in becoming successful in these mundane but extremely important aspects of their lives.

Acting-out behavior can occur sporadically in response to situational exacerbations of a chronic condition, or it can occur chronically as a manifestation of depression. Acting-out behavior can be viewed as one of the few ways a person who has not yet developed formal operational thought (i.e., a child) can express anxiety or depression. This kind of behavior is tolerated in small children, but it is disconcerting to adults when it comes from a young adolescent who, by physical appearance, looks more like an adult. This kind of behavior can be very damaging to a teenager because it manifests in ways that often are very harmful, such as inappropriate sexual behavior, substance abuse, school failure, and delinquent acts. Again, firm limits and early intervention can avoid much damage. Anticipation that these behaviors might occur and early intervention are the keys to avoiding potentially serious consequences.

TRANSITION ISSUES

Because most adolescents with chronic health conditions will enter adulthood [20], their need for care and resources will continue as well. The issues surrounding this "transition" into adulthood are called "transition issues." The major areas that need to be considered in this arena are:

- Medical care, both primary and specialty
- Sexuality
- Financial resources including health insurance
- Education and vocation
- Facilities for independent living

TABLE 4. *Rights of chronically ill or disabled adolescents*

The right to sexual expression
The right to privacy
The right to be informed
The right of access to needed services
The right to choose marital status
The right to choose whether to have children
The right to make decisions that affect one's own life
The right to develop one's fullest potential

Each of these areas should be considered and planned for at the beginning of care for any child or adolescent with a chronic condition [21]. One of the major problems is that there are not enough resources to allow a smooth transition for all affected adolescents. An example is the lack of adequate medical care by adult providers for adolescents with such conditions as cystic fibrosis or congenital heart disease. Pediatric providers end up caring for these patients well into their adulthood. Another area of concern is health insurance. How is an adolescent to pay for care if he or she cannot qualify for insurance because of a preexisting condition? This has been alleviated to some degree by recent federal legislation, but it still is a significant problem.

HEALTH CARE GOALS AND RIGHTS OF THE CHRONICALLY ILL OR DISABLED ADOLESCENT

Despite having to cope with the exigencies of a chronic health condition as well as with the challenges of normal adolescent growth and development, these youngsters do remarkably well in accepting their condition, adjusting to it, and in going on with their lives. Studies have shown that these teenagers are no more prone to psychological dysfunction than are their healthy peers [10,16,22–25]. What they do need is to be understood and accorded their rights (Table 4), and to receive specific assistance in managing practical issues and problems such as physical appearance, issues of sexuality [26,27], reintegrating into normal school activities, obtaining a driver's license, obtaining adequate insurance, getting a good job, and achieving success in relating to the opposite sex [28–30] (Table 5).

TABLE 5. *Goals of health care for adolescents with chronic health conditions*

Possession of enough information about one's disability to understand it
Opportunity to associate with nonhandicapped people of the same age
Opportunity to have some experience of living on one's own
Opportunity to learn about different occupations and careers
Chance to talk with someone about a personal problem
A work experience
Opportunity to participate in an educational program at each individual's level
Opportunity to do household tasks
Chance to talk with someone about physical abilities and disabilities
Opportunity to learn social graces
Opportunity to earn money
Opportunity to develop a hobby
Opportunity for a comprehensive sex education program

With help in these and other practical areas, adolescents with chronic health problems should be able to negotiate the transition into adult life with considerable success.

REFERENCES

1. Gode RO, Smith MS. Effects of chronic disorders on adolescent development: self, family, friends, and school. In: Smith MS, ed. *Chronic disorders in adolescence.* Littleton, MA: John Wright Publishing; 1983:31.
2. Newacheck PW, McManus MA, Fox HB. Prevalence and impact of chronic illness among adolescents. *American Journal of Diseases of Children* 1991;145:1367.
3. Newacheck PW. Adolescents with special health needs: prevalence, severity, and access to health services. *Pediatrics* 1989;84:872.
4. Stein REK, Bauman LJ, Westbrook LE, et al. Framework for identifying children who have chronic conditions: the case for a new definition. *J Pediatr* 1993;122:342.
5. Kaplan ME, Friedman SB. Reciprocal influences between chronic illness and adolescent developments. *Adolescent Medicine: State of the Art Reviews* 1994;5:211.
6. Caprio S, Pleeve G, Diamond MP, et al. Increased insulin secretion in puberty: a compensatory response to reduction in insulin sensitivity. *J Pediatr* 1989;114:963.
7. Okinow NA. Educational issues in adolescents with chronic illness. *Adolescent Medicine: State of the Art Reviews* 1994;5:223.
8. Rimel RW, Giordani B, Barth JT, et al. Disability caused by minor head injury. *Neurosurgery* 1981;9:221.
9. Gerring JP. Psychiatric sequelae of sever closed head injury. *Pediatr Rev* 1986;8:115.
10. Pless IB, Roghmann KJ. Chronic illness and its consequences: observations based on three epidemiologic surveys. *J Pediatr* 1971;79:351.
11. Boyle IR, di Sant Agnese PA, Sack S, et al. Emotional adjustment of adolescents and young adults with cystic fibrosis. *J Pediatr* 1976;88:318.
12. Kumar S, Powars D, Allen J, et al. Anxiety, self-concept, and personal and social adjustments in children with sickle cell anemia. *J Pediatr* 1963;88:859.
13. Macbriar BR. Self-concept of preadolescent and adolescent children with a meningomyelocele. *Issues in Comprehensive Pediatric Nursing* 1983;6:1.
14. McAnarney ER. Social maturation: a challenge for handicapped and chronically ill adolescents. *Journal of Adolescent Health Care* 1983;6:90.
15. Mulhern RK, Wasserman AL, Friedman AG, et al. Social competence and behavioral adjustment of children who are long-term survivors of cancer. *Pediatrics* 1989;83:18.
16. Lavigne JV, Faier-Routman J. Psychological adjustment to pediatric physical disorders: a meta-analytic review. *J Pediatr Psychol* 1992;17:133.
17. Kashani JH, Konig P, Shepperd JA, et al. Psychopathology and self-concept in asthmatic children. *J Pediatr Psychol* 1988;13:509.
18. Simmons RF, Corey M, Cowen L, et al. Emotional adjustment of early adolescents with cystic fibrosis. *Psychosom Med* 1985;47:111.
19. Ungerer JA, Horgan B, Chaitow J, et al. Psychosocial functioning in children and young adults with juvenile arthritis. *Pediatrics* 1988;81:195.
20. Blum RW. Transition to adult health care: setting the stage. *J Adolesc Health* 1995;17:3.
21. Rosen DS. Transition from pediatric to adult-oriented health care for the adolescent with chronic illness or disability. *Adolescent Medicine: State of the Art Reviews* 1994;5:241.
22. Cadman D, Boyle M, Szatmari, et al. Chronic illness, disability, and mental and social well-being: findings of the Ontario Child Health Study. *Pediatrics* 1987;79:805.
23. Seigel WM, Golden NH, Cough JW, et al. Depression, self-esteem, and life events in adolescents with chronic diseases. *Journal of Adolescent Health Care* 1990;11:501.
24. Weiland SK, Pless IB, Roghmann KJ. Chronic illness and mental health problems in pediatric practice: results from a survey of primary care providers. *Pediatrics* 1992;89:445.
25. Gortmaker SL, Walker DK, Weitzman M, et al. Chronic conditions, socioeconomic risks, and behavioral problems in children and adolescents. *Pediatrics* 1990;85:267.
26. Sawyer SM, Phelan PD, Bowes G. Reproductive health in young women with cystic fibrosis: knowledge, behavior and attitudes. *J Adolesc Health* 1995;17:46.
27. American Academy of Pediatrics Committee on Children with Disabilities. Sexuality education of children and adolescents with developmental disabilities. *Pediatrics* 1996;97:275.
28. Kellerman J, Zeltzer L, Ellenberg L, et al. Psychological effects of illness in adolescence: I. anxiety, self-esteem, and perception of control. *J Pediatr* 1980;97:126.
29. Stein REK, Jessop DJ, Russman CK. Health care services received by children with chronic illness. *American Journal of Diseases of Children* 1983;137:225.
30. Orr DP, Weller SC, Sattershite B, Pless IB. Psychological implications of chronic illness in adolescents. *J Pediatr* 1984;104:152.

SUGGESTED READING

American Academy of Pediatrics Committee on Children with Disabilities. Sexuality education of children and adolescents with developmental disabilities. *Pediatrics* 1996;97:275.

American Academy of Pediatrics Committee on Children with Disabilities and Committee on Adolescence. Transition of care provided for adolescents with special health care needs. *Pediatrics* 1996;98:1203.

Blum RW. Transition to adult health care: setting the stage. *J Adolesc Health* 1995;17:3.

Brown RT, Coupey SM, eds. Chronic and disabling disorders. *Adolescent Medicine: State of the Art Reviews* 1994;5:1.

5

Adolescent Sexuality And
Health-Related Problems

HISTORICAL PERSPECTIVE AND THE ROLE OF THE HEALTH PROFESSIONAL

No single aspect of adolescence alarms adult society more than the prospect of young people engaging in sexual activity, particularly sexual intercourse [1]. Complaints have been registered since the earliest recorded history: in the 8th century BC, the Egyptian historian Hesiod lamented, "I see no hope for the future of our people if they are dependent on the frivolous youth of today, for certainly all youth are reckless beyond words .... When I was a boy, we were taught to be discreet and respectful of elders, but the present youth are exceedingly wise and impatient of restraint " [2]. Several centuries later, Aristotle complained that "in regard to sexual desire, [teenagers] exercise no restraint" [3]. And in *The Winter's Tale*, Shakespeare wrote: "I wish there were no age between ten and three-and-twenty, or that youth would sleep out the rest; for there is nothing in the between but getting wenches with child, wronging the ancientry, stealing, fighting" [4].

Although adults—particularly physicians—are all too cognizant of the risks that premature sexual intercourse involves, teenagers often do not comprehend that pregnancy and sexually transmitted disease (STD) may follow even the first episode of intercourse. Their unique psychology and idiosyncratic thinking make them immune to such worries, but, unfortunately, not to the inevitable consequences of their sexual activity.

The United States has the highest rate of teenage pregnancy and abortion in the industrialized Western world (Fig. 1), despite the fact that American teenagers are no more sexually active than their European counterparts [5–7]. In fact, Sweden has one-third and The Netherlands one-sixth the U.S. teen pregnancy rate despite comparable levels of teenage sexual activity [8]. Overall, this amounts to over one million teenage pregnancies in the United States annually, with about 50% ending in live births, 35% in abortions, and 14% in miscarriages [9,10]. One in 10 female teenagers becomes pregnant each year in the United States and, at present rates, 4 in 10 will become pregnant while still in their teens [11]. This translates into 2,800 adolescents becoming pregnant each day, with 1,300 giving birth, 1,100 having an abortion, and 400 miscarrying [12]. Of concern is the number of births to girls younger than 15 years of age, which has risen to 12,554 in 1993 [10,13]. (Note that teenage pregnancy figures usually include young women up through the age of 19, an age when many of them are married.)

The figure of one million American teenagers is appallingly high, but not necessarily accurate [14]. In fact, the teenage pregnancy rate has either increased or decreased in the past two decades, depending on the method of calculation. If the rate is calculated using *all* teenage women aged 15 to 19 years, the rate has increased 23% from 1972 to 1990; but if only sexually experienced 15- to 19-year-olds are considered, the rate has decreased 19% [9]. Overall, the teen pregnancy rate was highest in the 1950s and has now levelled off (Table 1). The difference is that in 1960, only 15% of all teen births occurred outside of marriage, whereas in 1993 72% were nonmarital [13].

A number of important observations can be made concerning teenage sexual activity and its consequences:

- More than 80% of Americans first have sexual intercourse as teenagers, but most teens wait until middle or late adolescence [8] (Tables 2, 3).
- The average age at first intercourse is 15 to 16 for boys and approximately 1 year later for girls in the United States [9,15,16] (Tables 4, 5).

151

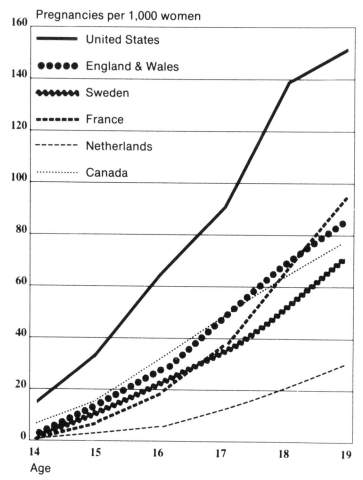

FIG. 1. Adolescent pregnancy rates: United States vs. other Western nations. The United States has the highest teenage pregnancy rate in the Western world, despite the fact that American teenagers' rate of sexual activity does not differ from that of their European peers. Lack of comprehensive sex education in schools, relative unavailability of birth control, and inappropriate portrayals of sexuality in the media are all important contributing factors. (Trussel J. Teenage pregnancy in the United States. *Fam Plann Perspect* 1988;20:264. Copyright 1988. Reprinted with permission of the Alan Guttmacher Institute.)

TABLE 1. *Teen birth rate (per 1,000 15- to 19-year-olds)*

1955	1975	1980	1985	1990	1991	1993	1994
90	56	53	51	60	62	60	59

From National Center for Health Statistics. *Advance report of final natality statistics, 1994.* Hyattsville, MD: NCHS; 1996.

TABLE 2. *Teenage sexual activity*

| | | Age | | | | | |
| | | 13 | | 15 | | 17 | |
	N	M	F	M	F	M	F
Zelnik and Kantner (1979)	1,717	14%	2%	35%	19%	52%	44%
Harris et al. (1986)	1,000	11%	10%	35%	22%	57%	53%
National Survey of Adolescent Males (Sonenstein FL, et al. 1988)	1,880	—	—	33%	—	66%	—
Minnesota (Blum, 1989)	36,284	17%	11%	29%	26%	57%	45%
National Household Survey (Leigh BC, et al. 1990)	536	6%	3%	29%	37%	67%	56%
National Longitudinal Survey of Youth (Mott FL, et al. 1992)	1,825	15%	3%	35%	27%	72%	66%
Youth Risk Behavior Survey (CDC, 1993)	16,296	—	—	44%	32%	60%	55%
Youth Risk Behavior Survey (CDC, 1995)	10,904	13%	5%	41%	32%	60%	57%

Adapted from Zelnik M, Kantner JF. Sexual activity, contraceptive use, and pregnancy among metropolitan-area teenagers: 1971–1979. *Fam Plann Perspect* 1980;12:230; Harris L, and Associates. *American teens speak: sex, myths, TV, and birth control*. New York: Planned Parenthood Federation of America; 1986; Sonenstein FL, Pleck JH, Leighton CK. Sexual activity, condom use and AIDS awareness among adolescent males. *Fam Plann Perspect* 1989;21:152; Blum RW. *The state of adolescent health in Minnesota*. Minneapolis: University of Minnesota; 1989; Leigh BC, Morrison DM, Trocki K, et al. Sexual behavior of American adolescents: results from a U.S. national survey. *J Adolesc Health* 1994; 15:117; Mott FL, Fondell MM, Hu PN, et al. The determinants of first sex by age 14 in a high-risk adolescent population. *Fam Plann Perspect* 1996;28:13; Centers for Disease Control and Prevention. Youth risk behavior surveillance: United States, 1993. *MMWR Morb Mortal Wkly Rep* 1995;44(SS-1):1; and Centers for Disease Control and Prevention. Youth risk behavior surveillance: United States, 1995. *MMWR Morb Mortal Wkly Rep* 1996;45(SS-4):1.

- Since the 1970s, the percentage of sexually active teens has climbed dramatically, from 29% to 52% for girls age 15 to 19 years, and from 55% to 83% for boys age 18 years [15,17] (see Table 3). For certain high-risk populations, the percentages are even higher (Table 6). Even more worrisome, some national data indicate that 9% of 12-year-olds and 16% of 13-year-olds are sexually active [9].
- However, during the 1990s, percentages of sexually active youth have stabilized [17–19] (Table 7). In addition, an increasing number of sexually active teens are using condoms (Fig. 2). Therefore, live birth rates have declined 2% and rates of gonorrhea have decreased 20% for boys and 13% for girls [17].

TABLE 3. *Sexual behavior among U.S. high school students, 1995 (N = 10,904)*

| | Ever had sexual intercourse | | Currently sexually active[a] | | Four or more lifetime sex partners | | Condom use at last sex | |
Grade	F	M	F	M	F	M	F	M
9th	32%	41%	22%	24%	7%	18%	59%	66%
10th	46%	50%	35%	32%	11%	20%	52%	68%
11th	60%	57%	48%	37%	17%	21%	49%	57%
12th	66%	67%	52%	48%	21%	25%	43%	57%

[a]Sexual intercourse during the 3 months before the survey.
From Centers for Disease Control and Prevention. Youth risk behavior surveillance: United States, 1995. *MMWR Morb Mortal Wkly Rep* 1996;45(SS-4):1.

TABLE 4. *Age at first sexual intercourse for rural and urban students (among adolescents ever having had sexual intercourse)*

	Girls	Boys
10–11 y	6.4%	14.5%
12–13 y	17.0%	22.0%
14–15 y	42.8%	37.6%
16–17 y	33.2%	25.0%
Median age at first intercourse	14.6 y	14.0 y

Adapted from Blum RW. *The state of adolescent health in Minnesota.* Minneapolis: University of Minnesota; 1989.

TABLE 5. *Age of first intercourse in an urban population (N =1,602)*

Ever had intercourse?	59%
Age at first intercourse	
<12 y	17%
12–13 y	24%
14–15 y	37%
≥16 y	22%
Total	100%

From Centers for Disease Control and Prevention. Miami youth risk behavior survey, 1993. *MMWR Morb Mortal Wkly Rep* 1994; 43:873.

TABLE 6. *Sexual behaviors in a high school versus a high-risk adolescent population*

Behavior	Regular high school sample (N = 1602)	Drop-out prevention school students (N = 77)
No. sex partners in past 3 mo		
0	33%	35%
1	47%	26%
≥2	20%	33%
Used condom at last intercourse	56%	43%
Used alcohol at last intercourse	14%	33%
Been pregnant or gotten someone pregnant		
1×	5.3%	24%
≥2×	1.6%	3%

From Centers for Disease Control and Prevention. Miami youth risk behavior survey, 1993. *MMWR Morb Mortal Wkly Rep* 1994; 43:873.

TABLE 7. *Trends in adolescent sexual activity during the 1990s*

Behavior	1990 (N =11,631, grades 9–12)	1993 (N =16,296, grades 9–12)
Ever had intercourse	54%	53%
Four or more partners	19%	19%
Intercourse in past 3 months	39%	38%
Used oral contraceptives at last intercourse	15%	18%
Used condoms at last intercourse	—	53%[a]

[a]46% in 1991.
From Centers for Disease Control and Prevention. Trends in sexual risk behavior among high school students: United States, 1990, 1991, and 1993. *MMWR Morb Mortal Wkly Rep* 1995;44:124.

- Despite some people's perceptions that teenagers want nothing more than to have babies and receive welfare checks, an estimated 85% to 95% of teen pregnancies are unintended [7,9].
- Teen pregnancies are expensive; they cost American taxpayers an estimated $30 billion a year in public funding support [12]. By contrast, all contraceptive methods are extremely cost effective compared with no contraception [20].

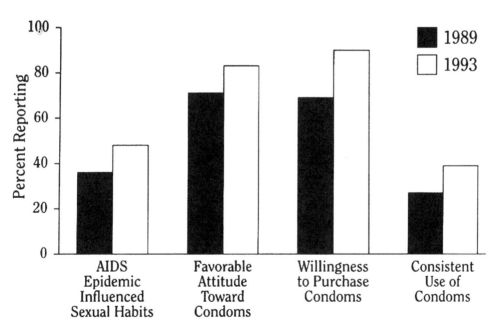

FIG. 2. Increased condom use among college students, 1989 to 1993, at one university. (Data from Nicholson ME, Wang MO, Mahoney BS, et al. Sexual behavior, contraception, condom use and intent to use condoms: five year trends. Presented at the 121st annual meeting of the APHA, October 25–27, 1993, San Francisco, California. Reproduced with permission from *The Contraception Report* 1994;IV(6):7.)

- New research indicates that adult men father more than 50% of babies born to women aged 15 to 17 years [13]. A California study put the figure even higher, at 70% [21].
- Although adolescent women account for one fifth of all abortions, their abortion rate (per 1,000 women aged 15–44 years) has dropped considerably, from 32.6 in 1972 to 20.2 in 1993 [22]. (These can be confusing data, however; the way they are computed is crucial. For example, if the abortion rate is calculated using abortions per 1,000 girls aged 15–19 years, then the rate rises from 22.8 in 1973 to a high of 43.5 in 1985, and drops to 37.6 in 1991 [13].) Expressed in a different way, young women's share of abortions to all women has dropped from 25.5% in 1987 to 21.5% in 1995 [23]. Women aged 20 to 24 years have the highest share, 33% of all abortions. Of particular note is that nearly 60% of women undergoing abortions have been using a contraceptive that failed [23.].

Epidemiology of Teen Sex

Accurate data about teenage sexual activity and sexual practices have always been difficult to find. For example, the pioneering work of Hopkins epidemiologists Zelnik and Kantner, in the 1970s, could not be continued in the 1980s because of lack of federal funding. Their 1979 survey revealed that by age 17 years, 52% of boys and 44% of girls had experienced sexual intercourse [24] (see Table 2). However, nearly 42% of the sexually active teens had *not* had intercourse within the 4 weeks before being interviewed for the survey, and another 25% of the girls had had intercourse only once or twice [13]. Hence, the episodic nature of teen sex was confirmed.

Several small surveys were conducted in the 1980s [5,6,24–31] (see Table 2). All except the 1988 National Survey of Adolescent Males and the 1989 Minnesota survey suffer from small numbers, and none was conducted exclusively to obtain sexual activity data.

In the 1990s, the Centers for Disease Control and Prevention's Youth Risk Behavior Survey (YRBS) added considerably to our knowledge of adolescent sexual behavior [17,19,32] (see Tables 2, 3, 5–7). This is a nationally selected sample, but individual communities have occasionally used the survey as well. However, the national YRBS includes high school youth only, so that our knowledge of very young teenagers is limited. In the Minnesota study, conducted in the late 1980s by Blum and colleagues [30], the age at first intercourse was extremely low (see Table 4). More recently, a Miami YRBS sample found similar results [32] (see Table 6). The Minnesota study also confirmed the sporadic nature of teen sexual activity, with 75% of teens reporting intercourse either rarely (a few times per year or less) or occasionally (one to four times per month) [30]. Likewise, in the YRBS study, the incidence of sexual intercourse drops from about one half of all high school teens in 1995 to one third if only the most recent 3 months preceding the survey are examined [17] (see Table 3).

A trend seems to be developing toward a leveling-off of rates for sexual intercourse among middle and older teens [18]. In addition, according to the YRBS, more teens are using condoms; however, this was due primarily to use among girls and African Americans only [17,18]. Sex with multiple partners also has leveled off at about 18% of all teens reporting having had sex, according to the YRBS data [17].

How sexually active are sexually active teenagers? Here, there seems to be a significant difference among girls versus boys. One study found that sexually experienced young women wait nearly 18 months between their first intercourse and the time they have a second partner [33]. However, several studies reveal a worrisome and significant increase in numbers of sexual partners for boys and, to a lesser extent, for female teens as well. From 1971 to 1988, the proportion of sexually active female teens reporting having had only one partner decreased from 62% to 39% [33]. Those reporting four to six partners or more increased from 14% to 31% [33]. In a second study of urban teens, most sexually active students had had two or more partners, with 36% of boys (but only 7% of girls) reporting six or more sexual partners [34]. In a third study, male adolescents aged 15 to 19 years reported having had an average of five sexual partners [35]. Apparently, if the term *promiscuity* is to be used, it is still best reserved for male adolescents, not female adolescents.

Teen Sexual Practices

Adolescent sexuality is not a problem, but rather a part of the human condition: sexuality is indigenous to all human beings and begins in utero, with the differentiation into male and female. In fact, ultrasonographs have demonstrated that male fetuses have spontaneous erections as early as the 18th week of gestation [36]. Only when sexuality becomes expressed in terms of intercourse at an early age do the medical and emotional risks begin to add up.

Not surprisingly, if data on sexual intercourse are difficult to find, data on other teenage sexual practices are even scarcer. Yet, a better understanding of sexual activities short of intercourse might enable health professionals to counsel teenagers more effectively about how to avoid pregnancies and STDs. A 1984 study of 1,067 teenagers nationwide found that [26]:

- Approximately 20% of 13-year-olds, 40% of 15-year-olds, and 60% of 17-year-olds of both sexes had engaged in vaginal play.
- Over 40% of 17- to 18-year-old girls reported performing fellatio; and nearly a third of 17- to 18-year-old boys reported performing cunnilingus.
- Interestingly, 72% of the boys enjoyed receiving oral sex, and 58% enjoyed giving it; whereas only 49% of girls similarly enjoyed receiving oral sex, and 28% enjoyed giving it. In addition, for 16% of the respondents, oral sex was not accompanied by subsequent intercourse.
- Ninety-three percent of boys and 70% of girls report enjoying intercourse "a large amount" or "a great deal"; but 36% of girls reported sometimes finding intercourse painful, 24% reported difficulties having orgasms, and 24% also reported difficulty with lubrication. (Only one other study has addressed the issue of whether female adolescents have orgasms—in Haas' study of 600 Southern Californian 15- to 18-year-olds in 1979, 42% of the girls surveyed reported having had an orgasm, 25% never had, and 33% were unsure [37].)

A more recent study of 366 San Francisco teenagers (mean age, 17 years) also found high rates of oral sex (80% of both sexes engaged in oral receptive sex; 71% of girls and 91% of boys engaged in giving oral sex) [38]. Such data seem to reflect that adolescents engage in a wide variety of experimental sexual behaviors and that simple petting or "outer-course" is not a very viable solution as an alternative to intercourse [39]. Although some groups of teenagers move through a logical progression from kissing to noncoital behaviors to intercourse, some lower-income teens move quickly from kissing to intercourse [40].

A 1994 national Roper telephone survey of 503 high school students in grades 9 to 12 found the following [16]:

- Nearly all the students had engaged in kissing (90%) or "deep kissing" (78%).
- Seven in 10 (72%) had engaged in touching above the waist; over half (54%) in touching below the waist.
- More than one in seven teens had engaged in mutual masturbation (15%).
- More than half of the seniors (55%) had experienced intercourse. The average age at first intercourse was just under 15 years of age, and 40% of all the sexually active teens had had sex at age 14 or younger.
- Three fourths of the students reported having sex in their parents' home.
- As in other studies [26,41,42], these teens felt that the ideal age to begin having sex (18.3 years) was considerably older than their average age for actually beginning relations (14.8 years).

Most recently, a 1996 study of more than 2,000 urban students in grades 9 to 12 examined the sexual activities of virginal teens. Many had engaged in heterosexual masturbation of a partner or oral sex [43] (Table 8).

TABLE 8. *Sexual practices of virginal high school teenagers*

Group	N	Masturbation of partner	Masturbation by partner	Fellatio with ejaculation	Cunnilingus	Anal intercourse
Male	385	30%	31%	11%	9%	1%
Female	432	29%	31%	8%	12%	<0.5%
Grade						
9th	255	25%	27%	7%	7%	1%
10th	242	33%	36%	12%	11%	1%
11th	176	30%	30%	8%	10%	0%
12th	135	31%	33%	10%	15%	1%

Adapted from Schuster MA, Bell RM, Kanouse DE. The sexual practices of adolescent virgins: genital sexual activities of high school students who have never had vaginal intercourse. *Am J Public Health* 1996;86:1570.

A few smaller American studies and one large Canadian study have highlighted other sexual practices that have important implications for preventing the spread of acquired immunodeficiency syndrome (AIDS). For example, a study of 74 affluent New York 12th grade students and 172 inner-city youth attending an adolescent clinic found that a surprising 27% of the latter group reported having had anal intercourse (vs. 7% of the upper middle class students). More important, 70% of the teenagers reported never using condoms during such intercourse [44]. The National Survey of Adolescent Males in 1988 and 1991 showed lower rates of anal intercourse (9% in the previous year), but, again, 60% of boys failed to use condoms [15]. A San Francisco study also confirmed sizeable rates of anal sex, with 20% of girls and 12% of boys reporting at least one episode of anal intercourse, and 7% of teens reporting sexual relations with someone who had had a same-sex encounter [38]. In a Baltimore survey of 351 African-American youth, 35% of the sexually active girls and 24% of the boys had experienced anal intercourse [39].

In Canada, a 1990 survey of over 5,500 first-year college students (mean age, 19.7 years) revealed that 14% of the men and 18% of the women had experienced anal intercourse, yet less than 25% of the men and 16% of the women used a condom regularly during intercourse. Even more alarming, the subgroup of both men and women who had more than 10 partners had higher rates of anal intercourse (27% and 35%, respectively), yet they had lower rates of condom use (21% and 7%, respectively). This group had also experienced a much higher rate of STDs—11% of the men and 24% of the women, compared with 5.5% of the less sexually promiscuous group [45].

How honest are young people with each other when it comes to divulging their sexual histories? Among college students in southern California, a 1990 survey revealed that many of the 665 men and women admitted to being dishonest in their dating practices, another factor that may have important implications for the spread of STDs [46] (Table 9).

One disturbing finding is that the younger a girl is at first intercourse, the greater the chances that she had involuntary or forced sex [47]. In the Guttmacher report, 74% of female teens having sex before age 14 years reported that it was involuntary [9]. In the Roper high school sample, 10% of teens reported a sexual experience in which they did not give consent [16]. Sexual assault is one of the fastest-growing crimes in the United States, with an annual incidence of 80 per 100,000 women and a peak incidence among 16- to 19-year-olds [48,49]. Acquaintance rape and date rape account for 70% to 80% of rape crisis center contacts [50]. Aside from the significant medical, legal, and moral aspects of sexual assault, data also indicate that girls who have been sexually abused as children or young teenagers may be more likely to become pregnant during adolescence [9,51,52] or begin having sex earlier [47].

Estimates of homosexuality among adolescents are notoriously scarce and probably unreliable. Although it is commonly stated that 10% of male and 5% of female teenagers are homosexual in orientation, these are figures originally derived from Kinsey and colleagues' 1940 survey of over 10,000 men and women [53]. Two conflicting factors make estimating homosexual behavior among teenagers difficult [54]: experimentation with the same sex is common during adolescence, but same-sex orientation probably begins even before then [55]. In the Minnesota study—which represents the largest sampling to date—90% of boys and 83% of girls viewed themselves as being exclusively heterosexual, and only 1% of 12th grade boys and less than 1% of 12th grade girls viewed themselves as being mostly or completely homosexual. At the same time, over 10% of the teens were unsure about their

TABLE 9. *College students and dating honesty*

	Men (N = 196)	Women (N = 226)
Have lied in order to have sex?	34%	10%
Sexually involved with more than one person	32%	23%
Partner did not know	68%	59%
Would lie about human immunodeficiency virus test	20%	4%
Would understate number of previous partners	47%	42%

Adapted from Cochran SD, Mays VM. Sex, lies and HIV. *N Engl J Med* 1990;322:774.

sexual orientation [30,56]. Similar results were found in the national Roper poll of high school students, with only 2% reporting that they had a sexual experience with someone of the same sex [16].

Why Teens Have Sex

Is teen sex a normal developmental milestone, a transition-marking behavior, or a risk-taking behavior? The answer is all three, depending on the kind of activity and the maturity of the individuals involved [57]. Ideally, sexual intercourse occurs in the context of a committed, mature emotional relationship—a developmental milestone normally not attained until late adolescence (18–21 years) or later. Female teenagers seem to subscribe to this philosophy, but, unfortunately, their concept of being "in love" does not coincide with the adult version: in Coles' survey, 52% of all the respondents believed that they had been in love by age 13, and 84% by age 18 years [26]! In the recent Roper poll, 71% of female adolescents claim that they were in love with their last sexual partner (compared with only 45% of boys) [16].

Popular media—especially soap operas and teen magazines—may contribute to these notions, and young girls are especially fond of both [42,58–60]. In a 1996 study of American soap operas, researchers found an average of six sexual behaviors depicted per hour, but only 10% involved discussion of consequences or birth control [59]. Most adults recognize the influence of peers on teenagers, but few appreciate that television and other media function as a kind of "super-peer" [58].

Alternatively, teenagers simply may have not met the right partner or been asked to have sex. In a small Connecticut study, only one third of 15-year-olds said that they did not feel emotionally ready for sexual intercourse [61].

Certainly, despite the perception that "everyone is doing it," teenagers have begun to display their own brand of conservatism about sex: in the Coles study, half of the girls wanted to be "virgins" at marriage, and a Baltimore study of 3,500 junior and senior high school students found that 32% of the boys and 39% of the girls thought that premarital sex is wrong [26,41]. Most recently, a national sample of teens cited 18 years of age as the ideal age to begin having sex (actually, the virgins suggested age 19, whereas the sexually experienced teens suggested age 17) [16]. Inevitably, teens seem to acknowledge that they (or their peers) are beginning to have sexual intercourse at too young an age.

Some Important Factors Affecting a Teenager's Choice

What are the important determinants of a teenager's decision to begin or delay having sexual relations? Sexual intercourse holds a number of possible attractions [57,61,62]:

1. Gaining a sense of physical attractiveness
2. Attaining more mature, adult status
3. Asserting a sense of independence and autonomy
4. Testing one's capability for intimacy
5. Testing one's "new" body
6. Flaunting social conventions
7. Providing a sense of "intimacy" and closeness for teens who cannot find it in other ways
8. Feeling good

Interestingly, teenagers with chronic disabilities are just as likely to be sexually active as their healthy peers, regardless of whether they have visible or invisible chronic conditions [63]. This makes perfect sense in light of the aforementioned reasons why teens begin to have sex in the first place.

In Jessor and Jessor's landmark study of 900 high school and college students, followed prospectively for 4 years to examine the transition from virginity to intercourse, the following characteristics emerged from the sexually active group [64]:

• Less expectation of and value attached to achievement
• More tolerance of differences between themselves and others
• Less religiosity
• Greater likelihood of having friends whose views differed from their parents' views
• Greater influence exerted by their peers
• More rigid parents
• Greater use of alcohol and marijuana

The overall picture adds up to increased nonconformity and influence by peers, lower academic expectations, and diminished parental influence (Tables 10, 11). Certainly, the notion of sexual intercourse—particularly unprotected intercourse—as a risk-taking behavior is appealing to many theorists and has much data to support it [61,65–75]. For example, one survey of over 12,000 young men and women, aged 14 to 22 years, confirmed the association between drug use and early onset of intercourse, particularly for marijuana [74]. In many studies, drug use seems to represent a particularly significant marker for early sexual activity and other high-risk sexual behavior [65,67,68,74,75].

In the most recent study, teens using drugs at an early age were found to be twice as likely to have sex before age 14 years, although the type of drug differed (cigarettes for girls; alcohol for boys) [74]. More frequent male users of cocaine or alcohol were also more likely to have caused a pregnancy [75].

Another recent finding is that high school students involved in fights are far more likely to engage in many other risky behaviors, including sex with multiple partners and unprotected sex [72]. Other researchers have found an association between very early sexual intercourse and academic risk, gang involvement, and a history of mental health treatment [69–71]. Only among African-American youth is this association in dispute [76]. Finally, a recent comprehensive study of adolescents' media consumption found a link between certain media (e.g., heavy metal music) and risk-taking behaviors [77].

The Influence of the Changing American Family

Early sexual activity must also be viewed in the context of the changing American family. Adolescents have a special need for closeness, and if that need is not being met at home, they may seek alternative ways of fulfilling it. Several studies have implicated divorce, family instability, poor communications with parents, and poverty [28,42,78–85]:

- In one study, white teenagers in fatherless families were 60% more likely to be sexually active [78]. In another study, daughters in white, single-parent (female) households were more likely to begin sex before age 15 years and have multiple partners [79].
- Beginning in the 1970s and extending now into the 1990s, black teenagers have had higher rates of sexual activity and pregnancy than white or Hispanic teens [28,74,86].
- Several studies have found that a teenager's unhappiness at home, or her feelings of alienation from her mother, have correlated with an earlier age at first intercourse and with having multiple partners [80,85]. Feeling misunderstood or ignored by one's parents may lead some teenagers to experiment with sex at a young age [82,87]. Conversely, good communication seems to have a protective effect. Many studies have found that teens who can communicate with their parents about sexual issues are less likely to have early intercourse [88–91], multiple partners [91–93], or unprotected sex [91–95].

TABLE 10. *Why teenagers do not delay sex*

Reasons given	Total teenagers ($N = 1,000$)	Boys ($n = 513$)	Girls ($n = 486$)
Social pressure	**61%**		
Peer pressure	30%	26%	34%
Everyone is doing it	12%	10%	14%
Boys talk/pressure girls into it	9%	2%	17%
Feelings	**55%**		
Curiosity	15%	16%	14%
In love with partner	8%	6%	11%
Sexual gratification	8%	10%	5%
Want to feel grown up	7%	7%	7%
Other			
Influenced by media	3%	4%	2%
Want to have baby	1%	1%	1%

Adapted from Harris L, and Associates. *American teens speak: sex, myths, TV, and birth control.* New York: Planned Parenthood Federation of America; 1986.

TABLE 11. *Sexually active teenagers and their perceived relationships with their parents*

Relationship	Sexually active
Mother + Father +	6.4%
Mother − Father −	37.5%
Mother + Father −	44.0%
Mother − Father +	66.7%

Adapted from Welches LJ. Adolescent sexuality. In Mercer R, ed. *Perspectives on adolescent health care.* Philadelphia: JB Lippincott, 1979:29.

This may have important implications for preventing not only early intercourse and pregnancy, but human immunodeficiency virus infection and other STDs.

- Rates of sexual intercourse increase among teens whose mothers had a teenage pregnancy themselves, were married young, or were divorced and remarried [74,81]. Such mothers seem to have more tolerant views about premarital sex (having experienced it themselves) and are therefore more likely to have children who are sexually active [42]. In fact, there may be a kind of intergenerational "tradition" of teen pregnancy, particularly within the African-American community [96–99]. In one study of the children of teen mothers, one fourth of the girls and 11% of the boys had become teen parents themselves, and half were sexually active before age 14 years [98].

- A new study found that both female and male siblings of parenting teenagers have fewer qualms about early childbearing and, for girls, greater intentions of having a child at a younger age [100].

Socioeconomic Level, Academic Ability, Religion, and Race

The 1986 Harris Report, which surveyed a representative national sample of 1,000 adolescents, found that sexual intercourse was highest among [27]:

- Teens whose parents were not college graduates
- Teens with poor school grades
- African-American teens

A later and larger national study of over 13,000 high school sophomores found that just three factors could explain teenagers' willingness to have children outside of marriage: 1) socioeconomic level, 2) academic ability, and 3) being raised in a single-mother household [101]. Sexual activity—and certainly, teenage pregnancy—may, in fact, be more determined by socioeconomic factors than personality, religion, or race. Clearly, poorer teens are more likely to begin having sex at an early age and less likely to use contraception [102].

Traditionally, religiosity and self-esteem have been implicated in early teenage sexual behavior [42], but this may represent adults' wishful thinking more than actual fact. Even conservative religious youth show surprisingly high rates of sexual intercourse: one study of 1,438 "born-again" teenagers found that 43% were sexually active by 18 years of age [103]. In the most recent study, church attendance was an important predictor of delayed sexual activity, but only when the teen's friends attended the same church [74]. Studies seem to indicate that school success and academic performance correlate negatively with early sexual activity, whereas risk-taking behaviors are more positively correlated [42,69,104]. However, "school self-esteem" seems to far outweigh "home self-esteem" or "peer self-esteem" as a predictive factor [105].

Peer Pressure

What role does that old adolescent bugaboo, peer pressure, play in teenage sexual activity? Many teenagers think that everyone is having intercourse except them. In the Roper poll, more than half of all the teens surveyed thought that their friends were sexually active [16]. Of course, this could represent more rationalization than actual etiology: in Coles and Stokes' study, for example, 78% of the virgins thought their friends were virgins, whereas 72% of the nonvirgins thought their friends were sexually active, too [26]. But some teens *do* report social pressure and peer pressure as being two key reasons for their beginning sexual intercourse early [27].

The Influence of the Media

Interestingly, in the Roper poll more teens felt pressure from the media to begin having sex (17%) than from friends (4%) or partners (6%) [16]. Television and movies may constitute a sort of super-peer pressure on adolescents. In the 1996 Kaiser study, one third of teenagers reported that they felt current media encouraged teenagers to become sexually active [106]. Some of the messages contained in the media include [58,60,107]:

• Sex is fun; seemingly everyone is doing it.
• Having sex has few if any risks.
• Extramarital sex and premarital sex are common.
• No one talks or worries much about contraception, or the risks of pregnancy or STD.

Every year, the average American teenager views nearly 14,000 sexual references, innuendoes, and behaviors, but less than 175 of these refer to birth control or abstinence [108]. Among prime-time TV characters, one in four interactions involves some aspect of sex [106]. Only four studies have examined the link between television and early or unprotected sexual activity, but all four have found an association [109–112]. When sex is used to sell everything from beer to perfume to hotel rooms, teenagers begin to think that having sex, even at a young age, is normative behavior [107]. At the same time, one "solution" to early sexual activity—contraception—is infrequently mentioned in prime-time programming and is not allowed to be advertised on network television [58]. This apparent hypocrisy may be responsible for untold numbers of teenage pregnancies and other complications, especially considering that other countries that incorporate healthier messages into their programming have far fewer teen pregnancies and much better contraceptive use [5,6,113]. Clearly, more research is needed in this crucial area of adolescent sexual behavior and psychology.

Biology: Is it Their Hormones?

Although this sounds like a facetious question, it is a legitimate one. For example, early maturation is associated with earlier sexual behavior, including intercourse [114,115]. For girls, there is a definite correlation between age at menarche and age at first intercourse [116]. Monozygotic twins reared apart tend to have first intercourse at similar ages [117]. However, most of the evidence for a biologic contribution to adolescent sexual behavior is indirect, extrapolating from adult hormone studies [83]. In men, a threshold level of testosterone seems to catalyze sexual interest and behavior; and small doses of the hormone have been given to adult women complaining of lack of libido [83]. The relationship between hormones, behavior, and social factors, however, is a far more complex one that remains to be elucidated.

Is Adolescent Abstinence a Reasonable Goal?

Many conservative critics feel that "Don't have sex when you're young, but if you do, use contraception" is a double message that is hypocritical, confusing, and ignores the importance of abstinence [118–123]. On the contrary, it is a message of crucial importance, easily understandable to most adolescents [107,124], and one that also acknowledges that adults no longer have complete control over adolescent behavior. In the Roper poll, nearly two thirds of teens thought that "Just Say No" is ineffective in preventing early sexual activity [16].

However, this does not mean that abstinence is not a worthy goal or that it should not be emphasized in sex education programs. Rather, it cannot be the sole goal or the only feature of such programs, or such efforts will inevitably fail [8,124–126]. As the National Commission on Adolescent Sexual Health states [8]:

"Society should encourage adolescents to delay sexual behaviors until they are ready physically, cognitively, and emotionally for mature sexual relationships and their consequences. This support should include education about intimacy; sexual limit setting; resisting social, media, peer, and partner pressure; benefits of abstinence from intercourse; and pregnancy and STD prevention (p. 20)."

Only three studies of abstinence-only programs have been published in the scientific literature [127–129], and none found any impact on delaying the age of first intercourse [125,130]. Similarly, there are no data to support the effectiveness of abstinence-only sex education programs or having young people sign pledges of abstaining from sex until marriage. On the other hand, teaching about abstinence can and should be incorporated into routine sex education programs and into teenage pregnancy prevention programs [8,130]. A thorough evaluation of five such programs found that several of the programs succeeded in delaying first intercourse by as much as 15%, increasing contraceptive use by as much as 22%, and decreasing the teen pregnancy rate [125] (Table 12). Whether the results are applicable to all teenagers is unclear, however, because these programs mostly involved inner-city, low-income, high-risk adolescents. Success was greatest when younger teenagers were targeted and when a variety of key elements were incorporated [125]:

• An emphasis on abstinence or delay of sexual initiation
• Training in decision-making and negotiation skills
• Education on sexuality and contraception
• Access to contraceptive services

The Role of Health Professionals

Despite the popular stereotype, modern teenagers are not sex-crazed "hormones-with-legs." Many appear to be highly conflicted about their sexual activities, especially young women, and largely ignorant of the repercussions involved. Adolescence can be a time of great and satisfying personal growth, but not if it is marred by a premature pregnancy or STD. The medical and social consequences of teen pregnancy are now well known:

• A 60% higher risk of death for teens younger than 15 years of age [12].
• Increased risks of anemia, toxemia, hypertension, and cephalopelvic disproportion, prematurity, and low–birth-weight babies, particularly in the under-15 age group [12,131]. Even older adolescents from higher socioeconomic groups have poorer pregnancy outcomes, with lower-weight and more premature babies, despite receiving good prenatal care [132].
• Nearly 70% of all teen pregnancies are to unmarried women. Nearly a third of teen marriages end in divorce within 5 years [9].
• Without intensive school-based programs and efforts at secondary prevention, 40,000 female adolescents drop out of school because of pregnancy. Only 30% eventually complete high school [133]. Compared with older mothers, teen mothers are far less likely to complete high school (90% vs.

TABLE 12. *Effectiveness of teen pregnancy prevention programs*[a]

Program	Delaying first sex		Contraceptive use		Pregnancy rate	
	Trtm.	Cntl.	Trtm.	Cntl.	Trtm.	Cntl.
Postponing Sexual Involvement	24%	39%	50%	33%	3%	4%
Reducing the Risk	29%	38%	100%	70%	NA	NA
Self Center	45%	60%	57%	53%	17%	37%
Teen Talk	30%	29%	35%	65%	9%	13%
School/community	NA	NA	NA	NA	4%	7%

NA, not applicable.
[a]Comparison of treatment (Trtm.) and control (Cntl.) groups in each of the five programs.
Adapted from Frost JJ, Forrest JD. Understanding the impact of effective teenage pregnancy prevention programs. *Fam Plann Perspect* 1995;27:188.

70%, respectively) [9]. Having a child before age 20 reduces the amount of schooling teenagers obtain by 1 to 3 years [134].

• Teenage pregnancy exacts a staggering socioeconomic toll, which includes lower levels of income and job success and satisfaction [135]. Society must also bear a major share of the impact (Table 13). Over half of all money dispersed by the Aid to Families with Dependent Children program goes to women who had teenage pregnancies [9].

• There are greater risks to the offspring of teen pregnancies, including lower levels of school achievement, more emotional problems, and the possibility of increased abuse [42,136,137].

Even if teenage pregnancy were not a factor, the risks of STD alone—especially AIDS—would well warrant the intervention of concerned health professionals. What should their approach be?

1. **Confidential health care must be guaranteed** [92,131,138–140]. In several studies, confidentiality is the primary issue for teenagers seeking health care [27,141,142]. A Canadian survey found that 57% of teens were afraid that their family doctors would inform their parents about the visit [141], and a 1986 Harris Poll found that guaranteeing confidentiality was the primary reason that 78% of teens preferred family planning clinics to their own doctors [27]. In private practice, the easiest way to avoid any potential problems is to meet with or send a letter to parents of 10- to 11-year-olds explaining that a new policy will be in effect once the child reaches age 12 (Fig. 3). Ensuring confidentiality may mean keeping separate files for those sensitive health visits that require it and not sending a bill home to parents. Studies show that many teenagers have the ability to pay for their own health care visits [143]. Or, parents may agree, prospectively, to pay for visits without knowing why the visit was made.

2. **Physicians should be interested in seeing teenagers and skilled in the basics of adolescent medicine.** Otherwise, the health visit becomes counterproductive for both the teenager and the professional [144]. Family practitioners, pediatricians, internists, nurse practitioners and physician assistants, and even gynecologists can all serve teenage patients well but only if they are interested, willing, and knowledgeable. Unfortunately, that is not always the case: a 1983 survey of pediatricians showed that 20% did not want to see adolescents in their practice, and an additional 26% admitted that their knowledge of adolescent medicine was inadequate [145]. Compared with gynecologists and family practitioners, pediatricians are the least likely to want to treat teenage patients or to prescribe oral contraceptives (OCs) to a sexually active 15-year-old [146,147] (Table 14). But even gynecologists may not be the ideal health care providers for adolescents. An Associated Press article profiled a 38-year-old gynecologist who began refusing to prescribe contraception for any of his patients who are sexually active and unmarried because he feels that premarital sex is morally wrong [148].

Despite the efforts of the Section on Adolescent Health of the American Academy of Pediatrics, the Society for Adolescent Medicine, and many other organizations, pediatricians still lag behind family practitioners in their residency training exposure to adolescent patients [149]. A 1992 study surveyed 3,000 pediatricians who have completed their residency training since the American Academy of Pediatrics' Task Force on Pediatric Education Report in 1978 [150]. Among the more recent graduates (completing training since 1984), the following percentages of pediatricians found their residency training experiences to be *insufficient*:

• Care of adolescents: 51%
• Psychosocial problems: 50%

TABLE 13. *Estimated economic consequences of teenage pregnancy, 1996*

Public program	Cost: all recipients (in billions)	Cost: teen mothers (in billions)
Aid to Families with Dependent Children	$19.5	$10.5
Food Stamps	7.8	4.2
Medicaid	11.7	6.3
Total	$39	$21

Adapted from Burt MR. Estimating the public costs of teenage childbearing. *Fam Plann Perspect* 1986;18:221; Elster AB, Kuznets NJ. *AMA guidelines for adolescent preventive services (GAPS): recommendations and rationale.* Baltimore: Williams & Wilkins; 1994; and Advocates for Youth. *Fact sheet: adolescent sexual behavior, pregnancy, and parenthood.* Washington, DC: Advocates for Youth; 1995.

HYMAN C. TOLMAS, M.D., F.A.A.P., F.S.A.M.

Adolescent Medicine and Pediatrics
2017 Metairie Road
Metairie, Louisiana 70005
(504) 833-2821

Dear Mr. & Mrs. Jones:

Now that Amy is eleven years old and has entered adolescence there are some things I would like to bring to your attention that are important to ensure the positive continuity of care.

As you are aware, in addition to the physical and sexual changes that are taking place, there are significant changes in attitudes and feelings at this age.

On future visits to the office I will address Amy relative to her reason(s) for the visit, and I will explain the treatment plan to her. It is most important that she understand that I regard her as my patient and respect her feelings, wishes and concerns. As an integral part of this new relationship we must all be cognizant of the confidential nature of our interactions. There will be some things that Amy will feel comfortable talking about only to me. I very much appreciate your understanding the effectiveness of this new adolescent/doctor relationship, and I think that Amy will appreciate it as well.

Another goal of this special relationship is to make Amy aware of the importance of her own role in accepting some of the responsibility for her health care. If there are some questions or problems you would like to discuss, I will be delighted to meet with you.

I enjoy treating your children and look forward to many more years of continuing medical care. It is important that we make your adolescent feel at ease. I know we will all continue to be proud of our budding young adult as we watch her grow.

Fondly,

Hyman C. Tolmas, M.D., FAAP, FSAM

FIG. 3. How to deal with the issue of confidentiality in a private practice: one method. (Tolmas HC, Long WA Jr, Grace E. The role of the private practitioner. *Adolescent Medicine: State of the Art Reviews* 1990;1:145, with permission.)

- Interviewing and counseling: 33%
- School health: 61%
- Child advocacy: 44%

In 1996, the Residency Review Committee revised its guidelines to mandate at least 1 month of exposure, and more longitudinal experience, in adolescent medicine during pediatric residency. However, given the current financial pressures on department chairmen, these guidelines are likely to be either ignored or unenforced [149].

Do all primary care clinicians *have* to see adolescent patients? Although this is a controversial question, the answer is "probably not." But adolescents make excellent and rewarding patients, their health needs are urgent, and nowhere else in the human life span can an interested and skilled practitioner make such an effective and lifelong impact on a patient's life [151–153].

3. **There is NO evidence that sex education increases levels of adolescent sexual activity** [86,122,154–158]. There is evidence that SOME sex education courses, in combination with intensive pregnancy prevention programs, can actually delay first intercourse and increase use of contraception [122,158,159]. To accomplish the latter, programs must incorporate several elements [158,159]:

TABLE 14. *How different specialists would treat a 15-year-old seeking contraceptives*

Specialty	Serve	Refer	Do neither
Ob-Gyn (*N* = 541)	92%	3%	5%
Family practitioner (*N* = 265)	66%	17%	17%
Pediatrician (*N* = 401)	32%	61%	7%

Adapted from Orr MT. Private physicians and the provision of contraceptives to adolescents. *Fam Plann Perspect* 1984;16:83.

- Use social learning theory (proven to work in various drug prevention programs)
- Keep a narrow focus on reducing specific high-risk behaviors
- Use experiential activities to convey and personalize information on the risks of unprotected sexual activity
- Acknowledge and discuss social pressures on teens (e.g., lines used to get someone to have sex, and possible responses)
- Reinforce individual and group values against high-risk sexual activity
- Increase social skills and model ways to say "no" or "not yet"
- Vary the emphasis according to the age of the students: for example, for young students, "Wait until you're older to begin having sex"; for older students, "Abstinence is the best protection, but if you have sex, always use protection."
- Provide access to contraceptive services

In the most recent study, researchers found that if contraceptive education occurs in the same year that an adolescent begins having intercourse, the odds of condom use are increased by 70% to 80% and the odds of OC use are more than doubled [122].

What most sex education programs seem to do is to make teenagers more knowledgeable about sexual matters and more tolerant of others. Teaching children about sex is no more likely to make them immediately become sexually involved than teaching them about geography is likely to make them drop out of school to join an expedition to Antarctica. One reason why sex education is not the panacea it was once thought to be is that a large number of teenagers are beginning sexual intercourse before they can be exposed to a sex education course (Tables 15, 16).

Although some parents claim that sex education belongs exclusively at home, one third of 15-year-old girls say that neither parent has talked to them about pregnancy and about half report that neither parent has discussed either STDs or contraception. Teenage boys receive even less sex education from

TABLE 15. *Content of school sex education programs*

	Teens with sex education at school (*N* = 582)
Reproduction	89%
Sexual development	79%
Kinds of birth control	66%
Sexual abuse	55%
Abortion	54%
Where to get birth control	51%
"Comprehensive sex education"	60%

Note: Of the 1,000 teenagers surveyed, 40% had never been offered a sex education program in school. Therefore, the overall availability of "comprehensive sex education" is 35%.

Adapted from Harris L, and Associates. *American teens speak: sex, myths, TV, and birth control.* New York: Planned Parenthood Federation of America; 1986.

TABLE 16. *Teenagers' knowledge about sex (N = 1,000 teens)*

Questions asked of teenagers	Percentage wrong or uncertain
A girl usually cannot become pregnant if she has intercourse during her menstrual period (TRUE)	76
It is possible for a girl to become pregnant even though her male partner's penis did not actually enter her vagina (TRUE)	65
The time when a girl is most likely to become pregnant is about two weeks after her menstrual period begins (TRUE)	59
A girl has to have an orgasm during intercourse to become pregnant (FALSE)	41
A girl cannot become pregnant if she douches with Coca-Cola after intercourse (FALSE)	28
A girl cannot become pregnant the first time she has intercourse (FALSE)	20
A girl can get pregnant only if she is lying flat on her back during intercourse (FALSE)	18

From Harris L, and Associates. *American teens speak: sex, myths, TV, and birth control.* New York: Planned Parenthood Federation of America, 1986. Reprinted by permission of the Planned Parenthood Federation of America.

their parents [9]. In the Kaiser study, 54% of teens felt that their parents had failed miserably in their sex education efforts at home [106].

Thus, for many teens school-based sex education is the only possibility. Yet, a 1984 national survey demonstrated that of sexually active teens at age 15, only 48% of the girls and 26% of the boys had received sex education at school. Even by age 18, only 61% of the girls and 52% of the boys had taken a course [154]. In the more recent Roper poll, one third of teens reported having had sex education classes in elementary school; however, only 5% of all teens report having had classes every year in school [16]. According to the 1994 Guttmacher report, most teenagers report having had some sex education; but again, the actual content and amount is less than ideal: an average of 5 hours total of instruction on birth control and 6 hours on STDs between grades 7 and 12 [9].

In 1988 the Alan Guttmacher Institute found that of the nearly $6.3 million spent on sex education by states in 1987 to 1988, $5.1 million was specifically targeted for AIDS education [160]. Nearly one third of sex education teachers felt that their biggest obstacle was pressure from parents and school administrators, particularly if they tried to address issues of homosexuality, condoms, or abortion [161]. Only two states, Delaware and Georgia, specifically mandate that the risks and benefits of all contraceptive methods be discussed [162] (Fig. 4).

Although 89% of adults support the concept of sex education being taught in schools and 73% support adolescents' access to birth control information and contraceptives in school clinics [163], sex education programs have come under increasing fire from conservative groups. Currently, most states [45] recommend that schools provide sex education, but all states recommend or mandate AIDS education [9]. Yet, 41 states still do not have teacher training requirements for sex education [164]. Increasingly, sex education programs are being limited to topics such as abstinence (27 of 28 states, in one study) and AIDS and omitting equally important topics such as contraception, sexual identity and orientation (only 13 of 29 states), or abortion (11 of 29 states) [164].

Overall, less than 10% of students are receiving comprehensive, kindergarten-through-12th-grade sex education; the percentage receiving effective training is probably smaller still [157]. Clearly, sex education is under attack by conservative elements in society who would have parents and school officials believe that teaching kids about sexuality is the prime cause of young adolescents' sexual activity [121,165]. It is up to health professionals who know better to set the record straight. Ideally, physicians should play a major catalytic role in the dissemination of sex education at home, in the office or clinic, and in schools.

4. **There is NO evidence that making contraception available to teenagers makes them sexually active at a younger age** [152,153,166,167]. Several studies have documented that most of the teenagers seeking contraceptives in clinics have already been sexually active for at least 6 to 24 months [6,9,168,169], and that giving teens OCs does not increase their frequency of intercourse or number of partners [6,9,158,170,171]. One study found that nearly three fourths of sexually active

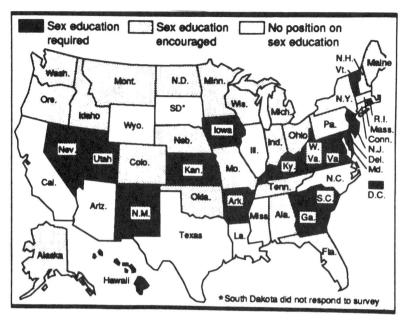

FIG. 4. State policies on sex education. (Alan Guttmacher Institute. *Risk and responsibility: teaching sex education in America's schools today.* New York: Alan Guttmacher Institute; 1989, with permission.)

young women wait an average of nearly 2 years after first intercourse before visiting a family planning clinic, whereas only 17% visit such a clinic before first intercourse [172]. On the other hand, an aggressive campaign to distribute to and promote the use of condoms by Latino youth increased the use of condoms without increasing baseline rates of sexual activity [166]. That giving teenagers access to birth control makes them more sexually active at a younger age is a myth that, unfortunately, still pervades a large part of American society. Teenagers' decisions about where, when, and with whom to begin having sex are far more complex than whether a fish-bowl full of condoms is displayed at a school-based clinic. The most persuasive scientific argument to counter such misinformation is the Guttmacher Report, which found that the United States has the highest teenage pregnancy rate in the Western world, despite the fact that many other countries' teens are having sex at younger ages or more frequently than ours [6,9]. In European countries and in Canada, the societal norm is that if teenagers are going to have sex, they must use contraception.

   5. **Even if physicians decide that they would rather not see adolescent patients, they must still learn routinely to ask "the sexual question" of any young woman or man they are asked to evaluate for other medical problems.** Female teens with abdominal pain are far more likely, statistically, to have pelvic inflammatory disease (incidence, one of eight 15- to 19-year-olds) [173] than appendicitis (7% lifetime incidence), for example [174]. Yet, a study of female teenagers presenting to the Stanford University Hospital Emergency Room with acute abdominal pain showed that a sexual history was elicited from 100% of minorities but only 44% of whites and only 27% of those younger than 15 years of age [175].

   A Massachusetts survey documented that only 22% of girls and 4% of boys coming to a private practitioner's office had ever previously been asked about their sexual activity, and of the teens who were sexually active, 62% had never been asked about it by their physician [176]. One report found that physicians say that they routinely ask new adolescent patients about cigarette smoking (84%), but far fewer ask about STDs (56%), condom use (52%), numbers of sex partners (34%), or sexual orientation (27%) [177]. Other studies have reported similar findings [178–180]. In the most recent study of 2,026 9th through 12th grade California students, only 39% reported having discussions with their physicians about how to avoid getting AIDS, 37% about using condoms for vaginal intercourse, 13% about how to use condoms, 15% about the teenager's sex life, 13% about how to say "no" to unwanted sex, and 8% about sexual orientation [180].

Practitioners need to be especially sensitive to the issue of sexual abuse and unwanted sexual experiences in adolescents. In one study, 40% of girls and 16% of boys reported having had at least one unwanted sexual experience before age 18 years, but the time to disclosure averaged over 2 years because of fear and embarrassment [181].

What appear to be "simple" medical problems may, in fact, be related to sexual activity and have significant future consequences. Studies have shown that female teens presenting with dysuria have as great a risk of having vaginitis as a urinary tract infection [182]. Two studies have documented that two thirds of teenagers who had a negative pregnancy test at one clinic returned within 18 to 24 months and were pregnant, and a national study of nearly 3,000 teenagers found that almost three of five teenage girls had had a negative pregnancy test at a clinic before they ever became pregnant [183,184].

Some physicians are using computers to elicit sensitive information from adolescents [185]. Regardless of how the information is obtained, *no medical history of a teenager—male or female—is complete without a sexual history, and teenagers who admit to being sexually active need careful counseling and follow-up* [138,152,153,183,184,186].

6. **Every health encounter with the adolescent—sports physicals, immunizations, job or camp physicals—should be seen as an opportunity to consolidate and update the sexual history.** What constitutes a complete sexual history? There are a variety of ways to obtain the necessary information (Tables 17, 18).

7. **The sex of the examiner is not nearly as important as the gentleness and sensitivity with which the examination is explained and completed** [138,144,187–189]. In a large national survey of teenagers, 69% said that the fear of having a pelvic examination kept them from seeking contraception. Unfortunately, the same percentage said that they still feared pelvic examinations after they had actually undergone one [27]. The indications for doing a pelvic examination are straightforward (Tables 19, 20), and the "basics" of pelvic examination have been extensively reviewed elsewhere [138,144,188–193]. Here are some hints that may prove useful, however:

- Telling a young teenager to "relax" on the examining table is akin to telling a small child that receiving a vaccination will not hurt. Showing them *how* to relax using "biofeedback" methods is far better: after inserting one finger into the vagina, the examiner presses on the pubococcygeus muscle and explains that this muscle is the one that is squeezed to stop the flow of urine. The patient often involuntarily contracts the muscle at this point. The examiner can then explain that this muscle should be allowed to go loose; and when the patient complies, the examiner should then comment on the relaxed muscle tone and how much easier it will be to do the examination. Alternatively, some examiners prefer to assess the tone of the patient's inner thigh muscles.

- Not everyone needs a "full" pelvic examination. A 13-year-old with dysfunctional uterine bleeding, for example, may require only a bimanual rectoabdominal examination, or no examination, if she is not sexually active. Doing a speculum examination would, in fact, be counterproductive if she is actively bleeding at the time. Likewise, teenagers who are not engaging in intercourse but who have severe enough dysmenorrhea to warrant a concerted effort at treatment might require some assessment of their pelvic anatomy (e.g., a rectoabdominal examination) but do not require a speculum examination. In general, speculum insertion is the most feared part of the examination, and if visualization of the cervix and a Pap smear are *not* required, dispensing with this part of the examination will be welcomed. Occasionally, young women will ask for OCs because they are about to initiate

TABLE 17. *Asking the sexual question*

Incorrect:	"Are you sexually active?"
	(Comic response: "No, I just lie there.")
	"Do you have any questions about sex?"
	(Inevitable response: "No.")
Correct:	
Indirect:	"Do you think many of your friends are involved sexually with their boyfriends/girlfriends?"
Direct:	"Are you having sex?" or "Are you doing *it*?"
	If answer is yes: "With whom (male, female, or both)?"

TABLE 18. *Screening history for contraception*

Please circle the appropriate answer or fill in the blank.

1. Have you ever been hospitalized?	Yes	No

Have you ever had:

2. Surgery	Yes	No
3. High blood pressure	Yes	No
4. Frequent headaches	Yes	No
5. Jaundice or hepatitis	Yes	No
6. Gallbladder disease	Yes	No
7. Diabetes	Yes	No
8. Phlebitis or blood clots	Yes	No
9. Heart murmur	Yes	No
10. Epilepsy or seizures	Yes	No
11. Any sexually transmitted disease: syphilis, gonorrhea, chlamydia, warts, or pelvic inflammatory disease	Yes	No

12. Family history of:

Heart trouble	Yes	No
Diabetes	Yes	No
Cancer	Yes	No

Please answer:

13. Do you wear contact lenses?	Yes	No

14. Please list any medicines taken regularly and what they are for:

15. Age of onset of first period. _____

16. How often do your periods come? _____

17. How long do they last? _____

18. Any discomfort with periods? _____

19. Any bleeding between periods? _____

20. What day did your last menstrual period start? _____

21. Age at time of your first intercourse. _____

22. Current frequency of intercourse. _____

23. Have you ever been pregnant? _____

24. Have you ever been sexually abused, raped, or pressured into having sex? _____

25. What type of contraception have you used? _____

26. Date of your last pelvic exam? _____

27. Do you smoke cigarettes? How many?

sexual intercourse with their boyfriends, but refuse a pelvic examination. Counseling them and giving them one package of OCs, until they can return for a complete baseline examination, is the wisest option and is recommended by the American College of Obstetricians and Gynecologists [192].

- No separate permission form is needed for a pelvic examination. Indeed, such a form is distasteful to those physicians who are already involved in doing adolescent gynecology. Because a separate permission form is not required to look in a patient's ears or down their throat, why should looking

TABLE 19. *Indications for doing a pelvic examination*

Sexual activity (past or current)
Unexplained abdominal pain
Unexplained dysuria
Abnormal vaginal discharge
Menstrual disorders
    Severe dysmenorrhea
    First- or second-degree amenorrhea
    Dysfunctional uterine bleeding
Routine: age 17 y or older

in their vagina be any different? However, it *does* require the informal verbal consent of the patient (a noncooperative patient cannot be adequately examined).

- Having a chaperon in the room makes good medicolegal sense and also is more practical—the examination is easier when specimens and supplies are being handed to the clinician, who is then free to concentrate on the patient and the findings.
- Some teenagers may prefer to have their mother, sister, or a friend in the room when the pelvic examination is done [194]. This option should be offered to younger teens, in particular.
- Physicians should familiarize themselves with the different kinds of specula: Huffman for the virginal patient, Pedersen for most teenagers, and Graves for young women who have children. In addition, a speculum that contains the light source in the handle (Welsh-Allyn) is often preferable and more straightforward to use than trying to visualize the cervix using an exterior light source.

8. **Providing gynecologic care to teenagers can be both challenging and rewarding, and is crucial if physicians are interested in meeting their patients' needs comprehensively.** Sending patients off to gynecologists for their routine care makes little sense—not all gynecologists are skilled with or interested in teenagers [148], and most prefer to do the specialty work associated with their field. Patients with STDs, contraceptive needs, or simple menstrual disorders can and should be managed by primary care physicians. More complicated patients, with chronic pelvic pain, primary amenorrhea, or hirsutism, either can be referred to gynecologist colleagues or worked up in conjunction with them. Several excellent and up-to-date references are available (see suggested readings).

Counseling Teenagers About Sex

Twenty-five years ago, Adele Hofmann wrote [195]:

"For an adolescent girl to have become pregnant because of ignorance about contraception, because she cannot bring herself to confide in parents, and because physicians have avoided their responsibility in taking the initiative in this area is indeed a harsh and cruel price for her and her consort to pay. It

TABLE 20. *Office materials for pelvic examinations*

Examination table with stirrups
Lighted speculum (Welsh-Allyn)
Culture/antigen tests
    Thayer-Martin (gonorrhea)
    Microtrak or Chlamydiazyme (*Chlamydia*)
    Nickerson (*Candida*)
Pap smear supplies
    Slides, spatulas or brushes, fixative
Microscope
    Normal saline
    KOH 10%
Pregnancy tests (e.g., Tandem-Icon, TestPack)

Adapted from Braverman PK, Strasburger VC. Why adolescent gynecology? Pediatricians and pelvic exams. *Pediatr Clin North Am* 1989;36:471.

TABLE 21. *Sources of information about birth control for adolescents*

Source	Percentage of teenagers (N = 1,000)
Parents	53
Television or movies	25 ⎫
Books or magazines	23 ⎭ 48
Friends	45
Doctor or nurse	**19**

From Harris L, and Associates. *American teens speak: sex, myths, TV, and birth control.* New York: Planned Parenthood Federation of America, 1986. Reprinted by permission of the Planned Parenthood Federation of America.

is time that all physicians and parents recognize the rights and needs of adolescents to receive health care for sensitive matters under the same terms as are afforded adults. The primary care physician who looks upon pregnancy prevention as being as much his responsibility as other facets of preventative medicine—and acts on this responsibility—will be welcomed by many of his adolescent patients as meeting an essential need."

Although sex education begins at home, there is no reason why it necessarily must be confined there. Traditionally, physicians have not been a major source of information for teenagers about sexual matters (Table 21). Physicians not only need to ask detailed sexual histories (and be prepared for the answers!), but should be able to do preventative and interventional counseling, tailored to fit the age, maturity, and sexual activity level of the patient. No longer can a practitioner assume that a teenager probably is or is not sexually active simply because of his or her ethnicity or socioeconomic status. In the past decade, rates of sexual activity have nearly equalized for non-Hispanic whites and African-American teens, as well as across socioeconomic lines [196].

From a practical viewpoint, discussing levels of sexual maturation with teenagers can prevent much anguish and frustration. For example, discovering that a 14-year-old is Sex Maturity Rating (SMR) II

TABLE 22. *Differences in the adolescent–physician agenda during office visits*

Topic	Teens interested (%)	Actually discussed (%)
Exercise	86	42
Nutrition	83	51
Sexually transmitted diseases	70	18
Contraception	66	22
Acne	64	30
Fear of cancer	65	12
Depression	59	16
Menses	55	49
Sexual functioning	53	24
Alcohol/other drugs	51	23
School	48	37
Smoking	47	30
Parents	46	19
Sexual abuse	36	6

From Malus M, LaChance PA, Lamy L, et al. Priorities in adolescent health care: the teenagers' viewpoint. *J Fam Pract* 1987; 25:159. Copyright © 1987. Reprinted by permission of Appleton & Lange, Inc.

TABLE 23. *Do adolescents understand medical terminology?*

Term	Correct (%)	Incorrect (%)	Don't know (%)	Example of incorrect answer
Sexually transmitted disease	41	15	44	"A disease you get from not being clean"
Confidential	43	35	22	"To have confidence in yourself"
Sexually active	46	37	17	"Urge for sex"
Sexual intercourse	64	14	22	"Having sex education"
Birth control	68	20	12	"To have self-control not to get pregnant"

Adapted from Ammerman SD, Perelli E, Adler N, et al. Do adolescents understand what physicians say about sexuality and health? *Clin Pediatr* 1992;31:590.

and telling him that his entire growth spurt is ahead of him can change his entire outlook on life. Likewise, informing a 14-year-old with slight gynecomastia that his hormones are not playing a cruel trick on him can be lifesaving. Such discussions naturally lead to the more difficult areas. Counseling teenagers about sex can be difficult, for the health professional and the teenager, and requires skills best learned through practice. Usually, the style of the conversation is equally as important as the substance [197] (Tables 22, 23). One eminent authority suggests [198]:

1. If you ask a teenager if they have any questions about sex, the answer will invariably be "no."
2. Avoid jargon.
3. Do not immediately assume that you are being understood.
4. Avoid lectures. Their parents do that. Give them credit for being capable of intelligence, thoughtfulness, and responsibility.
5. Do not be afraid to offer your opinions and counsel in a straightforward way. Teenagers will respond to this.
6. Do not try to talk to the teenager in the current adolescent vernacular unless this is your usual mode of speaking.

The content of such discussions can be far-ranging or confined, depending on the clinical situation, but at some time during adolescence, the following information should emanate from the practitioner:

- It is always okay to say "no"—whether you are male or female. Sex should never be used as a test of love. "If you love me, you'll have sex with me" is simply a line, and there are many easy and clever responses to it [199].
- Not all teenagers are sexually active.
- The decision to begin having intercourse places the teen at risk of pregnancy and STD. These risks can be lessened, but there is nothing as safe as abstinence.
- Sexual fantasies and masturbation are normal.
- Penis and breast size are variable and have no relationship to sexual functioning.
- Sexual fantasies about or experience with members of the same sex do not necessarily mean a teenager is homosexual.
- Taking OCs is 10 to 25 times safer than carrying a pregnancy to term.

There are numerous misconceptions about adolescent sexuality, and clinicians can serve as important sources of sound medical information, but only if they make a concerted effort to bring up the subject themselves. Most important, counseling young teenagers that they should avoid having intercourse at an early age, but that if they do engage in it, they should use contraception, is an easily understandable "double message" that most teenagers will appreciate. Promoting abstinence and responsible sexual behavior and encouraging the use of contraception are *not* mutually exclusive goals [123,193,200].

REFERENCES

1. Strasburger VC. *Getting your kids to say "no" in the '90s when you said "yes" in the '60s.* New York: Fireside/Simon & Schuster; 1993.
2. Hesiod, as quoted in Group for the Advancement of Psychiatry. *Normal adolescence.* Vol 6. New York: Brunner-Mazel; 1975:751.

3. Weldon JEC, ed. *The rhetoric of Aristotle.* New York: Oxford University Press; 1886:164.
4. Shakespeare W. *The winter's tale.* Act III, Scene 3, lines 58–62 Kermode F (ed). New York: New American Library, 1963.
5. Alan Guttmacher Institute. *Teenage pregnancy in developed countries.* New Haven: Yale University Press; 1986.
6. Trussell J. Teenage pregnancy in the United States. *Fam Plann Perspect* 1988;20:262.
7. Spitz A, Velebil P, Koonin LM, et al. Pregnancy, abortion, and birth rates among US adolescents—1980, 1985, and 1990. *JAMA* 1996;275:989.
8. Haffner DW, ed. *Facing facts: sexual health for America's adolescents.* New York: Sexuality Information and Education Council of the U.S. (SIECUS); 1995.
9. Alan Guttmacher Institute. *Sex and America's teenagers.* New York: Alan Guttmacher Institute; 1994.
10. Sells CW, Blum RW. Morbidity and mortality among US adolescents: an overview of data and trends. *Am J Public Health* 1996;86:513.
11. Centers for Disease Control and Prevention. State specific pregnancy and birth rates among teenagers: United States, 1991–92.*MMWR Morb Mortal Wkly Rep* 1995;44(37):677.
12. Advocates for Youth. *Fact sheet: adolescent sexual behavior, pregnancy, and parenthood.* Washington, DC: Advocates for Youth; 1995.
13. Moore KA, Snyder NO. *Facts at a glance.* Washington, DC: Child Trends; 1996.
14. Strasburger VC. Sex, drugs, rock 'n' roll: an introduction. *Pediatrics* 1985;76(Suppl):659.
15. Ku LC, Sonenstein FL, Pleck JH. Young men's risk behaviors for HIV infection and sexually transmitted diseases, 1988 through 1991. *Am J Public Health* 1993;83:1609.
16. Roper Starch Worldwise, Inc. *Teens talk about sex: adolescent sexuality in the 90's.* New York: SIECUS; 1994.
17. Centers for Disease Control and Prevention. Youth Risk Behavior Surveillance: United States, 1995. *MMWR Morb Mortal Wkly Rep* 1996;45(SS-4):1.
18. Centers for Disease Control and Prevention. *Adolescent health: state of the nation—pregnancy, sexually transmitted diseases, and related risk behaviors among U. S. adolescents.* DHHS publication no. (CDC) 099-4630. Atlanta: U.S. Department of Health and Human Services, 1995.
19. Centers for Disease Control and Prevention. Trends in sexual risk behavior among high school students—United States, 1990, 1991, and 119- 93.MMWR Morb Mortal Wkly Rep 1995;44:124.
20. Lee PR, Stewart FH. Editorial: failing to prevent unintended pregnancy is costly. *Am J Public Health* 1995;85:479.
21. Males M. School-age pregnancy: why hasn't prevention worked? *J Sch Health* 1993;63:429.
22. Centers for Disease Control and Prevention. Abortion surveillance: Preliminary data—United States, 1994. *MMWR Morb Mortal Wkly Rep* 1997;45:1123.
23. Henshaw SK, Kost K. Abortion patients in 1994–1995: characteristics and contraceptive use. *Fam Plann Perspect* 1996;28:140.
24. Zelnik M, Kantner JF. Sexual activity, contraceptive use, and pregnancy among metropolitan-area teenagers: 1971–1979. *Fam Plann Perspect* 1980;12:230.
25. Sonenstein FL, Pleck JH, Leighton CK. Sexual activity, condom use and AIDS awareness among adolescent males. *Fam Plann Perspect* 1989;21:152.
26. Coles R, Stokes G. *Sex and the American teenager.* New York: Harper & Row; 1985.
27. Harris L, and Associates. *American teens speak: sex, myths, TV, and birth control.* New York: Planned Parenthood Federation of America; 1986.
28. Hofferth SL, Kahn JR, Baldwin W. Premarital sexual activity among U.S. teenage women over the past three decades. *Fam Plann Perspect* 1987;19:46.
29. Mott FL, Haurin RJ. Linkages between sexual activity and alcohol and drug use among American adolescents. *Fam Plann Perspect* 1988;20:128.
30. Blum RW. *The state of adolescent health in Minnesota.* Minneapolis: University of Minnesota; 1989.
31. DeBuono BA, Zinner SH, Daamen M, et al. Sexual behavior of college women in 1975, 1986, and 1989. *N Engl J Med* 1990;322:821.
32. Centers for Disease Control and Prevention. Miami youth risk behavior survey, 1993. MMWR Morb Mortal Wkly Rep 1994;43:873.
33. Kost K, Forrest JD. American women's sexual behavior and exposure to risk of sexually transmitted diseases. *Fam Plann Perspect* 1992;24:244.
34. Barone C, Ickovics JR, Ayers TS, et al. High-risk sexual behavior among young urban students. *Fam Plann Perspect* 1996;28:69.
35. Sonenstein FL, Pleck JH, Ku L. Levels of sexual activity among adolescent males in the United States. *Fam Plann Perspect* 1991;23:162.
36. Calderone MS. Fetal erection and its message to us. *SIECUS Report* 1983;11(5/6):9.
37. Haas A. *Teenage sexuality: a survey of teenage sexual behavior.* New York: Macmillan; 1979.
38. Moscicki AB, Millstein SG, Broering J, et al. Risks of human immunodeficiency virus infection among adolescents attending three diverse clinics. *J Pediatr* 1993;122:813.
39. Stanton B, Li X, Black M, et al. Sexual practices and intentions among preadolescent and early adolescent low-income urban African-Americans. *Pediatrics* 1994;93:966.

40. Brooks-Gunn J, Furstenberg FF Jr. Coming of age in the era of AIDS: puberty, sexuality, and contraception. *Millbank Q* 1990;68(Suppl 1):59.

41. Zabin LS, Hirsch MB, Smith EA, et al. Adolescent sexual attitudes and behavior: are they consistent? *Fam Plann Perspect* 1984;16:181.

42. Braverman PK, Strasburger VC. Adolescent sexuality: I. adolescent sexual activity. *Clin Pediatr* 1993;32:658.

43. Schuster MA, Bell RM, Kanouse DE. The sexual practices of adolescent virgins: genital sexual activities of high school students who have never had vaginal intercourse. *Am J Public Health* 1996;86:1570.

44. Jaffe LR, Seehaus M, Wagner C, et al. Anal intercourse and knowledge of acquired immunodeficiency syndrome among minority-group female adolescents. *J Pediatr* 1988;112:1005.

45. MacDonald NE, Wells GA, Fisher WA, et al. High-risk STD/HIV behavior among college students. *JAMA* 1990;263:3155.

46. Cochran SD, Mays VM. Sex, lies, HIV. *N Engl J Med* 1990;322:774.

47. Miller BC, Monson BH, Norton MC. The effects of forced sexual intercourse on white female adolescents. *Child Abuse Negl* 1995;19:1289.

48. Hampton HL. Care of the woman who has been raped. *N Engl J Med* 1995;332:234.

49. Committee on Adolescence, American Academy of Pediatrics. Sexual assault in adolescents. *Pediatrics* 1994;94:761.

50. Advocates for Youth. *Fact sheet: health futures in jeopardy: young people and violence.* Washington, DC: Advocates for Youth; 1994.

51. Stevens-Simon C, Reichert S. Sexual abuse, adolescent pregnancy, and child abuse. *Arch Pediatr Adolesc Med* 1994;148:23.

52. Nagy S, DiClemente R, Adcock AG. Adverse factors associated with forced sex among southern adolescent girls. *Pediatrics* 1995;96:944.

53. Kinsey A, Pomeroy W, Martin C. *Sexual behavior in the human male.* Philadelphia: WB Saunders; 1948.

54. Committee on Adolescence, American Academy of Pediatrics. Homosexuality and adolescence. *Pediatrics* 1993;92:631.

55. Stewart DC. Sexuality and the adolescent: issues for the clinician. *Prim Care* 1987;14:83.

56. Remafedi G, Resnick M, Blum R, et al. Demography of sexual orientation in adolescents. *Pediatrics* 1992;89:714.

57. Cohen MW. Adolescent sexual activity as an expression of nonsexual needs. *Pediatr Ann* 1995;24:324.

58. Strasburger VC. *Adolescents and the media: medical and psychological impact.* Thousand Oaks, CA: Sage; 1995.

59. Heintz-Knowles KE. *Sexual activity on daytime soap operas: a content analysis of five weeks of television programming.* Menlo Park, CA: Kaiser Family Foundation; 1996.

60. Furno-Lamude D, Strasburger VC. Adolescent sexuality and the media: is there a connection? 1997 (unpublished manuscript).

61. Phillips SR. Turning research into policy: a survey on adolescent condom use. *SIECUS Report* 1995;24:9.

62. Strasburger VC. Current issues in adolescent sexuality. In: Strasburger VC, ed. *Basic adolescent gynecology: an office guide.* Baltimore: Urban & Schwarzenberg; 1990:1.

63. Suris J-C, Resnick MD, Cassuto N, et al. Sexual behavior of adolescents with chronic disease and disability. *J Adolesc Health* 1996;19:124.

64. Jessor SL, Jessor R. Transition from virginity to nonvirginity among youth: a social-psychological study over time. *Developmental Psychology* 1975;11:473.

65. Graves KL, Leigh BC. The relationship of substance abuse to sexual activity among young adults in the United States. *Fam Plann Perspect* 1995;27:18.

66. Millstein SG, Igra V. Theoretical models of adolescent risk-taking behavior. In: Wallander JL, Siegel LJ, eds. *Adolescent health problems: behavioral perspectives.* New York: Guilford Press; 1995:52.

67. Tubman JG, Windle M, Windle R. Cumulative sexual intercourse patterns among middle adolescents: problem behavior precursors and concurrent health risk behaviors. *J Adolesc Health* 1996;18:182.

68. Wendell DA, Onorato IM, McCray E, et al. Youth at risk: sex, drugs, and human immunodeficiency virus. *American Journal of Diseases of Children* 1992;146:76.

69. Resnick MD, Blum RW. The association of consensual sexual intercourse during childhood with adolescent health risk and behaviors. *Pediatrics* 1994;94:907.

70. Elster AB, Ketterlinus R, Lamb ME. Association between parenthood and problem behavior in a national sample of adolescents. *Pediatrics* 1990;85:1044.

71. Orr DP, Beiter M, Ingersoll G. Premature sexual activity as an indicator of psychosocial risk. *Pediatrics* 1991;87:141.

72. Sosin DM, Koepsell TD, Rivara FP, et al. Fighting as a marker for multiple problem behaviors in adolescents. *J Adolesc Health* 1995;16:209.

73. Millstein SG, Moscicki AB. Sexually-transmitted disease in female adolescents: effects of psychosocial factors and high risk behaviors. *J Adolesc Health* 1995;17:83.

74. Mott FL, Fondell MM, Hu PN, et al. The determinants of first sex by age 14 in a high-risk adolescent population. *Fam Plann Perspect* 1996;28:13.

75. Spingarn RW, DuRant RH. Male adolescents involved in pregnancy: associated health risk and problem behaviors. *Pediatrics* 1996;98:262.
76. Stanton B, Romer D, Ricardo I, et al. Early initiation of sex and its lack of association with risk behaviors among adolescent African-Americans. *Pediatrics* 1993;92:13.
77. Klein JD, Brown JD, Childers KW, et al. Adolescents' risky behavior and mass media use. *Pediatrics* 1993;92:24.
78. Gordon S, Scales P, Everly K. *The sexual adolescent.* 2nd ed. North Scituate, MA: Duxbury Press; 1979.
79. Akpom AC, Akpom KL, Davis M. Prior sexual behavior of teenagers attending rap sessions for the first time. *Fam Plann Perspect* 1976;8:203.
80. Fox GL. The family's influence on adolescent sexual behavior. *Child Today* 1979;8:21.
81. Thornton A, Camburn D. The influence on the family on premarital sexual attitudes and behavior. *Demography* 1987;24:323.
82. Whitbeck LB, Hoyt DR, Miller M, et al. Parental support, depressed affect and sexual experience among adolescents. *Youth and Society* 1992;24:166.
83. Morris NM. Determinants of adolescent initiation of coitus. *Adolescent Medicine: State of the Art Reviews* 1992;3:165.
84. Young WE, Jensen LC, Olsen JA, et al. The effects of family structure on the sexual behavior of adolescents. *Family Therapy* 1993;20:49.
85. Jaccard J, Dittus PJ, Gordon VV. Maternal correlates of adolescent sexual and contraceptive behavior. *Fam Plann Perspect* 1996;28:159.
86. Benson MD, Torpy EJ. Sexual behavior in junior high school students. *Obstet Gynecol* 1995;85:279.
87. Capaldi DM, Forgatch MS, Crosby L. Affective expression in family problem-solving discussions with adolescent boys. *Journal of Adolescent Research* 1994;9:28.
88. Newcomer SF, Udry JR. Parent–child communication and adolescent sexual behavior. *Fam Plann Perspect* 1985;17:169.
89. Furstenberg FF Jr, Moore KA, Peterson JL. Sex education and sexual experience among adolescents. *Am J Public Health* 1985;75:1331.
90. Moore KA, Peterson JL, Furstenberg FF Jr. Parental attitudes and the occurrence of early sexual activity. *Journal of Marriage and the Family* 1986;48:777.
91. Leland NL, Barth RP. Characteristics of adolescents who have attempted to avoid HIV and who have communicated with parents about sex. *Journal of Adolescent Research* 1993;8:58.
92. Walter HJ, Vaughn RD, Cohall AT. Psychosocial influences on acquired immunodeficiency syndrome: risk behaviors among high school students. *Pediatrics* 1991;88:846.
93. Holtzman D, Rubinson R. Parent and peer communication effects on AIDS-related behavior among U.S. high school students. *Fam Plann Perspect* 1995;27:235.
94. Furstenberg FF Jr. The social consequences of teenage parenthood. *Fam Plann Perspect* 1976;8:148.
95. Handelsman CD, Cabral RJ, Weisfeld GE. Sources of information and adolescent sexual knowledge and behavior. *Journal of Adolescent Research* 1987;2:455.
96. Zabin LS. Addressing adolescent sexual behavior and childbearing: self-esteem or social change? *Women's Health Issues* 1994;4:92.
97. Kahn JR, Anderson KE. Intergenerational patterns of teenage fertility. *Demography* 1992;29:39.
98. Horwitz SM, Klerman LV, Kuo HS, et al. Intergenerational transmission of school-age parenthood. *Fam Plann Perspect* 1991;23:168.
99. Alexander CS, Guyer B. Adolescent pregnancy: occurrence and consequences. *Pediatr Ann* 1993;22:85.
100. East PL. Do adolescent pregnancy and childbearing affect younger siblings? *Fam Plann Perspect* 1996;28:148.
101. Abrahamse AF, Morrison PA, Waite LJ. Teenagers willing to consider single parenthood: who is at greatest risk? *Fam Plann Perspect* 1988;20:13.
102. Forrest JD, Singh S. The sexual and reproductive behavior of American women, 1982–19 *Fam Plann Perspect* 1990;22:206.
103. Update. Kids will be kids. *Fam Plann Perspect* 1988;20:204.
104. Davis S. Pregnancy in adolescents. *Pediatr Clin North Am* 1989;36:665.
105. Young M. Self-esteem and sexual behavior among early adolescents. *Family Life and Education* 1989;7:16.
106. Kaiser Family Foundation. *The Kaiser Family Foundation survey on teens and sex: what they say teens today need to know, and who they listen to.* Menlo Park, CA: Kaiser Family Foundation; 1996.
107. Strasburger VC. Sex, teens, and the media. *Contemporary Pediatrics* 1996;13:29.
108. Harris L, and Associates. *Sexual material on American network television during the 1987–88 season.* New York: Planned Parenthood Federation of America; 1988.
109. Corder-Bolz C. Television and adolescents' sexual behavior. *Sex Education Coalition News* 1981;3:40.
110. Peterson RA, Kahn JR. Media preferences of sexually active teens. Presented at American Psychological Association meeting, Toronto, Ontario, Canada, August 26, 1984.
111. Brown JD, Newcomer SF. Television viewing and adolescents' sexual behavior. *J Homosex* 1991;21:77.
112. Peterson JL, Moore KA, Furstenberg FF Jr. Television viewing and early initiation of sexual intercourse: is there a link? *J Homosex* 1991;21:93.

113. Committee on Communications, American Academy of Pediatrics. Adolescent sexuality and the media (policy statement). *Pediatrics* 1995;95:298.

114. Chilman C. Family life education: promoting health adolescent sexuality. *Family Relations* 1990;39:123.

115. Paikoff R, Brooks-Gunn J. Do parent–child relationships change during puberty? *Psychol Bull* 1991;110:47.

116. Udry JR. Age at menarche, at first intercourse, and at first pregnancy. *J Biosoc Sci* 1979;11:433.

117. Martin NG, Eaves LJ, Eysenck HJ. Genetical, environmental and personality factors influencing the age of first sexual intercourse in twins. *J Biosoc Sci* 1977;9:91.

118. Khouzam HR. Promotion of sexual abstinence: reducing adolescent sexual activity and pregnancies. *South Med J* 1995;88:709.

119. Mondore PA. There's more than one way to skin a cat [letter]. *Contemporary Pediatrics* 1996;13:20.

120. Advocates for Youth. *Fact sheet: sexuality education curricula and programs*. Washington, DC: Advocates for Youth; 1994.

121. Whitehead BD. The failure of sex education. *The Atlantic Monthly* October, 1994:55.

122. Mauldon J, Luker K. The effects of contraceptive education on method use at first intercourse. *Fam Plann Perspect* 1996;28:19.

123. McGrath J, Strasburger VC. Preventing AIDS in teenagers in the 1990s. *Clin Pediatr* 1995;34:46.

124. Strasburger VC. There's more than one way to skin a cat: reply [letter]. *Contemporary Pediatrics* 1996;13:20.

125. Frost JJ, Forrest JD. Understanding the impact of effective teenage pregnancy prevention programs. *Fam Plann Perspect* 1995;27:188.

126. Dryfoos JG. School- and community-based pregnancy prevention programs. *Adolescent Medicine: State of the Art Reviews* 1992;3:241.

127. Christopher S, Roosa M. An evaluation of an adolescent pregnancy prevention program: is "just say no" enough? *Family Relations* 1990;39:68.

128. Roosa M, Christopher S. Evaluation of an abstinence-only adolescent pregnancy prevention program: a replication. *Family Relations* 1990;39:363.

129. Jorgensen SR, Potts V, Camp B. Project Taking Charge: six-month follow-up of a pregnancy prevention program for early adolescents. *Family Relations* 1993;42:401.

130. Howard M, Mitchell ME. Preventing teenage pregnancy: some questions to be answered and some answers to be questioned. *Pediatr Ann* 1993;22:109.

131. Rauh JL. The pediatrician's role in assisting teenagers to avoid the consequences of adolescent pregnancy. *Pediatr Ann* 1993;22:90.

132. Fraser AM, Brockert JE, Ward RH. Association of young maternal age with adverse reproductive outcomes. *N Engl J Med* 1995;332:1113.

133. Upchurch DM, McCarthy J. The timing of first birth and high school completion. *American Sociology Review* 1990;55:224.

134. Klepinger DH, Lundberg S, Plotnick RD. Adolescent fertility and the educational attainment of young women. *Fam Plann Perspect* 1995;27:23.

135. Hoffman SD, Foster EM, Furstenberg FF Jr. Reevaluating the costs of teenage childbearing. *Demography* 1993;30:1.

136. Zuravin S. Child maltreatment and teenage first births: a relationship mediated by chronic sociodemographic stress? *Am J Orthopsychiatry* 1988;58:91.

137. Kotagal UR. Newborn consequences of teenage pregnancies. *Pediatr Ann* 1993;22:127.

138. Braverman PK, Strasburger VC. Adolescent sexuality: IV. the practitioner's role. *Clin Pediatr* 1994;33:100.

139. Committee on Adolescence, American Academy of Pediatrics. Sexually transmitted diseases (policy statement). *Pediatrics* 1994;94:568.

140. Epner JEG, ed. *Policy compendium on reproductive health issues affecting adolescents*. Chicago: American Medical Association; 1996.

141. Herold ES, Goodwin MS. Why adolescents go to birth-control clinics rather than to their family physicians. *Can J Public Health* 1979;70:317.

142. Cheng TL, Savageau JA, Sattler AL, et al. Confidentiality in health care: a survey of knowledge, perceptions, and attitudes among high school students. *JAMA* 1993;269:1404.

143. Fisher M, Marks A, Trieller K, et al. Are adolescents able and willing to pay the fee for confidential care? *J Pediatr* 1985;107:480.

144. Braverman PK, Strasburger VC. Why adolescent gynecology? Pediatricians and pelvic exams. *Pediatr Clin North Am* 1989;36:471.

145. Comerci G. Adolescent medicine and the pediatrician: changes and controversies. Presented at the American Academy of Pediatrics annual meeting, San Francisco, California, October 24, 1983.

146. Chamie M, Eisman S, Forrest JD. Factors affecting adolescents' use of family planning clinics. *Fam Plann Perspect* 1982;14:126.

147. Orr MT. Private physicians and the provision of contraceptives to adolescents. *Fam Plann Perspect* 1984;16:83.

148. Armour N. *Doctor refuses birth control to singles*. Associated Press, January 15, 1995.

149. Strasburger VC. Adolescent medicine in the 1990s: no more excuses. *Clin Pediatr* 1997;36:87.

150. Wender EH, Bijur PE, Boyce WT. Pediatric residency training: ten years after the Task Force report. *Pediatrics* 1992;90:876.
151. Strasburger VC. Who speaks for the adolescent? *JAMA* 1983;249:1021.
152. Ringdahl EN. The role of the family physician in preventing teenage pregnancy. *Am Fam Physician* 1992;45:2215.
153. Gillett RC Jr. Adolescent sexuality and the family physician. *Am Fam Physician* 1992;45:2026.
154. Marsiglio W, Mott FL. The impact of sex education on sexual activity, contraceptive use and premarital pregnancy among American teenagers. *Fam Plann Perspect* 1986;18:151.
155. Stout JW, Rivara FP. Schools and sex education: does it work? *Pediatrics* 1989;83:375.
156. Juszcak L, Fisher M, eds. Health care in schools. *Adolescent Medicine: State of the Art Reviews* 1996;7:163.
157. Stout JW, Kirby D. The effects of sexuality education on adolescent sexual activity. *Pediatr Ann* 1993;22:120.
158. Kirby D, Short L, Collins J, et al. School-based programs to reduce sexual risk behaviors: a review of effectiveness. *Public Health Rep* 1994;109:339.
159. Kantor LM, Haffner DW. Responding to "The failure of sex education." *SIECUS Report* 1995;23:17.
160. Alan Guttmacher Institute. *Risk and responsibility: teaching sex education in America's schools today.* New York: Alan Guttmacher Institute; 1989.
161. Forrest JD, Silverman J. What public school teachers teach about preventing pregnancy, AIDS, and sexually transmitted diseases. *Fam Plann Perspect* 1989;21:65.
162. Kenny AM, Guardado S, Brown L. Sex education and AIDS education in the schools: what states and large school districts are doing. *Fam Plann Perspect* 1989;21:56.
163. Harris L, and Associates. *America speaks: America's opinions on teenage pregnancy, sex education and birth control.* New York: Planned Parenthood Federation of America; 1988.
164. Gambrell A, Haffner D. *Unfinished business: A SIECUS assessment of state sexuality education programs.* New York: SIECUS; 1993.
165. Ross S, Kantor LM. Trends in opposition to comprehensive sexuality education in public schools, 1994–95 school year. *SIECUS Report* 1995;23:9.
166. Sellers DE, McGraw SA, McKinlay JB. Does the promotion and distribution of condoms increase teen sexual activity? Evidence from an HIV prevention program for Latino youth. *Am J Public Health* 1994;84:1952.
167. American College of Obstetricians and Gynecologists. Condom availability for adolescents. *J Adolesc Health* 1996;18:380.
168. Zabin LS, Kantner JF, Zelnik M. The risk of adolescent pregnancy in the first months of intercourse. *Fam Plann Perspect* 1979;11:215.
169. Braverman PK, Strasburger VC. Adolescent sexuality: II. contraception. *Clin Pediatr* 1993;32:725.
170. Reichelt PA. Changes in sexual behavior among unmarried teenage women utilizing oral contraception. *Journal of Popular Behavior* 1978;1:57.
171. Berger DK, Perez G, Kyman W, et al. Influence of family planning counseling in an adolescent clinic on sexual activity and contraceptive use. *Journal of Adolescent Health Care* 1987;8:436.
172. Mosher WD, Horn MC. First family planning visits by young women. *Fam Plann Perspect* 1988;20:33.
173. Shafer MA, Sweet RL. Pelvic inflammatory disease in adolescent females. *Pediatr Clin North Am* 1989;36:513.
174. Sleisenger MH, Fordtran JS. *Gastrointestinal disease: pathophysiology, diagnosis, and management.* 3rd ed. Philadelphia: WB Saunders; 1983.
175. Hunt AD, Litt IF. Obtaining a sexual history and diagnostic labeling: the influence of ethnicity and age [abstract]. *Journal of Adolescent Health Care* 1982;3:139.
176. Fine JS, Jacobson MS. Physician assessment of adolescent sexual activity. *Fam Plann Perspect* 1986;18:233.
177. Centers for Disease Control and Prevention. HIV prevention practices of primary-care physicians: United States, 1992. *MMWR Morb Mortal Wkly Rep* 1994;42:988.
178. Marks A, Fisher M, Lasker S. Adolescent medicine in pediatric practice. *Journal of Adolescent Health Care* 1990;11:149.
179. Igra V, Millstein SG. Pediatrician AIDS/STD-related preventive service provision to adolescent patients [abstract]. *Pediatr Res* 1995;37(4, pt 2):6A.
180. Schuster MA, Bell RM, Petersen L, et al. Communication between adolescents and physicians about sexual behavior and risk prevention. *Arch Pediatr Adolesc Med* 1996;150:906.
181. Kellogg ND, Huston RL. Unwanted sexual experiences in adolescents: patterns of disclosure. *Clin Pediatr* 1995;34:306.
182. Demetriou E, Emans SJ, Masland RP. Dysuria in adolescent girls: urinary tract infection or vaginitis? *Pediatrics* 1982;70:299.
183. Stevens-Simon C, Beach R, Eagar R. Conception after a negative pregnancy test during adolescence. *Adolescent and Pediatric Gynecology* 1993;6:83.
184. Zabin LS, Emerson MR, Ringers PA, et al. Adolescents with negative pregnancy test results: an accessible at-risk group. *JAMA* 1996;275:113.
185. Paperny DM, Starn JR. Adolescent pregnancy prevention by health education computer games: computer-assisted instruction of knowledge and attitudes. *Pediatrics* 1989;83:742.

186. Task Force on Pediatric AIDS, American Academy of Pediatrics. Adolescents and human immunodeficiency virus infection: the role of the pediatrician in prevention and intervention (policy statement). *Pediatrics* 1993;92:626.
187. Magee J. The pelvic exam: a view from the other end of the table. *Ann Intern Med* 1975;83:563.
188. Wilson MD, Joffe A. Step-by-step through the pelvic exam. *Contemporary Pediatrics* 1988;5:92.
189. Rimsza ME. An illustrated guide to adolescent gynecology. *Pediatr Clin North Am* 1989;36:639.
190. Altemeier WA III, Robinson DP. "I refer all my adolescents who have behavioral or sexual problems." *Pediatr Ann* 1995;24:286.
191. Grace E, Pokorny SF. At what age should a virginal adolescent have her first pelvic examination? *Journal of Pediatric and Adolescent Gynecology* 1996;9:45.
192. Turetsky RA, Strasburger VC. Adolescent contraception: review and recommendations. *Clin Pediatr* 1983;22:337.
193. Elster AB, Kuznets NJ. *AMA guidelines for adolescent preventive services (GAPS): recommendations and rationale*. Baltimore: Williams & Wilkins; 1994.
194. Phillips S, Friedman SB, Seidenberg M, et al. Teenagers' preferences regarding the presence of family members, peers, and chaperones during examination of genitalia. *Pediatrics* 1981;68:665.
195. Hofmann AD. Identifying and counseling the sexually active adolescent is every physician's responsibility. *Clin Pediatr* 1972;11:625.
196. Advocates for Youth. *Fact sheet: adolescent contraceptive use*. Washington, DC: Advocates for Youth; 1995.
197. Ammerman SD, Perelli E, Adler N, et al. Do adolescents understand what physicians say about sexuality and health? *Clin Pediatr* 1992;31:590.
198. Gordon S. The doctor, the teenager, and sex. In: Lopez RI, ed. *Adolescent medicine*. Vol. 1. New York: Spectrum; 1976:1.
199. Gordon S. *Seduction lines heard 'round the world and answers you can give*. Fayetteville, NY: Ed-U-Press; 1987.
200. Ford CA, Millstein SG, Eyre SL, et al. Anticipatory guidance regarding sex: views of virginal female adolescents. *J Adolesc Health* 1996;19:179.

SUGGESTED READING

Alan Guttmacher Institute. *Sex and America's teenagers*. New York: Alan Guttmacher Institute; 1994.
Braverman PK, Strasburger VC. Update: adolescent sexuality. I. adolescent sexuality. IV. the practitioner's role. *Clin Pediatr* 1993;32:658; and 1994;33:100.
Braverman PK, Strasburger VC. Office-based adolescent health care: issues and solutions. *Adolescent Medicine: State of the Art Reviews* 1997;8:1.
Brown JD, Steele JR. Sexuality and the media: An overview. *SIECUS Report* 1996;24(4):3.
Brown RT. Adolescent sexuality. In: Goldfarb AF, ed. *Clinical problems in pediatric and adolescent gynecology*. New York: Chapman & Hall; 1996:71.
Cartoof VG. Adolescent abortion: correlates and consequences. *Adolescent Medicine: State of the Art Reviews* 1992;3:283.
Cohen MW. Adolescent sexual activity as an expression of nonsexual needs. *Pediatr Ann* 1995;24:324.
Committee on Adolescence, American Academy of Pediatrics. Homosexuality and adolescence. *Pediatrics* 1993;92:631.
Committee on Communications, American Academy of Pediatrics. Adolescent sexuality and the media (policy statement). *Pediatrics* 1995;95:298.
Coupey SM, Klerman LV, eds. Adolescent sexuality: preventing unhealthy consequences. *Adolescent Medicine: State of the Art Reviews* 1992;3:165.
Cromer B, Brown R. The pediatrician and the sexually active adolescent: I. sexual activity and contraception. *Pediatr Clin North Am* 1997 (in press).
Ellen JM, Irwin CE Jr. Primary care management of adolescent sexual behavior. *Curr Opin Pediatr* 1996;8:442.
Epner JEG, ed. *Policy compendium on reproductive health issues affecting adolescents*. Chicago: American Medical Association; 1996.
Fortenberry JD. Condom availability in high schools. *Adolescent Medicine: State of the Art Reviews* 1997;8:449.
Frost JJ, Forrest JD. Understanding the impact of effective teenage pregnancy prevention programs. *Fam Plann Persp* 1995;27:188.
Goldenberg RL, Klerman LV. Adolescent pregnancy: another look. *N Engl J Med* 1995;332:1161.
Haffner DW, ed. *Facing facts: sexual health for America's adolescents*. New York: Sexuality Information and Education Council of the U.S. (SIECUS); 1995.
Howard M. Abstinence-based sexuality education: does it work? *Adolescent Medicine: State of the Art Reviews* 1997;8:000 (in press).
Howard M, Mitchell ME. Preventing teenage pregnancy: some questions to be answered and some answers to be questioned. *Pediatr Ann* 1993;22:109.

Jaskiewicz JA, McAnarney ER. Pregnancy during adolescence. *Pediatr Rev* 1994;15:32.

Klerman LV. Adolescent pregnancy and parenting: controversies of the past and lessons for the future. *J Adolesc Health* 1993;14:553.

McGrath J, Strasburger VC. Preventing AIDS in teenagers in the 1990s. *Clin Pediatr* 1995;34:46.

Pipher M. *Reviving Ophelia: saving the selves of adolescent girls.* New York: Ballantine; 1994.

Ringdahl EN. The role of the family physician in preventing teenage pregnancy. *Am Fam Physician* 1992;45:2215.

Roper Starch Worldwise, Inc. *Teens talk about sex: adolescent sexuality in the 90's.* New York: SIECUS; 1994.

Ryan C, Futterman D, eds. Lesbian and gay youth: care and counseling. *Adolesc Medicine: State of the Art Reviews* 1997;8:207.

Selverstone R. Sexuality education for adolescents. *Adolescent Medicine: State of the Art Reviews* 1992;3:195.

Stout JW, Kirby D. The effects of sexuality education on adolescent sexual activity. *Pediatr Ann* 1993;22:120.

Strasburger VC. *Getting your kids to say "no" in the '90s when you said "yes" in the '60s.* New York: Fireside/Simon & Schuster; 1993.

Strasburger VC. *Adolescents and the media: medical and psychological impact.* Thousand Oaks, CA: Sage; 1995,

Strasburger VC. Sex, teens, and the media. *Contemporary Pediatrics* 1996;13:29.

Strasburger VC. Adolescent medicine in the 1990s: no more excuses. *Clin Pediatr* 1997;36:87.

Sugar M. Female adolescent sexuality. *Journal of Pediatric and Adolesc Gynecology* 1996;9:175.

Tsang RC, ed. Teenage pregnancy. *Pediatr Ann* 1993;22:81.

For Teenagers and Preteenagers

Akagi C. *Dear Larissa: sexuality education for girls ages 11–17.* Littleton, CO: Gylantic Publishing Company; 1994.

Bell R. *Changing bodies, changing lives: a book for teens on sex and relationships.* New York: Vintage Books; 1988.

Gordon S. *Seduction lines heard 'round the world and answers you can give.* Fayetteville, NY: Ed-U-Press; 1987.

Harris RH. *It's perfectly normal: changing bodies, growing up, sex and sexual health.* Cambridge, MA: Candlewick Press; 1994.

Harrison M. *The preteen's first book about love, sex, and AIDS.* Washington, DC: American Psychiatric Press; 1995.

Hein K, Digeronimo T. *AIDS: trading fears for facts.* New York: Consumer Reports Books; 1989.

Madaras L. *What's happening to my body book for boys.* New York: Newmarket Press; 1988.

Madaras L. *What's happening to my body book for girls.* New York: Newmarket Press; 1988.

Masland RP Jr. *What teenagers want to know about sex.* Boston: Little, Brown; 1988.

McCoy K, Wibbelsman C. *Growing and changing: a handbook for preteens.* New York: Putnam; 1986.

Planned Parenthood Federation of America. *That growing feeling: facts of life for teens and preteens.* New York: Planned Parenthood Federation of America; 1984.

National STD Hotline (800-227-8922)

National AIDS Hotline (800-342-2437)

For Parents

Committee on Adolescence, American Academy of Pediatrics. *Sex education: a bibliography of educational materials for children, adolescents, and their families.* Elk Grove Village, IL: American Academy of Pediatrics; 1993.

Bell R. *Changing bodies, changing lives: a book for teens on sex and relationships.* New York: Vintage Books; 1988.

Brown SS, Eisenberg L, eds. *The best intentions: unintended pregnancy and the well-being of children and families.* Washington, DC: National Academy Press; 1995.

Calderone MS, Ramey JW. *Talking with your child about sex.* New York: Ballantine; 1982.

Carrera MA. *Lessons for lifeguards: working with teens when the topic is hope.* New York: Donkey Press; 1996.

Cassell C. *Straight from the heart: how to talk to your teenagers about love and sex.* New York: Simon and Schuster; 1987.

Elkind D. *Parenting your teenager in the 90's.* Rosemont, NJ: Modern Learning Press; 1993.

Gordon S, Gordon J. *Raising a child conservatively in a sexually permissive world.* New York: Simon and Schuster, 1989.

Greydanus DE, ed. *Caring for your adolescent: ages 12–21.* New York: Bantam; 1991.

Haffner DW, ed. *Facing facts: sexual health for America's adolescents.* New York: Sexuality Information and Education Council of the U.S. (SIECUS); 1995.

Luker K. *Dubious conceptions: the politics of teenage pregnancy.* Cambridge, MA: Harvard University Press; 1996.

Pipher M. *Reviving Ophelia: saving the selves of adolescent girls.* New York: Ballantine; 1994.

Slap G. *Teenage health care.* New York: Pocket Books; 1994.

Strasburger VC. *Getting your kids to say "no" in the '90s when you said "yes" in the '60s.* New York: Simon and Schuster, 1993.

Winship EC. *Reaching your teenager.* Boston: Houghton Mifflin; 1982.

Organizations to Contact for Further Information

Advocates for Youth
[formerly: Center for Population Options]
1025 Vermont Avenue, N.W.
Suite 210
Washington DC 20005
(202) 347-5700
Association of Reproductive Health Professionals
2401 Pennsylvania Ave., N.W.
Suite 350
Washington, DC 20037-1718
(202) 466-3825
Children's Defense Fund
122 C Street, N.W.
Washington, DC 20001
(202) 628-8787
Sexual Information and Educational Council of the U.S. (SIECUS)
130 West 42nd Street, Suite 350
New York, NY 10036
(212) 819-9700
National Gay Health Coalition
26 N. 35th St.
Philadelphia, PA 19104
National Gay Task Force
80 Fifth Avenue, Suite 1601
New York, NY 10011
(212) 741-5800
Planned Parenthood Federation of America
810 Seventh Avenue
New York, NY 10019
(212) 541-7800
Protecting Sexually Active Youth Newsletter
Southwest Regional Laboratory
4665 Lampson Avenue
Los Alamitos, CA 90720

CONTRACEPTION AND THE ROLE OF THE PRACTITIONER

Teenagers rarely, if ever, come to a physician (or to their parents) to ask permission to begin having sexual intercourse. In fact, most teenagers have been having intercourse for 6 months to a year before ever seeking birth control from a health provider (yet half of all teenage pregnancies occur in the first 6 months after beginning intercourse, and 20% occur in the first month alone). Nevertheless, this is the area in which practitioners can make a great impact. A single act of unprotected sexual intercourse carries with it about a 3% risk of pregnancy (range, 0–30%, depending on the phase of the menstrual cycle), but a teenager who fails to use contraception has a 90% chance of becoming pregnant within a year [1].

Contraceptive counseling is an interesting and rewarding part of adolescent health care. Although many health providers shy away from this aspect of adolescent health care, they fail to realize that their patients may be far more willing to see them for gynecologic care than an unknown (adult) gynecologist. It takes only a few patients returning from college or a few invitations to former patients' weddings for practitioners to realize that they have made a tremendous difference in the health and well-being of their patients.

Prescribing contraceptives to teenagers remains a controversial area, although it really should not be. Teenagers decide on the timing of the sexual relations independently—apart from parents, physicians, and sometimes even peers. What the practitioner can offer is straightforward, nonjudgmental information, and a willingness to assist in avoiding pregnancies and sexually transmitted diseases (STD). *The availability of birth control does not make teenagers sexually active at any earlier age, or more sexually promiscuous* [2]. Parents and health professionals frequently think that there are three choices when a teenage girl begins having sex: 1) she can become pregnant, 2) she can use birth control, or 3) she can stop. In fact, the last choice is not actually on the menu. For parents, the real dilemma is whether to allow their daughters access to birth control, or to become grandparents. For health providers, the choice is between providing protection for their patients or not.

Teenage Contraceptive Habits

Because of their unique psychology, teenagers are not ideal contraceptors (Fig. 5). Teenagers view themselves egocentrically as being actors and actresses in their own personal fables in which the normal rules may apply to everyone but themselves [3]. Ask a 15-year-old what will happen if her best friend has intercourse, and the answer is: "She'll get pregnant." But ask her what will happen if *she* has intercourse, and the answer will be: "Nothing. It can't happen to me." This infuriates adults, but, in fact, is consistent with normal adolescent psychology. Even though 70% of teenagers are able to think logically and sequentially by age 16 years [4], they still may suffer from what Elkind terms "pseudo-stupidity"—"the capacity to conceive many different alternatives is not immediately coupled with the ability to assign priorities and to decide which choice is more or less appropriate than others" [5].

Many adults think that the fear of pregnancy (or, in the past decade, of acquired immunodeficiency syndrome [AIDS]) should be sufficient to deter teenagers from early initiation of sexual relations. But teenagers view themselves as being immune from such mundane afflictions. In the Johns Hopkins surveys during the 1970s, over 50% of teenage girls not using contraception thought that they could not become pregnant [6]. In the 1986 national survey by Harris, the leading reason for not using birth control was "no time to use" (Table 24). The 1994 Roper poll found that nearly 60% of teens who failed to use contraception did so because "they were not available at the time" [7]. Certainly, the amount of misinformation that today's teenagers have—despite their peers and the influence of the media—is as-

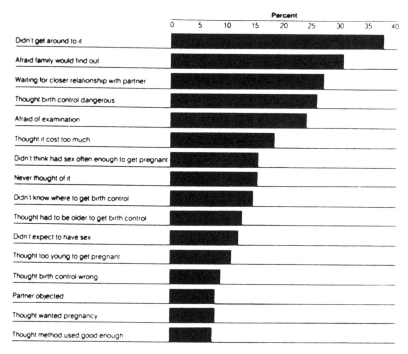

FIG. 5. Why teenagers do not use contraception. Reasons for not using contraception at last intercourse, of 337 female adolescents, aged 15 to 19 years, who were not trying to become pregnant. (Zenick M, Kantner JF. Reasons for nonuse of contraception by sexually active women aged 15–19. *Fam Plann Perspect* 1979;11:294. Copyright 1979. Reprinted with permission of the Alan Guttmacher Institute.

TABLE 24. *Reasons sexually active teenagers give for not using contraception*

Not available at the time (e.g., unexpected sex, didn't want to take time)	59%
Too embarrassing to buy	35%
Afraid parents would find the contraceptives	31%
Preferred not to use (e.g., it's unnatural, didn't think about it, against religion)	28%
Don't like the way contraceptives feel	25%
Lack of knowledge or access (e.g., couldn't get, couldn't afford, didn't know where to get)	14%
Fear or embarrassment (e.g., afraid parents would find out, afraid of side effects, embarrassed to ask for)	10%
No need (e.g., pregnancy won't happen to them, ineffective)	10%
Wanted to get pregnant	2%

Adapted from Harris L, and Associates. *American teens speak: sex, myths, TV, and birth control.* New York: Planned Parenthood Federation of America; 1986; and Roper Starch Worldwise, Inc. *Teens talk about sex: adolescent sexuality in the 90's.* New York: SIECUS; 1994.

tounding (see Table 16), but this is precisely where the practitioner can make the greatest difference [8]. Certain key myths about sexual activity and birth control must be dispelled; the facts are:

- You *can* get pregnant the first time you have intercourse.
- There is no absolutely safe time of the month to have sexual intercourse without using contraception.
- Contraception works! Nearly 40% of female adolescents not using contraception become pregnant within the first 6 months of beginning sexual relations, and two thirds are pregnant within 2 years [9].
- Pelvic inflammatory disease (PID) develops in one of eight sexually active 15- to 19-year-olds [10].
- Use of alcohol lowers normal inhibitions and may lead to activities the teenager may later regret. Female teens are generally more susceptible to alcohol's effects because they weigh less than male teens.
- Nothing is as safe as abstinence, but using birth control is approximately 10 to 25 times safer (and having a first-trimester abortion is approximately 10 times safer) than carrying a pregnancy to term.
- There is no one ideal contraceptive. Each person must make a decision about the ease, effectiveness, and safety of the various methods.
- There are virtually no medical risks associated with the use of either condoms or diaphragms, other than failure to prevent pregnancy if they are used improperly or malfunction. The risk of taking oral contraceptives (OCs) is minuscule compared with the overwhelming medical *and* social risks of having a teenage pregnancy. In fact, *in the world's medical literature, there is only one reported death of a teenager from taking OCs*—an 18-year-old, reported in the Swedish medical literature in 1968, who died from a subarachnoid hemorrhage [11]. And the OC preparation used was probably 80 to 100 μg—two to three times as potent as today's pills. It is imperative that practitioners put the risk of birth control into proper perspective (Tables 25, 26).
- Oral contraceptives do not stunt one's growth. The concentrations of estrogen and progesterone contained in OCs are far less than what is produced endogenously, and by menarche, most skeletal growth is finished. OCs can be started once a teenager has established her menarche and had three to six normal periods, or earlier if necessary.
- For the first time, new data [12,13] show that school-based educational programs *can* be effective in increasing rates of contraceptive use among teens by as much as 22%, but such programs must:
  - Provide access to birth control
  - Target younger adolescents
  - Target adolescents who are not yet sexually experienced

If contraceptive education occurs in the same year that a young woman becomes sexually active, her odds of condom use increase 70% to 80%, and those of pill use more than double [13].

A physician's ability to provide counseling may remove one of the biggest barriers to teenagers' effective use of birth control—inadequate access. In the Harris survey, over 75% of teens surveyed thought that "telling teenagers where they can get birth control without anyone else finding out" and "making birth control free of cost" would make them more likely to use contraception [14]. (Interestingly, only 48% thought that telling teenagers that using birth control was "healthy" would maximize use, and two thirds rejected the notion that telling teens that birth control is "cool" would be effective [14].) Clearly, for sexuality- and drug-related issues, confidentiality is one of the key issues for

TABLE 25. *Voluntary and involuntary risks in everyday life*

	Deaths/person/y, odds
Voluntary risks	
Smoking, 20 cigarettes/day	1 in 200
Drinking, 1 bottle wine/day	1 in 13,300
Motorcycling	1 in 1,000
Driving an automobile	1 in 6,000
Professional boxing	1 in 14,300
Playing football	1 in 25,000
Canoeing	1 in 100,000
Skiing	1 in 1,430,000
Involuntary risks	
Hit by automobile	1 in 20,000
Earthquake (California)	1 in 588,000
Tornados (Midwest)	1 in 455,000
Lightning	1 in 10 million
Falling aircraft	1 in 10 million
Leukemia	1 in 12,500
Influenza	1 in 5,000
Meteorite	1 in 100 billion

Adapted from Dinman BD. The reality and acceptance of risk. *JAMA* 1980;244:1226; and from Hatcher RA, Trussell J, Stewart F, et al. *Contraceptive technology.* 16th ed. New York: Irvington Publishers; 1994

most adolescents, and they do not tend to see their pediatrician or family physician as being willing or able to provide such services [15].

Other important barriers to adolescents' use of effective contraception include [1,2,14–18]:

- Lack of knowledge about services or methods and perceived side effects (Table 27)
- Cost of medical services and of contraceptives
- For girls, fear of a pelvic examination. (In the Harris report, more than two thirds of the young women said that having to undergo a pelvic examination was a deterrent to obtaining birth control. Prior experience did not alter this perception because 70% of those who had already used OCs and presumably already had a pelvic examination expressed fear of the examination [14].)

TABLE 26. *Risks of contraception and pregnancy*

Risk	Deaths/person/y, odds
Oral contraception (*all* women)	
Smoker	1 in 16,000
Nonsmoker	1 in 63,000
Intrauterine device	1 in 100,000
Barrier methods	None
Laparoscopic tubal ligation	1 in 67,000
Full-term pregnancy	1 in 11,000
Illegal abortion	1 in 3,000
Legal abortion	
Before 9 wk	1 in 260,000
Between 9–12 wk	1 in 100,000
Between 13–16 wk	1 in 34,000
After 16 wk	1 in 10,200

Adapted from Hatcher RA, Trussell J, Stewart F, et al. *Contraceptive technology.* 16th ed. New York: Irvington Publishers; 1994.

TABLE 27. *Teenagers' perceptions of the side effects of oral contraceptives*

Perceived side effect	Percentage of youth responding ($N = 426 + 99$)
Weight gain	82
Cancer	18
Nausea	12
Sterility	11
Can get pregnant despite use	8
Birth defects	6
Heart disease	5
Other	29
Not sure	17

Adapted from Harris L, and Associates. *American teens speak: sex, myths, TV, and birth control.* New York: Planned Parenthood Federation of America; 1986; and Grace E, Emans SJ, Havens KK, et al. Contraceptive compliance with a triphasic and a monophasic norethindrone-containing oral contraceptive pill in a private adolescent practice. *Adolescent and Pediatric Gynecology* 1994;7:29.

Teenagers' Use of Contraception in the 1990s

In 1997, the news still is decidedly mixed about adolescents and their use of contraception. On the positive side, programs aimed at increasing contraceptive use among American teens have worked (see Table 12). Among sexually active teens, pregnancy rates have decreased 19% since the mid-1970s [1]. More recently, birth rates decreased 2% between 1991 and 1992 and another 2% between 1992 and 1993 [19,20]. Numerous recent studies document that American teenagers are using contraception in increasing numbers (see Tables 3, 7; and 28, 29). In the most recent Youth Risk Behavior Survey of more than 16,000 high school students nationwide, 53% reported using condoms at their last sexual encounter, an increase from 46% in 1991 [21] (see Table 7). Some surveys report condom use at most recent intercourse at rates as high as 71% of all teenagers [22]. Increased awareness of and knowledge about human immunodeficiency virus (HIV) and AIDS seem to have catalyzed this increase [9,23,24], although not all studies demonstrate this linkage [25–27]. Two thirds of female adolescents use contraception the first time they have intercourse [1,28,29]. (The older the teenager at first intercourse, the greater the likelihood of contraception being used). And apparently increasing numbers of teenagers are now using two forms of birth control: OCs for pregnancy prevention and condoms for STD prevention [30].

Unfortunately, there is reason for continued concern. Several studies have documented that about one third of teens do not use any contraception at first intercourse [1,2,31] and that only one third of sexually active teens who say they use condoms use them *every* time they have intercourse [7,26,32]. Paradoxically, those teenagers at highest risk for STDs (e.g., substance abuse, multiple partners, early intercourse) are the least likely to use condoms [24,33,34]. In general, condom use decreases with

TABLE 28. *College women and condom use, 1975–1995*

Frequency of use	1975 ($N = 427$)	1986 ($N = 140$)	1989 ($N = 113$)	1995 ($N = 118$)
Always or almost always	11%	21%	41%	74%
Seldom or never	87%	71%	58%	24%

Adapted from Peipert JF, Domaglski L, Boardman L, et al. College women and condom use, 1975–1995. *N Engl J Med* 1996; 335:211.

TABLE 29. *Trends in young men's condom use*

Measure	Age (y)		
	17–18	19–20	21–22
Used condom at first intercourse	59%	56%	46%
Used condom at most recent intercourse	55%	42%	35%
Partner used pill at initial intercourse	21%	27%	35%
Average frequency of intercourse/month	3.9	6.1	7.4

Adapted from Ku L, Sonenstein F, Pleck JH. The dynamics of young men's condom use during and across relationships. *Fam Plann Perspect* 1994;26:246.

age, whereas OC use increases [1] (Table 30. To date, specific programs to increase condom use among high-risk youth have not always been successful beyond a few months [33,35,36].

What predicts which adolescents will use contraception? After age, the most important predictors of contracepting at first intercourse in one study were being white, having a mother with more than a high school education, delaying first relations until age 19 or later, and living in an intact family [37]. A sample of black Chicago teens showed that social class, neighborhood quality, and parental marital status were the most important predictors of first-time use—all of which may reflect the teenagers' "upward mobility" [38]. Other studies have found high self-esteem and positive attitudes toward birth control to be important [2,32], as well as communication with parents [2,39–41]. Early substance abusers are less likely to contracept [35,42,43]. Teenagers who are involved in longer relationships before intercourse and whose partners insist on condom use are more likely to use them [44].

Again, the media could be a powerful public health weapon here, encouraging sexually active teenagers to use contraception, but American media have shied away from mentioning birth control in advertising or in prime-time programming [45–47]. In Zaire, for example, use of the media to promote condom use increased sales from 900,000 to 18,000,000 in only 3 years [47].

Oral Contraceptives

In many ways, OCs represent an ideal form of pregnancy prevention for teenagers because they dissociate intercourse from the act of contracepting (Table 31). Female teenagers frequently like to think of sex as being "romantic and spontaneous" and of being "swept away by passion." Male teens, on the other hand, more closely resemble General Patton, eagerly eyeing enemy territory and plotting how to take it.

Despite the fact that OCs do not offer much protection against STDs, they do offer nearly 99.7% protection against pregnancy when taken as directed (Table 32). Therefore, they represent the easiest, most effective, and most rational form of pregnancy prevention for teenagers. The biggest disadvantages of OCs are that they are not readily available (a medical evaluation and prescription is required) and, as mentioned, they do not afford the kind of protection against STDs that barrier methods do. Currently, practitioners are recommending a "belt and suspenders" approach to contra-

TABLE 30. *Contraceptive habits of sexually active youth (Minnesota study)*

	Grades 7–8	Grades 9–10	Grades 11–12
Condom	33%	20%	12%
Oral contraceptives	8%	12%	30%
Withdrawal	9%	17%	18%
Other	4%	3%	2%
Do not use	46%	48%	39%

Adapted from Blum RW. *The state of adolescent health in Minnesota.* Minneapolis: University of Minnesota; 1989.

TABLE 31. *Adolescent contraception*

	Pill	Intrauterine device	Diaphragm	Condoms
Motivation required	+++	0	++++	++
Episodic sex	0	+	+	+
Frequent sex	++++	+++	+/−	+
Systemic side effects	++	+++	0	0
Messy	0	0	++++	++
Male cooperation required	0	0	+/−	++++
Secrecy possible	Difficult	Easy	Difficult	Possible

Adapted from Kreutner AK. Adolescent contraception. *Prim Care* 1987;14:121.

ception for adolescents: OCs for pregnancy prevention and condoms for STD prevention [48]. Asking a young teenager to use both OCs and a barrier method—while medically sound—may be overly optimistic, given normal adolescent psychology and the difficulty of using even one method. To date, about one fourth of sexually active teens seem able to combine both methods successfully [1,31].

Combination OCs are thought to work at several different levels of the reproductive system. Their primary action is to inhibit gonadotropin-releasing hormone, thereby blocking the mid-cycle surge of luteinizing hormone that produces ovulation. But at the ovarian level, they also inhibit follicular maturation; at the endometrial level, they cause thinning of the endometrium and a less hospitable environment for implantation; and at the cervical level, they thicken cervical mucus [49].

Practitioners also need to be cognizant of the many different effects OCs can have on various laboratory values (Table 33).

Formulation

There are 46 different name-brand OCs listed in the *1997 Physician's Desk Reference*; however, experience with just a handful of different types of pills is all that is required (Table 34).

Oral contraceptives in the United States contain one of two different estrogens and one of seven different progestins:

Estrogen
Ethinyl estradiol
Mestranol

TABLE 32. *Theoretical and actual effectiveness of various contraceptive methods*

Method	Perfect use	Actual use
Combination oral contraceptives	99.9%	90–97%
Depo-Provera	99.7%	99.7%
Norplant	99.9%	99.9%
Progesterone-only contraceptives	98%	90%
Condom + spermicide	99%	95%
Condom	97%	88%
Female condom	95%	79%
Spermicide	94%	79%
Diaphragm	94%	82%
Intrauterine device	98%	98%
Withdrawal	91%	75%
No method		85%

Adapted from Hatcher RA, Trussell J, Stewart F, et al. *Contraceptive technology.* 16th ed. New York: Irvington Publishers; 1994; and Choices of contraceptives. *The Medical Letter* 1995;37(941):9.

TABLE 33. *Laboratory changes in patients taking oral contraceptives*

Laboratory evaluation	Increased level	Decreased level
Plasma proteins	Prealbumin Immunoglobulins Transferrin Thyroid-binding globulin Fibrinogen	Albumin Haptoglobin Renin
Hormones	Thyroxine (T_4) Cortisol Prolactin Growth hormone Follicle-stimulating hormone	Triiodothyronine (T_3) resin uptake Urinary 17-OH and 17-keto steroids Luteinizing hormone
Other	Hematocrit Platelet count and cohesiveness Erythrocyte sedimentation rate Iron, TIBC Clotting factors II, VII, VIII, IX, X, and prothrombin Serum transaminases Antinuclear antibody	Urine THC Prothrombin time Vitamin B_{12} C-reactive protein Magnesium Folate Zinc

Adapted from Dickey RP. *Managing contraceptive pill patients.* 8th ed. Durant, OK: Creative Infomatics; 1996.

Progestin
Norethindrone
Norethindrone acetate
Ethynodiol diacetate
Norgestrel
Levonorgestrel
Norgestimate
Desogestrel

After being metabolized in the liver, the two estrogens are virtually identical, although ethinyl estradiol is thought to be slightly more potent on a microgram-for-microgram basis. However, the progestins are metabolized in different ways and may exert estrogenic, antiestrogenic, or androgenic effects in addition to their progestational effects (Table 35). The balance between the estrogens and progestins determines the overall effect on the endometrium and, to a large extent, the side effects of the particular preparation.

Estrogens were originally thought to be the culprit in producing the major morbidity of OCs. They increase levels of plasminogen and fibrinogen and consequently predispose toward the formation of clots (i.e., stroke, pulmonary embolism, thrombophlebitis). However, these risks are greatly diminished when the level of estrogen is reduced to 50 μg or less, and most current formulations use 30 to 35 μg of estrogen.

TABLE 34. *One physician's armamentarium: eight oral contraceptives*

Starting pills	Desogen or Ortho-Cyclen Ortho-Novum 1/35 Triphasil or Ortho-Tricyclen
Acne (estrogen-dominant)	Demulen 1/35 Desogen or Ortho-Cept
Pill amenorrhea or breakthrough bleeding (progestin-dominant)	Lo-Ovral
Postcoital contraception	Ovral

TABLE 35. *Relative potencies of progestins in oral contraceptives*

Class and compound	Progestational	Estrogenic	Androgenic
Gonane			
Levonorgestrel	5.3	0	8.3
Norgestrel	2.6	0	4.2
Norgestimate	1.3	0	1.9
Desogestrel	9.0	0	3.4
Gestodene[a]	12.6	0	8.6
Estrane			
Norethindrone	1.0	1.0	1.0
Norethindrone acetate	1.2	1.5	1.6
Ethynodiol diacetate	1.4	3.4	0.6

[a]Not currently available in the United States.
Adapted from Dickey RP. *Managing contraceptive pill patients.* 8th ed. Durant, OK: Creative Infomatics; 1996.

In the 1980s, progestins were implicated in creating certain risks, particularly in altering lipid profiles [50]. Pills containing levonorgestrel or norgestrel appear to have adverse effects on serum lipids, perhaps lowering the high-density lipoprotein (HDL_2) subfraction of cholesterol that is thought to be protective [51–53]. However, these lipid disturbances are probably *not* significant for the average adolescent taking OCs for a few years, and some animal studies suggest that OCs may have a protective effect against atherosclerosis, despite lowering HDL levels [54].

The New Progestins

In 1992 and 1993, two new progestins were introduced into OCs: norgestimate and desogestrel [55] (Table 36). Another new progestin, gestodene, is available in Europe and may become available in the United States soon [56]. These new progestins are more progestational and less androgenic in their effects and therefore have several theoretical and practical advantages over OCs containing older progestins [55,57,58]:

• Greater improvement in patients with acne
• More effectiveness in treating hirsutism, especially in combination with leuprolide (Lupron) [59]
• More favorable impact on lipoprotein profiles

Some of the benefits of the older OCs remain unchanged:

• Minimal or no weight gain: because weight gain is of prime concern to most adolescents (see Table 27), it is important to emphasize that low-dose OCs do not result in significant weight gain [60] (Tables 37, 38).
• Good cycle control: approximately 10% of patients experience breakthrough bleeding or spotting in the first 6 months' of OC use, and this number diminishes during the next 6 months [61].
• Improvement in dysmenorrhea: by 6 months, 90% of patients experience improvement [57].

However, there is a new controversy surrounding two of the new progestins, desogestrel and gestodene. In October, 1995, the United Kingdom Committee on the Safety of Medicines recommended that women taking OCs containing either progestin switch to another OC after completing their cur-

TABLE 36. *The later generation progestin pills*

Name	Estrogen	Progestin
Ortho-Cyclen	Ethinyl estradiol, 35 μg	Norgestimate, 0.25 mg
Ortho-TriCyclen	Ethinyl estradiol, 35 μg	Norgestimate, 0.18 mg, 0.215 mg, 0.25 mg
Ortho-Cept	Ethinyl estradiol, 30 μg	Desogestrel, 0.15 mg
Desogen	Ethinyl estradiol, 30 μg	Desogestrel, 0.15 mg

TABLE 37. *Side effects of later generation hormonal contraceptives*

Condition	New oral contraceptives	Depo-Provera	Norplant
Acne	++	−	−
Anemia	++	++	+
Dysmenorrhea	++	++	+
Hirsutism	++	−	−
Ovarian cancer	++	?	−
Endometrial cancer	++	++	−
Breast cysts	+	?	−

+, positive effect; −, no effect.
Adapted from Coupey SM. New hormonal contraceptive options for adolescents. In: Goldfarb AF, ed. *Clinical problems in pediatric and adolescent gynecology.* New York: Chapman & Hall; 1996:77.

rent pack [62]. The warning was based on three, large, then-unpublished studies that showed a two- to fourfold increased risk of venous thromboembolism for patients taking the new OCs (but not OCs containing norgestimate—there were too few norgestimate users to assess risk [63]). However, the Federal Food and Drug Administration (FDA) reviewed the preliminary data and concluded that the "risk is not great enough to justify switching to other products." According to the FDA, the risk of nonfatal venous thromboembolism is still twice as high in pregnancy as in women using OCs containing desogestrel [64]. Altogether, there are now five published studies dealing with this issue [65–69], and a number of conclusions can be drawn [62,70]:

1. Given that the overall risk of thromboembolism is quite small, the warning seemed like an overreaction to many observers.
2. This is especially true because the risk remains lower than during a full-term pregnancy [71].
3. Although large, most of the studies excluded adolescents, failed to factor in cigarette use, and were heavily weighted toward older women, so that the implications for teenagers are completely unknown.
4. Even if the studies were applicable to teenage women, a doubling of the risk of deep venous thrombosis translates into a increase from 1 to 2 per 100,000 per woman-years of contraceptive use. By comparison, the risk of thrombosis in pregnant women of all ages is 8/100,000 [72].
5. The studies all suffer from significant methodologic biases.
6. One study has actually found a significant protective effect of desogestrel-containing OCs against myocardial infarction [73]. Such a positive effect may outweigh other, smaller negative effects.
7. With proper informed consent, OCs containing desogestrel are still appropriate for most women desiring contraception, especially teenagers.

TABLE 38. *Actual side effects of oral contraceptives reported by adolescents (after 12 months' use)*

Side effect	Triphasic pill (N = 41)	Monophasic pill (N = 32)
Breakthrough bleeding	66%	28%
Weight gain	17%	0%
Breast soreness	12%	3%
Amenorrhea	5%	16%
Headaches	5%	0%
Total reported side effects	73%	44%

Adapted from Grace E, Emans SJ, Havens KK, et al. Contraceptive compliance with a triphasic and a monophasic norethindrone-containing oral contraceptive pill in a private adolescent practice. *Adolescent and Pediatric Gynecology* 1994;7:29.

Multiphasic Oral Contraceptives

The terminology used in describing OCs can often get confusing. Multiphasic pills can be either biphasic (two different concentrations of hormone) or triphasic (three). Furthermore, some multiphasic pills are "true" triphasic OCs—that is, they vary concentrations of both the estrogen and the progestin three separate times (e.g., Triphasil, Ortho-Tri-Cyclen). Others vary only the progestin content (e.g., Ortho 7/7/7, Tri-Norinyl). The goal of pill manufacturers is to mimic as closely as possible the hormonal changes in a normal menstrual cycle; however, changing the estrogen phase of the pill necessitates repeating expensive studies on pregnancy rates, whereas the progestin component can be changed more easily.

Triphasic OCs were introduced in 1984 and can now be recommended as pills of first choice because they contain the lowest average concentrations of estrogen and progestin [74]. Certain triphasic pills contain levonorgestrel, which may have a negative impact on lipoprotein profiles (e.g., Triphasil and Tri-Levlen), although their total progestin content is only 10% that of such pills as Ortho-Novum 7/7/7, which contains norethindrone. Practitioners should be aware of these differences and monitor serum lipid levels if patients have high coronary risk profiles. Ortho-Tri-Cyclen is the only triphasic OC which contains one of the new progestins (norgestimate).

Triphasic OCs are a little more difficult to use. Because of their low hormonal content, they must be taken at close to the same time each day; and missing even one pill in the second week can diminish effectiveness. For some patients, the multicolor pill sequences can be confusing. In addition, in one small study, triphasic pill-users reported a higher incidence of side effects after 12 months (but not after 3 months) compared with monophasic pill users [75]. Therefore, triphasic pills probably should be reserved for college-age women and selected younger teenagers who are likely to be highly compliant.

Contraindications

In many ways, female teens are the ideal population to be taking OCs [57]. Few of the absolute contraindications come into play for teenagers [52,76]:

- Thrombophlebitis, thromboembolic disease, or stroke
- Impaired liver function
- Breast cancer or estrogen-dependent neoplasia
- Undiagnosed abnormal vaginal bleeding
- Known or suspected pregnancy

Relative contraindications are far more numerous, and include [76,77]:

- Migraine headaches
- Hypertension
- Diabetes mellitus
- Seizure disorder
- Sickle cell anemia
- Systemic lupus erythematosus
- Hyperlipidemia
- Gallbladder or renal disease

In particular, the relationship between migraine headaches or hypertension and strokes has never been definitively proven. But because migraine may involve a vasoconstrictive phase, and the pill produces an increased tendency toward clotting and a decreased hemovascular ability to dissolve clots, some experts believe it is wisest to avoid it in such patients. In older studies, higher-dose OCs were found to increase the risk of stroke among women with a history of migraine headaches [78]. One compromise solution would be to reserve OCs to young women with nonvascular tension headaches and those with common migraine (without focal symptoms) [79]. However, because headaches are a major warning signal of cerebrovascular accidents—a rare but well known complication of all OCs—using OCs in a patient with any history of severe headaches may be problematic [76]. Other experts believe that a cautious trial of OCs can be used, particularly because many patients will experience less severe headaches. Certainly, the incidence of thrombotic stroke could probably be decreased if hypertensive patients were not given OCs. One alternative that is generally accepted is to treat patients who have either migraine or hypertension with the progestin-only minipill [80].

All patients taking OCs should be instructed to 1) discontinue them 2 to 4 weeks before elective surgery, 2) avoid taking medications that may interfere with their efficacy (Table 39), and 3) stop smoking. Teenagers who smoke should probably be counseled that their risks of serious complications are increased, although the confirmatory data all involve adult women, usually older than 35 years of age [81].

Risks

What should patients be told about the risk of taking OCs? Overemphasizing the complications may lead to a patient's reticence in beginning oral contraception or jeopardize her compliance. On the other hand, informed consent must be obtained, and this involves providing a realistic assessment of risks and benefits to the patient. Part of this dilemma is solved by putting the risks of OCs into proper perspective—they must be compared with the risks of everyday life and the risk of pregnancy or abortion (see Tables 25, 26). Although exact data are hard to come by, it is probably 10 to 25 times safer for a teenager to take the pill than to carry a pregnancy to term or have an abortion.

Mortality

Mortality is *not* a significant risk in teenagers taking the pill. Although the patient information packet lists such mortality figures as 1.2 deaths/100,000 users/year for nonsmokers and 1.4 deaths/100,000 users/year, in fact these are theoretical figures. In addition, they must be placed in perspective: the estimated risk of death during a full-term pregnancy is 11.1/100,000 during adolescence [82]. In a large, comprehensive study that encompassed 54,971 woman-years of OC use and looked at all age groups, only a slight excess mortality for OC users was demonstrated (1.3-fold) [83]. With only one reported death among teenagers taking the pill [11], it is completely appropriate to tell patients, "You probably have a greater chance of dying from a 747 aircraft landing on your head than from taking the pill."

Morbidity

Morbidity also must be placed in proper perspective. In general, it is worthwhile informing patients that they have an increased risk of forming clots while on the pill but that pregnancy would involve greater risks [71]. Unfortunately, the literature is replete with large studies of older women taking high-dose OCs (more than 50 μg, now no longer available). Teenagers have the lowest risk rate of any group of OC users. Overall, the vascular risks of OCs (e.g., venous thromboembolism, thrombotic stroke, hypertension, and subarachnoid hemorrhage) are increased approximately two- to fivefold, but this amounts to an occurrence rate of approximately 2 incidents per 100,000 users per year and, again, is far more common in older women [62,65–69,78]. A meta-analysis of 47 different studies found a relative risk of 1.8 for OC users, but high-dose pills were used by women in some of the studies [84]. Many observers believe that most, if not all, of this increased risk can be attributed to cigarette smoking [85]. Studies have failed to show an increased risk of myocardial infarction in either users of low-

TABLE 39. *Drugs that may interfere with oral contraceptives*

Drug	Mechanism of action	Solution
Anticonvulsants (phenobarbital, phenytoin, ethosuximide, carbamazepine)	Induction of microsomal liver enzymes; more rapid estrogen metabolism	Use another method, drug, or higher-dose oral contraceptive (50 μg)
Antibiotics (penicillin, ampicillin, metronidazole, tetracycline)	Enterohepatic circulation disturbance; induction of microsomal enzymes	Controversial: more data needed; consider another drug or backup method if long course
Sedatives (benzodiazepines, chloral hydrate, antimigraines)	Increased microsomal liver enzymes	Use another drug or back-up method

Adapted from Dickey RP. *Managing contraceptive pill patients.* 8th ed. Durant, OK: Creative Infomatics; 1996.

dose pills or in previous users [50,85,86]; the most recent study actually found a significant protective effect [73].

According to a 1993 Gallup Poll, a majority of men and women believe that taking OCs involves "substantial risks," and nearly two thirds of women thought that OC use was as risky as childbirth [79]. The risk most associated with OCs is cancer, although in fact OCs significantly *lower* the risk of ovarian cancer and endometrial cancer [87–91], as well as benign breast masses (fibroadenomas and cysts), uterine fibroids, and ovarian cysts [76,92]. Their effect on breast and cervical cancers remains unclear and controversial. Benign liver tumors, a rare occurrence in adult women only, are increased [76]; the risk for hepatocellular carcinoma is also unsettled [93,94].

Breast Cancer. Several years ago, an FDA panel reviewed all breast cancer studies to date and found that there is insufficient evidence to link OCs with breast cancer, except perhaps in certain sub-groups of former users [89,95]. There is continued concern that adolescents may constitute one of these subgroups [76,96]. The largest study to date, involving over 118,000 nurses, found no increased risk of breast cancer in former OC users. However, few of the subjects began using OCs as teens. The researchers plan to enroll another 100,000 nurses in a follow-up study and remedy this situation [97].

More recently, a study of 2,203 women aged 20 to 54 years with in situ or invasive breast cancer found that women who have used OCs for at least 6 months are 1.3 times more likely as others to have breast cancer, but that the risk increases to 1.7 for those younger than 35 years. Women reporting 10 or more years of OC pill use had a relative risk of 2.3. In addition, women who initiated pill use before age 18 years had a 2.2-fold increased relative risk of breast cancer [98]. If this more recent study holds up, it may have important implications for teenagers who have strong family histories of breast cancer [90].

Finally, in 1996, the Collaborative Group on Hormonal Factors in Breast Cancer published a re-markable study that identified all available studies involving breast cancer. They identified a total of 53,297 women with breast cancer and 100,239 control subjects from 54 different studies; these data were then reanalyzed. No evidence of an increased risk was found for women who had stopped using OCs 10 years or more previously, and only a slight increased relative risk was found during OC use, equivalent to one additional cancer per 20,000 women aged 16 to 19 years taking OCs. However, the risk increased more substantially for women in their third decade (an additional 9.4 cancers per 20,000 women aged 25–29 years taking OCs) [99].

Cervical Cancer. Several 1980s studies demonstrated an increased risk of cervical cancer of 1.3 to 1.8 for women taking OCs, with the higher figure applying to those who used the pill longer [100–103]. Three more recent studies all confirm this finding [104–106]:

- A case–control study in Los Angeles found that use of OCs doubles the risk for development of ade-nocarcinoma of the cervix, with long-term users having the highest risk [104].
- A Canadian study found that pill users are 40% more likely to have cervical intraepithelial neopla-sia. The risk doubles for long-term pill users [105].
- An international case–control study suggests that women who have ever used OCs are 30% more likely to have cervical carcinoma in situ, with long-term users having about twice the risk of those who never used [106].

Despite these studies, the link between cervical dysplasia and human papillomavirus (HPV) re-mains much stronger [107]. Along with cigarette smoking, OCs could function as a cocarcinogen in women already infected with HPV. In addition, the protective effects of OCs against endometrial and ovarian cancers could outweigh any increased risk for cervical or breast cancers [90].

Cervicitis and Pelvic Inflammatory Disease. Oral contraceptives may play a role in cervical infec-tions and PID [108]. Studies have found increased [109] and decreased [110] rates of gonococcal cer-vical infections, but by 1985, 15 of 17 published reports had described a positive association between OCs and chlamydial cervicitis [76,111]. A large 1995 report disputes these findings, however: a study of 1,779 Seattle women aged 15 to 34 years found no effect of OCs on the risk of chlamydial infection [112]. OC users tend to be younger and have a higher incidence of cervical ectopy than other contra-ceptors. Therefore, the authors suggest, previous researchers may have improperly adjusted for age, leading to the conclusion that OCs increase the risk of chlamydial infection by inducing cervical ec-topy [113]. The issue is also complicated by the fact that the presence of cervical ectopy provides eas-ier sampling of cervical tissue, making diagnosis easier [79], and young women on OCs tend to have more frequent check-ups. Paradoxically, researchers reason that although OCs may increase the colo-nization of the lower genital tract, they also may exert a protective effect against dissemination be-cause they thicken cervical mucus [111,114]. Consequently, OC users have 50% less hospitalizations for PID and lower rates of chlamydial salpingitis and endometritis [79].

Other effects of OCs are misunderstood or relatively minor. They do *not* inhibit skeletal growth because female teenagers have already attained 97% of their height potential by menarche [76]. They do *not* cause amenorrhea or infertility when discontinued: 98% of women are ovulatory by the third cycle after stopping OCs, and most women resume their normal prepill menstrual pattern, regardless of how long they have taken OCs [108,115]. Newer formulations have no adverse effects on glucose metabolism [58,116].

A report from the 1988 World Congress on AIDS in Stockholm [117] found that African prostitutes who used OCs were two to three times more likely to become infected with the AIDS virus than other prostitutes. This represents a preliminary finding and could be related to the virulence of the HIV strains or other factors [79]. Studies in developed countries have found no such increase in the risk of HIV transmission with OC use [79], but the pill does increase the vascularity of the cervical epithelium and alter local immune mechanisms [118], so overall the relationship between OCs and HIV remains ill defined [76].

Beneficial Effects

Oral contraceptives also have many beneficial effects, aside from their effectiveness in preventing pregnancy and lowering the incidence of endometrial and ovarian cancer [108,119] (Table 40). They represent the treatment of choice for teenagers with severe dysmenorrhea or moderate or severe dysfunctional uterine bleeding, and they decrease the incidence of iron deficiency anemia by decreasing blood loss. For female athletes experiencing amenorrhea, treatment with OCs could have a favorable impact on bone mineral density, although more research is needed [120]. Using any risk–benefit scheme, the benefits of OCs far outweigh the risks for most potential adolescent users [48,121].

How to Prescribe Oral Contraceptives for Teenagers (Fig. 6)

No physician has ever been successfully sued for prescribing OCs to a minor, nor has any lawsuit been filed in the past 30 years [122,123]. Yet many practitioners remain either reluctant to provide birth control to minors (see Table 14) or less knowledgeable than they should be. During the past decade, several studies have documented pediatricians' reluctance to deal with sexually active teenagers and their self-confessed deficits in knowledge [2,124–127]. In one study, only 32% of pediatricians said that they would be willing to prescribe OCs for a 15-year-old patient, and many would insist on parental consent [128], despite no legal requirement to do so [129]. In another, more recent study of pediatricians in private practice in Pittsburgh, less than one third offered gynecologic or family planning services, and only 36% of practices even had a gynecology table in their offices [125]. This is one area in which family practitioners clearly feel more comfortable and better trained than pediatricians.

TABLE 40. *Noncontraceptive benefits of contraceptives*

Benefit	Relative risk
Iron deficiency anemia	0.57
Menorrhagia	0.52
Endometrial cancer	0.50
Ovarian cancer	0.60
Breast cancer	0.96
Breast fibroadenoma	0.50
Fibrocystic breast disease	0.40
Functional ovarian cysts	0.07
Rheumatoid arthritis	0.49
Pelvic inflammatory disease	0.50
Ectopic pregnancy	0.01
Dysmenorrhea	0.37
Premenstrual syndrome	0.71
Acne	0.84

Adapted from Kulig JW. Adolescent contraception: an update. *Pediatrics* 1985;76(Suppl):675.

What is your first choice oral contraceptive?

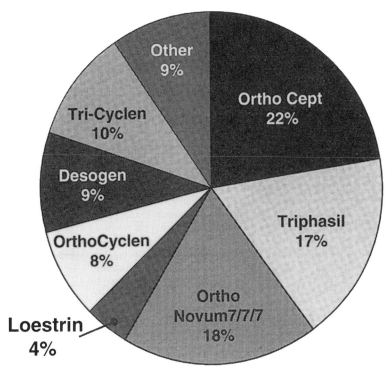

FIG. 6. Prescribing choices of oral contraceptives, as reported in a survey of nearly 300 physicians and nurse practitioners nationwide. (American Health Consultants, Depo-Provera and Norplant implants prove no competition for no. 1 choice OCs. *Contraceptive Technology Update* 1994;15(12):157, with permission.)

United States courts have given health professionals wide latitude in determining what constitutes a "mature minor," and such minors have the right to consent to confidential health care in most states, either by statutory law, public health policy, legal precedent, or common (judge-granted) law [129]. In general, "mature minors" should be near the age of majority and be able to give an informed consent (i.e., understand the risks and benefits of OCs; see Chapter 9 for further discussion). Although private practitioners may refuse to prescribe contraceptives for teenagers as a matter of conscience [129], this is ultimately counterproductive, and it does not represent ideal medical practice [123].

After an appropriate medical and sexual history (see Table 18), the health provider should do a thorough physical and pelvic examination. This screening examination should include measurement of blood pressure, Tanner staging, a Pap smear, a urine pregnancy test, tests for gonorrhea and chlamydial infection, a complete blood count, test for syphilis, and a urinalysis. Tests for cholesterol and triglycerides are also indicated if the patient's family fits a high cardiac risk profile [123].

Because the average cost of OCs is now $10 to $25 per pack (retail; Table 41), practitioners can maximize compliance by giving teenagers one or two sample packages. A 6-week visit is scheduled for follow-up, at which blood pressure is rechecked and side effects are discussed. If the teenager is initially informed that "there are many different kinds of birth control pills, and we need to find the right one for you," and that "most young women your age do not have any problems taking the pill," their compliance probably will be improved.

TABLE 41. *Costs of contraception*

Method	Cost
Oral contraceptives	$10–25/pack
Male condom	$0.50
Female condom	$2.50
Diaphragm	$20 + $50–150 for fitting
Cervical cap	$20 + $50–150 for fitting
Depo-Provera	$35/injection
Norplant	$350/kit + $150–250 for insertion/removal
Spermicides	$0.85 per application
Intrauterine device	$120 + $40–50 for insertion/lab tests

Adapted from Hatcher RA, Trussell J, Stewart F, et al. *Contraceptive technology.* 16th ed. New York: Irvington Publishers; 1994.

Although many teens have heard negative things about OCs ("they cause cancer, pregnancy, heart attacks" and the like), the *minor* side effects are what may result in discontinuation of the pill [2]. Chief among these are breakthrough bleeding (approximately 2–15%) and weight gain [75] (see Table 38). A little spotting in the first 3 months is not unusual, and the patient can be counseled that such bleeding is usually temporary, until her system adjusts to the exogenous hormones. Nausea can be minimized by taking OCs at bedtime. Weight gain on the pill is usually not more than 5 pounds, and some studies indicate that as many patients lose weight as gain weight on OCs [130]. Giving teenagers periodic "rests" from taking the pill achieves nothing more than increasing their risk of pregnancy.

Compliance is a key issue in adolescent contraception [48,131]. Having successfully identified a sexually active young woman, discussed her options with her, and convinced her to use an effective method, the practitioner still must brave the risk of incomplete compliance (Table 42). Various studies have shown low compliance rates for pill continuation among teenagers, ranging from 48% to 84% at 3 months to 34% to 56% at 12 months [132–139]. In general, only about half of teenagers who start OCs will still be using them 6 months later [48,140]. Perceived rather than actual weight gain results in poor compliance and must be addressed in advance of starting OCs [48,75]. As might be expected, teens who experience fewer side effects are also more likely to be compliant—68% versus 12% in one study [134]. However, even adult women have difficulty taking OCs regularly: in one 1995 study of

TABLE 42. *Checklist for contraceptive compliance*

1. How mature is this adolescent?
   - Independence
   - Self-esteem
   - Locus of control
   - Upward mobility
2. What is his or her sexual history?
   - Single or multiple partners
   - Length of current relationship
   - Age at first intercourse
   - Frequency of intercourse
   - Perceived risk of pregnancy
3. What are the teenager's previous experiences with birth control?
   - Side effects
   - Previous compliance
   - Parents' and peers' view of sex and contraception

Adapted from Jay MS, Bridges CE, Gottlieb AA, et al. Adolescent contraception: an overview. *Adolescent and Pediatric Gynecology* 1988;1:83.

1,555 women, 47% reported missing one or more pills in their cycle and 22% missed two or more [141].

What predicts compliance among adolescents? Good compliers tend to be older, suburban, "set the agenda" for the health visit, are happy with the pill at the first visit, engage in more frequent intercourse, and have a single partner. Poor compliers tend to be younger, urban, have no college plans, are dissatisfied with the health visit, have side effects from the pill, and have no parental involvement with the visit. Clinicians also need to be sensitive to cultural differences that may influence contraceptive compliance [137]. And, of course, side effects are a crucial issue—concern about them, actually experiencing them, even misinformation about them [48,134].

Pill Selection

Choosing a pill can be a difficult process when 46 different preparations are available and their potency cannot always be determined merely by reading the package or the *Physician's Desk Reference* (Table 43). Even the nomenclature is difficult to understand. For uniphasic pills, the first number refers to the concentration of progestin, the second to the concentration of estrogen. Ortho-Novum 1/35 contains 1 mg of norethindrone and 35 μg of ethinyl estradiol. For biphasic pills, the numbers refer to the sequence of changes in the progestin concentration. For example, Ortho 7/7/7 contains three 7-day allotments of 0.5 mg, 0.75 mg, and 1.0 mg of norethindrone. Triphasic pills can vary both the estrogen and progestin, and manufacturers wisely list no numbers.

Clinicians should always prescribe a 28-day pill, usually one that contains 30 to 35 μg of estrogen (e.g., Ortho 1/35, Triphasil, Desogen, Ortho-Cyclen, Ortho-Tri-Cyclen). There are no practical advan-

TABLE 43. *Choosing a low-dose oral contraceptive*

Desired characteristics	Pill	Estrogen dose	Biologic activity
Good initial choice New progestins	Desogen Ortho-Cept	30 μg Ethinyl estradiol	Proges: Int/high Andro: Low Endo: Int
	Ortho-Cyclen Ortho Tri-Cyclen (multiphasic)	35 μg Ethinyl estradiol	Proges: low Andro: Low Endo: Low
Fixed dose	Ortho 1/35 Norinyl 1/35	35 μg Ethinyl estradiol	Proges: Int Andro: Int
Multiphasic	Triphasil Tri-Levlen	32 μg Ethinyl estradiol (average)	Proges: Low Andro: Int Endo: Int
	Ortho 7/7/7	35 μg Ethinyl estradiol	Proges: Int Andro: Int Endo: Int
Good back-ups	Levlen Lo-Ovral Nordette	30 μg Ethinyl estradiol	Proges: Int Andro: Int Endo: Int
Postcoital	Ovral	50 μg Ethinyl estradiol	Proges: High Andro: High Endo: High
Good for acne	Desogen Ortho-Cept	35 μg Ethinyl estradiol	[see above]
	Demulen 1/35 or 1/50	35 μg Ethinyl estradiol 50 μg Ethinyl estradiol	Proges: High Andro: Low Endo: Low/Int
Minipills	Micronor Nor Q.D. Ovrette	No estrogen No estrogen No estrogen	Proges: Low Andro:Low Endo: Low

Proges, progestational; Andro, androgenic; Endo, endometrial; Int, intermediate.
Adapted from Dickey RP. *Managing contraceptive pill patients.* 8th ed. Durant, OK: Creative Infomatics; 1996.

tages to using a 50-μg pill other than Demulen 1/50 for severe acne patients or Ovral for postcoital contraception, and pills containing more than 50 μg of estrogen have now been completely phased out voluntarily by manufacturers [142]. A new 20 mg pill, Alesse, was released in 1997.

The type and amount of progestin may also be an important consideration. For example, Ortho 7/7/7 and Ortho 1/35 contain a weaker progestin (norethindrone) than Triphasil (levonorgestrel). But other factors are probably more important. For instance, a teenager with acne benefits from a pill with high estrogenic and low androgenic activity (e.g., Demulen 1/35, Desogen, or Ortho-Cept), whereas a high-androgenic pill exacerbates her problem (e.g., Lo-Ovral; Table 44). On the other hand, a pill with high progestational and endometrial effects, such as Lo-Ovral, which contains norgestrel, avoids breakthrough bleeding and can be used for the 5% of patients in whom pill amenorrhea develops on OCs with weaker progestins.

Certain side effects can be overcome, whereas others require discontinuation of the pill altogether (Table 45). The link between depression and OCs remains controversial, but pyridoxine hydrochloride, 25 mg once daily, can be tried before OCs are discontinued [143]. Because minor side effects may result in discontinuation of OCs, practitioners need to be careful in recommending certain formulations. For instance, pills with less than 30 μg of estrogen (e.g., Loestrin 1/20) are usually best avoided because of the risk of breakthrough bleeding.

Patients should always be instructed not to discontinue their pills without calling the physician. Warning signals that should be reported immediately include severe headache, unexplained chest pain, severe right upper quadrant pain, severe leg pains, and galactorrhea.

Starting the Pill

Taking the pill at nearly the same time every day minimizes the risks of failure or breakthrough bleeding. This can be accomplished best through linking the pill to some other routine activity (e.g., brushing teeth at night) [144]. OCs can be started on the first Sunday after menses begin, on day 5 of the menstrual cycle, or on day 1 of the menstrual cycle—whichever system the physician prefers. Triphasil and the new progestin OCs are designed specifically for a day 1 start (although the latter can be started using the first Sunday method as well). The advantage of a Sunday start is that menses usually occur during the week, making intercourse on weekends more feasible. The advantage of a day 1 start is a slightly greater chance of inhibiting ovulation during the very first cycle [143].

The pill's estimated effectiveness for the first cycle is still 95% to 97%, so requiring the teenager who has not been previously contracepting to use a second, back-up method to prevent pregnancy may be overly academic. Giving patients the information that they may be slightly less well protected for the first cycle will enable them to make their own decisions; however, emphasizing the need to use

TABLE 44. *Oral contraceptives, estrogenic effect, and androgenicity: implications for acne*

Pill	Relative estrogenic effect	Relative androgenic effect
Combination		
Ovcon-35	40	0.15
Ortho Tri-Cyclen	35	0.15
Desogen/Ortho-Cept	30	0.17
Demulen 1/35	19	0.21
Ortho 7/7/7	48	0.25
Triphasil	28	0.29
Ortho-Novum 1/35	38	0.34
Lo-Ovral	25	0.46
Loestrin 1.5/30	14	0.80
Ovral	42	0.80
Progestin-only		
Micronor/Nor-QD	1	0.13
Ovrette	0	0.13

Adapted from Dickey RP. *Managing contraceptive pill patients.* 8th ed. Durant, OK: Creative Infomatics; 1996.

TABLE 45. *Management of problems with oral contraceptives*

Problem	Management
Acne	Low-androgenic pill
	Try new progestin pill
Nausea	Take pill at bedtime or with meals
	Use 30- to 35-μg pill
Fluid retention	Low-estrogenic pill
Increased appetite	Low-androgenic pill
Hypertension	D/C pill
	Try Minipill
Headaches	Consider D/C pill
Breakthrough bleeding	Wait two to three cycles, then switch from a multiphasic to a constant-dose pill, or a moderate progestational pill
Depression	Try 20 mg pyridoxine twice daily; try 30-μg pill, new progestin pill, or Minipill
Dry eyes	Try progestin-dominant pill

OCs to prevent pregnancy and condoms to prevent STDs is crucial. Approximately 20% to 38% of adult women use OCs and condoms [31,76].

A urine pregnancy test is always advisable before starting a sexually active teenager on any form of contraception (or, indeed, evaluating any serious medical complaint). Fortunately, there is little to no risk of teratogenicity from taking low-dose OCs in the first trimester [76,143].

If patients miss one pill, they should be instructed to take it as soon as they remember, and they will probably remain protected (except with the triphasic OCs). A back-up method, however, is always advisable. Missing two or more pills usually results in breakthrough bleeding and loss of protection. Ordinarily, patients begin their menses while taking the placebo pills in the package.

Patients should be cautioned that OCs are a drug and need to be mentioned in the context of any health visit. In addition, certain antibiotics and other medications lower the pill's effectiveness and require use of a back-up method for the remainder of that month (see Table 39). Finally, although OCs decrease plasma levels of vitamins B_1, B_2, B_6, and B_{12}, folate, and zinc, there is no evidence that this is clinically significant and therefore no supplementation is required [143].

The Minipill

The minipill (e.g., Micronor, Nor Q.D., Ovrette) contains only the progestin half of regular OCs and is therefore problematic when used by adolescents. The incidences of failure and irregular bleeding are higher because of the weak endometrial and progestational effects. Practically, this means that a patient often requires frequent pregnancy tests to see if she is pregnant or is merely having irregular bleeding.

The minipill's mode of action is to make cervical mucus thicker and more impermeable to sperm. The minipill prevents ovulation in only 15% to 40% of cycles, has a pregnancy rate of 2.5% to 3.7%, and accounts for less than 8% of all OCs sold [76,108]. In fact, it is most effective when the normal menstrual bleeding pattern is maximally disrupted (i.e., amenorrhea). Consequently, 1-year continuation rates are less than 50% [108]. In certain patients, however, the minipill may be worth trying—particularly those with migraine headaches or hypertension who still prefer oral contraceptives to barrier methods. The minipill is also ideal for nursing mothers who want to use an oral contraceptive, because estrogens decrease lactation [145].

Postcoital Contraception

Significant advances have been made in the area of postcoital contraception since the mid-1970s. For many years, diethylstilbestrol was the only "morning-after" pill available and caused extreme nausea and a 10% risk of ectopic pregnancy. In the 1970s, Yuzpe and colleagues pioneered the use of

Ovral as a postcoital contraceptive, using two tablets within 72 hours of unprotected intercourse, followed by two additional tablets 12 hours later [146,147]. The pregnancy rate was only 1.6%—versus an estimated risk of 14% for a single episode of sexual intercourse at mid-cycle—and side effects were minimal. In one large study of 867 college women, Ovral averted 70% of anticipated pregnancies, but half of the patients did have either nausea or nausea with vomiting [147,148].

An estimated two million unplanned pregnancies and one million abortions could be prevented with maximal use of this regimen [149]. A 1995 national survey of adolescent medicine experts found that 80% prescribe postcoital contraceptives, but most do so only a few times a year, and only 16% counsel virginal teens about their availability [150]. On college campuses, awareness is high, but specific knowledge is lacking [151].

Although, in theory, any OC pill could be used in sufficient dosage (at least 100 μg of estrogen per dose), Ovral is the preferred pill because it has been tested so extensively [152–154]. Such a high dose of estrogen necessitates the use of an antiemetic, usually a Phenergan or Tigan suppository 1 hour before dosage [153]. Because this regimen merely represents a doubling-up of OCs, which is commonly done when a pill is missed, its safety and reliability are secure.

Other OCs, levonorgestrel, mifepristone, danazol, high-dose estrogens, and copper intrauterine devices (IUDs) have all been used for postcoital contraception as well, and a trial of vaginal hormones is being conducted in Mexico [154,155].

Medroxyprogesterone Acetate (Depo-Provera, DMPA)

In many ways, Depo-Provera represents an ideal form of contraception for adolescents—four shots a year, at a relatively low cost ($140 annually), are absolutely protective against pregnancy. In 1992, the FDA approved the use of Depo-Provera as a contraceptive [57]. For over 20 years, DMPA had been a subject of controversy because of its association with an increased frequency of mammary tumors in beagle dogs. Meanwhile, it had been used in developing countries for many years, where a community health worker visiting a village could administer the injections without awareness of the recipients' husbands, and protection was conferred for 3 months. Later studies demonstrated that the drug is not teratogenic or carcinogenic in humans [156]. Unfortunately, this issue is not yet resolved. The latest and largest study indicates that there may, indeed, be an increased risk of breast cancer in some women, including teenagers, as high as twice the relative risk [157]. This could be due to increased detection of tumors or stimulation of the growth of preexisting tumors. Women who had used DMPA more than 5 years previously had no increased risk, however [157].

The usual method of administration is by intramuscular injection, 150 mg every 3 months. Initial injection is best given during the first 5 days of a normal menstrual period, to ensure that a teenager is not pregnant. Side effects include spotting and mild breakthrough bleeding, especially in the first 3 to 6 months of use. By 1 year, most women are nearly or completely amenorrheic [145], although this can be an advantage for some adolescent patients [158]. Depo-Provera produces thinning and sometimes profound atrophy of the endometrium and increases the viscosity of cervical mucus [159]. Teens who choose DMPA have often had problems with previous forms of birth control [138].

Depo-Provera has several attractive features for use with teenagers:

- One shot actually inhibits ovulation for *14 weeks* [160], so even though patients are told to return every 3 months, they actually have a 2-week "grace" period (sometimes longer in some instances) [76]. This can be useful when dealing with teenagers who do not always remember appointments.
- Depo-Provera is an extremely effective form of birth control, with a failure rate of less than 1% [48].
- Because it causes endometrial atrophy and leads to amenorrhea, it is an ideal contraceptive agent for developmentally delayed teens who cannot cope with taking OCs or with the personal hygiene issues surrounding menstruation.
- Depo-Provera does not interfere with breast milk production, nor does it carry a significant risk of thromboembolism for use postpartum or postabortion [55].
- One size fits all: dosage does not need to be adjusted for obese or thin patients.
- There is no potential incompatibility with other concomitantly used medications, as there is with OCs. In fact, DMPA has anticonvulsant properties of its own and is an excellent choice for birth control in teens with a seizure disorder [57].

Depo-Provera is particularly useful when clinicians identify sexually active teenagers who are not using any form of birth control and are not coming in for contraception. Such teens are likely to be noncompliant, and a single injection of DMPA can buy 3 months of time before a definitive decision about birth control needs to be made. However, the drug is not without its disadvantages as well:

- Weight gain can be considerable, averaging 1 to 2 kg per year or more [161].
- Fertility may take longer to return after discontinuation than with other methods—an average of 18 to 24 months [48,162].
- All adolescent women who use DMPA experience some degree of menstrual irregularity [57]. In one study, 60% of teens were amenorrheic after 1 year of use [138]. This can be a major reason for discontinuing the drug [163].
- There is increasing concern about the effect of the drug on bone mineral density in teenagers [57,164–166]. In one study, long-term users had decreased bone density [167], but in another it increased after the drug was discontinued [168]. A small 1995 study of teenagers did find 1.5% decreases in bone mineral density among DMPA users, compared with increases of up to 2.9% for young women using either OCs, Norplant, or no hormones [158].
- There are many other clinically important side effects, including headaches, depression, worsening of acne, bloating, hypertension, dizziness, and nausea [161]. Two studies dispute that depression occurs more frequently with DMPA, however [138,169].
- Discontinuation rates can be high, 37% at 6 months and 58% at 1 year in one study [163], or 71% at 1 year in another study [170]. Patients who discontinued DMPA were more likely to have heavier and more frequent bleeding, cramping, weight gain, headaches, depression, nervousness, or amenorrhea. Concern with side effects expressed at the first injection seems to predict early discontinuation [170].
- There can be confusion about the preparation itself. DMPA comes in concentrations of 150 mg/ml and 400 mg/ml. The latter is not approved as a contraceptive—it is too difficult to provide the correct volume (0.37 ml), injection can be painful, and its efficacy is not ideal [76].

Norplant

Norplant—six small capsules containing levonorgestrel that are implanted into the skin—was approved for use by the FDA in 1991 [55]. A constant, low dose of progestin is released and provides effective contraception for 5 years, with an annual pregnancy rate of less than 1% [145]. Compliance is not an issue with Norplant, but teenagers are not always willing to tolerate the minor surgery or the sometimes major side effects. Although Norplant is a progestin-only contraceptive like Depo-Provera, it does not inhibit ovulation, which means that there is at least an increased theoretical risk of ovarian cysts or ectopic pregnancy—risks that do not exist with OCs or DMPA [57]. Implantation and removal require local anesthesia only, but the latter can sometimes be difficult [171]. After removal, return to fertility is immediate.

Continuation rates are high—80% after 1 year, 50% after 5 years [172]. Teenagers choosing Norplant tend to be older, previously pregnant, and frustrated previous OC users [138,173,174]. They often fail to return for scheduled follow-up visits, but no more so than teens using other methods [175]. In any comparison between Norplant and other contraceptive methods, inevitably Norplant produces far less pregnancies [140,173]. However, the side effects can sometimes be troublesome: irregular menses, headaches, mood swings, weight gain, nausea, amenorrhea, worsening acne, and hair loss [48]. In particular, heavy and irregular bleeding tends to plague some teens in the first few months after insertion [176]. Ibuprofen and small supplemental doses of estrogens may be useful [48]. Other teens sometimes experience rapid, excessive weight gain, also within several months after insertion [55]. Another significant disadvantage is cost: $375 for the kit, another $125 to $225 for insertion.

A similar implant, Capronor, which would dissolve rather than require surgical removal, has been tested [177]. Microimplants of norethindrone are also being developed and tested, with high rates of effectiveness [178]. A one- or two-rod system being tested in Europe might also be better tolerated by teenagers [171].

The development of Norplant demonstrates one of the primary difficulties in bringing new contraceptives to the marketplace. In 1994 alone, nearly 200 lawsuits were filed against Wyeth-Ayerst, one fourth of them class-action suits [178]. The suits allege a variety of problems, ranging from emotional distress to scarring to autoimmune disorders.

Barrier Methods

An ideal contraceptive for teenagers would be one that is [179]

- Easy to use
- Readily obtainable without a prescription
- Inexpensive
- Completely protective
- Reversible
- Separate from the coital act
- Without side effects or risks

Although OCs have the advantage of dissociating sex from contraception, they can have surprisingly high failure rates in actual use [108], whereas barrier methods offer greater protection against STDs and may be more attractive from a public health perspective. In addition, OCs and barrier methods are not mutually exclusive. Although some family planning experts despair of American teenagers ever using one contraceptive method, let alone two, experience in Europe suggests that adolescents are capable of very responsible sexual behavior when societal messages point them in the right direction [48].

One primary benefit of barrier methods is that most use spermicide. Nonoxynol-9 is a chemical surfactant that destroys the cell walls of sperm and offers some protection against bacterial and viral STDs [180]. In addition, women who use spermicides are only one third as likely to have cervical cancer as a control group [74]. Studies show *no* increased risk of congenital malformations in women who conceived while using spermicides [181]. However, using any medical form of contraception requires a high degree of motivation and advance planning, which many teenagers lack.

Unfortunately, studies have shown that teenagers are not enamored of the diaphragm, the cervical cap is not widely available, the contraceptive sponge was recently taken off the market [182], and the use of condoms remains inconsistent (see Tables 28, 29). However, studies do show that teenagers' use of condoms doubled during the 1980s [28].

Diaphragm

Three older reports have touted the use of diaphragms for teenage women. In the largest sample to date, 8% of a New York cohort of over 2,000 diaphragm users were teenagers, and 65% were still using their diaphragms 1 year later [183]. In a smaller study of middle-class teens, 27% chose the diaphragm and 72% were using it a year later [184]. In a suburban teen clinic, diaphragm users had similar rates of pregnancy (15%) and discontinuation (55%) as OC users after 1 year [185].

The news about the diaphragm is old and decidedly mixed: it is difficult for teens to use, and its protection against pregnancy is less than ideal (6% failure rate with perfect use, 18% with actual use) [145]. On the other hand, the diaphragm offers *some* protection against gonorrheal infection [186], tubal damage [187], cervical neoplasia [188], and HPV [189]. Use of the diaphragm *and* condoms represents nearly ideal protection against both pregnancy and STDs, but there are no data available about teenagers who are able to combine two barrier methods at once.

The amount of planning involved, the necessary self-manipulation, and the messiness of this method make this an option for only the best-motivated patients—usually, college students. Even then, the failure rate in women having frequent intercourse may be unacceptably high [76,190] (Table 46). This is probably because increased blood flow during intercourse results in pelvic dilatation, making the diaphragm relatively smaller, no matter how perfect the office fit was. One useful screening question is that teenagers who do not use tampons are unlikely to use diaphragms. Although there is a slightly increased risk of toxic shock syndrome, this is unlikely when the diaphragm is used properly [108,159,191].

Diaphragm fitting is a relatively easy office procedure. The practitioner should start with an "average" size, 75 mm, and proceed to the next smaller or larger size until the largest-size diaphragm is comfortably in place. Although diaphragms come in three different rim styles, the all-flex variety is usually preferred by most teenagers. The rim should fit snugly behind the symphysis pubis and extend to the posterior fornix, covering the cervical os. A diaphragm that is too large impinges on the membranous part of the urethra and leads to urinary tract infections [108,192,193]. One that is too small increases the risk of pregnancy. When properly fitted, the patient should not be able to sense that the di-

TABLE 46. *Intercourse frequency and diaphragm failure*

	Pregnancies per 100 women during first 12 mo of use
Consistent diaphragm users	
Intercourse <3–4×/week	3.4– 9.9
Intercourse >3–4×/week	9.7–20.7

Data from McIntyre SL, Higgins JE. Parity and use-effectiveness with the contraceptive sponge. *Am J Obstet Gynecol* 1986;155:796; and Trussell J, Strickler J, Vaughan B. Contraceptive efficacy of the diaphragm, sponge and cervical cap. *Fam Plann Perspect* 1993;25:101.
Adapted from Hatcher RA, Trussell J, Stewart F, et al. *Contraceptive technology.* 16th ed. New York: Irvington Publishers; 1994.

aphragm is in place. She should be instructed, however, to feel through the rubber dome to make sure that the cervix is covered and that "it feels like the tip of your nose." The patient should then be asked to insert the diaphragm herself, and the practitioner can check its placement. An instruction sheet is also useful. The diaphragm should be inserted no more than 2 hours before intercourse, unless additional contraceptive cream or jelly is added, and left in place for at least 6 hours afterward. Fitting should be rechecked a week later, in 6 months, and if the patient gains or loses 10 pounds or more.

Cervical Cap

The cervical cap is first cousin to the diaphragm and was approved in 1988 for use in the United States [76]. The Prentif Cavity-Rim Cervical Cap (Lamberts Ltd., England) is a rubber device that fits over the cervix like a thimble, comes in four sizes, may be inserted any time before intercourse, and can be left in place for up to 48 hours [194]. It is being distributed in the United States by Cervical Cap [(CxC) Ltd, P.O. Box 38003-292, Los Gatos, CA 95031, but only to practitioners who have attended a training seminar. Unfortunately, the cervical cap suffers from a high pregnancy rate—18% at 1 year, 38% at 2 years [145,195]—and may predispose to abnormal Pap smears, *Gardnerella* or *Monilia* infections, and dyspareunia [194]. In addition, the cap is more difficult to fit than a diaphragm and can be accidentally dislodged more easily. It does not appear to be a major form of contraception for teenagers [108].

Contraceptive Sponge/Contraceptive Gel

Any information about the sponge is "academic" only because its manufacture was discontinued in 1995. The makers of the Today sponge decided to cease production after an FDA inspection found evidence of substandard manufacturing practices [182]. The only other sponge-like product in development is the Protectaid sponge, which is being tested in Europe and incorporates three different spermicides [196].

The Today contraceptive sponge was a cup-shaped device manufactured from a polyurethane polymer and impregnated with the spermicide, nonoxynol-9. It cost approximately $2.50 per sponge (see Table 41). Unlike other barrier methods, the sponge did not have to be inserted into the vagina before each act of intercourse and remained effective for 24 hours. However, like other barrier methods, the sponge required self-insertion and planning and carried at least a theoretical risk of toxic shock syndrome, and its use resulted in a high failure rate (17% in the first year) [197]. It also was associated with allergic reactions in up to 5% of patients, odor if left in place for greater than 24 hours, and vaginal drying, because the sponge could absorb vaginal fluid during intercourse. Interestingly, pill users and diaphragm users are more influenced in their choice of method by their physician, whereas sponge users were more influenced by the media [198,199].

One possible replacement for the sponge is a contraceptive gel, Advantage 24, which claims to make use of "bioadhesive technology" to offer the same type of 24-hour protection against pregnancy [200]. Advantage 24 is not yet widely available and costs nearly twice as much as the sponge, $7.99 for a package of three. It, too, relies on the spermicide nonoxynol-9, but in lower concentrations than the sponge. According to a small, unpublished study, the gel has efficacy rates as high as 98% when applied 15 to 30 minutes before intercourse, dropping to 86% when used 24 hours beforehand [200].

As of early 1997, there is insufficient evidence to recommend Advantage 24 to patients, given that its protective efficacy against pregnancy and STDs is still unproven.

Condoms

In principle, the condom would seem to be the ideal contraceptive for adolescents: it can be furnished by either partner, prevents pregnancies, protects both male and female partners against STDs, is readily obtainable, inexpensive, easy to carry, and compatible with typical adolescent intercourse (hurried and unplanned), and does not require a visit to a health care facility [34,201]. However, in practice, condoms are not always as popular with teenagers as we would like. There are many varied reasons that teenagers give for this, and many appropriate and rational responses:

- *Purchasing condoms can be embarrassing.* Although they can be purchased by mail, condoms are usually obtained in drug stores (see Fig. 7), which often requires a young man or woman to confront an adult employee or pharmacist.
- *Condoms can break.* According to *Consumer Reports*, this occurs 1.5% to 10% of the time and is more likely if condoms are stored in wallets, are used after their expiration date, or are used with oil-based lubricants instead of K-Y jelly [202].
- *Condoms interrupt love-making.* Condoms must be applied when the male has developed an erection and before any pre-ejaculate is leaked. The only solution here is to make donning the condom part of foreplay.
- *Condoms may fall off.* Certain condoms offer a tighter fit (e.g., "hugger" style) or contain an inner adhesive band near the tip that prevents slippage (e.g., Mentor brand).
- *Condoms decrease sexual sensations during intercourse.* Although this may seem like a major disadvantage, it can also be a major advantage: decreased sensation allows for more prolonged sexual intercourse, particularly in young, inexperienced men.

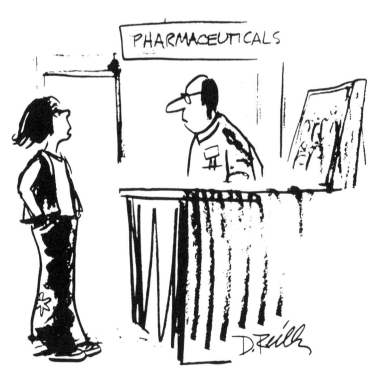

FIG. 7. "A package of condominiums . . . ." (Reproduced by special permission of *Playboy* magazine. Copyright © 1973 by *Playboy*.)

- *Condoms are messy.* Although lubricated condoms may be slightly moist, many teenagers find them far preferable to the discharge of semen from the vagina after intercourse.
- *Asking a partner to put on a condom is embarrassing.* Telling a partner a week later that he or she needs to be checked at the STD clinic is even more embarrassing, as is trying to inform one's parents that they are about to become grandparents. Female teenagers, in particular, must learn to say, "No condom, no sex."

The following points need to be emphasized in any discussion of condoms, whether with patients or with school boards considering approving condoms for school-based health centers [32]:

- Using a condom is 10,000 times safer than not using one during intercourse [203].
- Condoms are effective in preventing the transmission of *Chlamydia trachomatis, Neisseria gonor- rhoeae,* herpesvirus, and human papillomavirus [204,205]. Only latex condoms—*not* membrane condoms—offer protection against cytomegalovirus, hepatitis B virus, and HIV [205]. However, they must be used properly and with care. A coating of nonoxynol-9 may offer some additional protection if the condom breaks.
- When used properly, condoms are extremely effective (97%). However, their failure rate increases to 12% in actual practice [145]. Unprotected foreplay is the most common reason for failure, followed by careless removal of the condom and spillage of semen due to failure to remove the penis from the vagina immediately after ejaculation [206].
- Condoms offer the best protection for sexually active teenagers against HIV infection. Laboratory tests show that neither sperm (3 μm in diameter) nor STD-causing organisms (10–25% the size of sperm) can penetrate an intact latex condom [207,208]. Three studies of sexual pairings with one HIV-positive partner and one HIV-negative partner have proven that the latter does not become infected when condoms are used consistently and correctly [209–211]. Used incorrectly, 10% to 15% of the partners became infected [209,210]. Although an older report from UCLA found that 1 of every 200 condoms tested was defective and either allowed water or air to escape, failed durability tests, or allowed HIV to pass, the researchers still stated that even the worst-scoring condom was far better than no condom at all [212].

The latest development in the condom market has been the introduction of plastic (polyurethane) condoms [213] (Table 47). These are sold under the brand name Avanti and are available currently in 13 western states. In theory, plastic condoms have several significant advantages:

TABLE 47. *Types of condoms*

	Type of Condom			
	Latex	Plastic	Female	Natural skin
Brand name	Numerous	Avanti	Reality	Several
Material	Rubber	Polyurethane	Polyurethane	Lamb intestines
Failure rate (1 y)	3% if used properly; actual = 12%	No clinical trials	21%	Not adequately studied
Lubricants	Water-based only	Any	Any	Any
Cost	$0.50	$1.75	$2.75	$1.00
Pros and cons	• Cheap easy to obtain • Prevents STDs and pregnancy • Can break or tear • Cannot be used with oil-based lubricants	• Strong • Hypoallergenic • Claims to prevent STDs and pregnancy • Not well studied • Expensive • Not readily available	• Strong • Hypoallergenic • Prevents STDs and pregnancy • Can decrease sensation • Expensive • Not well studied	• Greater sensation • Does not prevent STDs • Unpleasant smell • More expensive

STD, sexually transmitted disease.
Adapted from Contraceptive Technology. Although condoms meet standards, complaints for brands differ. *Contraceptive Technology Update* 1995;16(3):29; with data from Hatcher RA, Trussell J, Stewart F, et al. *Contraceptive technology.* 16th ed. New York: Irvington Publishers; 1994; and Centers for Disease Control and Prevention. Update: barrier protection against HIV infection and other sexually transmitted diseases. *MMWR Morb Mortal Wkly Rep* 1993;42:589.

- Excellent for people allergic to latex
- Thinner and more sensitive than latex condoms
- Twice as strong as latex condoms
- Compatible with any type of lubricant

On the downside, Avanti sells for $5.95 for a three-pack and $10.95 for a six-pack and has not undergone thorough clinical efficacy trials [214]. At present, they should be reserved for teenagers allergic to latex [213].

The key issue in examining the role of condoms in adolescent contraception is, will teenagers use them? Here, the data are somewhat conflicting. On the one hand, many teenagers are ill informed about condoms, as in many aspects of sex: in the Harris survey, 39% thought condoms to be ineffective in preventing pregnancy [14]. A large Canadian study of over 5,500 college students (mean age, 19.7 years) showed that only 25% of the young men and 15% of the young women used a condom regularly and that a number of factors were associated with not using one: 1) a large number of sexual partners, 2) embarrassment about purchasing condoms, 3) use of OCs, 4) difficulty discussing condoms with partner, 5) insufficient knowledge about STDs, and 6) belief that condoms interfere with sexual pleasure [215]. Many studies show that although condom use has increased considerably since the 1970s and 1980s [21,22,24,34,108,216,217], most teenagers still do not use them *every* single time they have sex. Moreover, teenagers being surveyed in the 1990s about condom use now know what the "correct answer" is that they should be giving to researchers [218].

On the other hand, no other method is so readily available to teenagers, so relatively easy to use, so inexpensive, and so efficacious in preventing both pregnancy and STDs. And use has clearly increased: even comparing National Survey of Adolescent Males data from 1979 with 1993 YRBS data shows that for male 17- to 19-year-olds, condom use has nearly tripled in only 15 years [21,219]!

But, clearly, we can do better in this crucial area of public health. For example, a remarkable study conducted in 1971 seems to dispel the notion that male adolescents are reluctant to use condoms: during a 13-week period, over 18,000 free condoms were distributed to teens visiting nine commercial sites (e.g., barber shops, grocery stores, a pool hall). During this period, reported condom use at last intercourse rose from 20% to 91% [220]!

Accessibility is an important ingredient, and the availability of free condoms in school-based clinics can only help. New York City has condom availability programs mandated in each of its 130 high schools; Philadelphia has condoms available in one fourth of its high schools; and Seattle has condoms available in 10 of its public high schools [221,222]. In 1994, 420 schools were identified that made condoms available to sexually active students who requested them, and a 1991 Roper Poll found that two thirds of American adults support such availability [223]. Finally, partner insistence is a key factor in teenagers' condom use, and girls in particular must be counseled either to carry condoms themselves or insist on their use [44,224].

Aggressive national campaigns to increase condom use can work, but only if teenagers are targeted, widespread publicity is used, and the media are incorporated into the campaign [45]. Such a campaign was conducted in Switzerland over 5 years, and adolescents' use of condoms increased significantly without concomitant increases in sexual activity [225]. Mention of condoms has become more common on American television since the early 1990s, but, unfortunately, it has taken the threat of AIDS, not the continuing problem of teen pregnancy, to accomplish this [46]. Condom ads have not been well accepted by the media and are still not currently allowed on national network television [226]. In one well known campaign, a woman states, "I'll do a lot for love, but I'm not ready to die for it." This ad was dropped in favor of commercials that feature such characters as Robin Hood and the Phantom of the Opera, who are used to try to overcome the public's embarrassment about buying condoms. However, such ads may not be widely seen because many magazines, newspapers, and commercial television stations will only accept condom ads that emphasize disease prevention, not pregnancy prevention [225].

The Female Condom

In 1993, a new female condom (Reality) was approved by the FDA for over-the-counter marketing in the United States [76]. It consists of a loose polyurethane sheath with two flexible rings, one of which is inserted into the vagina like a tampon, with the other remaining outside to protect the labia [108]. With careful and consistent use, it affords 97.4% protection against pregnancy in the first 6 months; however, in actual use, the accidental pregnancy rate is quite high, 12% to 22% [145, 227–229]. Each condom costs $2.75 and can not be reused; however, 27 states have now approved the condom for Medicaid reimbursement [55]. No data exist regarding whether many adolescents actually use this form of birth control. Because the female condom is expensive and cumbersome, it seems destined to be ignored by most female adolescents.

Intrauterine Devices

Although four different IUDs are approved for use in the United States by the FDA, only two remain on the market: *Progestasert* (Alza) and *ParaGard* or *Copper T380A* (GynoPharma) [108]. The other two, the Copper-7 and Copper-T, were withdrawn from the market by their manufacturer in 1986 because of the increased cost of liability insurance [230]. The Levonorgestrel IUD (Leiras) may be approved soon [76].

The Progestasert is T-shaped and delivers 65 μg of progesterone per day and offers the advantages of less blood loss during menses and decreased dysmenorrhea. Unfortunately, it must be replaced annually [231]. The Paragard is also known as the Copper T380A because it contains 380 mm² of exposed copper, almost twice the amount of previous copper IUDs [212]. The Paragard carries a pregnancy risk of 3.7% in women younger than 20 years of age, expulsion rates of about 6% in the first year, and removal rates (for pain or bleeding) of 25% by the end of 4 years [231]. However, a single Paragard can be used for up to 8 years [76]. The Levonorgestrel IUD releases 20 μg per day of levonorgestrel directly into the uterus for up to 5 years. Supposedly, this low dosage reduces systemic side effects [76].

Although IUDs are theoretically appealing because compliance problems are eliminated, even in their heyday they did not represent a major contraceptive option for female adolescents. Older IUDs, particularly the Dalkon Shield, succeeded in giving this method of contraception a bad reputation [232]. Later studies found that the risk of IUD-associated salpingitis is limited to the first 4 months after insertion, which implicates contamination at the time of insertion as the precipitating factor [233–235]. Furthermore, the risk of infertility may be only slightly increased (1.3- to 1.6-fold) [74], or not increased at all for women with only one sexual partner [236].

Nevertheless, continued conservatism is warranted. In the latest World Health Organization (WHO) study, which re-examined 13 earlier studies [234], the risk of PID among IUD users was found to be most strongly correlated with the insertion process and their background risk of STDs (i.e., multiple partners). Teenagers, of course, seem nearly destined to have multiple partners during their early sexual careers. Moreover, women aged 15 to 24 years and nulliparous women still had PID rates that were increased two- to threefold [234]. Although it is entirely possible that IUDs will experience a renaissance in the 1990s as the product continues to be refined, current recommendations mandate *against* inserting one in any woman at high risk for salpingitis (i.e., women younger than 25 years of age, with a history of PID, or with multiple partners) or whose childbearing has not yet been completed [74,76,108,145,233].

Periodic Abstinence

Although periodic abstinence has been touted as a significant form of birth control, it inevitably results in a high rate of pregnancy [237]. Of those who report using abstinence as their main contraceptive method, 26% become pregnant each year [238]. It is worth remembering that 80% of all Americans have had sexual intercourse at least once before the age of 20 years [1,29].

Four approaches have been devised to assess when women are most fertile during their menstrual cycle: 1) calendar or rhythm method, 2) basal body temperature method, 3) cervical mucus method, and 4) symptothermal method [180]. Women with irregular cycles face the highest risk of pregnancy if they use one of these methods [76].

New and Experimental Methods

A number of new and experimental methods of birth control are in varying states of development [178,239,240]. A few may have direct applicability to teenage patients.

New Barrier Methods

Two new, disposable diaphragms, already impregnated with spermicide, will soon be entering clinical trials. A single diaphragm may confer up to 24 hours of protection against pregnancy.

A new contraceptive sponge, Protectaid, is being developed, containing three different spermicides [196]. In a very small, preliminary study, the new sponge was 100% effective for 1 year, with no side effects. In addition, it may inactivate STD organisms like HIV and *C. trachomatis* [240].

Several new spermicides are being developed. Some researchers speculate that strong spermicides or high concentrations may actually facilitate the risk of HIV transmission by increasing vaginal mucosal inflammation [241].

New Injectables

New combined injectables, adding estrogens to long-acting progestins, have been developed and used in other countries. In 1995, Upjohn announced that it would seek FDA approval for Cyclo-Provera (which combines DMPA with estradiol cypionate in an attempt to minimize menstrual irregularities. An injection is given once a month. Time-released microspheres containing either norethindrone or norgestimate and cholesterol are also being investigated and could provide 1 to 12 months of contraception, depending on the formulation and dose [240]. These will require several more years of testing before FDA approval [178].

New Implants

Norplant II, a two-rod system, is likely to become available in the United States in the next few years. A new drug application was submitted to the FDA in 1995 [178]. It would have an expected life span of 3 years. Three different types of single-rod progesterone implants, Uniplant (nomegestrol), Implanon (desogestrel), and Nestorone (ST-1435), are also being tested.

A new wrinkle is the development of biodegradable implants, such as Capranor. This is a single rod containing levonorgestrel in a biodegradable compound, thus eliminating the need for removal. However, thus far pregnancy rates have been unacceptably high (18% at 1 year) [177,242]. One alternative is the use of biodegradable pellets, about the size of a grain of rice. These release norethindrone over a 12- to 18-month period, but appear to induce the same menstrual problems as other progestin-only methods [242].

Vaginal Rings

Vaginal rings are impregnated with either progestins or a combination of estrogen and progestin, which leaches through the Silastic tubing directly into the vaginal epithelium, thus avoiding the portal circulation. Some rings can be removed after 3 weeks for menses to occur, others remain in the vagina for several months at a time. A vaginal ring containing levonorgestrel and developed by WHO has a pregnancy rate of 3% to 4%, but also the typical progestin-only side effects [243]. Other rings being tested contain megestrol, the synthetic progestin ST-1435 plus ethinyl estradiol, and norethindrone acetate plus estradiol [244].

Transdermal Contraceptives

A transdermal preparation of ST-1435 has been developed that inhibits ovulation but still maintains estradiol levels [245].

Male Methods

A large international study found that weekly injections of testosterone enanthate successfully suppressed spermatogenesis and provided good protection against pregnancy, with minimal side effects and full reversibility [246]. Do not expect long lines of male adolescents to begin congregating outside your office door.

REFERENCES

1. Alan Guttmacher Institute. *Sex and America's teenagers*. New York: Alan Guttmacher Institute; 1994.
2. Braverman PK, Strasburger VC. Adolescent sexuality: II. contraception. *Clin Pediatr* 1993;32:725.

3. Elkind D. Understanding the young adolescent. *Adolescence* 1978;13:127.

4. Piaget J. The intellectual development of the adolescent. In: Caplan G, Lebovici E, eds. *Adolescence: psychosocial perspectives*. New York: Basic Books; 1969.

5. Elkind D. Teenage thinking: implications for health care. *Pediatr Nurs* 1984;2:383.

6. Zelnik M, Kantner JF. Reasons for nonuse of contraception by sexually active women aged 15–19. *Fam Plann Perspect* 1979;11:289.

7. Roper Starch Worldwise, Inc. *Teens talk about sex: adolescent sexuality in the 90's*. New York: Sexuality Information and Education Council of the U.S. (SIECUS); 1994.

8. Adler NE, Kegeles SM, Irwin CE Jr, et al. Adolescent contraceptive behavior: an assessment of decision processes. *J Pediatr* 1990;116:463.

9. Advocates for Youth. *Fact sheet: adolescent contraceptive use*. Washington, DC: Advocates for Youth; 1995.

10. Shafer MA, Sweet RL. Pelvic inflammatory disease in adolescent females. *Pediatr Clin North Am* 1989;36:513.

11. Ask-Upmark E, Glas J, Stenram U. Oral contraceptives and cerebral arterial thrombosis. *Acta Med Scand* 1969;185:479.

12. Frost JJ, Forrest JD. Understanding the impact of effective teenage pregnancy prevention programs. *Fam Plann Perspect* 1995;27:188.

13. Mauldon J, Luker K. The effects of contraceptive education on method use at first intercourse. *Fam Plann Perspect* 1996;28:19.

14. Harris L, and Associates. *American teens speak: sex, myths, TV, and birth control*. New York: Planned Parenthood Federation of America; 1986.

15. Survey of knowledge, perceptions, and attitudes among high school students. *JAMA* 1993;269:1404.

16. Zabin LS, Stark HA, Emerson MR. Reasons for delay in contraceptive clinic utilization: adolescent clinic and non-clinic populations compared. *J Adolesc Health* 1991;12:225.

17. Winter L, Breckenmaker LC. Tailoring family planning services to the special needs of adolescents. *Fam Plann Perspect* 1991;23:24.

18. Brindis C, Starbuck-Morales S, Wolfe A, et al. Characteristics associated with contraceptive use among adolescent females in school-based family planning programs. *Fam Plann Perspect* 1994;26:160.

19. Ventura SJ, Martin JA, Taffel SM, et al. Advance report of final natality statistics, 1992. *Monthly Vital Statistics Report* 1994;43(Suppl 5):1.

20. Centers for Disease Control and Prevention. State specific pregnancy and birth rates among teenagers: United States, 1991–92. *MMWR Morb Mortal Wkly Rep* 1995;44(37):677.

21. Centers for Disease Control and Prevention. Trends in sexual risk behavior among high school students: United States, 1990, 1991, and 1993. MMWR Morb Mortal Wkly Rep 1995;44:124.

22. Barone C, Ickovics JR, Ayers TS, et al. High-risk sexual behavior among young urban students. *Fam Plann Perspect* 1996;28:69.

23. DiClemente RJ, Durbin M, Siegel D, et al. Determinants of condom use among junior high school students in a minority, inner-city school district. *Pediatrics* 1992;89:197.

24. Anderson JE, Brackbill R, Mosher WD. Condom use for disease prevention among unmarried U.S. women. *Fam Plann Perspect* 1996;28:25.

25. Brooks-Gunn J, Furstenberg FF Jr. Coming of age in the era of AIDS: Puberty, sexuality, and contraception. *Millbank Q* 1990;68(Suppl 1):59.

26. Leigh BC, Morrison DM, Trocki K, et al. Sexual behavior of American adolescents: results from a U.S. national survey. *J Adolesc Health* 1994;15:117.

27. Sikand A, Fisher M, Friedman SB. AIDS knowledge, concerns, and behavioral changes among inner-city high school students. *J Adolesc Health* 1996;18:325.15.Cheng TL, Savageau JA, Sattler AL, et al. Confidentiality in health care: a

28. Forrest JD, Singh S. The sexual and reproductive behavior of American women, 1982–1988. *Fam Plann Perspect* 1990;22:206.

29. Haffner DW, ed. *Facing facts: sexual health for America's adolescents*. New York: Sexuality Information and Education Council of the U.S. (SIECUS); 1995.

30. Santelli JS, Davis M, Celentano DD, et al. Combined use of condoms with other contraceptive methods among inner-city Baltimore women. *Fam Plann Perspect* 1995;27:74.

31. Holmbeck GN, Crossman RE, Wandrei ML. Cognitive development, egocentrism, self-esteem and adolescent contraceptive knowledge, attitudes and behavior. *Journal of Youth and Adolescence* 1994;23:169.

32. Phillips SR. Turning research into policy: a survey on adolescent condom use. *SIECUS Report* 1995;24(1):9.

33. DiClemente RJ, Lodico M, Grinstead OA, et al. African-American adolescents residing in high-risk urban environments do use condoms: correlates and predictors of condom use among adolescents in public housing developments. *Pediatrics* 1996;98:269.

34. Joffe A. Adolescents and condom use. *American Journal of Diseases of Children* 1993;147:746.

35. Orr DP, Langefeld CD, Katz BP, et al. Behavioral intervention to increase condom use among high-risk female adolescents. *J Pediatr* 1996;128:288.

36. Stanton BF, Li X, Ricardo I, et al. A randomized, controlled effectiveness trial of an AIDS prevention program for low-income African-American youths. *Arch Pediatr Adolesc Med* 1996;150:363.

37. Mosher WD, Bachrach CA. First premarital contraceptive use: United States, 1960-1982. *Stud Fam Plann* 1987;18:83.
38. Hogan D, Astone N, Kitagawa E. The impact of social status, family structure, and neighborhood on the fertility of black adolescents. *American Journal of Sociology* 1985;90:825.
39. Leland NL, Barth RP. Characteristics of adolescents who have attempted to avoid HIV and who have communicated with parents about sex. *Journal of Adolescent Research* 1993;8:58.
40. Shoop DM, Davidson PM. AIDS and adolescents: the relation of parent and partner communication to adolescent condom use. *Journal of Adolescence* 1994;17:137.
41. Jaccard J, Dittus PJ, Gordon VV. Maternal correlates of sexual and contraceptive behavior. *Fam Plann Perspect* 1996;28:159.
42. Ku LC, Sonenstein FL, Pleck JH. Young men's risk behaviors for HIV infection and sexually transmitted diseases, 1988 through 1991. *Am J Public Health* 1993;83:1609.
43. Orr DP, Langefeld CD. Factors associated with condom use by sexually active male adolescents at risk for sexually transmitted disease. *Pediatrics* 1993;91:873.
44. Rosenthal SL, Biro FM, Succop PA, et al. Reasons for condom utilization among high-risk adolescent girls. *Clin Pediatr* 1994;33:706.
45. McGrath J, Strasburger VC. Preventing AIDS in teenagers in the 1990s. *Clin Pediatr* 1995;34:46.
46. Strasburger VC. Sex, teens, and the media. *Contemporary Pediatrics* 1996;13:29.
47. Alter J. The power to change what's "cool." *Newsweek*, January 17, 1994, p. 23.
48. Hillard PJ. Contraception for the adolescent. In: Pokorny SF, ed. *Pediatric and adolescent gynecology.* New York: Chapman and Hall; 1996:117.
49. Blatzer FR. Formulation and noncontraceptive uses of the new, low-dose oral contraceptive. *J Reprod Med* 1984;29(Suppl):503.
50. Derman RJ. Oral contraceptives and cardiovascular risk: current perspectives. *J Reprod Med* 1989;34:747.
51. LaRosa JC. The varying effects of progestins on lipid levels and cardiovascular disease. *Am J Obstet Gynecol* 1988;158:1621.
52. World Health Organization Task Force on Oral Contraceptives. A multicentre comparative study of serum lipids and lipoproteins in four groups of oral combined contraceptive users and a control group of IUD users. *Contraception* 1988;38:605.
53. Patsch W, Brown SA, Gotto AM, et al. The effect of triphasic oral contraceptives on plasma lipids and lipoproteins. *Am J Obstet Gynecol* 1989;161:1396.
54. Clarkson TB, Shively CA, Morgan TM, et al. Oral contraceptives and coronary artery atherosclerosis of cynomolgus monkeys. *Obstet Gynecol* 1990;75:217.
55. Gold MA. New progestin oral contraceptives and the female condom. *Pediatr Ann* 1995;24:211.
56. Special Medical Report. ACOG issues report on hormonal contraception. *Am Fam Physician* 1995;51:543.
57. Coupey SM. New hormonal contraceptive options for adolescents. In: Goldfarb AF, ed. *Clinical problems in pediatric and adolescent gynecology.* New York: Chapman & Hall; 1996:77.
58. Grimes DA, ed. Metabolic effects of oral contraceptives. *The Contraception Report* 1996;6(6):4.
59. Elkind-Hirsch K. Oral contraceptives and leuprolide reverse hirsutism. *Am Fam Physician* 1995;51:204.
60. Emans SJ, Grace E, Woods ER, et al. Adolescents' compliance with the use of oral contraceptives. *JAMA* 1987;257:3377.
61. Rebar RN, Speroff L. The new progestins: Pharmacologic and clinical perspectives. *Dialogues in Contraception* 1993;4(1):1.
62. Grimes DA, ed. Venous thromboembolism and desogestrel- or gestodene-containing combination oral contraceptives: what are the facts? *The Contraception Report* 1996;7(1):2.
63. Klitsch M. New generation of progestins may raise oral contraceptive users' risk of blood clots. *Fam Plann Perspect* 1996;28:33.
64. Food and Drug Administration. Oral contraceptives and risk of blood clots. *FDA Talk Paper*, November 24, 1995.
65. World Health Organization Collaborative Study of Cardiovascular Disease and Steroid Hormone Contraception. Venous thromboembolic disease and combined oral contraceptives: results of international multicentre case-control study. *Lancet* 1996;346:1575.
66. World Health Organization Collaborative Study of Cardiovascular Disease and Steroid Hormone Contraception. Effect of different progestagens in low oestrogen oral contraceptives on venous thromboembolic disease. *Lancet* 1996;346:1582.
67. Hick H, Jick SS, Gurewich V, et al. Risk of idiopathic cardiovascular death and nonfatal venous thromboembolism in women using oral contraceptives with different progestagen components. *Lancet* 1995;346:1589.
68. Bloemenkamp KWM, Rosendaal FR, Helmerhorst FM, et al. Enhancement by factor V Leiden mutation of risk of deep-vein thrombosis associated with oral contraceptives containing a third-generation progestagen. *Lancet* 1995;346:1593.
69. Spitzer WO, Lewis MA, Heinemann LAJ, et al. Third generation oral contraceptives and risk of venous thromboembolic disorders: an international case-control study. *Br Med J* 1996;312:83.
70. Editorial. The desogestrel story. *NASPAG News* 1995;9(4):1.
71. Toglia MR, Weg JG. Venous thromboembolism during pregnancy. *N Engl J Med* 1996;335:108.

72. Kittner SJ, Stern BJ, Feeser BR, et al. Pregnancy and the risk of stroke. *N Engl J Med* 1996;335:768.
73. Lewis MA, Spitzer WO, Heinemann LAJ, et al. Third generation oral contraceptives and risk of myocardial infarction: an international case-control study. *Br Med J* 1996;312:88.
74. Mishell DR Jr. Contraception. *N Engl J Med* 1989;320:777.
75. Grace E, Emans SJ, Havens KK, et al. Contraceptive compliance with a triphasic and a monophasic norethindrone-containing oral contraceptive pill in a private adolescent practice. *Adolescent and Pediatric Gynecology* 1994;7:29.
76. Hatcher RA, Trussell J, Stewart F, et al. *Contraceptive Technology.* 17th ed. New York: Irvington; 1998.
77. Neinstein L, Katz B. Contraceptive use in the chronically ill adolescent female: parts I and II. *Journal of Adolescent Health Care* 1986;7:123, 350.
78. Bronner LL, Kanter DS, Manson JE. Primary prevention of stroke. *N Engl J Med* 1995;333:1392.
79. Burkman RT Jr. Oral contraceptives: an update. *Hosp Pract* 1995;30:85.
80. Hatcher RA, Guest F, Stewart F, et al. *Contraceptive Technology 1988–1989.* 14th ed. New York: Irvington; 1988.
81. Rosenfeld A. Oral and intrauterine contraception: a 1978 risk assessment. *Am J Obstet Gynecol* 1978;132:92.
82. Tyrer L. Teenagers and OCs. In: Dickey RP, ed. *Managing contraceptive pill patients.* 8th ed. Durant, OK: Creative Infomatics; 1996:58.
83. Porter JB, Jick H, Walker AM. Mortality among oral contraceptive users. *Obstet Gynecol* 1987;70:29.
84. Katerndahl DA, Realini JP, Cohen PA. Oral contraceptive use and cardiovascular disease: Is the relationship real or due to study bias? *J Fam Pract* 1992;35:147.
85. Grimes DA, ed. 30 Years of change: the current perspective on cardiovascular risks and oral contraceptives. *The Contraception Report* 1995;6(2):4.
86. Stampfer MJ, Willett WC, Colditz GA, et al. A prospective study of past use of oral contraceptive agents and risk of cardiovascular disease. *N Engl J Med* 1988;319:1313.
87. Centers for Disease Control and Prevention. The reduction in risk of ovarian cancer associated with oral-contraceptive use. *N Engl J Med* 1987;316:650.
88. Centers for Disease Control and Prevention. Combination oral contraceptive use and risk of endometrial cancer. *JAMA* 1987;257:796.
89. Golin M. O.C. pill/cancer decision "on hold" awaiting new, longterm research. *Adolescent Medicine Newsletter* 1989;16(1):2.
90. Chilvers C. Oral contraceptives and cancer. *Lancet* 1994;344:1378.
91. Rose PG. Endometrial carcinoma. *N Engl J Med* 1996;335:640.
92. Brinton LA, Vessey MP, Flavel R, et al. Risk factors for benign breast disease. *Am J Epidemiol* 1981;113:203.
93. Neuberger J, Forman D, Doll R, et al. Oral contraceptives and hepatocellular carcinoma. *Br Med J* 1986;292:1355.
94. World Health Organization Collaborative Study of Neoplasia and Steroid Contraceptives. Combined oral contraceptives and liver cancer. *Int J Cancer* 1989;43:254.
95. Johnson JH. Weighing the evidence on the pill and breast cancer. *Fam Plann Perspect* 1989;21:89.
96. Wingo PA, Lee NC, Ory HW, et al. Age-specific differences in the relationship between oral contraceptive use and breast cancer. *Obstet Gynecol* 1991;78:161.
97. Romieu I, Willett WC, Colditz GA, et al. Prospective study of oral contraceptive use and risk of breast cancer in women. *J Natl Cancer Inst* 1989;81:1313.
98. Brinton LA, Daling JR, Liff JM, et al. Oral contraceptives and breast cancer risk among younger women. *J Natl Cancer Inst* 1995;87:827.
99. Collaborative Group on Hormonal Factors in Breast Cancer. Breast cancer and hormonal contraceptives: collaborative reanalysis of individual data on 53,297 women with breast cancer and 100,239 women without breast cancer from 54 epidemiological studies. *Lancet* 1996;347:1713.
100. Beral V, Hannaford P, Kay C. Oral contraceptive use and malignancies of the genital tract. *Lancet* 1988;2:1331.
101. Vessey MP, Lawless M, McPherson K, et al. Neoplasia of the cervix uteri and contraception: a possible adverse effect of the pill. *Lancet* 1983;2:930.
102. World Health Organization Collaborative Study of Neoplasia and Steroid Contraceptives. Invasive cervical cancer and combined oral contraceptives. *Br Med J* 1985;290:961.
103. Brinton LA, Huggins GR, Lehman H, et al. Long-term use of oral contraceptives and risk of invasive cervical cancer. *Int J Cancer* 1986;38:339.
104. Ursin T, Peters RK, Henderson BE, et al. Oral contraceptive use and adenocarcinoma of cervix. *Lancet* 1994;344:1390.
105. Brisson J, Morin C, Fortier M, et al. Risk factors for cervical intraepithelial neoplasia: differences between low- and high-grade lesions. *Am J Epidemiol* 1994;140:700.
106. Ye Z, Thomas DB, Ray RM, et al. Combined oral contraceptives and risk of cervical carcinoma *in situ. Int J Epidemiol* 1995;24:19.
107. Gutman LT. Human papillomavirus infections of the genital tract in adolescents. *Adolescent Medicine: State of the Art Reviews* 1995;6:115.

108. Rosenfeld WD, and Swedler JB. Role of hormonal contraceptives in prevention of pregnancy and sexually transmitted diseases. *Adolescent Medicine: State of the Art Reviews* 1992;3:207.
109. Louv WC, Austin H, Perlman J et al. Oral contraceptive use and the risk of chlamydial and gonococcal infections. *Am J Obstet Gynecol* 1989;160:396.
110. Wolner-Hanssen P, Svensson L, Mardh P-A, et al. Laparoscopic findings and contraceptive use in women with signs and symptoms suggestive of acute salpingitis. *Obstet Gynecol* 1985;66:233.
111. Washington AE, Gove S, Schachter J, et al. Oral contraceptives, *Chlamydia trachomatis* infection and pelvic inflammatory disease: a word of caution about protection. *JAMA* 1985;253:2246.
112. Park BJ, Stergachis A, Scholes D, et al. Contraceptive methods and the risk of *Chlamydia trachomatis* infection in young women. *Am J Epidemiol* 1995;142:771.
113. Hollander D. Barrier methods may protect some women against cervical *Chlamydia*, but pill use does not affect risk. *Fam Plann Perspect* 1996;28:37.
114. Wolner-Hanssen P, Eschenbach DA, Paavonen J, et al. Decreased risk of symptomatic chlamydial pelvic inflammatory disease associated with oral contraceptive use. *JAMA* 1990;263:54.
115. Tyrer LB. Oral contraception for the adolescent. *J Reprod Med* 1984;29(Suppl):551.
116. Van Der Vange N, Kloosterboer HJ, Haspels AA. Effect of seven low-dose combined oral contraceptive preparations on carbohydrate metabolism. *Am J Obstet Gynecol* 1987;156:918.
117. Associated Press. Pill use raises AIDS risk. *Albuquerque Journal*, June 17, 1988.
118. Cates W Jr, Stone KM. Family planning, sexually transmitted diseases and contraceptive choice: a literature update, part II. *Fam Plann Perspect* 1992;24:122.
119. Mastroianni L Jr. Noncontraceptive benefits of oral contraceptive agents. *Postgrad Med* 1993;93:193.
120. Hergenroeder AC. Bone mineralization, hypothalamic amenorrhea, and sex steroid therapy in female adolescents and young adults. *J Pediatr* 1995;126:683.
121. Grimes DA. The safety of oral contraceptives: epidemiologic insights from the first 30 years. *Am J Obstet Gynecol* 1992;166:1950.
122. Holder AR. *Legal issues in pediatrics and adolescent medicine.* 2nd ed. New Haven: Yale University Press; 1985.
123. Braverman PK, Strasburger VC. Adolescent sexuality: IV. the practitioner's role. *Clin Pediatr* 1994;33:100.
124. Graves CE, Bridge MD, Nyhuis AW. Residents' perception of their skill levels in the clinical management of adolescent health problems. *Journal of Adolescent Health Care* 1987;8:413.
125. Bradford BJ, Lyons CW. Adolescent medicine practice in urban Pittsburgh: 1990. *Clin Pediatr* 1992;31:471.
126. Strasburger VC. Adolescent medicine: batteries not included. *Clin Pediatr* 1992;31:478.
127. Wender EH, Bijur PE, Boyce WT. Pediatric residency training: ten years after the Task Force report. *Pediatrics* 1992;90:876.
128. Orr MT. Private physicians and the provision of contraceptives to adolescents. *Fam Plann Perspect* 1984;16:83.
129. Holder AR. Legal issues in adolescent sexual health. *Adolescent Medicine: State of the Art Reviews* 1992;3:257.
130. Carpenter S, Neinstein LS. Weight gain in adolescent and young adult oral contraceptive users. *Journal of Adolescent Health Care* 1986;7:342.
131. Oakley D, Parent J. A scale to measure microbehaviors of oral contraceptive pill use. *Soc Biol* 1990;37:215.
132. Litt IF, Cuskey WR, Rudd S. Identifying adolescents at risk for non-compliance with contraceptive therapy. *J Pediatr* 1980;96:742.
133. Sher PW, Emans SJ, Grace EA. Factors associated with compliance to oral contraceptive use in an adolescent population. *Journal of Adolescent Health Care* 1982;3:120.
134. Jay MS, DuRant RH, Litt IR. Female adolescents' compliance with contraceptive regimens. *Pediatr Clin North Am* 1989;36:731.
135. Balassone ML. Risk of contraceptive discontinuance among adolescents. *Journal of Adolescent Health Care* 1989;10:527.
136. Cromer B, Brown RT. The pediatrician and the sexually active adolescent: I. sexual activity and contraception. *Pediatr Clin North Am* 1997 (in press).
137. Wiemann CM, Berenson AB. Contraceptive discontinuation among white, black, and Hispanic adolescents. *Adolescent and Pediatric Gynecology* 1993;6:75.
138. Cromer BA, Smith RD, Blair JA, et al. A prospective study of adolescents who choose among levonorgestrel implant (Norplant), medroxyprogesterone acetate (Depo-Provera), or the combined oral contraceptive pill as contraception. *Pediatrics* 1994;94:687.
139. Bearss N, Santelli JS, Papa P. A pilot program of contraceptive continuation in six school-based clinics. *J Adolesc Health* 1995;17:178.
140. Dinerman LM, Wilson MD, Duggan AK, et al. Outcomes of adolescents using levonorgestrel implants vs oral contraceptives or other contraceptive methods. *Arch Pediatr Adolesc Med* 1995;149:967.
141. Titus K. Even as new options emerge, gynecologists urge women to find older contraceptives user-friendly. *JAMA* 1996;276:440.
142. United States Department of Health and Human Services. Manufacturers phase out high-dose oral contraceptives. *FDA Drug Bulletin* 1988;18(2):19.

143. Dickey RP. *Managing contraceptive pill patients.* 8th ed. Durant, OK: Creative Infomatics, 1996.
144. Oakley D. Rethinking patient counselling techniques for changing contraceptive use behavior. *Am J Obstet Gynecol* 1994;170:1585.
145. The Medical Letter. Choice of contraceptives. *The Medical Letter* 1995;37(941):9.
146. Yuzpe AA, Lancee WJ. Ethinylestradiol and DL-norgestrel as a postcoital contraceptive. *Fertil Steril* 1977; 28:932.
147. Percival-Smith RKL, Abercrombie B. Post-coital contraception with DL-Norgestrel/ethinyl estradiol combination: six years experience in a student medical clinic. *Contraception* 1987;36:287.
148. Trussell J, Stewart F. The effectiveness of postcoital hormonal contraception. *Fam Plann Perspect* 1992; 24:262.
149. Trussell J, Stewart F, Guest F, et al. Emergency contraceptive pills: a simple proposal to reduce unintended pregnancies. *Fam Plann Perspect* 1992;24:269.
150. Gold MA, Schein A, Coupey SM. Emergency contraception: a national survey of adolescent health experts. Presented at the annual meeting of the North American Society for Pediatric and Adolescent Gynecology, Toronto, Ontario, Canada, April 22,1995.
151. Harper C, Ellertson C. Knowledge and perceptions of emergency contraceptive pills among a college-age population: A qualitative approach. *Fam Plann Perspect* 1996;28:149.
152. Buttermore S, Nolan C. Six years of clinical experience using postcoital contraception in college women. *J Am Coll Health* 1993;42:61.
153. Trussell J, Ellertson C, Stewart F. The effectiveness of the Yuzpe regimen of emergency contraception. *Fam Plann Perspect* 1996;28:58.
154. Ellertson C. History and efficacy of emergency contraception: beyond Coca-Cola. *Fam Plann Perspect* 1996;28:44.
155. Glasier A, Thong KJ, Dewar M, et al. Mifepristone (RU 486) compared with high-dose estrogen and progestogen for emergency postcoital contraception. *N Engl J Med* 1992;327:1041.
156. World Health Organization Collaborative Study of Neoplasia and Steroid Contraceptives. Breast cancer and depot-medroxyprogesterone acetate: a multinational study. *Lancet* 1991;338:833.
157. Skegg CG, Noonan EA, Paul C, et al. Depot medroxyprogesterone acetate and breast cancer: a pooled analysis of the World Health Organization and New Zealand Studies. *JAMA* 1995;273:799.
158. Smith RD, Cromer BA, Hayes JR, et al. Medroxyprogesterone acetate (Depo-Provera) use in adolescents: uterine bleeding and blood pressure patterns, patient satisfaction, and continuation rates. *Adolescent and Pediatric Gynecology* 1995;8:24.
159. Jay MS, Bridges CE, Gottlieb AA, et al. Adolescent contraception: an overview. *Adolescent and Pediatric Gynecology* 1988;1:83.
160. World Health Organization Task Force on Long-acting Systemic Agents for Fertility Regulation. A multicentered phase III comparative clinical trial of depo-medroxyprogesterone acetate given three-monthly at doses of 100 mg or 150 mg: I. contraceptive efficacy and side effects. *Contraception* 1986;34:223.
161. Cromer BA. Depo-Provera: wherefore art thou? *Adolescent and Pediatric Gynecology* 1992;5:155.
162. Pardthaisong T. Return of fertility after use of the injectable contraceptive Depo-Provera: updated analysis. *J Biosoc Sci* 1984;16:23.
163. Polaneczky M, Guarnaccia M, Alon J, et al. Early experience with the contraceptive use of depot medroxyprogesterone acetate in an inner-city clinic population. *Fam Plann Perspect* 1996;28:174.
164. Hergenroeder AC. Bone mineralization, hypothalamic amenorrhea, and sex steroid therapy in female adolescents and young adults. *J Pediatr* 1995;126:683.
165. Kreipe RE. Bone mineral density in adolescents. *Pediatr Ann* 1995;24:308.
166. Blair JM, Cromer B, Mahan J, et al. Bone density in adolescent girls on Depo-Provera and Norplant. *J Adolesc Health* 1995;16:164.
167. Cundy T, Evans M, Roberts H, et al. Bone density in women receiving depot medroxyprogesterone acetate for contraception. *Br Med J* 1991;303:12.
168. Cundy T, Cornish J, Evans, MC, et al. Recovery of bone density in women who stop using medroxyprogesterone acetate. *Br Med J* 1994;308:247.
169. Westhoff C, Wieland D. Depression in users of depot-medroxyprogesterone acetate. Contraception 1995;51: 351.
170. Sangi-Haghpeykar H, Poindexter AN III, Bateman L, et al. Experiences of injectable contraceptive users in an urban setting. *Obstet Gynecol* 1996;88:227.
171. Hatcher RA, Trussell J. Contraceptive implants and teenage pregnancy. *N Engl J Med* 1994;331:1229.
172. Cullins VE, Remsburn RE, Blumenthal PD, et al. Comparison of adolescent and adult experiences with Norplant levonorgestrel contraceptive implants. *Obstet Gynecol* 1994;83:1026.
173. Polanecsky M, Slap G, Forke C, et al. The use of levonorgestrel implants (Norplant) for contraception in adolescent mothers. *N Engl J Med* 1994;331:1201.
174. Wiemann CM, Berenson AB. An investigation into why adolescents may reject Norplant. *Pediatrics* 1996; 97:185.
175. Rainey DY, Parsons LH, Kenney PG, et al. Compliance with return appointments for reproductive health care among adolescent Norplant users. *J Adolesc Health* 1995;16:385.

176. Harel Z, Biro FM, Kollar LM, et al. Adolescents' reasons for and experience after discontinuation of the long-acting contraceptives Depo-Provera and Norplant. *J Adolesc Health* 1996;19:118.
177. Darney PD, Klaisle CM, Monroe SM, et al. Evaluation of a 1-year levonorgestrel-releasing contraceptive implant: side effects, release rates, and biodegradability. *Fertil Steril* 1992;58:137.
178. Klitsch M. Still waiting for the contraceptive revolution. *Fam Plann Perspect* 1995;27:246.
179. Hofmann AD. Contraception in adolescence: a review. *Bull World Health Org* 1984;62:151.
180. The Medical Letter. Choice of contraceptives. *The Medical Letter* 1988;30:105.
181. Einarson TR, Koren G, Mattice D, et al. Maternal spermicide use and adverse reproductive outcome: a meta-analysis. *Am J Obstet Gynecol* 1990;162:655.
182. Contraceptive Technology. FDA inspection sounds death knell for sponge. *Contraceptive Technology Update* 1995;16(3):42.
183. Lane ME, Arceo R, Sobrero AJ. Successful use of the diaphragm and jelly by a young population: report of a clinical study. *Fam Plann Perspect* 1976;8:81.
184. Marks A, Mueller M. The diaphragm: An appealing and effective contraceptive for many teenagers. *Pediatr Res* 1979;12:328.
185. Fisher M, Marks A, Trieller K. Comparative analysis of the effectiveness of the diaphragm and birth control pill during the first year of use among suburban adolescents. *Journal of Adolescent Health Care* 1987;8:393.
186. Stone KM, Grimes DA, Magder LS. Personal protection against sexually transmitted diseases. *Am J Obstet Gynecol* 1986;155:180.
187. Cramer DW, Goldman MB, Schiff I, et al. The relationship of tubal infertility to barrier method and oral contraceptive use. *JAMA* 1987;257:2446.
188. Wright NJ, Vesey MP, Kenward B, et al. Neoplasia and dysplasia of the cervix uteri and contraception: a possible protective effect of the diaphragm. *Br J Cancer* 1978;38:273.
189. Celentano DD, Klassen AC, Weisman CS, et al. The role of contraceptive use in cervical cancer: the Maryland cervical cancer case–control study. *Am J Epidemiol* 1987;126:592.
190. Klitsch M. FDA approval ends cervical cap's marathon. *Fam Plann Perspect* 1988;20:137.
191. Foxman B. Recurring urinary tract infection: incidence and risk factors. *Am J Public Health* 1990;80:331.
192. Fihn SD, Latham RH, Roberts P, et al. Association between diaphragm use and urinary tract infection. *JAMA* 1986;254:240.
193. Strom BL, Collins M, West SL et al. Sexual activity, contraceptive use, and other risk factors for symptomatic and asymptomatic bacteriuria. *Ann Intern Med* 1987;107:816.
194. The Medical Letter. The cervical cap. *The Medical Letter* 1988;30:93.
195. Powell MG, Mears BJ, Deber RB, et al. Contraception with the cervical cap: effectiveness, safety, continuity of use, and user satisfaction. *Contraception* 1986;33:215.
196. Psychoyos A, Creatsas G, Hassan E, et al. Spermicidal and antiviral properties of cholic acid: contraceptive efficacy of a new vaginal sponge (Protectaid) containing sodium cholate. *Hum Reprod* 1993;8:866.
197. North BB, Vorhauer BW. Use of the Today contraceptive sponge in the United States. *Int J Fertil* 1985;30:81.
198. Harvey SM, Beckman LJ, Murray J. Factors associated with use of the contraceptive sponge. *Fam Plann Perspect* 1989;21:179.
199. Jones EF, Beringer JR, Westoff CF. Pill and IUD discontinuation in the United States, 1970–1975: the influence of the media. *Fam Plann Perspect* 1980;12:293.
200. Contraceptive Technology. New Advantage 24 contraceptive gel claims 24-hour effectiveness. *Contraceptive Technology Update* 1995;16(4):45.
201. Trussell J, Leveque JA, Koenig JD, et al. The economic value of contraception: a comparison of 15 methods. *Am J Public Health* 1995;85:494.
202. Can you rely on condoms? *Consumer Reports* March, 1989, p. 135.
203. Carey RF, Herman WA, Retta SM, et al. Effectiveness of latex condoms as a barrier to human immunodeficiency virus-sized particles under the conditions of simulated use. *Sex Transm Dis* 1992;19:230.
204. Richardson AC, Lyon JB. The effect of condom use on squamous cell cervical intraepithelial neoplasia. *Am J Obstet Gynecol* 1981;140:909.
205. Condoms for prevention of sexually transmitted diseases. *MMWR Morb Mortal Wkly Rep* 1988;37:133.
206. Parrish SK Jr. Barrier contraceptives. In: Strasburger VC, ed. *Adolescent gynecology: an office guide.* Baltimore: Urban & Schwarzenberg; 1990:45.
207. Rietmeijer C, Krebs JW, Feorino PM, et al. Condoms as physical and chemical barriers against human immunodeficiency virus. *JAMA* 1988;259:1851.
208. Shaw EJ, Rienzo BA. Permeability of latex condoms: do latex condoms prevent HIV transmission? *Journal of Health Education* 1995;26:372.
209. Saracco A, Musicco M, Nicolosi A, et al. Man-to-woman sexual transmission of HIV: longitudinal study of 343 steady partners of infected men. *Journal of Acquired Immune Deficiency Syndromes.* 1993;6:497.
210. DeVincenzi IA, for the European Study Group on Heterosexual Transmission of HIV. A longitudinal study of human immunodeficiency virus transmission by heterosexual partners. *N Engl J Med* 1994;331:341.
211. Guimaraes M, Munoz A, Boschi-Pinto C, et al. HIV infection: female partners of seropositive men in Brazil. *Am J Epidemiol* 1995;142:538.
212. Associated Press. Some condoms leak AIDS. *Chicago Sun-Times*, September 17, 1989;.

213. Davis AJ. Plastic condoms. *NASPAG News* 1995;9(2):1.
214. Contraceptive Technology. FDA: polyurethane condom carries "extremely misleading" label. *Contraceptive Technology Update* 1995;16(2):17.
215. MacDonald NE, Wells GA, Fisher WA, et al. High-risk STD/HIV behavior among college students. *JAMA* 1990;262:3155.
216. Peipert JF, Domaglski L, Boardman L, et al. College women and condom use, 1975–1995. *N Engl J Med* 1996;335:211.
217. Nelson KE, Celentano DD, Eiumtrakol S, et al. Changes in sexual behavior and a decline in HIV infection among young men in Thailand. *N Engl J Med* 1996;335:297.
218. Zenilman JM, Weisman CS, Rompalo AM, et al. Condom use to prevent incident STDs: the validity of self-reported condom use. *Sex Trans Dis* 1995;22:15.
219. Sonenstein FL, Pleck JH, Ku LC. Sexual activity, condom use and AIDS awareness among adolescent males. *Fam Plann Perspect* 1989;21:152.
220. Arnold CB, Cogswell BE. A condom distribution program for adolescents: the findings of a feasibility study. *Am J Public Health* 1971;61:739.
221. Stryker J, Samueles SE, Smith MD. Condom availability in schools: the need for improved program evaluations. *Am J Public Health* 1994;84:1901.
222. American Medical Association. HIV impact on adolescents advances prevention and treatment initiatives. *Target 2000 Newsletter* 1995;5(2):1.
223. Advocates for Youth. *Fact sheet: school condom availability.* Washington, DC: Advocates for Youth; 1995.
224. Santelli JS, Kouzis AC, Hoover DR, et al. Stage of behavior change for condom use: the influence of partner type, relationship and pregnancy factors. *Fam Plann Perspect* 1996;28:101.
225. Hausser D, Michaud PA. Does a condom-promoting strategy (the Swiss STOP-AIDS) campaign modify sexual behavior among adolescents? *Pediatrics* 1994;93:580.
226. Committee on Communications, American Academy of Pediatrics. Adolescent sexuality and the media (policy statement). *Pediatrics* 1995;95:298.
227. Trussell J, Sturgen K, Strickler J, et al. Contraceptive efficacy of the Reality female condom: comparison with other barrier methods. *Fam Plann Perspect* 1994;26:66.
228. Farr G, Gabelnick H, Sturgen K, et al. Contraceptive efficacy and acceptability of the female condom. *Am J Public Health* 1994;84:1960.
229. Contraceptive Technology. New data found on failure rates for female condom. *Contraceptive Technology Update* 1995;16(4):54.
230. Kreutner AK. Adolescent contraception. *Prim Care* 1987;14:121.
231. The Medical Letter. New copper IUD. *The Medical Letter* 1988;30:25.
232. Burnhill MS. The rise and fall and rise of the IUD. *American Journal of Gynecologic Health* 1989;III(35):6.
233. Grimes DA. Reversible contraception for the 1980s. *JAMA* 1986;255:69.
234. Farley TMM, Rosenberg MJ, Rowe PJ, et al. Intrauterine devices and pelvic inflammatory disease: an international perspective. *Lancet* 1992;339:785.
235. Editorial. Does infection occur with modern intrauterine devices? *Lancet* 1992;339:783.
236. Cramer DW, Schiff I, Schoenbaum C, et al. Tubal infertility and the intrauterine device. *N Engl J Med* 1985;312:941.
237. Hatcher RA. Little white lie: abstinence is 100% effective. *Contraceptive Technology Update* 1995;16(2):27.
238. Jones E, Forrest J. Contraceptive failure rates based on the 1988 NSFG. *Fam Plann Perspect* 1992;24:21.
239. Grimes DA, ed. Developments in male contraception: a review of potential male contraceptive agents. *The Contraception Report* 1992;2(6):12.
240. Mastroianni L Jr. Future contraceptive methods. *The Contraception Report* 1994;5(4):4.
241. Elias CJ, Heise LL. Challenges for the development of female-controlled vaginal microbiocides. *AIDS* 1994;8:1.
242. Darney PD. Hormonal implants: contraception for a new century. *Am J Obstet Gynecol* 1994;170:1536.
243. Koetsawang S, Ji G, Krishna U, et al. Micro-dose intravaginal levonorgestrel contraception: a multicentre clinical trial: I. contraceptive efficacy and side effects. *Contraception* 1990;41:105.
244. Mishell DR Jr. Vaginal contraceptive rings. *Ann Med* 1993;25:191.
245. Laurikka-Routti M, Haukkamaa M, Lahteenmaki P. Suppression of ovarian function with the transdermally given synthetic progestin ST-1435. *Fertil Steril* 1992;58:680.
246. World Health Organization Task Force on Methods for the Regulation of Male Fertility. Contraceptive efficacy of testosterone-induced azoospermia and oligozoospermia in normal men. *Fertil Steril* 1996;65:821.

SUGGESTED READING

Adler NE, Kegeles SM, Irwin CE Jr, et al. Adolescent contraceptive behavior: an assessment of decision processes. *J Pediatr* 1990;116:463.
Alan Guttmacher Institute. *Sex and America's teenagers.* New York: Alan Guttmacher Institute; 1994.
American College of Obstetricians and Gynecologists. Condom availability for adolescents (position paper). *J Adolesc Health* 1996;18:380.

Beach RK. Contraception for adolescents I and II. *Adolescent Health Update* 1994;7(1):1 and 1995;7(2):1.

Braverman PK, Strasburger VC. Adolescent sexuality, parts I–IV. *Clin Pediatr* 1993–1994: I. Adolescent sexual activity. 1993;32:658. II. Contraception. 1993;32:725. III. Sexually transmitted diseases. 1994;33:26. IV. The practitioner's role. 1994;33:100.

Burkman RT Jr. Oral contraceptives: an update. *Hosp Pract* 1995;30:85.

Chilvers C. Oral contraceptives and cancer. *Lancet* 1994;344:1378.

Coupey SM. New hormonal contraceptive options for adolescents. In: Goldfarb AF, ed. *Clinical problems in pediatric and adolescent gynecology.* New York: Chapman & Hall; 1996:77.

Coupey SM, Klerman LV, eds. Adolescent sexuality: preventing unhealthy consequences. *Adolescent Medicine: State of the Art Reviews* 1992;3:165.

Cromer BA. Depo-Provera: wherefore art thou? *Adolescent and Pediatric Gynecology* 1992;5:155.

Cromer BK, Brown RT. The pediatrician and the sexually active adolescent: I. sexual activity and contraception. *Pediatr Clin North Am* 1997 (in press).

Darney P.D. Hormonal implants: Contraception for a new century. *Am J Obstet Gynecol* 170:1536, 1994;.

Dickey RP. *Managing contraceptive pill patients.* 8th ed. Durant, OK: Creative Infomatics; 1996.

Emans SJH, Goldstein DP. *Pediatric and adolescent gynecology.* 4th ed. Boston: Little, Brown; 1996.

Fortenberry JD. Condom availability in high schools. *Adolescent Medicine: State of the Art Reviews* 1997;8(3): 449.

Gold MA. Contraception update: implantable and injectable methods. *Pediatr Ann* 1995;24:203.

Gold MA. New progestin oral contraceptives and the female condom. *Pediatr Ann* 1995;24:211.

Gold MA. Emergency contraception. *Adolescent Medicine: State of the Art Reviews* 1997;8(3) (in press).

Gold MA, Schein A, Coupey SM. Emergency contraception: a national survey of adolescent health experts. *Fam Plann Perspect* 1997;29:15.

Grimes DA. A 17-year-old mother seeking contraception. *JAMA* 1996;276:1163.

Hatcher RA, Trussell J. Contraceptive implants and teenage pregnancy. *N Engl J Med* 1994;331:1229.

Hatcher RA, Trussell J, Stewart F, et al. *Contraceptive technology.* 17th ed. New York: Irvington; 1998.

Heaton C, Smith M. The diaphragm. *Am Fam Physician* 1989;39:231.

Hillard PJ. Contraception for the adolescent. In: Pokorny SF, ed. *Pediatric and adolescent gynecology.* New York: Chapman and Hall; 1996:117.

Holder AR. Legal issues in adolescent sexual health. *Adolescent Medicine: State of the Art Reviews* 1992;3:257.

Huwitt GD. Should adolescents have over the counter access to oral contraceptive pills and antibiotics? *Adolescent Medicine: State of the Art Reviews* 1997;8(3):443.

Joffe A. Adolescents and condom use. *American Journal of Diseases of Children* 1993;147:746.

The Medical Letter. Choice of contraceptives. *The Medical Letter* 1995;37(issue 941):9.

Mishell DR Jr. Correcting misconceptions about oral contraceptives. *Am J Obstet Gynecol* 1989;161:1385.

Mishell DR Jr. Contraception. *N Engl J Med* 1989;320:777.

Neinstein L. *Issues in reproductive management.* New York: Thieme; 1994.

Rosenfeld WD, Swedler JB. Role of hormonal contraceptives in prevention of pregnancy and sexually transmitted diseases. *Adolescent Medicine: State of the Art Reviews* 1992;3:207.

Sikand A, Fisher M. The role of barrier contraceptives in prevention of pregnancy and disease in adolescents. *Adolescent Medicine: State of the Art Reviews* 1992;3:223.

Stevens-Simon C. Reproductive health care for your adolescent female patients. *Contemporary Pediatrics* 1997;14:35.

Strasburger VC. Prescribing oral contraceptives. In: Strasburger VC, ed. *Adolescent gynecology: an office guide.* Baltimore: Urban & Schwarzenberg; 1990:23.

Sulak PJ, Haney AR. Unwanted pregnancies: understanding contraceptive use and benefits in adolescents and older women. *Am J Obstet Gynecol* 1993;168:2042.

PREGNANCY TESTING AND COUNSELING

Physicians can make a critical difference in young teenagers' lives, and nowhere is this more apparent than in pregnancy counseling. Such visits represent a kind of crisis intervention and, done well, can avoid such impulsive and drastic teenage behavior as running away or making a suicide attempt. On the other hand, clinicians must be aware of their own limitations in such situations:

• Many studies document that physicians rarely, if ever, talk teenagers "into" or "out of" any of the three options after pregnancy (i.e., carrying to term, abortion, adoption).
• A nonjudgmental attitude is crucial.
• Physicians may represent the only adult contact that the patient has. As such, they must carefully balance the teenager's right to confidential health care; her need for emotional, moral, and financial support; and her parents' need or "right" to know about her situation. In fact, the teenagers' initial inclination often dictates the practitioner's approach. For instance, a decision to carry the pregnancy

to term almost inevitably will mean that the teen's parents will find out. Offering to inform one or both of them may greatly relieve the teenager. Teenagers choosing abortion require emotional support and, ideally, a family member is best suited for this. Even in states that have no abortion notification statute, parental involvement is almost always desirable, particularly with teenagers younger than 15 years.

Diagnosis

Any female teenager who presents with an acute health problem should be questioned about her sexual activity and the possibility that she could be pregnant. In particular, a confidential sexual history *must* be elicited from teenage girls with acute abdominal pain, dysuria, menstrual irregularities, or vaginal symptoms [1]. Most teenagers will give an accurate sexual history if confidentiality is ensured, and they understand the need for such questioning. But if any doubt remains, the clinician should always make liberal use of pregnancy testing—especially before scheduling major diagnostic procedures or surgery. An estimated 40% of female teens become pregnant at least once before their 20th birthday, and over 75% of these pregnancies are unplanned [2]. So teenage pregnancy is not a rare diagnosis: over one million teen pregnancies occur every year in the United States.

Normal Intrauterine Pregnancy

Clinically, pregnancy symptoms include nausea and vomiting (usually in the 2nd–12th weeks), urinary frequency, breast tenderness or engorgement, and fatigue. Although a hallmark of pregnancy is amenorrhea, physicians should never be misled by a history of continued menstrual periods because implantation bleeding can often mimic menstrual flow. On examination, softening of the cervix occurs by the beginning of the second month (Goodell's sign) and a bluish hue to the cervix and vagina appears between 6 and 8 weeks (Chadwick's sign), but neither of these signs is completely reliable. The size of the uterus may approximate either a lemon (normal, nonpregnant), an orange (6 weeks), or a grapefruit (8–10 weeks).

Since the early 1980s, urine pregnancy tests have been revolutionized and virtually have replaced serum tests in all but a few instances. Both tests measure human chorionic gonadotropin (hCG), usually in milli-international units (mIU per milliliter). hCG is produced by trophoblastic cells within 1 day of implantation—8 days after ovulation and approximately 5 days before the first missed menstrual period. Normally, the hCG concentration doubles every 1 to 3 days during the first 8 weeks of pregnancy: $\leq$ 5 mIU 24 hours after implantation; 70 to 100 mIU at 1 week; and > 250 mIU at 2 weeks. A peak hCG level of 100,000 mIU is reached during the third month of gestation. It then falls to 3,000 to 10,000 mIU between days 100 to 130, and remains steady thereafter (Fig. 8).

Ectopic Pregnancy

Although more common among women aged 35 years and older [3], ectopic pregnancies account for 2% of all pregnancies and are the leading cause of pregnancy-related death in the first trimester [4]. Women who have one ectopic pregnancy are at increased risk for a second, as well as for future infertility [5]. It is the only life-threatening condition for which the prevalence has increased as the mortality has decreased [6]. Between 1970 (when surveillance of ectopic pregnancy began) and 1987, the rate increased nearly fourfold, presumably related to an increase in sexually transmitted diseases, especially chlamydial infection [7,8]. Since 1987, that rate has leveled off and is now decreasing [5]. Teenagers have the lowest rate of ectopic pregnancies, but they have the highest reported death rate [3].

Ectopic pregnancy can be difficult to diagnose. Indeed, physicians misdiagnose more than 40% of ectopic pregnancies on the initial visit, primarily because of an inadequate history or physical examination [8]. The "classic" triad of amenorrhea, pelvic pain, and pelvic mass is not so classic (14% of patients in one study) [9] and may be more commonly associated with pelvic inflammatory disease, ovarian cysts, or spontaneous abortion. However, most patients have menstrual irregularity (76%), vaginal bleeding (68%), pelvic pain (91%), or an adnexal mass (55%) [9] (Table 48). If undetected, an ectopic pregnancy can produce hypotension, bleeding, and shock [6].

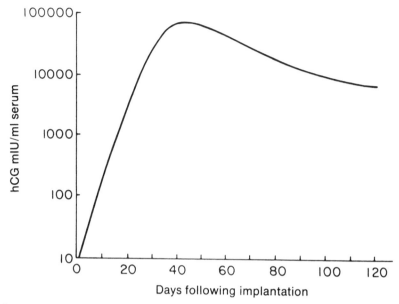

FIG. 8. Serum human chorionic gonadotropin (hCG) levels during normal pregnancy. (Reprinted with permission from Stephenson JN. Pregnancy testing and counseling. *Pediatr Clin North Am* 1989;36: 681.)

With newer, more sophisticated techniques, ectopic pregnancies can be diagnosed before menses have been absent for 6 weeks. The algorithm pictured in Figure 9 correctly diagnosed 100% of ectopic pregnancies when tested randomly against confirmatory laparoscopy [6].

Human Chorionic Gonadotropin

Virtually all teenagers with ectopic pregnancies have a positive β-hCG serum test, although the levels of hCG are much lower than in intrauterine pregnancies. If two serum hCG levels, drawn 24 hours apart, have not shown an increase of at least 66%, an ectopic pregnancy should be suspected (although this rule is too high for 15% of normal pregnancies and misses 13% of ectopic pregnancies) [10,11]. In normal pregnancies, hCG levels double every 2 to 3 days during the first 60 to 70 days of the pregnancy, whereas ectopic pregnancies generate lower levels of hCG [12]. Quantitative serum hCG determinations are most useful in considering this diagnosis.

Serum Progesterone

Progesterone is produced by a corpus luteum that is stimulated by a viable pregnancy. During the first 8 to 10 weeks of gestation, concentrations do not change much, but if the pregnancy is not viable, the levels diminish. Thus, serum levels less than 5 ng/ml exclude a viable pregnancy with 100% sensitivity; levels of 25 ng/ml or higher rule out an ectopic pregnancy with 97.5% sensitivity [12]. Although a level less than 5 ng/ml does not distinguish between an ectopic pregnancy and a spontaneous intrauterine abortion, a diagnostic uterine evacuation can then be performed [6].

Transvaginal Ultrasound

Using the newer form of ultrasound [13], intrauterine pregnancies can be diagnosed earlier than with transabdominal ultrasound, and many ectopic gestations can be detected [8].

TABLE 48. *Common features of ectopic pregnancy*

Feature	Frequency (Range)
Symptoms	
Lower abdominal pain	100% (95–100%)
Generalized	44%
Unilateral	33%
Radiating	23%
Amenorrhea	75% (75–95%)
Vaginal bleeding/spotting	75% (50–80%)
Signs	
Vital signs	Usually stable
Fever	5% (5–10%)
Abdominal tenderness	90% (80–95%)
Pelvic tenderness	85% (75–90%)
Cervical motion tenderness	85%
Pelvic mass	50% (40–60%)
Uterine enlargement	50% (25–70%)
Laboratory features	
Leukocyte count	Normal or slightly elevated
Quantitative hCG, serum	Elevated
Qualitative hCG, urine	Usually increased but can be decreased

hCG, human chorionic gonadotropin.
Adapted from Ammerman S, Shafer MA, Snyder D. Ectopic pregnancy in adolescents: a clinical review for pediatricians. *J Pediatr* 1990;117:677; and from Neinstein LS. *Adolescent health care: a practical guide.* 3rd ed. Baltimore: Williams and Wilkins, 1996.

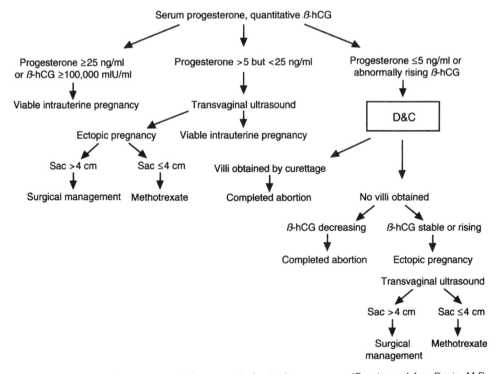

FIG. 9. Diagnosis and management of a suspected ectopic pregnancy. (Courtesy of Ann Davis, M.D., with permission.)

Increasing numbers of women with ectopic pregnancies are being treated with medical regimens, as outpatients [5,6,14]. Systemic methotrexate (50 mg/m^2 intramuscularly) can be used in stable patients with unruptured ectopic sacs measuring 4 cm or less by ultrasound [14]. Actively proliferating trophoblastic cells, as found in an ectopic pregnancy, are susceptible to methotrexate. In 306 cases reported since 1982, the outcome compares well with laparoscopic surgery: 94% successfully treated; 81% with tubal patency; 71% subsequently became pregnant, with 11% of those pregnancies ectopic. Methotrexate by direct injection into the sac has not been as successful (83% success rate) [6]. If laparoscopy is needed for diagnosis, then new microsurgical techniques can be used to perform a salpingostomy. Otherwise, methotrexate is the treatment of choice [6].

Primary care clinicians need to recognize that any teenager presenting with signs or symptoms of an ectopic pregnancy warrants immediate consultation with a gynecologist. Liberal use of transabdominal or transvaginal ultrasonography avoids many misdiagnoses [8].

Pregnancy Tests

The variety of tests that are available may be confusing [1,10,15,16] (Table 49). Both serum and urine tests detect the presence of hCG, which is present 7 to 9 days after ovulation. For most purposes, a simple qualitative urine hCG test is sufficient. It uses a double monoclonal antibody sandwich technique that is highly specific for hCG. In a normal intrauterine pregnancy, the hCG level doubles every 2 to 3 days and reaches a level of 50 to 250 mIU within 14 days after conception [1]. Urine tests are now extremely sensitive (to as little as 25 mIU of hCG), cheap ($20), and easy to run (5 minutes). One of the ultrasensitive tests turns positive 3 to 5 days postimplantation (i.e., even before the first missed period). The only disadvantage is an occasional false-negative test due to very dilute urine if the patient has had a high fluid intake. Alternatively, a qualitative serum hCG test can be done for the same price, with sensitivity as low as 20 mIU.

Quantitative serum hCG determinations are made by radioimmunoassay and are most useful in diagnosing ectopic pregnancies or threatened abortions (cost = $35). They measure the β-subunit of the hCG molecule, which is the unique part of the hormone. (The α-subunit, by comparison, may cross-react with luteinizing hormone or thyroid-stimulating hormone.) Use of the more highly sensitive urine tests eliminates many of the previously encountered problems with false-negative tests in early pregnancies. However, teenagers have been known to substitute tapwater or a friend's urine for their own, yielding a false-negative test. For that reason, clinicians may still want to use the qualitative serum test, especially if they have to obtain blood for other tests. Conversely, these urine hCG tests are now sufficiently sensitive that many early pregnancies that may be diagnosed will spontaneously

TABLE 49. *Selected serum and urine pregnancy tests*

Product	Sensitivity (mIU/ml hCG)	Test time (mins)	Type
Icon II hCG (Hybritech)	25	4	Urine
	20	5	Serum
One Step (Wampole)	25	5	Urine
Quick Vue (Quidel)	25	3	Urine
Surcell hCG	30	1	Urine
	30	2	Serum
Tandem Icon QSR (Hybritech)	<5	7	Serum
Target (V-Tech)	50	4	Urine
	50	5	Serum
Testpack plus hCG combo (Abbott)	50	4	Urine
	25	7	Serum
Over-the-counter tests			
Pregnosticon (Organon)	1,000–2,000	2	
Pregnosis (Roche)	1,500–2,500	2	
Wampole UCG (Wampole)	1,500–2,500	2	

hCG, human chorionic gonadotropin.
Adapted from Hatcher RA, Trussell J, Stewart F, et al. *Contraceptive technology.* 16th ed. New York: Irvington Publishers; 1994.

terminate without any clinical repercussions. Tests may also remain positive for up to 4 weeks after a therapeutic abortion. Rarely, several endocrinologically active or inactive tumors may produce hCG as well.

Home pregnancy tests use monoclonal hCG antibodies and can detect a pregnancy as early as days 31 to 34 of the menstrual cycle. Although accuracy is claimed as high as 98% to 99%, such a figure depends on the collection of a first morning urine in a clean container, free of detergent, at room temperature, along with correct interpretation of the test. Even so, few women trust the results of the test and usually seek confirmation from a physician or clinic. Such tests also miss low levels of hCG produced by an ectopic or threatened pregnancy. Therefore, home pregnancy testing cannot be recommended in the adolescent population.

Pregnancy Scare

Pregnancy scares provide a unique opportunity for clinicians to intervene with teenagers who are sexually active but are not yet pregnant. About 60% of teenagers conceive within 18 to 24 months after an initial negative pregnancy test [17,18]. Sometimes teenagers ask for pregnancy tests even though they are quite certain they are not pregnant [18]. This represents a unique opportunity to discuss contraception, negotiating sexual relationships, and factors related to the decision to become pregnant. Role-playing may help to help the adolescent "reality test" about what having a baby would actually be like [1].

Options Counseling

Much misinformation exists regarding teenagers and abortion. As mentioned previously, it is extremely rare for a physician to talk a patient "into" or "out of" having an abortion. At the same time, teenagers have a legal, moral, and medical right to know exactly what their options are. A kind, nonjudgmental, sensitive practitioner can make a tremendous difference in the life of a young woman who is pregnant, scared, and does not know what to do next.

Teenagers should be told calmly of their three options: 1) carrying the pregnancy to term, 2) abortion, or 3) carrying to term and placing the infant for adoption. For many teenagers, this may represent the first autonomous decision in their lives, and it is certainly one that may have lifelong repercussions. In general, 20% of teens initially desire the pregnancy, 20% want an abortion, and the rest are undecided, although this does *not* mean that the physician will heavily influence the eventual decision [10]. Rather, the clinician can help the teen deal with the variety of emotions she may be experiencing—ranging from anger and guilt to fear and disbelief—and with the crisis at hand. An immediate decision is neither needed nor desirable. Instead, the physician needs to help identify support for the teenager as well as catalyzing her own decision-making processes. Open-ended questions and a focus on the issue of this pregnancy help serve this purpose. Use of neutral words—"partner" instead of "father," "fetus" instead of "baby"—will be helpful in not prejudicing the teen. Her own choice of words may then reveal much of her initial inclinations.

Term Pregnancy

Although teenagers frequently have unrealistic ideas about parenting a child, it is difficult, if not impossible, to disabuse them of their notions [19]. In particular, teens age 15 and younger require referral to a high-risk maternity program and more frequent prenatal care. Carrying the pregnancy to term usually means that the mother or father of the teen will eventually have to know the situation. The teen's mother especially may have strong feelings, negative or positive, about being a grandmother and substitute caregiver. It is essential that pregnant adolescents do not delay prenatal care (or an abortion decision) because they fear parental reprisal. Often, a physician's offer to inform the teen's mother will be met with great relief. Involving the male partner in the process also may be constructive.

Studies indicate that a teenager's satisfaction with the outcome of her pregnancy depends on whether she has made her own decision and received parental support for her decision [20], which makes sense in terms of normal adolescent psychology. In one study, more than 90% of pregnant teens have spoken with either a parent or a parent surrogate [20]. Similarly, the relationship with the prospective father is often long term, an average of 2 years in one study [21], and perhaps half of all teen fathers are closely involved with the baby [21–23]. However, teen fathers are also more likely to have lower educational and job aspirations and to drop out of school [22,24].

Adoption

Only an estimated 2% of female teenagers give up their babies for adoption, and this figure has decreased since the 1970s [25]. Although adults on both sides of the abortion issue frequently agree that adoption is one ideal solution to the problem of teen pregnancy, unfortunately, teens who do place their children for adoption may have to face peers who view their behavior as selfish and unloving [26]. Such teens also may continue to fantasize about the babies they have given up, although the use of open adoptions could help to alleviate this problem [27]. Research indicates that those choosing this option tend to be unusually mature or upwardly mobile teenagers who were either adopted themselves or who know someone in their own family or group of friends who was also adopted [26,28]. Adolescents choosing adoption are also more likely to have mothers who support their decision [29]. Given the lack of healthy newborns for potential adult parents, such teenagers need to be encouraged vigorously and put in contact with local adoption agencies [30].

Abortion

In 1994 (the last year for which data are available), nearly 1.3 million American women had abortions [31]. Not only has the overall abortion rate decreased about 2% a year during the 1990s, but the percentage of abortions obtained by women younger than 19 years has steadily decreased as well, from 26% in the mid-1980s to 21% in 1991 [31,32]. These decreases could be the result of better use of contraception and fewer teenage pregnancies, or of more restrictive laws, more limited availability of abortion services, and decreased public funding for abortion [33].

Of all adolescent pregnancies, about half end in birth, slightly over a third in abortion, and the rest in miscarriage [2]. Still, most *unintended* pregnancies (53%) among adolescents end in abortion [2]. And a surprising 58% of all women who have abortions report that they had been using a contraceptive method during the month they became pregnant [32].

Although most Americans continue to support abortion (60% in a 1995 poll) [34], teenagers often see this issue in the absolute moral terms indigenous to their age group. But their ambivalence is also clear: they are less likely than older women to approve of abortions, in general, but they are perfectly willing to tolerate them for friends or even for themselves. In addition, younger women tend to delay their abortions until late in the first trimester or into the second trimester, and they have a disproportionate number of second-trimester abortions, especially teenagers younger than 15 years of age [31]. This is especially significant because the medical and psychological complications of abortion increase with each week of gestational age [35].

Factors that may delay the abortion decision include [1,36,37]:

- Psychological denial of the pregnancy
- Ambivalence about pregnancy or pregnancy options
- Fear of discovery
- Fear of side effects from an abortion
- Lack of money
- Negative impact of parental notification and consent laws

Teenage pregnancy is far more socioeconomically than racially determined [2]. A decision to have an abortion usually indicates a more independent teenager who is upwardly mobile and has a more realistic view of pregnancy and parenting [38,39]. By contrast, teenagers who carry to term sometimes have a poor concept of their future, an immature view of parenting, and are less upwardly mobile [1,40,41]. Either group may be influenced strongly by their mothers or boyfriends, either in favor of keeping the pregnancy ("I love the idea of having another baby around the house") or having an abortion ("If you keep this baby, I'm breaking up with you"). One crucial question in pregnancy and abortion counseling is, "Who wants this pregnancy?/Who wants this abortion?"

Adolescents have the lowest mortality and morbidity of any women undergoing abortion [16,37]. First-trimester abortions carry very slight medical risks: 0.06 cases/100 suction procedures require transfusion [42], uterine perforation occurs in approximately 0.9 cases/1,000 abortions [43], and injury to the cervix occurs in 1.03/100 first-trimester curettage procedures [43]. The risk of death from abortion is lower than in any other surgical procedure—0.5 per 100,000 procedures, which is 15 times less than the mortality associated with giving birth, 7.5 per 100,000 [43,44]. Most of the morbidity and mortality of abortion occurs in the second trimester, often associated with hypertonic saline infusion (secondary to amniotic fluid, clot, or air embolism). Fortunately, this method has been largely replaced by the safer infusion of prostaglandins [16]. Finally, although one study found a weak positive relationship between abortion and the risk of breast cancer (relative risk, 1.12–1.35) [45], a large-scale, 1997 Danish study that examined the incidence of breast cancer associated with 370,715 abortions found no such risk [46,47].

In general, teenagers can be counseled that abortions are safe, especially in the first trimester, and involve a far lower risk of death or complications than carrying to term. Younger teenagers may face a slightly higher risk of cervical laceration because the nulliparous cervix is less easily dilated. General anesthesia carries greater risks than local anesthesia. A review of 10 studies found that one abortion does not compromise future fertility, although repeated abortions (particularly later in gestation) may [48]. First-trimester abortions cost $250 to $450 and are an outpatient procedure; second-trimester abortions cost $500 to $600 and may involve an overnight hospital stay [34].

Far more significant than the medical risks of abortion are the psychological sequelae, although the overall incidence of severe negative reactions is low [1,49,50]. Teenagers may feel guilty, isolated, or depressed—especially with second-trimester procedures (which mimic normal pregnancy and delivery)—but often these feelings can be worked through if their mothers or partners are supportive [51]. Teenagers at high risk for psychological difficulties include those who felt pressured by their families to terminate the pregnancy, those with limited coping skills, limited support, or strong religious beliefs, and those undergoing second-trimester procedures [36]. Most teenagers inform at least one of their parents about their intent to have an abortion [52] (Table 50).

Practitioners should be aware that late reactions do occur, even when teenagers receive good family and social support, and should see the teen back for frequent, postabortion counseling—especially around the anniversary date of the abortion and the date when the pregnancy would have been delivered (peak suicide risks). Teens undergoing abortions usually make good contraceptors subsequently [1,53].

TABLE 50. *Teenagers, parents, and abortions*
(N = 1,519 teens who had abortions)

Who knew about the abortion?	
One or both parents	61%
Mother knew	59%
Mother told by daughter	43%
Father knew	26%
Father told by daughter	12%
Why daughters told parents	
Wouldn't have felt right not telling	48%
Needed parent to help decide	41%
Thought parent would be sympathetic	34%
Helped most with the decision	
Mother	20%
Boyfriend	25%
Didn't need help	25%
Teens who did not tell parents	
Didn't want to hurt or disappoint them	73%
Thought parent would be angry with them	55%
Didn't need parent to help decide	23%
Thought parent would make them leave home	18%
Thought parent would try to make them continue with the pregnancy	14%
Thought they would be beaten	6%

Adapted from Henshaw SK, Kost K. Parental involvement in minors' abortion decisions. *Fam Plann Perspect* 1992;24:196.

Mifepristone (RU-486)

Mifepristone (RU-486) is an antiprogesterone that works at the receptor level to interrupt pregnancy early, primarily by interfering with implantation and decidua functioning. In women at up to 9 weeks of gestation, a single dose of 600 mg results in complete expulsion of the products of conception in 60% to 85% of cases [54]. When a single 600-mg dose is followed 36 to 48 hours later by administration of a prostaglandin analogue (gemeprost or sulprostone), efficacy increases to 96% [55]. It is currently being used in France, where approximately 450 centers use it more than 2,000 times per month. A single dose is given, followed by an intramuscular dose of a synthetic prostaglandin analog 36 to 48 hours later. In 7-week pregnancies, the procedure is successful in over 95% of cases. Expulsion usually occurs within 4 hours of prostaglandin administration, and bleeding occurs on day 2 or 3—usually no more than 70 to 80 ml. Ten percent of patients require analgesics, and less than 1% require dilatation and curettage or blood transfusion, although patients must be carefully monitored [56].

In a 1995 study, researchers tried following RU-486 with a dose of misoprostol, a prostaglandin E_1 analogue, given vaginally or orally. The combination was 95% effective during the first trimester, with few side effects [57]. A similar success rate has been achieved using a single dose of methotrexate (50 mg/m^2 intramuscularly), followed 5 to 7 days later by a dose of misoprostol administered intravaginally [58–60]. No serious complications occurred in either study. Misoprostol alone is not nearly as effective [61].

RU-486 is currently being tested for use in this country, and Food and Drug Administration (FDA) approval is pending, but it remains surrounded by considerable controversy [62,63]. Methotrexate, however, is already an FDA-approved drug. Within the next decade, primary care practitioners may need to decide if they are willing to induce first-trimester medical abortions in their adolescent patients.

Societal Considerations

Teenage sexual activity, pregnancy, and abortion are currently "hot" topics in the United States. Unfortunately, teenagers get trapped in the middle of the debate. Adults frequently blame teenagers for becoming sexually active prematurely, not recognizing or understanding that teenagers are simply responding to the cues they see all around them in the adult world—cues that say that sex is fun, easy, and carries no attendant risks [64]. Although parental notification laws for teen abortions are becoming increasingly discussed around the United States, there is no evidence that they actually discourage teenagers from having abortions or decrease the number of teenage abortions [65–67]. Giving teenagers easy access to contraceptives and to abortions will not encourage them to become sexually active at younger ages or increase their numbers of partners. It *will* prevent the needless tragedies of teen pregnancy and sexually transmitted disease [68].

REFERENCES

1. Braverman PK, Strasburger VC. Update: adolescent sexuality: IV. the practitioner's role. *Clin Pediatr* 1994;33:100.
2. Alan Guttmacher Institute. *Sex and America's teenagers*. New York: Alan Guttmacher Institute; 1994.
3. Ammerman S, Shafer MA, Snyder D. Ectopic pregnancy in adolescents: a clinical review for pediatricians. *J Pediatr* 1990;117:677.
4. Ory S. New options for diagnosis and treatment of ectopic pregnancy. *JAMA* 1992;267:534.
5. Centers for Disease Control and Prevention. Ectopic pregnancy: United States, 1990–1992. *MMWR Morb Mortal Wkly Rep* 1995;44:46.
6. Carson SA, Buster JE. Ectopic pregnancy. *N Engl J Med* 1993;329:1174.
7. Centers for Disease Control and Prevention. Ectopic pregnancy: United States, 1988–1989. *MMWR Morb Mortal Wkly Rep* 1992;41:591.
8. Kaplan BC, Dart RG, Moskos M, et al. Ectopic pregnancy: prospective study with improved diagnostic accuracy. *Ann Emerg Med* 1996;28:10.
9. Schwartz RO, DiPietro DL. β-HCG as a diagnostic aid for suspected ectopic pregnancy. *Obstet Gynecol* 1980;56:197.
10. Stephenson JN. Pregnancy testing and counseling. *Pediatr Clin North Am* 1989;36:681.

11. Kadar N, DeVore G, Romero R. Discriminatory HCG zone: its use in the sonographic evaluation for ectopic pregnancy. *Obstet Gynecol* 1981;58:156.
12. McKennett M, Fullerton JT. Vaginal bleeding in pregnancy. *Am Fam Physician* 1995;51:639.
13. Deluca SA. Transvaginal ultrasonography. *Am Fam Physician* 1995;52:875.
14. Slaughter JL, Grimes DA. Methotrexate therapy for unruptured ectopic pregnancy. *West J Med* 1995;162:225.
15. Bluestein D. Should I trust office pregnancy tests? *Postgrad Med* 1990;87:57.
16. Hatcher RA, Trussell J, Stewart F, et al. *Contraceptive technology*. 17th ed. New York: Irvington; 1998.
17. Stevens-Simon C, Beach R, Eagar R. Conception after a negative pregnancy test during adolescence. *Adolescent and Pediatric Gynecology* 1993;6:83.
18. Zabin LS, Emerson MR, Ringers PA, et al. Adolescents with negative pregnancy test results: an accessible at-risk group. *JAMA* 1996;275:113.
19. Gordon DE. Formal operational thinking: the role of cognitive developmental processes in adolescent decision-making about pregnancy and contraception. *Am J Orthopsychiatry* 1990;60:346.
20. Zabin LS, Hirsch M, Emerson MR, et al. To whom do inner-city minors talk about pregnancies? Adolescents' communication with parents and parent surrogates. *Fam Plann Perspect* 1992;24:148.
21. Toledo-Dreves V, Zabin LS, Emerson MR. Durations of adolescent sexual relationships before and after conception. *J Adolesc Health* 1995;17:163.
22. Rivara FP, Sweeney PJ, Henderson BF. Black teenage fathers: what happens when the child is born? *Pediatrics* 1986;78:151.
23. Resnick MD, Chambliss SA, Blum RW. Health and risk behaviors of urban adolescent males involved in pregnancy. *Families in Society* 1993;74:366.
24. Hardy JB, Duggan AK. Teenage fathers and the fathers of infants of urban teenage mothers. *Am J Public Health* 1988;78:919.
25. Bachrach CA, Stolley KS, London KA. Relinquishment of premarital births: evidence from national survey data. *Fam Plann Perspect* 1992;24:27.
26. Bose J, Resnick MD, Smith M. *Adoption and parenting decision making among adolescent females: final report to the office of adolescent pregnancy prevention*. Washington, DC: U.S. Department of Health and Social Services; 1987.
27. Kallen DJ, Griffore RJ, Popovich S, et al. Adolescent mothers and their mothers view adoption. *Family Relations* 1990;39:311.
28. Resnick MD, Blum RW, Bose J, et al. Characteristics of unmarried adolescent mothers: determinants of child rearing versus adoption. *Am J Orthopsychiatry* 1990;60:577.
29. Kalmuss D, Namerow PB, Cushman LF. Adoption versus parenting among young pregnant women. *Fam Plann Perspect* 1992;23:17.
30. Mech EV. Pregnant adolescents: communicating the adoption option. *Child Welfare* 1986;65:555.
31. Centers for Disease Control and Prevention. Abortion surveillance: preliminary data—United States, 1994. *MMWR Morb Mortal Wkly Rep* 1997;45:1123.
32. Henshaw SK, Kost K. Abortion patients in 1994–1995: characteristics and contraceptive use. *Fam Plann Perspect* 1996;28:140.
33. Moore KA, Miller BC, Glei D, et al. *Adolescent sex, contraception and childbearing: a review of recent research*. Washington, DC: Child Trends; 1995.
34. Rosoff J, Henshaw S, Van Vort J. *What's happening to abortion rates?* Menlo Park, CA: Henry J. Kaiser Family Foundation; 1996.
35. Cates W Jr. Adolescent abortions in the United States. *Journal of Adolescent Health Care* 1980;1:18.
36. Biro FM, Wildey LS, Hillard PJ, et al. Acute and long-term consequences of adolescents who choose abortions. *Pediatr Ann* 1986;15:667.
37. Henshaw SK, Binkins NJ, Blaine E, et al. A portrait of American women who obtain abortions. *Fam Plann Perspect* 1985;17:90.
38. Advocates for Youth. *Fact sheet: adolescent pregnancy and childbearing*. Washington, DC: Advocates for Youth; 1996.
39. Udry JR, Kovenock J, Morris NM. Early predictors of nonmarital first pregnancy and abortion. *Fam Plann Perspect* 1996;28:113.
40. Morin-Gonthier M, Lottie G. The significance of pregnancy among adolescents choosing abortion as compared to those continuing pregnancy. *J Reprod Med* 1984;29:255.
41. Blum RW, Resnick MD. Adolescent sexual decision-making: contraception, pregnancy, abortion, motherhood. *Pediatr Ann* 1982;11:797.
42. Grimes DA, Cates W. Complications from legally-induced abortions: a review. *Obstet Gynecol Surv* 1979;34:177.
43. Centers for Disease Control and Prevention. *Abortion surveillance 1981*. Atlanta: Centers for Disease Control and Prevention; 1985.
44. Tietze C. The public health effects of legal abortion in the United States. *Fam Plann Perspect* 1984;16:26.
45. Newcomb PA, Storer BE, Longnecker MP, et al. Pregnancy termination in relation to risk of breast cancer. *JAMA* 1996;275:283.
46. Melbye M, Wohlfahrt J, Olsen JH, et al. Induced abortion and the risk of breast cancer. *N Engl J Med* 1997;336:81.

47. Hartge P. Abortion, breast cancer, and epidemiology. *N Engl J Med* 1997;336:127.
48. Hogue CJR, Cates W, Tietze C. Impact of vacuum aspiration abortion on future childbearing: a review. *Fam Plann Perspect* 1983;15:119.
49. Adler NE, David HP, Major BN, et al. Psychological responses after abortion. *Science* 1990;248:41.
50. Dagg P. The psychological sequelae of therapeutic abortion: denied and completed. *Am J Psychiatry* 1991; 148:578.
51. Robbins JM, deLamater JD. Support from significant others and loneliness following induced abortion. *Soc Psychiatry* 1985;20:92.
52. Henshaw SK, Kost K. Parental involvement in minors' abortion decisions. *Fam Plann Perspect* 1992;24:196.
53. Abrams M. Birth control use by teenagers. *Journal of Adolescent Health Care* 1985;6:196.
54. Ulmann A. Uses of RU 486 for contragestion: an update. *Contraception* 1987;36:27.
55. Silvestre L, Dubois C, Renault M, et al. Voluntary interruption of pregnancy with mifepristone (RU 486) and a prostaglandin analogue. *N Engl J Med* 1990;322:645.
56. Baulieu E-E. RU-486 as an antiprogesterone steroid: from receptor to contragestion and beyond. *JAMA* 1989; 262:1808.
57. El-Refaey H, Rajasekar D, Abdalla M, et al. Induction of abortion with mifepristone (RU 486) and oral or vaginal misoprostol. *New Engl J Med* 1995;332:983.
58. Creinin MD, Vittinghoff E. Methotrexate and misoprostol vs. misoprostol alone for early abortion. *JAMA* 1994;272:1190.
59. Hausknecht RU. Methotrexate and misoprostol to terminate early pregnancy. *New Engl J Med* 1995;333: 537.
60. The Medical Letter. Methotrexate and misoprostol for abortion. *The Medical Letter* 1996;38(issue 973):39.
61. Koopersmith TB, Mishell DR Jr. The use of misoprostol for termination of early pregnancy. *Contraception* 1996;53:237.
62. Kolata G. RU 486: it isn't just popping a pill. *New York Times*, July 28, 1996, p. E14.
63. Neergaard L. Safety, education at core of RU-486: abortion pill debate rages on. Associated Press, *Albuquerque Journal*, July 21, 1996, p. A9.
64. Strasburger VC. Sex, teens, and the media. *Contemporary Pediatrics* 1996;13:29.
65. Blum RW, Resnick MD, Stark TA. The impact of a parental notification law on adolescent abortion decision-making. *Am J Public Health* 1987;77:619.
66. Henshaw SK. The impact of requirements for parental consent on minors' abortions in Mississippi. *Fam Plann Perspect* 1995;27:120.
67. Committee on Adolescence, American Academy of Pediatrics. The adolescent's right to confidential care when considering abortion (policy statement). *Pediatrics* 1996;97:746.
68. Haffner DW, ed. *Facing facts: sexual health for America's adolescents*. New York: Sex Information and Education Council of the United States; 1995.

SUGGESTED READING

Alan Guttmacher Institute. *Sex and America's teenagers*. New York: Alan Guttmacher Institute, 1994.

Ammerman S, Shafer M-A, Snyder D. Ectopic pregnancy in adolescents: a clinical review for pediatricians. *J Pediatr* 1990;117:677.

Braverman PK, Strasburger VC. Update: adolescent sexuality: I. Adolescent sexuality. IV. The practitioner's role. *Clin Pediatr* 1993;32:658, and 1994;33:100.

Braverman PK, Strasburger VC. Why adolescent gynecology? Pediatricians and pelvic exams. *Pediatr Clin North Am* 1989;36:471.

Cartoof VG. Adolescent abortion: correlates and consequences. *Adolescent Medicine:* State of the Art Reviews 1992;3:283.

Committee On Adolescence, American Academy of Pediatrics. Adolescent pregnancy: Current trends and issues [Policy statement]. *Pediatr.* 1997, in press.

Coupey SM, Klerman LV, eds. Adolescent sexuality: preventing unhealthy consequences. *Adolescent Medicine: State of the Art Reviews* 1992;3:165.

Crenin M. Abortion in adolescents: should pediatricians perform medical abortions? *Adolescent Medicine: State of the Art Reviews* 1997;8 (in press).

Goldenberg RL, Klerman LV. Adolescent pregnancy: another look. *New Engl J Med* 1995;332:1161.

Haffner DW, ed. *Facing facts: sexual health for America's adolescents*. New York: Sexuality Information and Education Council of the U.S. (SIECUS); 1995.

Howard M. Delaying the start of intercourse among adolescents. *Adolescent Medicine: State of the Art Reviews* 1992;3:181.

Howard M, Mitchell ME. Preventing teenage pregnancy: some questions to be answered and some answers to be questioned. *Pediatr Ann* 1993;22:109.

Klerman LV. Adolescent pregnancy and parenting: controversies of the past and lessons for the future. *J Adolesc Health* 1993;14:553.

Stephenson JN. Pregnancy testing and counseling. *Pediatr Clin North Am* 1989;36:681.

MENSTRUAL DISORDERS

The Practitioner as Gynecologist

Many primary care professionals are reluctant to do adolescent gynecology, either because of a lack of interest, lack of experience, or fear of not being a fully trained gynecologist [1]. Yet, many interested primary clinicians can and do perform significant gynecologic services for their teenage patients. In fact, the primary care physician or nurse practitioner is uniquely situated to be the ideal person for the young woman to turn to: they have an established rapport with the patient, are familiar with other aspects of her medical care, and are nonsurgical in their approach to patients. Most gynecologists probably would prefer to have their primary care colleagues deal with the "routine" aspects of gynecologic care. This section discusses fundamental aspects of adolescent gynecology. The key for clinicians is to know when to treat, when to refer, and when to do both, and this we discuss for each situation mentioned.

Normal Menstrual Physiology

Onset of Puberty

The average age of menarche (first menses) in the United States is 12.8 ± 1.2 years and has remained constant since the 1950s [2]. Before that, it had declined approximately 2 to 3 years in the past century, probably because of improved nutrition, with an earlier accumulation of total body fat, and improved socioeconomic standards [3,4]. Although the sequence of pubertal changes is well understood (Table 51; also see Chapter 1), its etiology remains unclear. Several theories exist [5].

- The *"gonadostat" theory* contends that decreased sensitivity of the hypothalamus to levels of estrogen result in increased release of gonadotropin-releasing hormone (GnRH), resulting in augmented levels of luteinizing hormone (LH) and follicle-stimulating hormone (FSH) and stimulation of the prepubescent ovaries. Low levels of the sex hormones are known to exist from 12 weeks of gestation on, and they remain low until perhaps some weak adrenal hormones, such as dehydroepiandrosterone (DHEA) and its sulfate act on the hypothalamus to decrease its sensitivity to negative feedback.
- According to the *critical weight* or *body fat theory*, in many young girls, a mean weight of 47.8 ± 0.5 kg, or a body fat composition of at least 17%, must be reached before menarche is triggered (and 22% body fat to maintain regular cycles) [6,7]. This theory remains largely unsubstantiated, although it does seem to have some rough predictive value clinically [8].
- The *basal hypothalamic release theory* is predicated on experimental work in primates that seems to indicate that this part of the brain may provide the origin for puberty, with the release of pulses of GnRH [9].
- Most recently, a theory has been proposed that puberty occurs as the result of either a *derepression of the arcuate nucleus in the hypothalamus* (with resultant increases in LH-releasing hormone [LHRH]) or *increasing amplitude in LHRH cycles*, leading to increases in LH and FSH [10].

Of course, all four theories may in fact be operative: at puberty, decreased sensitivity of the "gonadostat" could induce sleep-associated pulses of GnRH, resulting in greater levels of LH and FSH, pro-

TABLE 51. *Incidence of menarche by Tanner stage*

Stage I	0%
Stage II	0%
Stage III	25%
Stage IV	65%
Stage V	10%

Kulig JW. Adolescent menstrual disorders. In: Strasburger VC, ed. *Adolescent gynecology: an office guide.* Baltimore: Urban & Schwarzenberg; 1990. With permission.

duction of estradiol (E_2), and the normal sequence of female puberty. Perhaps a critical body mass is required to provoke this derepression of the hypothalamic arcuate nucleus [11].

Initiation of puberty may also be linked to neurotransmitters in the central nervous system that initiate release of GnRH [5,12]. Dopamine inhibits GnRH; epinephrine stimulates GnRH. GnRH may also be affected by the release of beta-endorphins, as in stress, which diminish the pulses of hormone needed for menstruation and ovulation.

The Menstrual Cycle

The normal adolescent menstrual cycle lasts 28 ± 4 days, with a range of 21 to 35 days, a flow of 3 to 7 days, and an estimated average blood loss of 30 to 40 ml (range, 25–70 ml) [4]. Nearly 90% of girls will have experienced menarche by Tanner stage 4 breast and pubic hair development, and normally the sequence from breast budding to menarche averages 2.3 years [13]. Although 55% of cycles are anovulatory in the first year, 45% are not—meaning that teenagers can and do become pregnant the first time they have intercourse. In fact, 10% of all teenage pregnancies occur in the first month after beginning sexual relations, and half occur within the first 6 months [14]. (More recent work suggests that a lower percentage of teens have ovulatory cycles: 15% in the first year postmenarche, 40% by 2 years, 70% by 3 years, and 100% by 5–6 years [10].)

Menstrual periods can be highly irregular in the first year or two after menarche, with long pauses in between periods and unpredictable duration and amount of flow. "Normal menses" require a complex relationship between the hypothalamus, pituitary, and ovary—one that often takes a year or two to mature. The later menarche occurs, the longer it takes to establish regular ovulatory cycles.

The normal menstrual cycle can be subdivided into follicular (or proliferative), ovulatory, and luteal (or secretory) stages (Fig. 10).

- In the *follicular stage*, a chosen ovarian follicle matures, with stimulation from FSH. Estradiol (E_2) levels rise, exerting both a negative feedback on FSH and LH secretion and a positive feedback on the latter once sufficiently high levels are attained. The choice of one follicle over others seems to be exclusively an ovarian event and permits the other follicles to be "recycled." Meanwhile, the endometrium is regenerating, from 0.5 to 5.0 mm in depth, as development of endometrial glands and secretory activity occurs [15].
- *Ovulation* requires a rapid rise in LH concentration—usually in surges, over a period of 36 to 48 hours—leading to final maturation of the follicle and release of the ovum. Increasing levels of progesterone (aided by E_2's enhancing effect on granulosa cells) may act synergistically with estradiol to incite the LH surge. *Spinnbarkeit*, or stringiness of the cervical mucus, usually precedes the LH surge by 24 hours, whereas ovulation usually occurs 24 hours afterward. The basal body temperature rises 0.2° to 0.5° (because of the thermogenic effect of progesterone). How the ovum breaks free is still not well understood, but it may be caused by a prostaglandin-induced thinning of surrounding connective tissue in the follicle. Fertilization must occur within the next 24 hours, usually in the fallopian tube, and the fertilized ovum may remain in the tube for 48 hours before beginning implantation in the uterus as an embryo.
- The *luteal phase* is a constant 14 ± 2 days, the life span of the corpus luteum, which forms at the site of the previously released ovum and is responsible for progesterone production. Under this hormone's influence, endometrial glands become coiled and secretory, with increased vascularity of the stroma. Normally, levels of estrogen and progesterone decline in the late luteal phase, triggering endometrial and blood vessel necrosis and bleeding. However, if fertilization occurs, human chorionic gonadotropin functions to protect the corpus luteum and keep levels of steroid hormones high.

Adolescents can have a slower rise in FSH, a lower LH peak, and occasionally ovulate as late as day 20. Their peak progesterone levels may also be lower, compared with adult women.

The Pap Smear

In 1988 and 1991, a workshop of experts was convened by the National Cancer Institute to refine the old system of reporting Pap smear results, which suffered from being outmoded and subject to multiple interpretations [16,17]. The Bethesda system (TBS) is outlined in Table 52, and its nomenclature is translated into the previous systems in Table 53 [18].

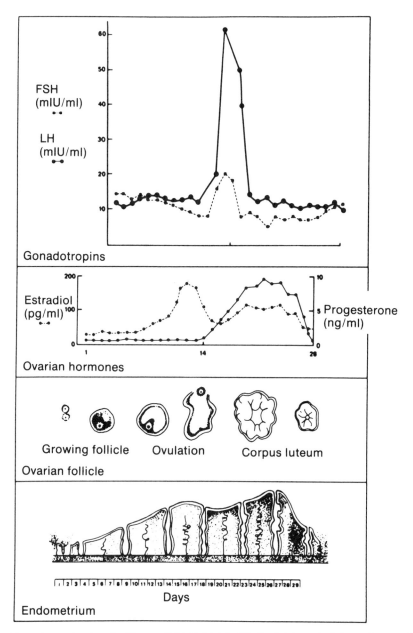

FIG. 10. Normal menstrual cycle. (Emans SJH, Goldstein DP. *Pediatric and adolescent gynecology.* 4th ed. Philadelphia: Lippincott–Raven Publishers, 1997, with permission.)

Pap smears have always been intended to be a *screening* test, not a means of making a specific diagnosis [19], and the prevalence of abnormal cervical cytology has indeed increased since the mid-1970s [20,21]. An incidence of abnormal Pap smears ranging from 2% to 18% has been reported, depending on the population examined [20]. The two key factors related to Pap smear abnormalities are 1) young age at first coitus, and 2) multiple sexual partners. In addition, both smoking and the use of

TABLE 5-52. *The Bethesda system for cytologic diagnosis*

Adequacy of the specimen

General categorization
Within normal limits
Benign cellular changes
Epithelial cell abnormality

Descriptive diagnoses
• Infection
    Protozoan
    Fungal
    Bacterial
    Viral
• Reactive changes
    Inflammation (includes repair)
• Epithelial cell abnormalities
    Squamous cell
        Atypical squamous cells of undetermined significance
        (ASCUS)
        Low-grade squamous intraepithelial lesion (includes
        human papillomavirus infection, CIN-1, mild dysplasia)
        High-grade squamous intraepithelial lesion (CIN-2 and
        CIN-3, moderate and severe dysplasia)
        Squamous cell carcinoma
    Glandular cell
        Presence of endometrial cells
        Atypical glandular cells
        Endocervical adenocarcinoma
        Endometrial adenocarcinoma

CIN, cervical intraepithelial neoplasia.
Adapted from Broder S. The Bethesda system for reporting cervical/vaginal cytologic diagnoses: report of the 1991 Bethesda workshop. *JAMA* 1992;267:1892.

TABLE 53. *Comparison of four major Pap smear reporting systems*

Papanicolaou classification	Cervical intraepithelial neoplasia system	Bethesda system	World Health Organization system
Class I	Normal	Within normal limits	Normal
Class II	—	Other:	Inflammation
		Infection	
		Reactive and reparative	
Class III		Squamous intraepithelial lesions	Dysplasia
	CIN-1	Low grade	Mild
	CIN-2	High grade	Moderate
			Severe
Class IV	CIN-3	—	Carcinoma in situ
Class V	Invasive squamous cell carcinoma	Squamous cell carcinoma	Invasive squamous cell carcinoma
	Adenocarcinoma	Adenocarcinoma	Adenocarcinoma

Adapted from Miller KE, Losh DP, Folley A. Evaluation and follow-up of abnormal Pap smears. *Am Fam Physician* 1992;45:143; and Roye CF. Pap smear screening for adolescents: rationale, technique, and follow-up. *Journal of Pediatric Health Care* 1993;7:199.

oral contraceptives (or failure to use a barrier method) seem to be related to abnormalities, but only for older women. Their effects require several years to become manifest [20]. False-negative rates range from 0% to 30% [22].

With a few exceptions, abnormalities on adolescents' Pap smears require referral for colposcopy and treatment [23]. This may involve observation and repeat sampling, biopsy, or use of the loop electrosurgical excision procedure [19,24,25]. Authors in the adult medical literature make a case for repeat Pap screening for atypical or low-grade lesions based on the following evidence [26–28]:

- Infection and repair can mimic cytologic changes.
- Spontaneous regression is well documented in up to 50% of low-grade squamous intraepithelial lesions (SIL).
- Patients with minor abnormalities on Pap smear have a high rate of normal findings on colposcopy.
- Even if high-grade lesions do develop, the rate of progression is slow.

However, adolescent patients differ significantly from adult women. In one study, only half of teens kept their referral appointment for a colposcopy after having an abnormal Pap smear [29]. Teens also tend to be unreliable in reporting previous Pap smears [30]. Finally, teenagers tend to have the highest rates of human papillomavirus (HPV) infection, and epithelial cell changes produced by HPV may be indistinguishable from neoplastic changes [19,23].

In the new Pap smear reports, atypical squamous cells of undetermined significance (ASCUS) and low-grade SIL constitute the majority of abnormalities, with high-grade SIL and cancer comprising less than 5% [26]. ASCUS was designed as a category to encourage clinicians to ask the pathologist for clarification of the reading. Many of these Pap smears show inflammation of unknown origin. In such cases, clinicians need to be highly suspicious of infection (*Chlamydia trachomatis*, *Neisseria gonorrhoeae*, or *Trichomonas vaginalis*), perform further testing, and treat accordingly [31,32]. In adolescent women who show significant inflammation on either Pap smear or saline preparation, without an identifiable source of infection, we recommend a course of treatment for chlamydial infection and rescreening afterward.

Dysmenorrhea

Pathophysiologic Features and Presentation

The menstrual disorder most often encountered by primary practitioners is dysmenorrhea. In female teens, it is the leading cause of short-term absence from school; several surveys have documented that nearly three quarters of all female adolescents experience some menstrual discomfort and that in 20% to 50% the symptoms are either moderate or severe [33–35]. Only 15% of female teens, however, specifically consult a physician for their dysmenorrhea [33], so practitioners must elicit this information as part of their normal sexual and menstrual history-taking (Table 54). Operationally, dysmenorrhea may be defined as follows:

Mild: pain occurs on the first day of menses only; few associated symptoms
Moderate: pain on the first 2 to 3 days, often associated with other symptoms
Severe: intense, crampy pain that lasts 2 to 7 days, usually disabling and accompanied by gastrointestinal symptoms

Typically, the pains are sharp, spasmodic, suprapubic abdominal pains that may radiate to the upper thighs or back and begin a few hours before the onset of menstrual flow. In more severe cases, the pain may be accompanied by gastrointestinal or vascular symptoms (e.g., vomiting, diarrhea, headache, fatigue).

It is extremely important to understand the division of dysmenorrhea into primary and secondary [13,36] (Table 55). In adolescents, *primary dysmenorrhea* accounts for 95% of all cases and signifies that there is no gross pelvic lesion. Because many teenagers are anovulatory for the first year or two, primary dysmenorrhea actually increases later in adolescence and seems to diminish after the first pregnancy. *Secondary dysmenorrhea* is more common in older women and results from other disease processes—chiefly, pelvic inflammatory disease, endometriosis, ovarian cysts, and congenital anomalies.

Although teens with primary dysmenorrhea do not have gross pelvic disease, they do have real biochemical events causing their pain: the fall in progesterone levels at the end of the luteal phase causes lysosomal membranes to become unstable and enzymes to be released, activating phospholipid A_2,

TABLE 54. *History for common menstrual disorders*

Menstrual specific
  Age at menarche
  Frequency of menses
  Quantity and duration of flow
  Presence of cramps
  Use of tampons or pads
  Last menstrual period
  Last normal menstrual period

Family history
  Family history of age at menarche
  Family history of gynecologic problems

Past medical history
  Hospitalizations or surgery
  Chronic illness
  Bleeding disorders

Medication/substance use[a]
  Contraceptives
  Drugs of abuse
  Medications

Related health issues[a]
  Weight change
  Nutrition
  Exercise/sports
  Emotional symptoms
  Eating disorders

Sexual behavior[a]
  Sexual activity
  Use of contraception
  Sexually transmitted diseases
  Number of sexual partners
  Last sexual contact
  Pregnancies
  Sexual abuse
  Types of sexual contact

[a]Interview alone with patient.
Adapted from Blythe MJ. Common menstrual problems of adolescence. *Adolescent Medicine: State of the Art Reviews* 1997; 8:87.

which converts phospholipids to arachidonic acid and then to elevated amounts of prostaglandins E_2 (PGE_2) and $F_{2\alpha}$ ($PGF_{2\alpha}$) [13]. PGE_2 and $PGF_{2\alpha}$ then act to produce uterine ischemia, excessive and dysrhythmic uterine contractions, and increased resting muscle tone in the uterus—all hallmarks of menstrual pain. In fact, clinical symptoms correlate with the amount of prostaglandins produced. Prostaglandins can also stimulate smooth muscle contractions in the gastrointestinal tract, which may account for the associated symptoms of nausea, vomiting, diarrhea, and irritability [37].

Management

A good menstrual history includes the following information: age at menarche, date of last period, length and regularity of periods, amount of flow, number and type of pad or tampon used, and presence or absence of cramps and other symptoms. Clinicians may be surprised at the number of teenagers they diagnose as having dysmenorrhea, even though it is rarely a presenting complaint. When cramps are present, it is important to ask when in the menstrual cycle they occur—before, during, or after the menstrual flow has begun. The degree of disability should be documented, as well as a family history (mothers and sisters frequently also have a positive history).

TABLE 55. *Comparison of primary versus secondary dysmenorrhea*

Feature	Primary	Secondary
Incidence	Very common	Rare
Onset	Near menarche	Usually after age 20 y
Character of pain	Intermittent, sharp, colicky	Constant, dull
Location of pain	Suprapubic; occasional radiation to thighs or back	Diffuse, low abdominal
Associated symptoms	Gastrointestinal, cardiovascular	—
Response to oral contraceptives or antiprostaglandins	Excellent	Poor

Simmons PS. Common gynecological problems in adolescents. *Prim Care* 1988;15:629. With permission.

Certainly, not every teenager with dysmenorrhea requires a complete pelvic examination. If that were true, 36% of 12-year-olds and 72% of 17-year-olds would qualify [38]. Teenagers with no history of sexual intercourse and with mild symptoms can be given a trial of therapy [13]. Sexually active teens always need a full speculum examination (to obtain a Pap smear and cultures), but virginal teens with moderate to severe symptoms may only require some assessment of their internal pelvic anatomy—either a bimanual vaginal examination or a rectoabdominal examination—as well as a careful inspection of their external genitalia. Failure to respond to a therapeutic trial in any patient should lead to a renewed search for pelvic disease. Some experts believe that as many as half of all teenagers who fail to respond to treatment with nonsteroidal antiinflammatory drugs (NSAIDs) or oral contraceptives (OCs) have endometriosis [5,39].

Nonsteroidal antiinflammatory drugs have become the standard treatment for dysmenorrhea; they inhibit the enzyme prostaglandin synthetase and therefore diminish levels of the offending chemicals [40]. As with OCs or antihistamines, there are several different types of NSAIDs, and each one has its proponents and responders (Table 56). Each of these drugs is likely to induce a significant clinical response in 75% to 90% of patients treated [13,36]:

- Ibuprofen (Motrin, Advil) is available without prescription in 200-g tablets. Its usual dose is 400 to 600 mg every 4 to 6 hours. As an over-the-counter medication, however, ibuprofen lacks any potential "placebo effect."
- Naproxen sodium (Anaprox) is rapidly absorbed and has a long half-life, making twice-a-day dosage possible (550 mg loading, followed by 275 mg bid). Naproxen (Naprosyn) is similar, with a 500-mg loading dose followed by 250 mg every 6 to 8 hours, or 500 mg every 12 hours.
- Mefenamic acid (Ponstel) is unique in not only blocking prostaglandin synthetase but in blocking the action of prostaglandins that are already formed. It, too, requires a loading dose, 500 mg, followed by 250 mg qid.

TABLE 56. *Treatment of dysmenorrhea with prostaglandin inhibitors*

Agent	Dosage
Nonprescription	
Advil (ibuprofen)	Two 200-mg tablets PO qid
Prescription	
Anaprox (naproxen sodium)	550 mg PO initially, then 275 mg bid–qid
Orudis (ketoprofen)	75 mg PO tid
Motrin (ibuprofen)	400–800 mg PO qid
Naprosyn (naproxen)	500 mg PO initially, then 250–500 mg bid
Ponstel (mefenamic acid)	500 mg PO initially, then 250 mg tid–qid

Patients should be counseled initially that there are several different NSAIDs, and if a trial of one drug fails, another one should be tried before moving on to OCs. Although there is no advantage in beginning treatment before menses, NSAIDs must be started at the first sign of pain. Because they are used for only a few days each month, prostaglandin inhibitors have few significant side effects (occasional gastrointestinal symptoms, at most) and have the additional advantage of decreasing the amount of menstrual flow. Therefore, they may be useful in treating dysfunctional uterine bleeding (DUB) as well. NSAIDs are contraindicated in teenagers with known aspirin hypersensitivity, peptic ulcer disease, hepatic or renal disease, or bleeding disorders. Because similar drugs are used to close a patent ductus arteriosus in neonates, they should also be avoided if there is a possibility of pregnancy. Although aspirin is a weak synthetase inhibitor, it must be taken 3 days before the onset of menses (600 mg qid) and leads to increased menstrual bleeding and gastrointestinal upset. In addition, it does not have the theoretical placebo effect of a prescription medication. Use of transdermal glyceryl trinitrate (a uterine relaxant) was successful in a small, placebo-controlled trial [41].

In sexually active teenagers, OCs may be preferable to NSAIDs because they provide contraception as well as treatment for dysmenorrhea [42]. However, because they may take 2 to 3 months to have an effect on the latter, NSAIDs should be used initially as well. OCs not only prevent ovulation but result in a thinning of the endometrium, therefore decreasing prostaglandin production as well. About 90% of patients experience a decrease in their symptoms [43]. For nonsexually active patients who are reluctant to take "birth control pills," OCs can be repackaged by pharmacists into regular medication bottles. Because it is the progestin part of OCs that is most effective, patients using Depo-Provera or Norplant also can experience some relief in their symptoms [13].

Secondary dysmenorrhea may develop into or be a function of chronic pelvic pain (see section on Chronic Pelvic Pain) and usually requires consultation with or referral to a gynecologist skilled with adolescent patients. A 1985 report describes using 30 mg of a calcium channel blocker, nifedipine, to help differentiate primary from secondary dysmenorrhea. Nine of 12 adolescents experienced relief of their cramps within 20 to 30 minutes of taking the drug. Of the other three studied, two were found to have pelvic disease on laparoscopy [44]. With more experience, this could become a useful diagnostic and therapeutic aid.

Dysfunctional Uterine Bleeding

An old saying in medicine states, "Bleeding always stops." Nowhere is this more true than in DUB, which can be life threatening to the female adolescent. Although early adolescent menstrual cycles are notoriously irregular, they usually are not associated with excessive duration, flow, or frequency and do not cause significant disability or anemia [13]. In addition, normal cycles should always be 21 to 45 days long. Cycles that last longer, with heavy bleeding when periods do occur, are anovulatory and may be the result of an immature hypothalamic–pituitary–ovarian axis in the early postmenarcheal years or a harbinger of disorders such as polycystic ovary disease in older adolescents [45].

Dysfunctional uterine bleeding can be defined operationally as painless menstrual bleeding heavy or frequent enough to cause clinical problems. Ninety-five percent of women experience a monthly blood loss less than 60 ml; recurrent menstrual losses of over 80 ml are associated with a high risk of anemia [46]. Unfortunately, DUB is a difficult diagnosis to make by historical data alone because teenagers frequently overreport amount of blood loss during menses or numbers of pads used. But practically, a simple determination of hematocrit (Hct) and hemoglobin (Hgb) alerts the clinician to those teenagers with moderate or severe DUB requiring more immediate assessment and treatment.

Pathophysiologic Features and Presentation

As with dysmenorrhea, DUB can be subdivided into primary and secondary. Most teenagers—perhaps 95%—have the primary form: an immaturity in the hypothalamic–pituitary–ovarian axis leading to anovulation, the build-up of an overestrogenized endometrium, and an insufficient production of progesterone to initiate normal menstrual sloughing (Fig. 11). Instead, the endometrium sloughs irregularly, stimulated only by estrogen, until the follicle finally involutes. Small arterioles may become exposed and, rarely, patients have been known to exsanguinate [47,48]. Primary DUB can also be complicated by the presence of a bleeding disorder—the odds of which increase with the severity of the bleeding: approximately one of five patients requiring hospitalization, one of four patients with

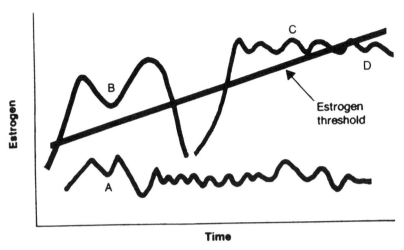

FIG. 11. Schematic representation of dysfunctional uterine bleeding. **A:** Superficial endometrial slough-ing is manifested as spotting. **B,C:** Amount of spotting increases as larger amounts of the developing en-dometrium are exposed and shed. **D:** Erosion of the basal endometrium exposes myometrial arteries and causes profuse hemorrhage. (Strickler RC. Dysfunctional uterine bleeding. *Postgrad Med* 1979;66:138, with permission.)

a Hgb less than 10 g/dl, one of three patients requiring transfusion, and one of two patients presenting at menarche have a concomitant coagulation problem [49] (Fig. 12).

The remaining 5% of patients who have secondary DUB may have a more local lesion, including a complication of pregnancy such as an ectopic pregnancy or threatened abortion. *A negative history of sexual activity (and a negative pregnancy test) and a lack of pain are crucial to defining primary DUB, because it is essentially a diagnosis of exclusion* [45,50]. Vaginitis, cervicitis, salpingitis, or en-dometriosis may also present with abnormal bleeding, although this is not their typical pattern and other symptoms are frequently present. Occasionally, an endocrine abnormality presents with heavy bleeding—most commonly, hypothyroidism or polycystic ovary syndrome (PCOS). The latter most

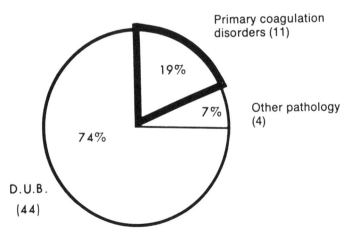

FIG. 12. Etiology of acute adolescent menorrhagia in 59 cases. (Claessens EA, Cowell CA. Acute ado-lescent menorrhagia. *Am J Obstet Gynecol* 1979;139:277, with permission.)

often presents with secondary amenorrhea, but periods may abruptly become reestablished in one third of patients with an episode of menorrhagia.

Clinically, such teenagers usually present in the first few years after menarche with *painless bleeding*, occurring irregularly and unpredictably. This is an important differentiating point between primary and secondary DUB, because patients with the latter usually have significant pain associated with their bleeding. Heavy menstrual bleeding lasting more than 5 days, occurring more frequently than every 21 days, and associated with more than six full-sized soaked pads per day usually becomes significant clinically. Associated symptoms may include syncope, light-headedness, palpitations, headache, and fatigue. A history should include the patient's age at menarche, usual menstrual pattern, sexual activity, use of contraception, previous history of excessive bleeding during surgical or dental procedures, and recent use of aspirin.

Management

Management of DUB is straightforward and depends largely on the pregnancy test and the degree, if any, of anemia [51]. Patients who are virgins and have mild DUB may require treatment only and do not require referral to a gynecologist [52]. In moderate or severe cases, a rectoabdominal examination can suffice to assess pelvic anatomy, if necessary. Patients who are sexually active require appropriate cultures to rule out vaginitis or cervicitis, although this can be done "blindly" if they are actively bleeding.

The physical examination should concentrate on ruling out signs of hypothyroidism, PCOS (e.g., hirsutism, virilism, obesity), or a bleeding disorder. A pregnancy test should be done routinely. In either group, a negative pregnancy test allows the primary clinician to assume medical management of the patient. A positive pregnancy test (or continued suspicion of an ectopic pregnancy) warrants immediate and urgent referral to a gynecologist. In general, patients with ectopic pregnancies present with painful vaginal bleeding, whereas DUB is usually painless.

Patients with mild to moderate DUB should have a complete blood cell count, platelet count, pregnancy test, and thyroid function studies. Those requiring hormonal treatment should also have a clotting profile performed, including prothrombin time, partial thromboplastin time, and bleeding time. Patients with suspected von Willebrand's disease may need specialized tests (e.g., factor VIII-related antigen, ristocetin cofactor) because the clotting profile can still be normal [47,48]. The prognosis for these patients is bleaker than in the more typical patient, who has a 50% chance of reverting to normal menses within 4 years [43]. If the patient has any signs of hyperandrogenism, a DHEA sulfate and testosterone level should also be obtained [50]. A pelvic ultrasound can sometimes be useful if pelvic disease is a concern.

Unlike adult women, adolescents rarely have endometrial disease accounting for their bleeding and therefore virtually never require dilatation and curettage (D&C). However, the bleeding must be stopped expeditiously.

Treatment is neatly divided by level of the initial hematocrit and hemoglobin (Table 57). Transfusion is indicated *only* if the patient's cardiovascular status becomes unstable, because even severe anemias can be reversed within a month on high-dose iron therapy.

Mild Dysfunctional Uterine Bleeding

Patients with a normal Hgb and Hct do not require intensive hormonal therapy but do benefit from reassurance that their reproductive system is intact. In addition, prophylactic iron therapy is indicated. All menstruating teenagers should ingest adequate amounts of iron (e.g., 18 mg of elemental iron a day, as contained in most over-the-counter, one-a-day multiple vitamins). One easy regimen for teens with mild DUB is to take 325 mg of ferrous sulfate each day that they are menstruating. Close follow-up should include periodic rechecking of Hgb and Hct levels. Most teenagers should "mature out" of this condition by 2 to 3 years postmenarche.

Patients using one of the long-acting progestins, Depo-Provera or Norplant, may also experience irregular and mild dysfunctional bleeding. For these teens, a supplemental dose of oral estrogens may be useful, either estradiol 1 mg/day for 7 days, or conjugated estrogens (Premarin), 0.625 mg/day for 7 days [53].

TABLE 57. *Management of dysfunctional uterine bleeding (DUB)*

Mild (Hgb normal)	Moderate (Hgb >10)	Severe (Hgb <10)
1. Counsel and reassure	1. Progestin-dominant OCs, 1–2 pills daily (e.g., Ovral, Lo-Ovral)	1. Progestin-dominant OCs, 1 pill qid × 4d; 1 pill tid × 3d; 1 pill bid × 7d; 1 pill qd × 7–14 d[a] *OR:* Premarin 25–40 mg IV q4–6h. Transfuse only if necessary.
2. Routine iron supplements	2. Ferrous sulfate 325 mg tid or sustained-release preparation	2. Ferrous sulfate 325 mg tid or sustained-release preparation
3. Follow-up in 2 months	3. Follow-up weekly, then monthly	3. Follow-up daily, then weekly, then monthly

Hgb, hemoglobin; OC, oral contraceptive.

[a]Initial 3–4 weeks of therapy should be with a standard 30- to 50-μg pill; thereafter, any OC pill, including a triphasic pill, can be used for cycling if bleeding is controlled.

Adapted from Coupey SM, Ahlstrom P. Common menstrual disorders. *Pediatr Clin North Am* 1989;36:551; and Braverman PK, Sondheimer SJ. Menstrual disorders. *Pediatr Rev* 1997;18:17.

Moderate Dysfunctional Uterine Bleeding

Patients with an anemia but with a Hgb in excess of 10 g/dl and a Hct in excess of 30% fall into this category. Patients who are actively bleeding and initially are considered "mild" may, in fact, belong in this category as well. Therapy is aimed at stopping the bleeding, restoring the serum blood values to normal levels, and "buying time" for the hypothalamic–pituitary–ovarian axis to mature. This can be accomplished through the use of combination OCs, particularly those that are progestin dominant, now that high-dose OCs have been removed from the market.

Many regimens work: basically, a progestin-dominant OC (e.g., Ovral, Lo-Ovral) is started immediately and given once or twice a day, depending on how active the bleeding is. Up to one OC pill every 4 to 6 hours can be administered, although this regimen requires antinausea medication as well. Bleeding should stop within 24 to 48 hours. The patient should then continue taking the OCs until the first 21 days of pills are completed. After this, if she takes the seven placebo pills, she will have a heavier-than-usual withdrawal bleed; or, she can immediately be switched to a second package of 28-day pills and allow the endometrium time to regenerate. Another popular regimen is one pill qid for 2 days, tid for 2 days, bid for 2 days, and qd for 3 days, after starting a new package of pills. A total of three to six cycles of OCs are usually given, then the patient is allowed to cycle on her own. By this time, it is hoped that her endocrine axis has matured sufficiently to avoid dysfunctional problems.

Unfortunately, the teenager's parents may object to the use of OCs. To avoid this, the wise practitioner always refers to the medication as "hormones" or "estrogen and progesterone," rather than "oral contraceptives" or "birth control pills." Frequently, parents believe that putting their daughters on OCs provides them with a license to become sexually involved or even begin taking multiple partners. The life-threatening nature of this disorder often requires emphasis. Occasionally, separate hormones may need to be prescribed: ethinyl estradiol, 50 to 100 μg daily, and either norethindrone, 5 to 20 mg daily, or norethindrone acetate, 2.5 to 10 mg daily. Alternatively, the birth control pills can be placed in an ordinary medication container, with a standard label. An alternative regimen—Provera (medroxyprogesterone acetate) only, taken as 10 mg daily on the first 5 days of every other month, or on the first 14 days of each month, to induce withdrawal flow and prevent endometrial hyperplasia—is usually not nearly as successful as using combination OCs.

All patients with moderate DUB require intensive iron therapy. Ferrous sulfate 325 mg tid can be used, but a long-acting iron preparation given twice daily and combined with a stool softener is often better tolerated. Normal blood values should be restored within a month, but the therapy should be continued for 2 to 3 months afterward to replenish total body stores of iron.

Severe Dysfunctional Uterine Bleeding

Patients with a Hgb of less than 10 g/dl and a Hct of less than 30 mg% who continue to bleed actively ordinarily require hospitalization for observation and treatment. A pelvic examination to rule out trauma or rape should also be done. If patients who are actively bleeding become unstable hemodynamically, they may require a blood transfusion, but this is best avoided whenever possible. In addition, patients have been known to restore their normal blood volume within a month, on appropriate therapy, even with Hcts low as 15 to 20%. Initially, maximum oral therapy can be tried (one OC pill every 4 to 6 hours), together with antinausea medication, but the patient may require intravenous administration of Premarin (conjugated estrogen), 25 to 40 mg, every 4 to 6 hours. High-dose estrogen helps heal the ragged endometrium and stop the bleeding, but progesterone is needed as well to ensure a smooth slough. Therefore, a combination OC should be given simultaneously as well. A gynecologist can be consulted on admission to help follow the patient while in hospital. However, a therapeutic D&C should be considered only if this medical regimen fails after 48–72 hours. (Note: in adult women, a D&C would be done immediately, for diagnostic as well as therapeutic reasons.) Iron therapy can be delayed a few days until high-dose estrogens are no longer required, in deference to the patient's gastrointestinal system. Further testing for a bleeding disorder may be necessary.

Primary and Secondary Amenorrhea and Oligomenorrhea

The occurrence of primary and secondary amenorrhea in teenagers represents medical verification of Murphy's Law that "anything that can go wrong, will." In that sense, evaluating this group of disorders requires a basic expertise in both adolescent gynecology and endocrinology. For patients with primary amenorrhea, in particular, clinicians may need to call on their endocrine and gynecology colleagues. On the other hand, patients with secondary amenorrhea easily can be evaluated initially by the primary practitioner and may not need subsequent referral. Although these are discussed as though they were separate disorders, they probably represent a spectrum of dysfunction. Moreover, considerable overlap may exist, depending on the timing and manifestations of problems. For example, heavy athletic training undertaken before menarche can result in primary amenorrhea, but after menarche may result in secondary amenorrhea.

Primary Amenorrhea

Primary amenorrhea indicates that the patient has never begun menstruating, or is unlikely to before age 15–16 years (or 4 years after onset of pubertal development). This age limit represents two standard deviations beyond the mean age of menarche in the United States, 12.8 years. Thus, given the normal pubertal sequence, a teenager who has not developed breast buds by age 13 years would merit an evaluation [54] (Table 58).

Clinicians are far more likely to see patients with secondary amenorrhea than primary amenorrhea. The latter is relatively rare and can be complicated to evaluate and manage [36]. Basically, the initial workup is dictated by the history, physical examination, pelvic examination or pelvic ultrasound, and

---

TABLE 58. *Indications for evaluation of primary amenorrhea*

- Absence of menses by age 15 y
- Absence of breast budding or development by age 13 y
- Absence of menses more than 3–4 y after onset of breast development
- Height or weight below the third percentile for age
- Cyclic lower abdominal pain or midline suprapubic pain without onset of menses

Adapted from Kulig JW. Adolescent menstrual disorders. In: Strasburger VC, ed. *Adolescent gynecology: an office guide.* Baltimore: Urban & Schwarzenberg; 1990.

TABLE 59. *Sequential evaluation of primary amenorrhea*

1. Complete history
   Includes family background, chronic illness, stress, diet, exercise, drugs, sex, contraception
2. Complete physical examination
   Includes Tanner staging of secondary sexual development, visualization of hymen, and assessment of pelvic anatomy
3. Ultrasound to define pelvic anatomy, if necessary
4. Follicle-stimulating hormone, luteinizing hormone, prolactin, testosterone
5. Bone age film
6. Karyotype

Kulig JW. Adolescent menstrual disorders: In: Strasburger VC, ed. *Adolescent gynecology: an office guide.* Baltimore: Urban & Schwarzenberg; 1990. With permission.

skillful interpretation of LH and FSH levels (Table 59). Unfortunately, the literature is replete with such terms as "hypergonadotropic and hypogonadotropic hypogonadism," which really serve no useful purpose except to confuse the clinician! The defect can exist at any level of the hypothalamic–pituiary–ovarian axis, and carefully thinking about and evaluating each level of the reproductive system is far easier to remember and makes more common sense (Table 60).

In a large study of 252 patients with delayed sexual development, the following types of problems were represented [55]:

- Primary ovarian failure 43%. Nearly two thirds of these had chromosomal abnormalities.
- Failure of ovarian stimulation by sex hormones 31%. These included patients with physiologic delay (14%) and congenital deficiency syndromes (8%).
- Normal sex hormone levels with anatomical problems 26%. This included anatomic malformations of the lower reproductive system (18%) and PCOS (7%).

One simplified way of approaching these patients is from "the ground up," as outlined in the following sections.

TABLE 60. *Causes of Primary Amenorrhea*

Physiologic site	Condition[a]
Hypothalamus	*Stress*
	Competitive athletics; ballet
	Physiologic delay, often familial
	Anorexia nervosa
	Obesity
	Kallman's syndrome
	Drugs (e.g., phenothiazines)
Pituitary	Idiopathic hypopituitarism
	Tumor
Adrenal cortex	Congenital adrenal hyperplasia
	Tumor
Ovary	*Turner's syndrome and mosaicism*
	Gonadal dysgenesis or failure
	Polycystic ovary syndrome
	Testicular feminization syndrome
Uterus	Agenesis
	Asherman's syndrome
Vagina	Mayer-Rokitansky-Kuster syndrome
	Transverse vaginal septum
	Imperforate hymen
Systemic	Severe malabsorption
	Crohn's disease

[a]The more common diagnoses are italicized.

Local or Anatomic Problems in the Outflow Tract

Any obstruction to menstrual flow prevents menarche. Thus, patients with an imperforate hymen or a transverse vaginal septum present with primary amenorrhea. Mayer-Rokitansky-Kuster syndrome—congenital absence of the vagina, a rudimentary uterus, and normally functioning ovaries—requires reconstructive surgery. Testicular feminization (or androgen insensitivity syndrome) is a rare disorder in which phenotypic females lack a uterus, fallopian tubes, or upper vagina. The clue to the diagnosis is the presence of normal breast development, absence of pubic and axillary hair, and absence of uterus on pelvic examination. Genetically, they are XY, with male levels of testosterone, although their cells have an end-stage insensitivity to it. Inguinal or abdominal testes are present and require surgical removal after breast development is complete, followed by sequential estrogen and progesterone therapy [56]. Postabortion synechiae that impede menstrual flow constitute Asherman's syndrome.

This group of problems is best diagnosed through careful attention to the physical and genital examinations. A careful rectoabdominal examination and complete pelvic ultrasound are usually necessary to define the anatomy adequately.

Ovarian Failure

The ovaries may be understimulated by appropriate cycles of LH and FSH, or they may be incapable of manufacturing mature levels of estradiol. In the first situation, a family history of pubertal delay is frequently found. An adolescent's menarche tends to correlate closely with her mother's and sisters', usually within a year. Patients with constitutional delay have normal, prepubertal levels of LH and FSH and delayed bone ages. Patients in the second category comprise the largest single group—those with gonadal dysgenesis. Although the classic Turner's syndrome is well known (XO karyotype, with short stature, webbed neck, shield chest, cubitus valgus), mosaicism or a structurally abnormal X chromosome also occur and may have widely variable physical findings. In either case, levels of LH and FSH are extremely high after puberty. Very rarely, patients can also have ovarian failure secondary to radiation, chemotherapy, autoimmune disease, or infiltrative disease. Such patients may actually be taller than normal because their epiphyses remain open in the absence of normal levels of sex hormones.

Here again, the history and physical examination may yield important clues to the eventual diagnosis. Certainly, any amenorrheic teenager less than 5 feet tall deserves karyotyping, and the practitioner should always be alert to the possibility of XO/XX mosaicism.

Hypothalamic Failure

Various systemic diseases may act, through the hypothalamus, to delay normal puberty: hypothyroidism, congenital adrenal hyperplasia, Cushing's syndrome, anorexia nervosa, and inflammatory bowel disease, to name a few. Pituitary tumors may interfere with the normal feedback of LH and FSH on the hypothalamus and production of GnRH. Intensive athletic training may delay menarche for up to 2 years, probably as a result of the stress of training and its interaction with catecholamines and GnRH [57,58]. Rarely, GnRH may be congenitally absent, as in Kallman's syndrome, which is associated with anosmia [12]. And still rarer, hyperprolactinemia and galactorrhea may delay puberty, even in the absence of pituitary tumors [59].

Debilitating systemic diseases should be readily apparent by history, physical examination, and careful inspection of the growth chart. Close attention should be paid to the funduscopic examination, and the ability to smell may require testing using increasing molar concentrations of pyridine. Congenital adrenal hyperplasia may be suspected by family history, presence of hirsutism or virilism, or hypertension. Provocative testing using dexamethasone suppression may be required (2 mg orally of dexamethasone at midnight before testing, then adrenocorticotropic hormone as an intravenous bolus of 10 μg/m^2 body surface area; a 17-hydroxyprogesterone level of greater than 3 ng/ml 15 minutes after adrenocorticotropic hormone administration indicates 21-hydroxylase deficiency, the most common form of congenital adrenal hyperplasia).

Secondary Amenorrhea

The primary clinician is far more likely to encounter cases of secondary amenorrhea—the prolonged absence (for 4–6 months) of menstrual bleeding after menarche has already been established.

TABLE 61. *Causes of secondary amenorrhea*

Common
Pregnancy
Stress
Exercise
Weight loss/eating disorders
Polycystic ovary syndromes

Rarer
Systemic disease
  • Inflammatory bowel disease
  • Hyperthyroidism
  • Congenital adrenal hyperplasia
  • Cushing's syndrome
  • Diabetes
  • Renal failure
Drugs
  • Sex steroids
  • Phenothiazines
  • Amphetamines
  • Isotretinoin (Accutane)
  • Opiates
Pituitary adenoma/hyperprolactinemia
Partial gonadal dysgenesis/ovarian failure
Adrenal or ovarian tumor
Post-oral contraception

Adapted from Kulig JW. Adolescent menstrual disorders. In: Strasburger VC, ed. *Adolescent gynecology: an office guide.* Baltimore: Urban & Schwarzenberg; 1990.

Unfortunately, secondary amenorrhea is all too common among adolescents—secondary to pregnancy. *Even in the absence of a positive sexual history, a urine or serum pregnancy test should always be performed before embarking on a more elaborate laboratory evaluation* [60].

The differential diagnoses in this disorder are a little easier to understand, and management tends to be far more straightforward (Tables 61, 62). After pregnancy has been ruled out, a diagnostic challenge with Provera, 10 mg once or twice daily for 5 to 10 days, or 100 to 200 mg of progesterone-in-

TABLE 62. *Sequential evaluation of secondary amenorrhea*

Initial evaluation
  1. Complete history
     Includes family background, chronic illness, stress, diet, exercise, drugs, sex, contraception
  2. Complete physical examination
     Includes Tanner staging of secondary sexual development and pelvic examination
  3. Pregnancy test—urine or serum human chorionic gonadotropin
  4. If pregnancy test is negative, then additional laboratory tests:
     Luteinizing hormone, follicle-stimulating hormone, prolactin, thyroid function tests
  5. Induction of menses trial, using either:
     Provera, 10 mg p.o. bid × 5–10 days *or* Progesterone-in-oil, 100–200 mg IM

If no withdrawal flow occurs after induction:
  5. Complete blood count, sedimentation rate, urinalysis, serum carotene
  6. Androgens: free testosterone, androstenedione, DHEA, DHEA sulfate, 17-OH progesterone
  7. Pelvic ultrasound
  8. Computed tomography or magnetic resonance imaging if necessary
  9. Consultation with adolescent gynecologist or pediatric endocrinologist if needed

DHEA, dehydroepiandrosterone.
Adapted from Kulig JW. Adolescent menstrual disorders. In: Strasburger VC, ed. *Adolescent gynecology: an office guide.* Baltimore: Urban & Schwarzenberg; 1990; and Polaneczky MM, Slap GB. Menstrual disorders in the adolescent: amenorrhea. *Pediatr Rev* 1992;13:43.

oil intramuscularly, can help determine whether the hypothalamic–pituitary–ovarian axis is adequately "primed." Initial laboratory tests can include serum LH, FSH, and prolactin levels, erythrocyte sedimentation rate, and thyroid function tests. Prolactin should be measured routinely because only one third of patients with elevations report having galactorrhea. As many as 5% to 10% of patients with amenorrhea and elevated prolactin levels have pituitary adenomas; however, mild elevations in prolactin levels are more commonly associated with medications, stress, breast stimulation, hypothyroidism, or other factors [61,62].

Situational stress, intensive athletic training, weight loss, and eating disorders comprise most of the problems in patients with secondary amenorrhea who are not pregnant. Less commonly, this disorder parallels primary amenorrhea, with chronic illnesses, PCOS, and pituitary adenomas being included in the differential diagnosis.

The hypothalamus probably serves as the focal point for most cases of secondary amenorrhea. Stress may affect levels of central nervous system neurotransmitters, which in turn affect the pulsatile secretion of GnRH. In a normal individual, a 15% weight loss or a drop below 22% total body fat may cause menses to cease [63]. Interestingly, in patients with anorexia nervosa, the cessation of menses may actually precede or coincide with the weight loss and behavioral abnormalities in up to 71% of patients [64]. Even after patients regain their normal weight, if they persist in abnormal eating behavior, their LH release pattern may remain prepubertal. Teenage girls, who are extremely weight conscious to begin with, may also have growth failure and secondary amenorrhea secondary to inadequate caloric intake, recurrent dieting, and poor calcium intake in a picture that stops just short of full-blown anorexia nervosa [63]. In addition, secondary amenorrhea can develop in normal or above-weight teens if they engage in fasting or purging behaviors [65].

Increasingly, practitioners are seeing extremely athletic young women with secondary amenorrhea [58,66]. (As with other teenagers, athletes with amenorrhea should be considered pregnant until proven otherwise.) Runners, gymnasts, and ballet dancers have the highest incidence of menstrual dysfunction, and runners have twice the prevalence of amenorrhea as swimmers or cyclists [67]. The prevalence of secondary amenorrhea in women is estimated at 5% overall, but 20% in athletic women and 50% in competitive female athletes [37]. In runners, the prevalence increases with number of miles of training per week. For all athletes, as the percentage of body fat diminishes, the prevalence of amenorrhea increases. One study found a higher incidence of eating disorders and affective disorders among runners with amenorrhea [68].

Pituitary microadenomas are a rare cause of hyperprolactinemia and secondary amenorrhea, even in the absence of a history of galactorrhea. In one series, galactorrhea had to be expressed in 50% of patients and was spontaneous in the other 50%. Headaches may be prominent, and visual field defects may be present on examination. Over half of the patients had either recently been pregnant or used OCs. A random serum prolactin level serves as a useful screening test, because adenomas greater than 1 cm in diameter usually produce levels above 100 ng/dl. Microadenomas may only slightly elevate the serum prolactin level. The clinical course is usually benign, and patients do not require surgery unless the adenoma grows beyond the sella turcica [69]. Bromocriptine has also been used for medical management.

Again, treatment depends on etiology. Stress-related amenorrhea, whether environmentally or athletically induced, should remain a diagnosis of exclusion. Certainly, a positive response to progesterone challenge is reassuring in patients with suggestive histories. Athletes' amenorrhea may be reversed by decreasing training or increasing caloric intake, but this may be asking too much of a competitor. However, estrogen deficiency in amenorrhea may predispose to increased bone resorption of calcium and decreased bone mineral density [58,70,71]. Therefore, these young women should be counseled to increase their calcium intake to 1,500 mg per day (four to five glasses of milk) and require cycling with hormones. An exact replacement regimen is still controversial [70]. Estrogen replacement therapy stabilizes cortical bone density [72], but adolescents should have increasing bone density [58]. Combination OCs are useful, particularly in the sexually active teenager, or a combination of Premarin, 0.625 to 1.25 mg/day for days 1 to 25 each month, and Provera, 10 mg daily for days 13 to 25, can be tried [63].

Oligomenorrhea

Oligomenorrhea refers to scanty, irregular bleeding. It can also be defined as only one to six cycles per year in a young woman at least 2 years past menarche, or as cycles occurring more than 45 days apart [73]. Patients with PCOS, as well as up to 25% of teenagers with congenital adrenal hyperplasia, can have either secondary amenorrhea or oligomenorrhea. Androgen excess is at the root of both disorders. The "classic" PCOS presentation of a teenager who is hirsute, obese, and virilized is not always found. Indeed, oligomenorrhea may be a variant of normal development in some teens and a transition to full-blown PCOS in others [74].

All patients with oligomenorrhea do not necessarily have androgen excess, however. One study found that over 50% of patients had hypothalamic suppression and normal androgen levels [73]. Such patients may have mean LH levels that are three times higher than in normal adolescents. These patients usually require the expertise of an experienced gynecologist or endocrinologist.

Polycystic Ovary Syndrome

Polycystic ovary syndrome is a fascinating disorder that is currently undergoing major reassessment and scrutiny [75–77]. There are few disorders in adolescent gynecology about which so much is known and yet so little is understood [78]! Multiple biochemical abnormalities are known, but not all patients have them [75]:

- Increased total and free testosterone
- Decreased serum sex hormone-binding globulin
- Increased LH
- Hyperinsulinemia

The fundamental problem seems to be hyperinsulinism and an increased ovarian production of androgens, particularly testosterone. Excess testosterone then causes premature follicular atresia, anovulation, and systemic effects. Levels of LH are also greatly increased, and this hormone drives the growth of theca cells and the production of androgens. Likewise, higher levels of insulin increase testosterone production in stromal tissue. Insulin also decreases levels of sex hormone-binding globulin produced by the liver, allowing more unbound testosterone to produce androgenic side effects [77].

Clinically, the cardinal manifestations of PCOS are hirsutism, anovulation, and either oligomenorrhea or amenorrhea. About half of teenagers with PCOS are obese, and one fourth are either hirsute or virilized [77] (Table 63). The exact degree of hirsutism can be assessed by using the Ferriman-Gallwey score (see Gilchrist and Hecht [79]). Although ultrasonography of the ovaries is usually abnormal, with multiple thickened follicles, it can be completely normal. However, most patients have elevations in serum testosterone levels and a high LH-to-FSH ratio (greater than $2 \times$).

Many disorders involving androgen excess can overlap with PCOS, including HAIR AN syndrome (*h*yperandrogenism, *i*nsulin *r*esistance, and *a*canthosis *n*igricans), Cushing's disease, congenital adrenal hyperplasia, a virilizing ovarian tumor, an arrhenoblastoma, or simple obesity [53].

First-line treatment involves the use of combination OCs, which lower androgen levels, provide effective contraception, and help produce more regular cycles. OCs with the newer progestins, norgestimate and desogestrel, may be especially useful because they are potent progestins without androgenic side effects [61,80]. Weight reduction in obese adolescents is also a crucial part of initial therapy. Other treatments have included the use of antiandrogens such as spironolactone (for hirsutism) or, more recently, flutamide, a nonsteroidal drug [75]. Patients refractory to medical treatment have also undergone laparoscopic surgery, with some success [76]. Most recently, obese adult women with PCOS were successfully treated with metformin, a drug used in non–insulin-dependent diabetics that inhibits production of hepatic glucose, enhancing peripheral sensitivity to insulin and thereby decreasing insulin secretion [81].

TABLE 63. *Clinical features of polycystic ovary syndrome*

Feature	Frequency
Hirsutism	61–69%
Obesity	35–41%
Infertility	29–74%
Amenorrhea	26–51%
Oligomenorrhea	29–52%
Regular menses	15–25%
Acne	24–27%

Adapted from Franks S. Polycystic ovary syndrome. *N Engl J Med* 1995;333:853.

Premenstrual Syndrome

Premenstrual syndrome (PMS) remains a scientific "black box." To date, it lacks a uniform definition, and its etiology, pathogenesis, and treatment remain uncertain [82–84]. In France, PMS is considered a form of insanity, and in Canada, the United States, and Great Britain, the diagnosis has resulted in shortened sentences in several murder and assault cases [85].

Scientists cannot even agree on the proper terminology: in the American Psychiatric Association's *Diagnostic and Statistical Manual* (4th edition), PMS is relabeled premenstrual dysphoric disorder (PDD), with emphasis on the dysphoric mood as the most important feature [86]. However, no matter what term is applied, the diagnosis of PMS must focus on three key elements [84]:

- Symptoms must occur during the luteal phase and resolve within 1 to 2 days after onset of menses.
- Symptoms must be documented for several menstrual cycles.
- Symptoms must be recurrent and not caused by other medical or psychological disorders.

Because its first cousin, dysmenorrhea, has been found to have a solid biochemical base where previously it was believed to be psychogenic, the tendency now exists to discount all psychological theories of PMS and concentrate on physiologic mechanisms. Depressed women have been found more likely to report premenstrual symptoms, but this may be effect rather than cause [87]. At present, it is probably unwise to ignore behavioral theories of causation in favor of hormonal theories, or vice versa [38].

Premenstrual syndrome is characterized by recurring symptoms during the luteal phase of the menstrual cycle. Such symptoms may include weight gain, bloating, breast engorgement, edema, constipation, headaches, food cravings, anxiety, fatigue, tension, depression, and inability to concentrate. Typically, patients with PMS do *not* have dysmenorrhea; their symptoms usually disappear within the first day or two of blood flow. The full-blown syndrome is probably rare among adolescents, although many do report premenstrual symptoms—nearly two thirds of female teens in one study (42% weight gain or bloating, 30% mood changes, 19% cramps) [35]. In adult women, prevalence rates range from 3% to 10% [88,89]. One study of nearly 400 female adolescents reported a prevalence of 14% [90].

Etiologic Theories

Although a variety of etiologies have been discussed and investigated, there is no known cause [84,91]. Progesterone has been suspected as the main culprit, although the evidence is not at all conclusive [92]. PMS usually occurs only with ovulatory cycles, but affected women have normal estrogen and progesterone levels [38]. In addition, placebo-controlled trials of oral or vaginal progesterone have shown no therapeutic benefit [92,93]. As of 1997, there are no known abnormalities of either gonadal steroids or menstrual cycle physiology that characterize PMS [94,95].

Secondary hyperaldosteronism has been suggested because women have such symptoms as weight gain, edema, and bloating, but these symptoms are not consistent, and plasma aldosterone levels are normal in PMS patients [37]. Vitamin deficiency has also been suggested, especially B_6 (pyridoxine). Again, there have been no consistent findings or responses to treatment [84]. The most prominent environmental variable study has been diet [96]. Heavy consumption of chocolate or alcoholic beverages has been linked to PMS in college women [97]. Another college study found that severe PMS symptoms increased 3-fold in young women consuming two caffeinated beverages per day and 7.5-fold in those who averaged six such beverages per day [98].

Most recently, research has focused on the role of neurotransmitters like serotonin, which is known to mediate such mood and behavioral traits as depression, irritability, and aggression [96]. The effectiveness of serotonin reuptake inhibitors like fluoxetine (Prozac) [89] has revived interest in PMS as a form of atypical depression [95].

Management

A menstrual cycle diary is crucial to establishing the diagnosis of PMS (Fig. 13). But because the etiology is completely unknown, the treatment tends to be a smorgasbord of methods. In addition, therapeutic trials are plagued by the fact that the response to placebo is quite high, 50% to 94% [96]. To date, only three double-blinded, placebo-controlled studies have documented effectiveness of any one treatment [95]:

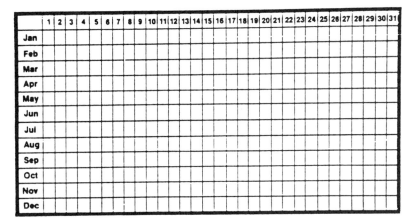

FIG. 13. Sample menstrual calendar. Days of bleeding are recorded with a dot and days of spotting with an *x*. (Kulig JW. Menstrual disorders. In: Strasburger VC, ed. *Basic adolescent gynecology: an office guide.* Baltimore: Urban and Schwarzenberg; 1990:141, with permission.)

- Alprazolam (a benzodiazepine with anxiolytic and antidepressant properties) reduced symptoms by 50% or more in one third of women studied, whereas oral progesterone had no effect [93]. An earlier but much smaller trial in Britain had found similar results [99].
- Fluoxetine (Prozac), a serotonin reuptake inhibitor, was highly effective at a dose of 20 mg/day throughout the menstrual cycle in reducing symptoms of tension, irritability, and dysphoria [89]. This is probably the drug of choice for young women with predominantly emotional symptoms [91].

Attempted treatments have included hormones, vitamins, counseling, and dietary change. A practical approach to treatment is probably best, given the current lack of answers concerning PMS (Table 64). Initial management needs to include education, emotional support, and reassurance. Regular exercise and careful diet are also important and may result in a lessening of symptoms [84]. Some experts recommend cautious vitamin and mineral supplementation: calcium, 1 g/day, magnesium, 360 mg/day, and pyridoxine 50 mg/day [84]. Certainly, if PMS represents a disorder of menstrual cyclicity, then a trial of overriding that cyclicity by using OCs seems reasonable [84,100]. However, data

TABLE 64. *Guidelines for management of adolescent premenstrual syndrome*

- Confirm the cyclicity of symptoms using a menstrual calendar. Symptoms should disappear with onset of menses and be followed by a symptom-free week.
- Identify the symptoms of greatest concern and severity to the patient.
- Provide education and reassurance about current knowledge of premenstrual syndrome. Relieve fears about cancer or adverse reproductive outcome.
- Maintain ideal body weight.
- Encourage aerobic exercise.
- Decrease or eliminate use of caffeinated beverages, chocolate, and tobacco.
- Encourage dietary change, including increased protein, vegetables, fruits, and fish. Increase calcium and decrease sodium intake.
- A variety of medications to consider:
  Pyridoxine, 50 mg daily
  Progestin-dominant oral contraceptives
  Fluoxetine (Prozac), 20 mg/d, for symptoms of dysphoria
  Mefenamic acid (Ponstel), 500 mg tid, for pain
  Bromocriptine, 5 mg nightly, or danazol, 200 mg/d, for severe breast pain or swelling
  Spironolactone, 50 mg/d, for fluid retention

Adapted from Kulig JW. Adolescent menstrual disorders. In: Strasburger VC, ed. *Adolescent gynecology: an office guide.* Baltimore: Urban & Schwarzenberg; 1990; and Steiner M, Steinberg S, Stewart D, et al. Fluoxetine in the treatment of premenstrual dysphoria. *N Engl J Med* 1995;332:1529.

concerning OCs and their impact on PMS are quite variable, and although some patients' symptoms may improve, others may worsen [91]. Other drugs that have been tried include transdermal estradiol (Estraderm), danazol (Danocrine), and GnRH agonists such as leuprolide (Lupron) and histrelin (Supprelin). Use of Depo-Provera to eliminate cycles altogether would also seem to be a reasonable (but as yet untested) alternative.

Chronic Pelvic Pain

Chronic pelvic pain must be differentiated from chronic abdominal pain in teenagers (see section on Psychosomatic Disorders in Chapter 7) [101–103]. It is usually defined as pain within the pelvic brim, or below the level of the iliac crests, lasting 3 months or more (constantly or intermittently). In perhaps half of the patients, the pains may have some relation to menstrual periods. In one study of 140 adolescents, two thirds had pelvic tenderness, 29% had cul-de-sac nodularity, 19% had a distinct mass, and 17% had adnexal thickening; and less than one fourth had normal pelvic examinations [104]. The differential diagnosis tends to be extensive, and ordering appropriate diagnostic tests requires great skill and restraint [105]. Among the most common diagnoses that should be considered are:

- Pregnancy
- Pelvic inflammatory disease
- Dysmenorrhea, primary or secondary
- Endometriosis
- Mittelschmerz
- Ovarian cyst, torsion, or tumor
- Adhesions
- Sexual abuse
- Nongynecologic causes (e.g., functional, irritable bowel syndrome, inflammatory bowel disease)

Endometriosis

Half of adolescents, or more, with refractory dysmenorrhea or chronic pelvic pain eventually are found to have endometriosis [106–108] (Table 65). Pelvic pain is the most common presenting symptom, and pelvic tenderness is the most common finding on physical examination, although the pelvic examination can be entirely normal (Table 66). Other symptoms may include abnormal vaginal bleeding, dyspareunia, and bladder or gastrointestinal symptoms, depending on the location of the implants [109]. A number of theories have been suggested concerning endometriosis, the most current of which are retrograde menstruation or defective immunoregulation [107,109,110].

Making the diagnosis is the most difficult and significant aspect of this disorder. Clearly, laparoscopy is warranted in patients with severe and restricting pains who are refractory to other treatments. The diagnostic yield is high, ranging from 60% to 94% [107,108,111,112]. The remaining patients may have psychogenic or functional bowel disease, but three fourths of them improved

TABLE 65. *Surgical findings at laparoscopy/laparotomy in 67 female adolescents with chronic pelvic pain*

Finding	Patients with finding
Endometriosis	73%
Adhesions	51%
Benign ovarian cyst	18%
Peritoneal pocket	13%
Chronic pelvic inflammatory disease	11%
Dermoid cyst	3%
Ovarian torsion	2%
Appendicitis	2%
No lesion found	6%

Adapted from Reese KA, Reddy S, Rock JA. Endometriosis in an adolescent population: the Emory experience. *Journal of Pediatric and Adolescent Gynecology* 1996;9:125.

TABLE 66. *Clinical presentation of 67 female adolescents with chronic pelvic pain*

Symptoms	
Pelvic pain	95%
Dysmenorrhea	95%
Abdominal pain	43%
Dyspareunia	29%
Irregular menses	25%
Constipation or diarrhea	3%
Physical examination findings	
Diffuse tenderness	95%
Localized tenderness	78%
Adnexal mass	22%
Nodularity in cul-de-sac	2%

Adapted from Reese KA, Reddy S, Rock JA. Endometriosis in an adolescent population: the Emory experience. *Journal of Pediatric and Adolescent Gynecology* 1996;9:125.

symptomatically after laparoscopy in one study [111]. Treatment by operative laparoscopy and suppression of ovulation with OCs has been successful in up to 84% of patients [106]. GnRH agonists have also been used successfully in refractory cases [113].

Ovarian Cysts

Most ovarian cysts—certainly ones less than 4 cm—do not cause pelvic pain [114]. However, simple cysts are extremely common in adolescents and frequently may be seen on routine ultrasonography [115]. Usually, cysts represent the failure of maturing follicles to ovulate or involute, and sometimes the ovary can appear to be polycystic because of multiple follicles developing at different rates [116]. Transvaginal ultrasonography can be extremely useful in differentiating simple cysts from malignancies, which are relatively rare in the adolescent age group [115].

Simple follicular cysts are often treated with either "watchful waiting" or the use of OCs for "hormonal suppression," although the latter is unproven [115]. Monophasic OCs seem to be preferable to multiphasic formulations [117], and progestin-only OCs increase the incidence of cyst formation [118]. Rarely, laparoscopy is required to treat a persistent or complex cyst [115].

Toxic Shock Syndrome

Although toxic shock syndrome (TSS) is included in the menstrual disorders section, clinicians should be aware that the epidemiology of the disorder has changed dramatically since 1980 and that there are now as many nonmenstrual as menstrual cases [119]. In 1980, 890 cases of TSS were reported (91% menstrually related), whereas only 61 cases were reported in 1989 (74% menstrually related) [120]. Currently, the risk of acquiring TSS is estimated to be 6.2 per 100,000 women, a risk that can be lowered even further if women avoid tampon use or use them only intermittently [121,122].

Todd et al. first reported TSS in 1978, describing three men and four women who had acute fever, hypotension, rash, and multisystem disease in association with phage group I staphylococci [123]. At first, TSS was associated with menstruation in young women, particularly with tampon use. A report in 1980 implicating Rely tampons resulted in their removal from the market [124]. However, the incidence of TSS did not decrease in some areas after Rely was removed, and increasing numbers of cases in men were described [121,125,126].

Women who use high-absorbency tampons continue to be at increased risk of TSS, but so are women who use contraceptive sponges (currently off the market) or diaphragms [127,128]. In addition, postpartum women, and *any* patients with either surgical wound infections, focal staphylococcal infections including sinusitis, or nasal surgery are also at increased risk [129,130] (Table 67). Menstruation or tampon use is *not* part of the case definition for the syndrome, and TSS still represents a significant risk to children and young adults, presumably because they have not previously encoun-

TABLE 67. *Conditions associated with nonmenstrual toxic shock syndrome*

Burns	Postoperative wound infection
Cellulitis	Postpartum infection
Empyema	Insect bites or abrasions
Lung abscess	Diaphragm use
Osteomyelitis	Sinusitis
Lymphadenitis	Influenza
Impetigo	Tracheitis

Adapted from Strausbaugh LJ. Toxic shock syndrome: are you recognizing its changing presentations? *Postgrad Med* 1993;94: 107.

tered the toxins involved [131]. One epidemiologist has speculated that the great plague of Athens from 430 to 420 BC may have been caused by a TSS epidemic [132].

Pathophysiologic Features

Toxic shock syndrome is clearly associated with certain strains of *Staphylococcus aureus*. Toxic shock syndrome toxin 1 (TSST-1) was isolated in 1981 and was thought to be the sole culprit. Now, the pathogenesis of TSS is thought to be a bit more complicated. For instance, many people carry antibodies to TSST-1 and have no history of TSS. TSST-1-producing strains of *S. aureus* may require special in vivo conditions to create the full-blown picture of TSS [121,133]. Favorable growth conditions include an environment with a neutral pH, high in protein, with an increased PCO_2—conditions best found in focal soft tissue *S. aureus* infections and in the vagina during menstruation and tampon use or with barrier contraceptive use. Ordinarily, menstruation is a time of acidic pH and an increased PO_2 in the vaginal environment. However, introducing a tampon into this environment raises the PCO_2 dramatically and makes the pH more neutral—ideal conditions for the elaboration of TSST-1 if *S. aureus* is present. The toxin (or toxins) produced ultimately impair capillary integrity, causing leakage, hypotension, shock, erythema, and multisystem involvement [121,133] (Fig. 14).

A TSS-like picture has been described in adults infected with group A streptococci that produces a pyrogenic erythrotoxin as in scarlet fever [134]. These patients tend to be older, between the ages of 20 and 50 years, with a greater incidence of extensive soft tissue infection and a case fatality rate (30%) that is five times that seen with staphylococcal TSS [135].

Signs and Symptoms

Toxic shock syndrome presents as an acute illness, with abrupt onset of fever and a viral-like picture. However, within 48 hours hypotension and repeated syncopal episodes occur, and the patient may appear severely ill. Decreased urine output and poor capillary perfusion are common manifestations of the hypotension. On examination, bilateral conjunctivitis, pharyngitis, a strawberry tongue, a sunburn-like rash (erythroderma), muscle tenderness, and joint edema are characteristic. The rash is similar to the rash of scarlet fever, but not as intense or rough. Compared with scalded skin syndrome, the TSS rash is rarely bullous, and Nikolsky's sign is negative (no peeling with abrasion of the skin). Patients may also be either jaundiced or semicomatose at initial presentation. If the TSS is menstrually related, there may be vaginal hyperemia and a malodorous cervical discharge.

A number of laboratory abnormalities are typically present and reflect the multiorgan involvement: a leukocytosis with left shift, normocytic anemia, decreased platelet count, sterile pyuria, prolonged prothrombin and partial thromboplastin times, hyponatremia, hypokalemia, metabolic acidosis, and increases in serum bilirubin, creatinine, blood urea nitrogen, and transaminases.

Diagnosis and Treatment

A strict definition for TSS has been devised (Table 68). To have TSS, a patient must have four of the five major criteria and exclusionary evidence for related disorders. Menstruation is *not* mentioned in the criteria for diagnosis, nor is a focus of *S. aureus* infection or its isolation from any site a requisite.

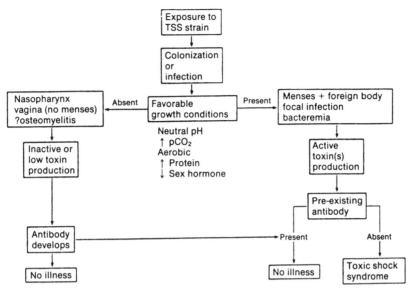

FIG. 14. Pathophysiology of toxic shock syndrome. (Todd JK. Toxic shock syndrome. *Clin Microbiol Rev* 1988;1:432. Copyright 1988, The American Society for Microbiology, with permission.)

TABLE 68. *Toxic shock syndrome: criteria for diagnosis*

Major criteria (four of five must be present)
- Temperature >102°F (38.9°C)
- Rash (diffuse, macular erythroderma, or maculopapular)
- Desquamation of palms or soles 1–2 wk after onset of illness
- Hypotension
    Adults: systolic pressure <90 mm Hg
    Children: systolic pressure <5th percentile
    or orthostatic syncope
- Involvement of three or more of the following organ systems:
    Gastrointestinal (vomiting, diarrhea)
    Muscular (severe myalgia or creatine phosphokinase more than twice normal)
    Mucous membrane (hyperemia of conjunctivae, pharynx, or vagina)
    Renal (elevated blood urea nitrogen or creatinine; >5 white blood cells per hpf in the absence of
      a urinary tract infection)
    Hepatic (elevated bilirubin or transaminases)
    Hematologic (platelets <100,000/mm³)
    Central nervous system (altered consciousness or disorientation)

plus

Reasonable evidence to exclude other causes of the illness
- Blood or cerebrospinal fluid cultures must be negative for organisms other than *Staphylococcus aureus.*
- Serologic tests must be negative for Rocky Mountain spotted fever, leptospirosis, and measles, if obtained.

Adapted from Todd JD. Toxic shock syndrome. *Clin Microbiol Rev* 1988;1:432; and from Committee on Infectious Diseases. *1997 red book: report of the Committee on Infectious Diseases.* 24th ed. Elk Grove Village, IL: American Academy of Pediatrics; 1997;481–482.

Similar diseases that may require excluding tests include bacterial sepsis, meningococcemia, staphylococcal scaled skin syndrome, Stevens-Johnson syndrome, group A streptococcal disease, Rocky Mountain spotted fever, leptospirosis, and measles. Undoubtedly, cases with less severe manifestations exist. Probable cases include those where some of the major criteria are missing without other explanations for the illness [121].

Treatment of TSS is mainly supportive, but that does not minimize its importance. Approximately 2% to 5% of patients die with TSS, but mortality has decreased since the mid-1980s. The pathophysiology of the disease suggests a high-output, low–peripheral-resistance state, with capillary leakage and poor venous return [121]. Therefore, patients may require extremely large amounts of fluid to counteract loss into the interstitial space. Because of leaky capillaries, edema is common—but is *not* a sign of fluid overload, and should not deter the clinician from aggressive fluid management.

Antistaphylococcal therapy is prescribed, primarily to avoid the 30% recurrence risk (which, to date, have all been in menstruating women) [136]. A vigorous search must be made for potential foci of staphylococcal infection. *It is imperative surgically to drain even small amounts of infection, including wounds that may look relatively innocuous* [121]. In addition, there is increasing evidence that corticosteroid therapy may be useful if given early in the course of the disease [137].

Sequelae include reversible loss of hair and nails, vocal cord paralysis, paresthesias, prolonged weakness and fatigue, amenorrhea, coronary artery aneurysms, and recurrence of TSS [122]. Recurrence rates in menstrual cases have been in the range of 30% to 60%, often within the first 2 months. Use of aggressive antistaphylococcal treatment has lessened this risk, but so too can avoidance of tampon use. In fact, some experts would counsel all menstruating women to use low-absorbency tampons, change them frequently, and alternate their use with pads at night.

REFERENCES

1. Braverman PK, Strasburger VC. Adolescent sexuality: IV. the practitioner's role. *Clin Pediatr* 1994;33:100.
2. Zacharias L, Rand WM, Wurtman RJ. A prospective study of sexual development and growth in American girls: the statistics of menarche. *Obstet Gynecol Surv* 1976;31:325.
3. Baker ER. Body weight and the initiation of puberty. *Clin Obstet Gynecol* 1985;28:573.
4. Merritt DF. Menstrual problems within the first three years of menarche. In: Pokorny S, ed. *Pediatric and adolescent gynecology*. New York: Chapman & Hall; 1996:55.
5. Rosenfeld RL, Barnes RB. Menstrual disorders in adolescence. *Endocrinol Metab Clin North Am* 1993; 22:491.
6. Frisch RE, McArthur JW. Menstrual cycles: Fatness as a determinant of minimum weight for height necessary for their maintenance of onset. *Science* 1974;185:949.
7. Frisch RE. Body fat, puberty, and fertility. *Biol Rev* 1984;59:161.
8. Gonzales GF, Villena A. Critical anthropometry for menarche. *Journal of Pediatric and Adolescent Gynecology* 1996;9:139.
9. Knobil E. The neuroendocrine control of the menstrual cycle. *Recent Prog Horm Res* 1980;36:53.
10. Apter D. Endocrine developments during female puberty with some implications for adult life. Presented at the 4th Annual Conference on Pediatric and Adolescent Gynecology, Costa Mesa, California, January 12–13, 1990.
11. Kustin J, Rebar RW. Menstrual disorders in the adolescent age group. *Prim Care* 1987;14:139.
12. Soules MR. Adolescent amenorrhea. *Pediatr Clin North Am* 1987;34:1083.
13. Braverman PK, Sondheimer SJ. Menstrual disorders. *Pediatr Rev* 1997;18:17.
14. Zabin LS, Kantner JF, Zelnik M. The risk of adolescent pregnancy in the first months of intercourse. *Fam Plann Perspect* 1979;11:215.
15. Franz WB. Basic review: endocrinology of the normal menstrual cycle. *Prim Care* 1988;15:607.
16. National Cancer Institute Workshop. The 1988 Bethesda System for reporting cervical/vaginal cytological diagnoses. *JAMA* 1989;262:931.
17. Broder S. The Bethesda System for reporting cervical/vaginal cytologic diagnoses: report of the 1991 Bethesda Workshop. *JAMA* 1992;267:1892.
18. Shepherd JC, Fried RA. Preventing cervical cancer: the role of the Bethesda System. *Am Fam Physician* 1995;51:434.
19. Chacko MR, and Rosenfeld WD. The uterine cervix: diagnostic opportunities. *Pediatr Ann* 1995;24:317.
20. Roye CF. Abnormal cervical cytology in adolescents: a literature review. *J Adolesc Health* 1992;13:643.
21. Roye CF. Pap smear screening for adolescents: rationale, technique, and follow-up. *Journal of Pediatric Health Care* 1993;7:199.
22. Koss LG. Cervical (Pap) smear: new directions. *Cancer* 1993;71(Suppl 4):1406.
23. Rosenfeld WD. Genital human papillomavirus infection in adolescents. In: Goldfarb AF, ed. *Clinical problems in pediatric and adolescent gynecology* New York: Chapman & Hall; 1996:89.
24. Miller KE, Losh DP, Folley A. Evaluation and follow-up of abnormal Pap smears. *Am Fam Physician* 1992;45:143.

25. Crane S. Abnormal Pap smears in the adolescent: the role of LEEP. *NASPAG News* 1995;9(1):1.
26. Nuovo J, Melnikow J, Paliescheskey M. Management of patients with atypical and low-grade Pap smear abnormalities. *Am Fam Physician* 1995;52:2243.
27. Brotzman GL, and Julian TM. The minimally abnormal Papanicolaou smear. *Am Fam Physician* 1996;53: 1154.
28. Zuber TJ. The minimally abnormal Pap smear: a conservative approach. *Am Fam Physician* 1996;53:1042.
29. Lavin C, Goodman E, Perlman S, et al. Follow-up of abnormal Pap smears in a hospital based adolescent clinic [Abstract]. *Journal of Pediatric and Adolescent Gynecology* 1996;9:156.
30. Biro FM, Rosenthal SL, Kollar LM, et al. Abnormal Pap smears as a screening question in young adolescent girls [Abstract]. Journal of Pediatric and Adolescent Gynecology 1996;9:157.
31. Eckert LO, Koutsky LA, Kiviat NB, et al. The inflammatory Papanicolaou smear: what does it mean? *Obstet Gynecol* 1995;86:360.
32. Eltabbakh GH, Eltabbakh GD, Broekhuizen FF, et al. Value of wet mount and cervical cultures at the time of cervical cytology in asymptomatic women. *Obstet Gynecol* 1995;85:499.
33. Klein JR, Litt IF. Epidemiology of adolescent dysmenorrhea. *Pediatr* 1981;68:661.
34. Andersch B, Milsom I. An epidemiologic study of young women with dysmenorrhea. *Am J Obstet Gynecol* 1982;144:655.
35. Wilson C, Emans SJ, Mansfield J, et al. The relationships of calculated percent body fat, sports participation, age, and place of residence on menstrual patterns in healthy adolescent girls at an independent New England high school. *Journal of Adolescent Health Care* 1984;5:248.
36. Blythe MJ. Common menstrual problems of adolescence. *Adolescent Medicine: State of the Art Reviews* 1997;8:87.
37. Kulig JW. Adolescent menstrual disorders. In: Strasburger VC, ed. *Adolescent gynecology: an office guide.* Baltimore: Urban & Schwarzenberg; 1990:141.
38. Coupey SM, Ahlstrom P. Common menstrual disorders. *Pediatr Clin North Am* 1989;36:551.
39. Altchek A. Pediatric and adolescent gynecology. *Compr Ther* 1995;21:235.
40. Mortensen ME, Rennebohm RM. Clinical pharmacology and use of nonsteroidal anti-inflammatory drugs. *Pediatr Clin North Am* 1989;36:1113.
41. Pittrof R, Lees C, Thompson C, et al. Crossover study of glyceryl trinitrate patches for controlling pain in women with severe dysmenorrhoea. *Br Med J* 1996;312:884.
42. Robinson JC, Plichta S, Weisman CS, et al. Dysmenorrhea and use of oral contraceptives in adolescent women attending a family planning clinic. *Am J Obstet Gynecol* 1992;166:578.
43. Polaneczky MM, Slap GB. Menstrual disorders in the adolescent: dysmenorrhea and dysfunctional uterine bleeding. *Pediatr Rev* 1992;13:83.
44. Ulmsten U. Calcium blockage as a rapid pharmacological test to evaluate primary dysmenorrhea. *Gynecol Obstet Invest* 1985;20:78.
45. Jaffe SB, Jewelewicz R. Dysfunctional uterine bleeding in the pediatric and adolescent patient. *Adolescent and Pediatric Gynecology* 1991;4:62.
46. Rosenfeld J. Treatment of menorrhagia due to dysfunctional uterine bleeding. *Am Fam Physician* 1996;53:165.
47. Ward CL. Hemorrhaging at menarche: a case report. *J Fam Pract* 1992;34:351.
48. Duflos-Cohade C, Amandruz M, Thibaud E. Pubertal metrorrhagia. *Journal of Pediatric and Adolescent Gynecology* 1996;9:16.
49. Claessens EA, Cowell CA. Dysfunctional uterine bleeding in the adolescent. *Pediatr Clin North Am* 1981;28:369.
50. Bayer SR, DeCherney AH. Clinical manifestations and treatment of dysfunctional uterine bleeding. *JAMA* 1993;269:1823.
51. Goldfarb AF. Dysfunctional uterine bleeding. In: Goldfarb AF, ed. *Clinical problems in pediatric and adolescent gynecology.* New York: Chapman & Hall; 1996:61.
52. Hillard PA. Abnormal uterine bleeding in adolescents. *Contemporary Pediatrics* 1995;12:79.
53. Merritt DF. Menstrual problems within the first three years of menarche. In: Pokorny S, ed. *Pediatric and adolescent gynecology.* New York: Chapman & Hall; 1996:55.
54. Layman LC. An update on the treatment of hypogonadism: I. hyper-gonadotropic hypogonadism. *Adolescent and Pediatric Gynecology* 1994;7:183.
55. Reindollar RH, McDonough PG. Adolescent menstrual disorders. *Clin Obstet Gynecol* 1983;26:690.
56. Harkins JL, Gysler M, Cowell CA. Anatomical amenorrhea: the problem of congenital vaginal agenesis and its surgical correction. *Pediatr Clin North Am* 1981;28:345.
57. Frisch RE, Gotz-Welbergen AV, McArthur JW, et al. Delayed menarche and amenorrhea of college athletes in relation to age of onset of training. *JAMA* 1981;246:1559.
58. Morgan A, London S. Effects of excessive exercise and weight loss on adolescent menstrual cyclicity. *Adolescent and Pediatric Gynecology* 1993;6:63.
59. Hughes EG, Garner PR. Primary amenorrhea associated with hyperprolactinemia: four cases with normal sellar architecture and absence of galactorrhea. *Fertil Steril* 1987;47:1031.
60. Kiningham RB, Apgar BS, Schwenk TL. Evaluation of amenorrhea. *Am Fam Physician* 1996;53:1185.
61. Polanecsky MM, and Slap GB. Menstrual disorders in the adolescent: amenorrhea. *Pediatr Rev* 1992;13:43.
62. Shulman DI. Hyperprolactinemia in adolescents. *Adolescent and Pediatric Gynecology* 1995;8:213.
63. Mansfield MJ, Emans SJ. Anorexia nervosa, athletics, and amenorrhea. *Pediatr Clin North Am* 1989;36:533.

64. Fears WB, Glass AR, Vigersky RA. Role of exercise in the pathogenesis of the amenorrhea associated with anorexia nervosa. *Journal of Adolescent Health Care* 1983;4:22.
65. Selzer R, Caust J, Hibbert M, et al. The association between secondary amenorrhea and common eating disordered weight control practices in an adolescent population. *J Adolesc Health* 1996;19:56.
66. Marshall LA. Clinical evaluation of amenorrhea in active and athletic women. *Clin Sports Med* 1994;13:371.
67. Sanborn CF, Martin BJ, Wagner WW. Is athletic amenorrhea specific to runners? *Am J Obstet Gynecol* 1982;143:859.
68. Gadpaille WJ, Sanborn CF, Wagner WW. Athletic amenorrhea, major affective disorders, and eating disorders. *Am J Psychiatry* 1987;144:939.
69. Koppelman MCS, Jaffe MJ, Rieth KG, et al. Hyperprolactinemia, amenorrhea, and galactorrhea: a retrospective assessment of twenty-five cases. *Ann Intern Med* 1984;100:115.
70. Hergenroeder AC. Bone mineralization, hypothalamic amenorrhea, and sex steroid therapy in female adolescents and young adults. *J Pediatr* 1995;126:683.
71. Rencken ML, Chestnut CH III, Drinkwater BL. Bone density at multiple skeletal sites in amenorrheic athletes. *JAMA* 1996;276:238.
72. Emans SJ, Grace E, Hoffer FA, et al. Estrogen deficiency in adolescents and young adults: impact on bone mineral content and effects of estrogen replacement therapy. *Obstet Gynecol* 1990;76:585.
73. Emans SJ, Grace E, Goldstein DP. Oligomenorrhea in adolescent girls. *J Pediatr* 1980;97:815.
74. Siegberg R, Nilsson CG, Stenman UH, et al. Endocrinologic features of oligomenorrheic adolescent girls. *Fertil Steril* 1986;46:852.
75. Franks S. Polycystic ovary syndrome. *N Engl J Med* 1995;333:853.
76. Udoff LC, and Adashi EY. Polycystic ovarian disease: current insights into an old problem. *Journal of Pediatric and Adolescent Gynecology* 1996;9:3.
77. Utiger RD. Insulin and the polycystic ovary syndrome. *N Engl J Med* 1996;335:657.
78. Winter JSD. Hyperandrogenism in female adolescents. *Curr Opin Pediatr* 1993;5:488.
79. Gilchrist VJ, Hecht BR. A practical approach to hirsutism. *Am Fam Physician* 1995;52:1837.
80. Siegel SF, Lee PA. Polycystic ovary syndrome. *Curr Opin Pediatr* 1993;5:400.
81. Nestler JE, Jakubowicz DJ. Decreases in ovarian cytochrome P450c17a activity and serum free testosterone after reduction of insulin secretion in polycystic ovary syndrome. *N Engl J Med* 1996;335:617.
82. Mortola JF. Assessment and management of premenstrual syndrome. *Curr Opin Obstet Gynecol* 1992;4:877.
83. DeMonico SO, Brown CS, Ling FW. Premenstrual syndrome. *Curr Opin Obstet Gynecol* 1994;6:499.
84. Parker PD. Premenstrual syndrome. *Am Fam Physician* 1994;50:1309.
85. Lewis JW. Premenstrual syndrome as a criminal defense. *Arch Sex Behav* 1990;19:425.
86. American Psychiatric Association. *Diagnostic and statistical manual of mental disorders, fourth edition.* Washington, DC: American Psychiatric Association; 1994:714.
87. Logue CM, Moos RH. Perimenstrual symptoms: prevalence and risk factors. *Psychosom Med* 1986;48:388.
88. Nader S. Premenstrual syndrome: tailoring treatment to symptoms. *Postgrad Med* 1991;90:173.
89. Steiner M, Steinberg S, Stewart D, et al. Fluoxetine in the treatment of premenstrual dysphoria. *N Engl J Med* 1995;332:1529.
90. Raja SN, Feehan M, Stanton WR, et al. Prevalence and correlates of the premenstrual syndrome in adolescence. *J Am Acad Child Adolesc Psychiatry* 1992;31:783.
91. Severino SK, Moline ML. Premenstrual syndrome: identification and management. *Drugs* 1995;49:71.
92. Freeman E, Rickels K, Sondheimer SJ, et al. Ineffectiveness of progesterone suppository treatment for premenstrual syndrome. *JAMA* 1990;264:349.
93. Freeman EW, Rickels K, Sondheimer SJ, et al. A double-blind trial of oral progesterone, alprazolam, and placebo in treatment of severe premenstrual syndrome. *JAMA* 1995;274:51.
94. Rubinow DR, Schmidt PJ. Premenstrual syndrome: A review of endocrine studies. *The Endocrinologist* 1992;2:47.
95. Rubinow DR, Schmidt PJ. The treatment of premenstrual syndrome: forward into the past. *N Engl J Med* 1995;332:1574.
96. Mortola JF. Issues in the diagnosis and research of premenstrual syndrome. *Clin Obstet Gynecol* 1992;35:587.
97. Rossignol AM, Bonnlander H. Prevalence and severity of the premenstrual syndrome: effects of foods and beverages that are sweet or high in sugar content. *J Reprod Med* 1991;36:131.
98. Rossignol AM. Caffeine-containing beverages and premenstrual syndrome in young women. *Am J Public Health* 1985;75:1335.
99. Menkes DB, Taghavi E, Mason PA, et al. Fluoxetine treatment of severe premenstrual syndrome. *Br Med J* 1992;305:346.
100. Smith S, Schiff I. *Modern management of premenstrual syndrome.* New York: Norton; 1993.
101. Rosenthal RH. Psychology of chronic pelvic pain. *Obstet Gynecol Clin North Am* 1993;20:627.
102. Cavanaugh RM Jr. Nongynecologic causes of unexplained lower abdominal pain in adolescent girls. *Clin Pediatr* 1996;35:337.
103. Gidwani GP. Chronic pelvic pain: steps to take before and after operative intervention. In: Pokorny S, ed. *Pediatric and adolescent gynecology.* New York: Chapman & Hall; 1996:41.
104. Goldstein DP, deCholnoky C, Emans SJ, et al. Laparoscopy in the diagnosis and management of pelvic pain in adolescents. *J Reprod Med* 1980;24:251.

105. McGrath JW, Strickland JL. Chronic pelvic pain in the adolescent. *Adolescent and Pediatric Gynecology* 1995;8:107.
106. Davis GD, Thillet E, Lindemann J. Clinical characteristics of adolescent endometriosis. *J Adolesc Health* 1993;14:362.
107. Durinzi KL, DeLeon FD. Endometriosis in the adolescent and and teenage female. *Adolescent and Pediatric Gynecology* 1993;6:3.
108. Reese KA, Reddy S, Rock JA. Endometriosis in an adolescent population: the Emory experience. *Journal of Pediatric and Adolescent Gynecology* 1996;9:125.
109. Hurd SJ, Adamson GD. Pelvic pain: endometriosis as a differential diagnosis in adolescents. *Adolescent and Pediatric Gynecology* 1992;5:3.
110. Lu PY, Ory SJ. Endometriosis: Current management. *Mayo Clin Proc* 1995;70:453.
111. Goldstein DP. Acute and chronic pelvic pain. *Pediatr Clin North Am* 1989;36:573.
112. Vercellini P, Fedele L, Arcaini L, et al. Laparoscopy in the diagnosis of chronic pelvic pain in adolescent women. *J Reprod Med* 1989;34:827.
113. Hornstein MD, Yupze AA, Burry KA, et al. Prospective randomized double-blind trial of 3 versus 6 months of nafarelin therapy for endometriosis associated pelvic pain. *Fertil Steril* 1995;63:955.
114. Kozlowski KJ. Acute and chronic pelvic pain. In: Goldfarb AF, ed. *Clinical problems in pediatric and adolescent gynecology.* New York: Chapman & Hall; 1996:99.
115. Murray S, London S. Management of ovarian cysts in neonates, children, and adolescents. *Adolescent and Pediatric Gynecology* 1995;8:64.
116. Seigel M. Pediatric gynecologic sonography. *Radiol* 1991;179:593.
117. Lanes S, Birmann B, Walker A, et al. Oral contraceptive type and functional cysts. *Am J Obstet Gynecol* 1992;166:956.
118. Tayob Y, Adans J, Jacobs H, et al. Ultrasound demonstration of increased frequency of functional ovarian cysts in women using progestogen only oral contraception. *Br J Obstet Gynaecol* 1985;92:1003.
119. Strausbaugh LJ. Toxic shock syndrome: are you recognizing its changing presentations? *Postgrad Med* 1993;94:107.
120. Centers for Disease Control and Prevention. Reduced incidence of menstrual toxic shock syndrome: United States, 1980–1990. *MMWR Morb Mortal Wkly Rep* 1990;39:421.
121. Todd JD. Toxic shock syndrome. *Clin Microbiol Rev* 1988;1:432.
122. Pandit S. Index of suspicion. *Pediatr Rev* 1996;17:319.
123. Todd J, Fishaut M, Kapral F, et al. Toxic-shock syndrome associated with phage group-1 staphylococci. *Lancet* 1978;2:116.
124. Schlech WF III, Shands KN, Reingold AL, et al. Risk factors for development of toxic shock syndrome: association with a tampon brand. *JAMA* 1982;248:835.
125. Petitti DB, Reingold A, Chin J. The incidence of toxic shock syndrome in Northern California 1972 through 1983. *JAMA* 1986;255:368.
126. Kniffin WD, Smith R, Stashwick CA. Toxic shock syndrome in three adolescent males. *Journal of Adolescent Health Care* 1990;11:166.
127. Faich G, Pearson K, Fleming D, et al. Toxic shock syndrome and the vaginal contraceptive sponge. *JAMA* 1986;255:216.
128. Wilson CD. Toxic shock syndrome and diaphragm use. *Journal of Adolescent Health Care* 1983;4:290.
129. Ferguson MA, Todd JK. Toxic shock syndrome associated with *Staphylococcus aureus* sinusitis in children. *J Infect Dis* 1990;161:953.
130. Mansfield CJ, Peterson MB. Toxic shock syndrome: associated with nasal packing. *Clin Pediatr* 1989;28:443.
131. Todd JK, Weisenthal AM, Ressman M, et al. Toxic shock syndrome: II. estimated occurrence in Colorado as influenced by case ascertainment methods. *Am J Epidemiol* 1985;122:857.
132. Langmuir AD, Worthen TD, Solomon J, et al. The Thucydides syndrome: a new hypothesis for the cause of the plague of Athens. *N Engl J Med* 1986;313:1027.
133. Resnick SD. Toxic shock syndrome: recent developments in pathogenesis. *J Pediatr* 1990;116:321.
134. Stevens DL, Tanner MH, Winship J. Severe group A streptococcal infections associated with a toxic shock-like syndrome and scarlet fever toxin A. *N Engl J Med* 1989;321:1.
135. Wolf JE, Rabinowitz LG. Streptococcal toxic shock-like syndrome. *Arch Dermatol* 1995;131:73.
136. Bryner CL Jr. Recurrent toxic shock syndrome. *American Family Physician* 1989;39:157.
137. Todd JK, Ressman M, Caston SA, et al. Corticosteroid therapy for patients with toxic shock syndrome. *JAMA* 1984;252:3399.

SUGGESTED READING

General

Arbel-DeRose Y, Tepper R, Rosen DJ, et al. The contribution of pelvic ultrasonography to the diagnostic process in pediatric and adolescent gynecology. *Journal of Pediatric and Adolescent Gynecology* 1997;10:3;.

Bacon JL. Menstrual problems in the older adolescent. In: Pokorny S, ed. *Pediatric and adolescent gynecology.* New York: Chapman & Hall; 1996:77.

Blythe MJ. Common menstrual problems of adolescence. *Adolescent Medicine: State of the Art Reviews* 1997;8:87.

Braverman PK, Sondheimer SJ. Menstrual disorders. *Pediatr Rev* 1997;18:17.

Braverman PK, Strasburger VC. Why adolescent gynecology? Pediatricians and pelvic exams. *Pediatr Clin North Am* 1989;36:471.

Emans SJ. Menarche and beyond: do eating and exercise make a difference? *Pediatr Ann* 1997;26(Suppl):137.

Kulin HE, Muller J. The biologic aspects of puberty. *Pediatr Rev* 1996;17:75.

Lee PA. Normal pubertal development. In: Goldfarb AF, ed. *Clinical problems in pediatric and adolescent gynecology.* New York: Chapman & Hall; 1996:49.

Merritt DF. Menstrual problems within the first three years of menarche. In: Pokorny S, ed. *Pediatric and adolescent gynecology.* New York: Chapman & Hall; 1996:55.

O'Connell B. The pediatrician and the sexually active adolescent: II. treatment of common menstrual disorders. *Pediatr Clin North Am* 1997 (in press).

Rosenfeld RL, Barnes RB. Menstrual disorders in adolescence. *Endocrinol Metab Clin North Am* 1993;22:491.

Pap Smear Screening

Brotzman GL, Julian TM. The minimally abnormal Papanicolaou smear. *Am Fam Physician* 1996;53:1154.

Chacko MR, Rosenfeld WD. The uterine cervix: diagnostic opportunities. *Pediatr Ann* 1995;24:317.

Roye CF. Abnormal cervical cytology in adolescents: a literature review. *J Adolesc Health* 1992;13:643.

Miller KE, Losh DP, Folley A. Evaluation and follow-up of abnormal Pap smears. *Am Fam Physician* 1992;45:143.

National Cancer Institute Workshop. The 1988 Bethesda System for reporting cervical/vaginal cytological diagnoses. *JAMA* 1989;262:931.

Nuovo J, Melnikow J, Paliescheskey M. Management of patients with atypical and low-grade Pap smear abnormalities. *Am Fam Physician* 1995;52:2243.

Roye CF. Pap smear screening for adolescents: rationale, technique, and follow-up. *Journal of Pediatric Health Care* 1993;7:199.

Shepherd JC, Fried RA. Preventing cervical cancer: the role of the Bethesda System. *Am Fam Physician* 1995;51:434.

Dysmenorrhea

Gidwani G, Kay M. Dysmenorrhea and pelvic pain. In: Sanfilippo JS, Muram D, Lee PA, et al, eds. *Pediatric and adolescent gynecology.* Philadelphia: WB Saunders; 1994:233.

Hesla JS. Dysmenorrhea. In: Carpenter SEK, Rock JA, eds. *Pediatric and adolescent gynecology.* New York: Raven Press; 1992:205.

Polanecsky MM, Slap GB. Menstrual disorders in the adolescent: dysmenorrhea and dysfunctional uterine bleeding. *Pediatr Rev* 1992;13:83.

Smith RP. Cyclic pelvic pain and dysmenorrhea. *Obstet Gynecol Clin North Am* 1993;20:753.

Dysfunctional Uterine Bleeding

Bayer SR, DeCherney AH. Clinical manifestations and treatment of dysfunctional uterine bleeding. *JAMA* 1993; 269:1823.

Blythe M, Orr D. Common menstrual problems: III. abnormal uterine bleeding. *Adolescent Health Update* 1992;4(2):1.

Duflos-Cohade C, Amandruz M, Thibaud E. Pubertal metrorrhagia. *Journal of Pediatric and Adolescent Gynecology* 1996;9:16.

Goldfarb AF. Dysfunctional uterine bleeding. In: Goldfarb AF, ed. *Clinical problems in pediatric and adolescent gynecology.* New York: Chapman & Hall; 1996:61.

Hillard PA. Abnormal uterine bleeding in adolescents. *Contemporary Pediatrics* 1995;12:79.

Levin C. Dysfunctional uterine bleeding in adolescents. *Curr Opin Pediatr* 328;1996;8:.

Polanecsky MM, Slap GB. Menstrual disorders in the adolescent: dysmenorrhea and dysfunctional uterine bleeding. *Pediatr Rev* 1992;13:83.

Rosenfeld J. Treatment of menorrhagia due to dysfunctional uterine bleeding. *Am Fam Physician* 1996;53:165.

Wathen PI, Henderson MC, Witz CA. Abnormal uterine bleeding. *Med Clin North Am* 1995;79:329.

Amenorrhea and Oligomenorrhea

Blythe M, Orr D. Common menstrual problems: II. amenorrhea and oligomenorrhea. *Adolescent Health Update* 1991;4(1):1.

Emans SJ. Menarche and beyond: Do eating and exercise make a difference? *Pediatr. Ann.* 26(suppl.):S137, 1997.

Gidwani GP. Menstruation and the athlete. *Contemporary Pediatrics* 1997;14:27.
Hergenroeder AC. Bone mineralization, hypothalamic amenorrhea, and sex steroid therapy in female adolescents and young adults. *J Pediatr* 1995;126:683.
Kiningham RB, Apgar BS, Schwenk TL. Evaluation of amenorrhea. *Am Fam Physician* 1996;53:1185.
Marshall LA. Clinical evaluation of amenorrhea in active and athletic women. *Clin Sports Med* 1994;13:371.
Polanecsky MM, Slap GB. Menstrual disorders in the adolescent: amenorrhea. *Pediatr Rev* 1992;13:43.
Saenger P. Turner's syndrome. *N Engl J Med* 1996;335:1749.
Shulman DI. Hyperprolactinemia in adolescents. *Adolescent and Pediatric Gynecology* 1995;8:213.
Skolnick AA. "Female athlete triad" risk for women. *JAMA* 1993;270:921.

Polycystic Ovary Syndrome

Franks S. Polycystic ovary syndrome. *N Engl J Med* 1995;333:853.
Gilchrist VJ, Hecht BR. A practical approach to hirsutism. *Am Fam Physician* 1995;52:1837.
Siegel SF, Lee PA. Polycystic ovary syndrome. *Curr Opin Pediatr* 1993;5:400.
Udoff LC, Adashi EY. Polycystic ovarian disease: current insights into an old problem. *Journal of Pediatric and Adolescent Gynecology* 1996;9:3.
Utiger RD. Insulin and the polycystic ovary syndrome. *N Engl J Med* 1996;335:657.
Winter JSD. Hyperandrogenism in female adolescents. *Curr Opin Pediatr* 1993;5:488.

Premenstrual Syndrome

DeMonico SO, Brown CS, Ling FW. Premenstrual syndrome. *Curr Opin Obstet Gynecol* 1994;6:499.
Fisher M, Trieller K, Napolitano B. Premenstrual syndrome in adolescents. *Journal of Adolescent Health Care* 1989;10:369.
Mortola JF. Assessment and management of premenstrual syndrome. *Curr Opin Obstet Gynecol* 1992;4:877.
Nader S. Premenstrual syndrome: tailoring treatment to symptoms. *Postgrad Med* 1991;90:173.
Osofsky HJ. Efficacious treatments of PMS: a need for further research. *JAMA* 1990;264:387.
Parker PD. Premenstrual syndrome. *Am Fam Physician* 1994;50:1309.
Rubinow DR, Schmidt PJ. The treatment of premenstrual syndrome: forward into the past. *N Engl J Med* 1995;332:1574.
Severino SK, Moline ML. Premenstrual syndrome: identification and management. *Drugs* 1995;49:71.
Steiner M, Steinberg S, Stewart D, et al. Fluoxetine in the treatment of premenstrual dysphoria. *N Engl J Med* 1995;332:1529.

Chronic Pelvic Pain

Arbel-DeRowe Y, Tepper R, Rosen DJ, et al. The contribution of pelvic ultrasonography to the diagnostic process in pediatric and adolescent gynecology. *J. Pediatr. Adolesc. Gyn.* 10:3,1997.
Cavanaugh RM Jr. Nongynecologic causes of unexplained lower abdominal pain in adolescent girls. *Clin Pediatr* 1996;35:337.
Davis GD, Thillet E, Lindemann J. Clinical characteristics of adolescent endometriosis. *J Adolesc Health* 1993; 14:362.
Durinzi KL, DeLeon FD. Endometriosis in the adolescent and and teenage female. *Adolescent and Pediatric Gynecology* 1993;6:3.
Gidwani GP. Chronic pelvic pain: steps to take before and after operative intervention. In: Pokorny S, ed. *Pediatric and adolescent gynecology*. New York: Chapman & Hall; 1996:41.
Hurd SJ, and Adamson GD. Pelvic pain: endometriosis as a differential diagnosis in adolescents. *Adolescent and Pediatric Gynecology* 1992;5:3.
Kozlowski KJ. Acute and chronic pelvic pain. In: Goldfarb AF, ed. *Clinical problems in pediatric and adolescent gynecology*. New York: Chapman & Hall; 1996:99.
Lu PY, Ory SJ. Endometriosis: current management. *Mayo Clin Proc* 1995;70:453.
Magrina JF, Cornella JL. Office management of ovarian cysts. *Mayo Clin Proc* 1997;72:653.
McGrath JW, Strickland JL. Chronic pelvic pain in the adolescent. *Adolescent and Pediatric Gynecology* 1995;8:107.
Murray S, London S. Management of ovarian cysts in neonates, children, and adolescents. *Adolescent and Pediatric Gynecology* 1995;8:64.
Reese KA, Reddy S, Rock JA. Endometriosis in an adolescent population: the Emory experience. *Journal of Pediatric and Adolescent Gynecology* 1996;9:125.
Rosenthal RH. Psychology of chronic pelvic pain. *Obstet Gynecol Clin North Am* 1993;20:627.
Ryder RM. Chronic pelvic pain. *Am Fam Physician* 1996;54:2225.

Toxic Shock Syndrome

Bryner CL Jr. Recurrent toxic shock syndrome. *American Family Practice* 1989;39:157.
Centers for Disease Control. Toxic shock syndrome–United States. *MMWR* 1997;46:492.
Reingold AC. Nonmenstrual toxic shock syndrome. *JAMA* 1983;249:932.
Resnick SD. Toxic shock syndrome: recent developments in pathogenesis. *J Pediatr* 1990;116:321.
Sagraves R. Menstrual toxic shock syndrome. *Am Pharm* 1995;NS35:12.
Strausbaugh LJ. Toxic shock syndrome: are you recognizing its changing presentations? *Postgrad Med* 1993;94:107.
Todd JD. Toxic shock syndrome. *Clin Microbiol Rev* 1988;1:432.
Wolf JE, Rabinowitz LG. Streptococcal toxic shock-like syndrome. *Arch Dermatol* 1995;131:73.

SEXUALLY TRANSMITTED DISEASES AND RELATED DISORDERS

Of any sexually active age cohort, teenagers have the highest rate of contracting sexually transmitted diseases (STDs) [1]. Approximately one fourth of sexually active teens become infected each year, accounting for 3 million cases [2,3]. People younger than the age of 25 years account for two thirds of all STDs in the United States [4]. Adolescence is a time of risk-taking behavior for many (Table 69), and the consequences can be dire:

- An estimated 10% of all sexually active young women are currently infected with *Chlamydia trachomatis* [5].
- Human papillomavirus (HPV) has become the most common viral STD, and as many as 15% of young women may be infected with it [6].
- From 1981 until 1992, gonorrhea was the most frequently reported STD in the United States, and 15- to 19-year-old women had the highest rate [7].
- During the same time period, syphilis rates among 15- to 19-year-old women rose 112%, and 41% among men in the same age group [7].
- Acquired immunodeficiency syndrome (AIDS) is now the sixth leading cause of death among young people aged 15 to 24 years [8]. However, because of the 8- to 10-year incubation period between human immunodeficiency virus (HIV) infection and AIDS, it is likely that most 20- to 24-year-olds were infected during their teens (Fig. 15).

Teenagers are unique in their risk factors for a number of reasons [3,9]. The adolescent cervix is more prone to infection because of its exposed columnar epithelium (ectropion) and the active squamous metaplasia occurring at the transformation zone. Local cervical protective antibodies are also diminished in young women [10]. Early sexual activity is especially correlated with an increased risk of multiple partners and decreased discrimination in selection of those partners. Use of alcohol and other drugs correlates with early and high-risk sexual activity, such as multiple partners or unprotected sex. Finally, there are particular subgroups of adolescents who are at increased risk for STDs: male homosexuals, street youth, incarcerated youth, and teenage prostitutes.

Vaginitis: General Considerations

During early puberty, increased levels of estrogen produce thickening of the vaginal mucosa with many layers of superficial, glycogen-rich cells. Lactobacilli use the new glycogen-rich environment to produce lactic acid and acetic acid, giving a new vaginal pH of 3.5 to 5.0. These two factors

TABLE 69. *Adolescents' risk factors for sexually transmitted diseases*

Behavior	Boys	Girls
Had sexual intercourse (lifetime)	54.0%	52.1%
Had sexual intercourse during the past 3 months (currently sexually active)	35.5%	40.4%
Had sexual intercourse with four or more people (lifetime)	20.9%	14.4%
First sexual intercourse before age 13 y	12.7%	4.9%
Used a condom during last sexual intercourse (among currently sexually active)	60.5%	48.6%
Injected illegal drugs (lifetime)	3.0%	1.0%

Centers for Disease Control and Prevention. Youth risk behavior surveillance: United States, 1995. *MMWR Morb Mortal Wkly Rep* 1996;45(SS-4):1.

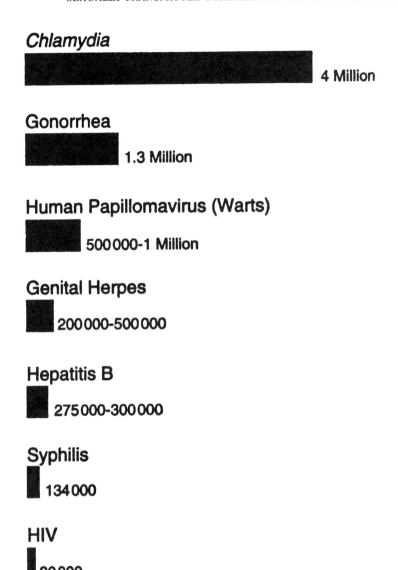

Chlamydia

4 Million

Gonorrhea

1.3 Million

Human Papillomavirus (Warts)

500 000-1 Million

Genital Herpes

200 000-500 000

Hepatitis B

275 000-300 000

Syphilis

134 000

HIV

80 000

FIG. 15. Estimated annual incidence of common sexually transmitted diseases in the United States. (Reproduced with permission from the American Medical Association. Randall T. News item. *JAMA* 1993;269:2716.)

alone—lactobacilli and an acidic pH—represent major defense mechanisms. Normally, 90% of the 10^5 to 10^7 organisms per milliliter present in the vagina are facultative lactobacilli (Fig. 16). Any disruption of this physiology (e.g., coital microtrauma, antibiotics, tight jeans or underwear, or sexually acquired pathogens) may produce vaginitis. A number of organisms normally comprise the vaginal flora that, given the proper conditions, can become pathogenic (e.g., *Candida albicans, Staphylococcus epidermidis,* diphtheroids, streptococci, *Escherichia coli, Gardnerella vaginalis,* various anaerobic bacteria; Table 70). In some pathologic conditions, such as bacterial vaginosis, the total concentration of bacteria increases 100- to 1,000-fold above normal.

Normally, an increase in vaginal discharge may be noticed 6 months to a year before menarche. At times, the discharge may be copious. Often a yellow stain is produced on the underpants because the discharge is mostly proteinaceous debris from lactobacilli that, when heated during washing, leaves a

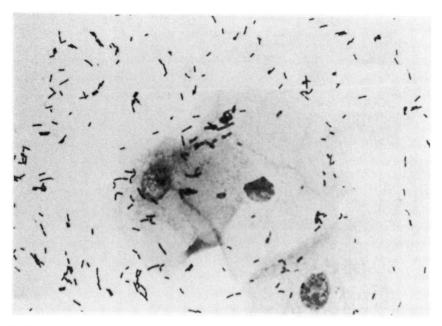

FIG. 16. Normal lactobacilli. Gram stain of vaginal discharge from a patient with a normal lactobacillus-dominant flora. (Courtesy of Sharon Hillier, Ph.D. From Eschenbach DA. Bacterial vaginosis. *Obstet Gynecol Clin North Am* 1989;16:593, with permission.)

yellowish stain on fabric. Patients should be reassured that menarche is impending, all is proceeding normally, and no cultures or treatment are necessary.

As estrogen stimulation increases, patients may continue to notice some pearly white vaginal discharge, so-called *physiologic leukorrhea*. This may represent the normal sloughing of superficial cells, mucus secretion from cervical columnar epithelium, or fluid transudation through the vaginal wall. The diagnosis can be made on visual inspection and requires no treatment other than reassurance and advice about proper hygiene and use of cotton underwear.

All adolescents with complaints of vaginal discharge deserve at least a visual inspection of the external genitalia. A history of sexual intercourse greatly expands the differential diagnosis and makes a complete pelvic examination necessary. In patients who are virginal, a speculum examination is not always necessary as long as adequate material can be obtained for culture and wet preparations (10% KOH and normal saline; Table 71). More recently, using polymerase chain reaction (PCR) tests and self-sampling with minimally invasive introital swabs, researchers demonstrated a high sensitivity for detecting both trichomonal and chlamydial infections [11]. In a related study, researchers have tried using leukocyte esterase dipsticks to test vaginal or cervical secretions for STD organisms, with only moderate success [12].

TABLE 70. *Normal vaginal flora of adolescents*

Lactobacilli	Diphtheroids
Bacteroides fragilis	Mycoplasmas
Enterobacteriaceae	*Gardnerella vaginalis*
Neisseria sicca	*Ureaplasma urealyticum*
Streptococcus sp.	*Staphylococcus* sp.
Candida albicans and other yeasts	Anaerobic bacteria

Adapted from Rosenfeld WD, Clark J. Vulvovaginitis and cervicitis. *Pediatr Clin North Am* 1989;36:489.

TABLE 71. *Use of wet preparations in diagnosis of vaginitis*

10% KOH: ⊕ in approximately 50% of *Candida* infections
Normal saline, 400× power (high, dry)
  <5 WBCs/hpf = Normal
        Rule out: bacterial vaginosis
  5–15 WBCs/hpf = Significant inflammation
        Rule out: candidiasis, *Trichomonas* infection,
            cervicitis
  >15 WBCs/hpf = Significant inflammation: suspect for
            Trichomonas infection or cervicitis
  Clue cells: Suspect for bacterial vaginosis if 20% or more of
        epithelial cells involved

WBCs/hpf, white blood cells per high-power field.

Finally, clinicians should be alert to the fact that a presenting complaint of dysuria may, in fact, represent vaginitis rather than a urinary tract infection. In one study of adolescents with dysuria, approximately one third had vaginitis, one third had urinary tract infection, and one third had both [13]. Patients with dysuria and vaginitis do not necessarily notice or complain of having a vaginal discharge. The easiest option is to screen the urine first and perform a pelvic examination if the urine is negative or if the teenager has a history of sexual activity.

The following general principles should be observed in evaluating and treating adolescents for STDs [1,3,14]:

- *Confidentiality must be ensured.* This is mandated, by law, in every state in the United States, primarily because of public health concerns. Yet, physicians sometimes breach confidentiality unintentionally by sending bills for laboratory tests or office visits home to parents or to insurance companies.
- *Every health encounter with an adolescent should be seen as an opportunity to elicit and update his or her sexual history.* This includes visits for acute illnesses and immunizations, and sports physicals.
- *Sexually active teenagers—both female and male—should be screened for STDs at least annually.*
- *Sexually active teenagers should be counseled appropriately about contraception.* In particular, the usefulness of barrier contraceptives in preventing STDs should be emphasized.
- *Sexual partners must be evaluated and treated.* The risk of multiple sexual partners should be emphasized strongly and repeatedly.
- *A Pap smear finding of dense inflammation has a strong correlation with the presence of an STD and should be followed up carefully with further testing.* Gonococcal, chlamydial, herpes simplex virus, or trichomonal infection all are possible causes [15]. However, the Pap smear is *not* an adequate screen for the presence of an STD [16].
- *When treating a patient for an STD, abstinence until the therapy is completed should be strongly urged.*
- *Efforts to maximize patient compliance should be made,* including education, reducing frequency of dosage, and avoiding painful treatments (e.g., intramuscular penicillin for gonorrhea).
- *A test of cure should be obtained for STDs.*
- *Female adolescents who have been raped have a high prevalence of preexisting STDs and a lower but still substantial risk of acquiring such diseases from the assault* [17]. Careful screening is therefore important.

Candidiasis

Although it is not an STD, Candidiasis is extremely common among young women—representing perhaps 50% of all cases of vaginitis—and may be shared by sexual partners. Most (85%) cases represent infection with *C. albicans* [18]. An estimated 75% of women will experience at least one episode of candidal vulvovaginitis during their lifetime, and 40% to 45% will have two or more episodes [19]. Antibiotics, oral contraceptives (OCs) [20], and microabrasions from sexual intercourse all may disrupt the normal vaginal homeostasis and therefore predispose to candidal overgrowth. So, too, may frequent intercourse [21]. Yeast have special endocrine receptors and a fondness for glycogen, which may explain the increased risk for OC users and girls with diabetes [18,20].

Signs and Symptoms

Infected women often complain of burning, itching, and a feeling of vaginal fullness. Occasionally, urinary symptoms may be present. On examination, the "classic" cottage-cheese–like discharge, with clumps adherent to the vaginal wall, is present in less than half of patients. If antibiotics are the precipitating factor, less discharge and more pruritus may be noticeable [22]. One reason for avoiding the casual administration of antibiotics for upper respiratory infections or viral pharyngitis in female adolescents is to avoid this unpleasant complication. Premenstrual onset of a vaginal discharge is typical, with improvement during menses. A certain subgroup of women seems prone to recurrent candidal infections. Unlike prepubertal girls, where *Candida* may represent the first sign of diabetes mellitus, adolescents normally have other physiologic reasons for such recurrences—for example, tight jeans, nylon underwear, or frequent use of antibiotics.

Diagnosis

Diagnostic wet preparations may demonstrate hyphae or spores, either on the KOH or the saline slides. However, the yield of positive KOH preparations may be 50% or lower [18]. Therefore, a high clinical suspicion should be maintained. Candidal infection is usually associated with a normal vaginal pH (≤4.5). Culturing the discharge on Nickerson's medium may be useful. Typically, brownish colonies form within 24 to 72 hours when incubated in the office at room temperature. Rapid in-office tests for candidal antigens are also commercially available and require only 3 to 5 minutes to process. Identifying yeasts and mycelia in the *absence* of symptoms should not lead to treatment because 10% to 20% of women normally harbor various *Candida* species and other yeasts in their vaginas [19].

Treatment

A variety of broad-spectrum antifungal agents (imidazoles and, more recently, terconazole, a triazole compound) are currently available and have cure rates in the 85% to 95% range. These include single-dose treatment, 3-day regimens, and 7-day regimens (Table 72). However, the latest and easiest method of treatment is to use a single oral dose of fluconazole (Diflucan), which is as effective as 3 days of intravaginal clotrimazole and is preferred by many patients [23,24]. Even a single dose of fluconazole can cause side effects, however: nausea, vomiting, abdominal pain, or headache in about 15% of patients [23]. In addition, the drug's safety for use during pregnancy or breast-feeding is unknown. Recurrences are quite common with all regimens. Associated vulvitis may require the use of sitz baths, baking soda, and hydrocortisone ointment.

For persistent or recurrent infection, a variety of methods can be tried [19,25]:

- A single prolonged course of Diflucan (e.g., 7–14 days days)
- Treatment through an entire menstrual cycle
- Use of an acidifying douche (e.g., Acijel)
- Use of a *Lactobacillus acidophilus* douche or tampon
- Treatment of the male partner with an antifungal ointment
- Use of a condom by the male partner
- Use of prophylactic oral ketoconazole, 100 mg daily, for up to 6 months, or oral fluconazole, 150 mg, once weekly or monthly, has been effective in some patients [26].
- Use of oral Nystatin (500,000 units bid–tid for 10 days) to eliminate the gastrointestinal reservoir in both partners may be tried, but its efficacy remains unproven.

Trichomoniasis

Trichomonas vaginalis is a flagellated protozoan that is a frequent cause of vaginitis (38% of STD clinic patients in one study [27]). Despite the fact that this organism can survive in wet towels for a few hours, it is almost exclusively sexually transmitted and is frequently associated with other STDs

TABLE 72. *A variety of treatments for vaginal candidiasis*

Drug	Trade name	Form	Prescription	Cost[a]
Oral				
Fluconazole	Diflucan (Roerig)	150-mg tab	1 tablet PO once	1 tab = $10.62
Intravaginal				
Over-the-counter				
Clotrimazole	Gyne-Lotrimin (Schering)	1% cream	5 g at bedtime × 7d	45 g = $12.00
	Mycelex-7 (Miles)	1% cream	5 g at bedtime × 7d	45 g = $11.77
Miconazole	Monistat-7 (Ortho)	2% cream	5 g at bedtime × 7d	45 g = $12.85
		100-mg supps	1 supp at bedtime ×7d	7 supps = $12.85
Prescription				
Butoconazole	Femstat (Syntex)	2% cream	5 g at bedtime × 3d	28 g = $18.35
Miconazole	Monistat-3 (Ortho)	200-mg supps	1 supp at bedtime × 3d	3 supps = $23.22
Terconazole	Terazol-7 (Ortho)	0.4% cream	5 g at bedtime × 7d	45 g = $22.26
	Terazol-3 (Ortho)	0.8% cream	5 g at bedtime × 3d	20 g = $22.26
		80-mg supps	1 supp at bedtime × 3d	3 supps = $22.26
Tioconazole	Vagistat (Mead Johnson)	6.5% ointment	4.6 g at bedtime × 1d	4.6 g = $24.20

[a]Cost to the pharmacist for package size necessary for a required course of therapy.
From The Medical Letter. Oral fluconazole for vaginal candidiasis. *The Medical Letter* 1994;36 (931):81.

[1,18]. In men, infection tends to be asymptomatic up to 90% of the time [1]. As with most STDs, the man is a more effective transmitting agent than the woman: trichomoniasis develops in 30% to 40% of men having intercourse with infected women, versus in 80% to 85% of female partners of infected men. Colonization during pregnancy is high, with rates ranging from 25% to 40%, and there is some evidence of an association with premature rupture of the membranes and preterm delivery [19]. Incubation period is 4 to 30 days.

Signs and Symptoms

In women, infection can be asymptomatic, but about half of women manifest a vaginal discharge—classically, yellowish-green, frothy, malodorous, with a pH greater than 5.0. Also "classic" is the appearance of punctate hemorrhages on the cervix ("strawberry cervix"), even though this is a finding in less than 5% of cases. Patients frequently complain of intense vaginal pruritus, dyspareunia, and urinary symptoms. Organisms may be found in the urine, although it remains unclear whether this represents actual urethral or bladder infection.

Sexually transmitted diseases frequently "travel in pairs," and nowhere is this more true than with *Trichomonas* infection. *T. vaginalis* can be found in 8% to 62% of women and nearly 20% of men with gonorrhea [28], and candidal infections coexist with it in as many as 97% of symptomatic women [29]. Unfortunately, symptoms of trichomoniasis often mimic other STDs, and the protozoan can be difficult to spot microscopically.

Diagnosis

Three tests are clinically useful for confirming *Trichomonas* infection: the saline wet preparation, a Pap smear, and culture. Saline wet preparations are the easiest and most cost-effective means of diagnosis, although they may miss up to 40% of infections, particularly in asymptomatic patients. Pap smears carry a false-negative rate up to 30% compared with culture [30], but some experts believe that the diagnosis of trichomoniasis by Pap smear is unreliable anyway [18]. Diamond's and Feinberg-Whittington media can be used for culture. When incubated for 1 to 3 days at 36° to 37°C, they each demonstrate an in vitro recovery rate of 100%, even for a small inoculum of trichomonads. One new development is the use of monoclonal antibodies against the protozoan's outer membrane protein that can detect both viable and nonviable organisms [27].

Generally, *Trichomonas* infection stimulates an abundant inflammatory response. Therefore, a saline wet preparation showing more than 15 white blood cells (WBCs) per high-power field (hpf) should alert the examiner to search carefully for trichomonads. These pear-shaped, flagellated, motile organisms are a few microns larger than white cells (Fig. 17). Although gentle warming may increase their motility, they are also prone to lose their motility or die under the heat of the microscope, especially if insufficient saline is used. An ideal saline wet mount is prepared by putting several drops of normal saline on a slide, mixing in a small amount of the vaginal discharge, adding a cover slip, and observing under the microscope (high dry, 400×) no more than 5 minutes later. An alternative is to collect a sample of discharge and add it to a small test tube containing normal saline. This has the advantage of giving the examiner more time and additional material if more than one preparation is necessary.

Vaginal pH may also be elevated (>5.0), although this occurs in bacterial vaginosis as well. An easy way to determine pH is to place a piece of nitrazine paper in the well of the vaginal speculum after it is withdrawn.

Treatment

Metronidazole is the treatment of choice, either as a single oral 2-g dose (four 500-mg tablets or eight 250-mg tablets) or 7-day course, 500 mg two times a day [19,31]. Patients with treatment failures can be given a repeat single dose or a longer course. Either the partner should be seen as well, or a double prescription written, because he will require treatment as well. Clearly, the single-dose regimen is easier and preferable for compliance.

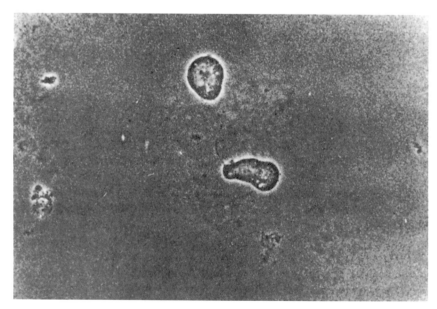

FIG. 17. Trichomonads. (Hammill HA. *Trichomonas vaginalis. Obstet Gynecol Clin North Am* 1989;16: 531, with permission.)

Side effects, such as gastrointestinal upset, metallic aftertaste, and candidal vaginitis, may be minimized with single-dose treatment as well. When combined with alcohol, metronidazole has a disulfiram-like (Antabuse) effect; therefore, alcohol should be assiduously avoided during the course of treatment. Cure rates approach 95% if the partner is treated simultaneously [1]. Resistant organisms are rare and may respond to higher doses of metronidazole or use of the intravaginal gel [18]. A few metronidazole-resistant strains of *Trichomonas* have been reported, and optimal treatment for these is undetermined [31].

Pregnant or lactating women require special consideration because a metabolite of metronidazole interacts with DNA, and the drug crosses the placenta and achieves high levels in breast milk. The risk of teratogenicity is probably more theoretical than actual, according to many studies [32]. Nevertheless, metronidazole is contraindicated in the first trimester [19]. Thereafter, it can be used in a single dose. In the first trimester, standard treatment is the use of clotrimazole, one 100-mg tablet intravaginally for 7 nights. This therapy has a cure rate of only 20%, but symptoms diminish in nearly 50% of patients. Betadine cream and douches may also be helpful. For lactating young women, metronidazole 2 g orally can be given in a single dose, with a 24-hour interruption in breast-feeding [18].

Patients with recurrent infections should be treated with a higher dose of metronidazole, either 2 g orally for 3 days or 500 g twice daily for 14 days, and have their urine and their partner's urine examined as a possible hidden reservoir. Poor compliance with the 7-day regimen and reinfection from an untreated sexual partner are by far the most likely causes of treatment failure, not resistant organisms.

Bacterial Vaginosis

Previously known as *Hemophilus vaginalis, G. vaginalis, Corynebacterium vaginalis,* or nonspecific vaginitis, bacterial vaginosis is one of the most common, least understood, and most significant causes of vaginitis. As many as 35% of women attending STD clinics and 15% to 20% of pregnant women have this vaginal disorder [33]. Since 1955, attention has been focused on *G. vaginalis*—a gram-negative facultative anaerobe named after Dr. Gardner—as the sole culprit [33,34]. Current thinking is that bacterial vaginosis involves a complex chain of events in the normal vaginal ecology, with *G. vaginalis* playing a co-starring role with facultative anaerobes, *Mycoplasma hominis,* and *Mobiluncus* species [31,35]. However, culturing for any of these organisms is not useful in establishing or confirming the diagnosis [36]. Some researchers now believe that pathogens involved in bacterial vaginosis may be responsible for up to 50% of upper tract disease (e.g., pelvic inflammatory disease [PID]) [33,37].

As illustrated in Figure 16, normal women have a lactobacillus-dominant flora with an acidic pH. For unknown reasons, patients with bacterial vaginosis experience a decreased oxidation–reduction potential with an increase in anaerobic metabolism, encouraging an overgrowth of *G. vaginalis,* anaerobic peptostreptococci, gram-negative bacteria, *M. hominis,* and *Mobiluncus.* Factors associated with the disorder include multiple sexual partners, use of an intrauterine device (IUD), lack of contraception, and the presence of another STD [18].

Bacterial vaginosis has also been implicated in preterm births [38].

Signs and Symptoms

Young women with bacterial vaginosis may have no signs or symptoms, but up to 50% have a grayish-white ("flour paste"), malodorous, frothy vaginal discharge. Vaginal pH is often 5.0 or greater. As the term *vaginosis* implies, there are few signs or symptoms of active inflammation, or *vaginitis.* Therefore, symptoms like dysuria and pruritus are uncommon, and the vulva, vagina, and cervix usually appear normal except for the presence of the discharge adherent to the vaginal walls. Frequently, a characteristic "fishy" odor during menstruation or after sexual activity may bring the patient in for attention. With ejaculation, seminal fluid transiently increases the vaginal pH, liberating amines from their protein attachment. These then become volatilized in the air and smell "fishy."

Diagnosis

The presence of three or more of the following criteria allows the diagnosis of bacterial vaginosis to be made [19,36]:

- *Homogeneous gray-white adherent discharge.* This discharge is different from the normal, thick, milky-appearing physiologic leukorrhea. Vaginal walls should not be erythematous (candidiasis) or have a punctate, strawberry appearance (trichomoniasis). In addition, a yellow or foamy quality suggests other forms of vaginitis or cervicitis.
- *Vaginal pH > 4.5.* Virtually all affected patients have an abnormally high pH, but the reverse does not hold true: normal women frequently have a pH > 4.5, as do patients with trichomoniasis or cervicitis. Black teenagers have a slightly higher vaginal pH (4.7 ± 0.6), which may make them more susceptible to common vaginal infections [39].
- *Clue cells comprising at least 20% of epithelial cells.* Clue cells are vaginal epithelial cells that are studded with many small bits of refractile bacteria. Originally believed to be *G. vaginalis* covering the epithelial cells, these bacteria actually represent a variety of anaerobes. Under high dry power magnification, a clue cell's border has a serrated appearance and is indistinct because of the large amount of adherent bacteria (Fig. 18). Large numbers of lactobacilli are typically absent, as are increased numbers of white blood cells per high-power field. Presence of clue cells is probably the single most important diagnostic criterion in bacterial vaginosis.
- *Fishy amine odor when vaginal fluid is mixed with 10% KOH.* An amine odor may also be present in patients with *Trichomonas* infections.

Gram-stain criteria have also been developed for the diagnosis of bacterial vaginosis. An increase in *G. vaginalis* and at least one other bacteria (e.g., gram-positive cocci, gram-negative rods, fusiform bacilli) to five or more per oil immersion field, and five or fewer lactobacilli per oil immersion field, constitute an easy and accurate test. Cultures are not useful because this disorder represents an overgrowth phenomenon involving many different organisms. Although virtually all patients with bacterial vaginosis have *G. vaginalis,* 40% to 50% of normal women harbor the organism as well, and it can still be isolated in a similar percentage of women who have been cured of bacterial vaginosis [19].

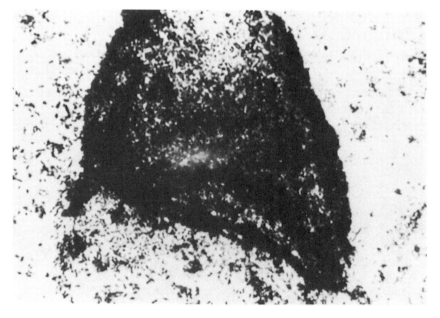

FIG. 18. Clue cell, a vaginal epithelial cell with attachment of many bacteria. Note the loss of the cell border margins. (Courtesy of Sharon Hillier, Ph.D. From Eschenbach DA. Bacterial vaginosis. *Obstet Gynecol Clin North Am* 1989;16:593, with permission.)

Treatment

Only young women who are symptomatic require treatment (half of those who meet the clinical criteria are asymptomatic) [19]. Typical therapy consists of metronidazole, 500 mg twice daily for 7 days, with cure rates of 80% to 95% (Table 73) [36]. A single dose of 2 g has a slightly lower cure rate, 84%, but may be preferable to a 7-day course, especially considering the ease of treating partners [31,40]. Another acceptable regimen is clindamycin, 300 mg orally, twice a day for 7 days.

Alternative regimens include vaginal metronidazole 0.75% gel (5 g intravaginally once or twice a day for 5 days) or vaginal clindamycin 2% cream (5 g intravaginally at bedtime for 7 days). These products are probably safe for use during pregnancy and may be better tolerated than 7 days of oral metronidazole [31].

During pregnancy, treatment of women with bacterial vaginosis with oral metronidazole and erythromycin can significantly decrease preterm deliveries, according to one study. The rate of preterm delivery was 31% with treatment, versus 49% with placebo [41].

Asymptomatic patients do *not* require treatment because the imbalance may spontaneously correct itself within several months [18,42]. Therapy during pregnancy with oral metronidazole is not advocated, although clindamycin or vaginal metronidazole can be used [31,43,44]. Treatment of the male partner remains controversial because it does not seem successful in preventing recurrent infection in the woman or even in eradicating *G. vaginalis* in the male urethra [36].

Vaginitis and Cervicitis

Herpes Simplex Infections

Genital herpes is one of the most common STDs in the United States, with more than 30 million people infected according to serologic studies [19]. Ten percent of herpes genital infections involve herpes simplex virus type I (HSV-I) and 90% type II (HSV-II) [45]. In a high-risk population, as many as 20% of sexually active female teens are seropositive for HSV-II [46]; in a more typical population, the incidence of positive cultures is 1% to 12% [47,48]. Not only is this a devastating infection for many adolescents, who view it as a "life sentence"—far worse than gonorrhea or syphilis—but it also has significant implications for pregnant teenagers and in its possible status as a cofactor in cervical cancer. HSV infection is the only STD that can recur without any further sexual contact.

A 15-fold increase has occurred in genital HSV infections since the early 1970s [9,49]. More than 60% of adult women have HSV antibodies [50], and the clinical history is often a poor indicator of HSV infection. In one study, only one fourth of patients with HSV-II antibodies had positive clinical histories [51]. Patients with asymptomatic infection may serve as reservoirs for both HSV-I and HSV-II infections [52,53]. Infection results from direct viral contact with susceptible mucous membranes,

TABLE 73. *Treatment regimens for bacterial vaginosis*

Antimicrobial agent		Cure rate
Effective		
Metronidazole	500 mg bid × 7d or 2 g × 1 dose	79–100%
	0.75% intravaginal gel, 1 applicatorful intravaginally bid × 5d	65–69%
Ampicillin	500 mg qid × 7d	33–43%
Clindamycin	2% cream × 7d	93%
Not effective		
Triple sulfa vaginal cream		
Betadine vaginal preparations		
Oral erythromycin		
Oral tetracycline		

From Eschenbach DA. Bacterial vaginosis: emphasis on upper genital tract complications. *Obstet Gynecol Clin North Am* 1989;16:593. Adapted, with permission.

with type II transmitted by sexual intercourse and type I probably by orogenital contact. As with *T. vaginalis*, HSV theoretically can survive on fomites (e.g., unchlorinated hot tubs, plastic seats), but this is not thought to be a major pathway for dissemination [54,55].

Herpes simplex virus lesions are extremely infectious, with 30% to 60% of exposed partners acquiring the disease. However, studies show a great deal of variation in the duration of viral shedding, from an average of 2 days [53] to 8 to 18 days [56]. Subclinical shedding can occur as well [53]. Consequently, many cases of genital herpes are acquired from people who do not know at the time that they have a genital infection or who are asymptomatic at the time of the sexual encounter.

Neonatal infections can be acquired transplacentally or postnatally, but most occur during vaginal delivery through an infected maternal genital tract. Estimated incidence is 1 in 2,000 to 10,000 deliveries, and mortality is greater than 50% [57]. HSV-II can transform host cells in vitro and has been associated with abnormal cervical cytology, but the exact nature of this relationship remains unclear.

Signs and Symptoms

Primary infection with HSV is often quite dramatic and painful. The incubation period is 3 to 7 days. Typically, the patient notices an area of pruritus or hyperesthesia, followed by an outbreak of painful vesicles, 1 to 3 mm in diameter, on an indurated, erythematous base. These remain for 3 to 15 days and may break down or coalesce into shallow, tender, grayish ulcers, but they heal without scarring. Lesions can be located anywhere on the genitalia, and a cervicitis with mucopurulent discharge is often present as well. Dysuria is often prominent, and acute urinary retention secondary to either extreme pain or a neurogenic bladder is not unusual.

Systemic symptoms include fever, malaise, headache, and enlarged, tender inguinal nodes. Between 40% and 75% of patients report constitutional symptoms [56]. Significant complications include viral meningitis and lower motor neuron or autonomic nervous system dysfunction [58], and are more common in women [45]. In addition, herpetic lesions may develop in extragenital sites in 10% of men and 25% of women (e.g., thorax, fingers, thighs), probably because of autoinoculation.

Between one third and one half of patients experience a recurrence within 6 months of the primary episode. Recurrences are more likely with HSV-II infection than HSV-I [58]. The neurotropic HSV reactivates within the nuclei of sensory ganglia and travels along nerve axons to the body surface. This occurs despite the production of lifelong complement-fixing antibodies within a week after primary infection in immunocompetent patients. Recurrences are frequently heralded by prodromal symptoms such as paresthesias, pruritus, and burning. Constitutional symptoms are not common. Exactly what causes recurrences is unknown. Stress seems to play a role [45,59]. Painful papules and vesicles develop within the first few days, but the entire course—including shedding—lasts only several days and is not nearly as severe as the primary episode. Viral shedding (usually HSV-II) has been demonstrated between clinically apparent recurrences [53,60]. One study found that subclinical shedding occurs frequently and accounts for nearly one third of the total days of HSV reactivation [53].

Diagnosis

The clinical picture of HSV primary infection is usually diagnostic in itself, but the presence of the virus can be confirmed in uncertain cases with the use of cytology or culture. Either a Tzank preparation or a Pap smear can be a useful office technique. A vesicle is unroofed, the base is scraped, and the material is smeared on a slide and either stained with a Giemsa or Wright stain or sprayed with Pap fixative. Multinucleated giant cells suggest infection. However, this technique may be positive only 50% of the time. A negative smear does not rule out HSV infection. Consequently, viral culture remains the definitive test, although it, too, may remain negative 20% to 30% of the time even in the presence of HSV infection [45]. Up to 6 days may be required to document cytopathic changes in tissue culture. Vesicles yield a much higher rate of positive cultures than ulcers or crusted lesions. Serologic testing is of limited value except in primary infections if the patient is initially seronegative. Antibody levels persist for life, but most laboratories cannot discriminate between HSV-I and HSV-II. A newer enzyme immunoassay (EIA), Herpcheck (Dupont, Wilmington, DE) is 97% sensitive and 100% specific in detecting HSV in genital samples, but requires a good deal of technical skill [61]. New PCR assays also show promise [45,62].

Treatment

There is no cure for genital herpes. Acyclovir, a synthetic purine nucleoside that HSV (but not normal cells) incorporates into its DNA, has become the mainstay of symptomatic treatment. Once acyclovir is phosphorylated and becomes incorporated into the viral genome, DNA synthesis ceases. However, clinical trials show that acyclovir provides only partial control of the initial outbreak and does not eradicate the latent virus nor prevent subsequent risk, frequency, or severity of recurrences once the drug is discontinued [19]. Daily suppressive therapy is effective, however, in reducing recurrences by at least 75% in patients who have six or more episodes per year [19]. Daily treatment can also suppress subclinical shedding, which may have important implications in preventing transmission of the virus to noninfected partners [63].

Acyclovir can be used topically, orally, or intravenously (Table 74). However, topical acyclovir is now being discouraged because it is minimally effective and may produce pain because of its polyethylene glycol base [45]. Primary infections warrant oral treatment, with intravenous use reserved for severe cases. Treatment has been shown to decrease the duration of viral shedding and to hasten the healing of lesions. Because long-term effects on the fetus are unknown, oral acyclovir is not usually recommended during pregnancy. Nevertheless, severe disease may necessitate the use of intravenous acyclovir [19].

Recurrences may be diminished with long-term oral acyclovir [64,65], but the drug should be reserved for those with six or more episodes per year [19]. Its safety and efficacy have now been documented for up to 5 years [66]. If acyclovir is used during the prodrome or within 2 days of a recurrence, patients may benefit from oral therapy. However, recurrent episodic treatment is not beneficial for most patients [45].

Side effects of short-term oral therapy include gastrointestinal upset, headache, diarrhea, dizziness, and fatigue [67]. Adjunctive treatment with oral analgesics, topical use of viscous lidocaine jelly or ointment, warm water sitz baths, and gentle douches with Betadine solution are often useful for symptomatic relief and prevention of secondary bacterial infection.

New drugs for genital herpes infections include famciclovir (Famvir), a twice-a-day drug that decreases viral shedding and is well tolerated, and topical penciclovir [55,68].

Patients with HSV genital infections should be advised to abstain from sexual activity until all lesions are healed, to avoid autoinnoculation, to inform their sexual partners so that they can seek treatment, and to use latex condoms [45].

Human Papillomavirus Infection

Human papillomavirus infection is the most common viral STD in the United States today [69], with adolescents probably at greatest risk [70–72]. Since the mid-1980s, knowledge of HPV infection has increased dramatically, although many clinicians may still be unaware of its manifestations or significance. Since the early 1970s, the prevalence of HPV has apparently increased severalfold [9,73]. Rates of infected adolescent women range from 5% to 46% in various studies, depending on the pop-

TABLE 74. *Use of acyclovir in treating first-episode and recurrent herpes simplex virus infections*

Mode of administration	Dose	Frequency	Duration
First clinical episode			
Oral	200 mg	Five times daily	7–10 d, or until resolution
Intravenous	5–10 mg/kg	Every 8 hours	5–7 d, or until resolution
Daily suppressive therapy (six or more recurrences per year)			
Oral	400 mg	Twice daily	
or	200 mg	Three to five times daily	

Adapted from Centers for Disease Control and Prevention. 1993 Sexually transmitted diseases treatment guidelines. *MMWR Morb Mortal Wkly Rep* 1993;42(no. RR-14):22.

ulation studied and the diagnostic method used [69,74–79]. An excellent 1989 study of nearly 250 female adolescents in New York revealed an overall prevalence rate for HPV of 38%. Those teenagers with multiple lifetime partners showed a prevalence rate of 54% [80]. In general, the prevalence of HPV increases as the sensitivity of the test for HPV DNA increases. For example, in a large study of college-aged women, a commercially available dot hybridization test (ViraPAP; Life Technologies, Gaithersburg, MD) found an 11% prevalence of HPV, whereas PCR techniques identified a 46% infection rate [78].

Not surprisingly, abnormal Pap smears among adolescents are increasing dramatically as well because most, if not all, are linked to HPV [81,82]. One study of over 230,000 Pap smears in all women found that 1.7% had evidence of HPV infection. Although 21- to 25-year-old women had the highest rate (2.5%), women aged 16 to 20 years were next (2.1%) [83]. Because not all female adolescents are sexually active, those who *are* probably represent the group at highest risk for HPV infection [84]. In the New York study, for example, 17% of adolescents harboring HPV had cytologic abnormalities, versus 2.7% of uninfected patients [80]. The younger a teenager is when she begins having intercourse, the greater the likelihood of progression from HPV infection to a dysplastic lesion [85].

Human papillomavirus is clearly associated with certain risk factors [71,72,77,86,87]:

- Multiple partners
- Having multiple partners who, themselves, have had multiple partners
- Increased sexual activity at a younger age
- Early menarche
- First intercourse within 18 months of menarche
- Other STDs, especially chlamydial infection

Other factors (cigarette smoking, type of contraception used, impaired immune response) may also play a significant role, but have been more difficult to delineate. Clearly, the two most important factors are younger age and number of partners. In one study, women with five or more sexual partners in the previous two years had a 12-fold increased risk of HPV [88].

Not all HPV subtypes are created equal. Molecular hybridization techniques—so-called "DNA probes"—have identified more than 60 types of HPV, with one third associated with genital tract infection. Some cause trivial or benign disease, some have moderate risk of oncogenicity, and some have high malignant potential (Table 75) [72]. The evidence for the link between HPV and certain genital tract cancers, especially cervical, is now compelling [82,89–96]. Along with *C. trachomatis*, HPV shares a predilection for the adolescent cervix because the maturing cervix contains an area of columnar cells in the ectocervix that is eventually be replaced or transformed into squamous cells—a process known as squamous metaplasia—which results in a relative increase in resistance to external forces. On pelvic examination, this zone is seen as an ectropion (*not* a "cervical erosion"). This "transformation zone" may be a target site for both neoplastic changes and certain infections.

After contact with an infected partner, a viral reservoir is established, and the virus enters a latent phase. Once reactivated, the virus produces DNA, capsid proteins, and viral particles [72]. In low-grade lesions, the HPV genome remains in an episomal (circular, nonintegrated) form, whereas in invasive cervical cancer, the genome is integrated into the host DNA [82].

TABLE 75. *Clinically significant human papillomavirus types*

Type number	Clinical manifestations
1–4, 7, 10, 28	Plantar and common warts
6, 11	Juvenile laryngeal papillomatosis
6, 11, 16, 18, 31, 33, 35, 39, 41–45, 51–56, 59	**Genital tract infection**
16, 18	High malignant potential; type 16 common in adolescents
31	Intermediate malignant potential
6, 11	External anogenital infection; low malignant potential

Adapted from Davis AJ, Emans SJ. Human papilloma virus infection in the pediatric and adolescent patient. *J Pediatr* 1989;115:1; and Mayeaux EJ, Harper MB, Barksdale W, et al. Noncervical human papillomavirus genital infections. *Am Fam Physician* 1995;52:1137.

The entire genital tract of men and women is at risk, including the vulva, vagina, cervix, penis, urethra, and perianal tissue. However, the middle third of the vagina is often spared. The infection easily may be recognizable as venereal warts (*condylomata*) or visualized only on application of acetic acid and use of magnification (subclinical disease). Half of patients with vulvar disease also have cervical involvement, and one third have vaginal disease [73]. Nearly half of patients with involvement at more than one site (multicentric disease) are infected with more than one HPV type [97].

One of the great mysteries of HPV disease is how, when, and why patients should be treated. Prevalence rates are extremely high, yet rates of cervical cancer are relatively low. Other than being infected with an HPV subtype that is highly oncogenic (subtypes 16 and 18, in particular), little is known about the factors surrounding progression or regression. Indeed, in one study of 51 sexually active 13- to 21-year-old women, using Southern blot hybridization DNA techniques, 39% of patients were initially infected, and 26% were found to be infected at a second visit 6 to 36 months later. However, only 8% were infected at both visits, and only one patient had the same HPV subtype [98]!

Signs and Symptoms

Human papillomavirus infection develops in approximately two thirds of exposed sexual partners, with a latency period ranging from 1 to 20 months (average, 2–3 months) [99]. Condylomata may have incubation periods as short as 3 weeks. Yet, many patients with subclinical HPV infection but without condylomata can have no obvious signs or symptoms. Some female patients may have symptoms of dyspareunia or vaginitis.

Overt clinical disease—condylomata, erythematous or pigmented macules, and flat papules—is most commonly seen on the external genitalia, where coital friction has occurred. Genital warts may be polypoid masses, with irregular or verrucous surfaces, or fleshy, pink, sessile tumors with capillary loops inside. Women frequently show condylomata on the posterior part of the introitus and adjacent labia; men frequently have involvement of the shaft, frenulum, coronal sulcus, and glans. Male homosexuals and women engaging in anal sex commonly have involvement of the perianal area. Half of women with external vulvar disease have cervical disease as well [100].

Men represent a large reservoir of subclinical and unsuspected disease [101]. Usually, their infection is not diagnosed until the diagnosis is made in their female partner. In one study, 41% of male partners of infected women had grossly visible disease, yet only 16% were aware of their infection [102].

Given the frequency of this infection and its relative "silent" nature, clinicians must maintain a high index of suspicion in any sexually active teenager, male or female (male teens seem to have a lower prevalence rate, about 1% to 8%) [103]. Some physicians are encouraging sexually active female adolescents to have twice-yearly pelvic examinations.

Diagnosis

The detection of subclinical disease can be maximized through the application of acetic acid in a 3% to 5% solution, followed by magnification with either a hand lens or colposcope. With HPV infection, small, white plaques, so-called "acetowhite" tissue, are seen. Acetic acid causes protein in the nuclei and cytoplasm of cells to coagulate. Cells with abnormal DNA content have a higher density and appear white. The degree of whiteness can be amplified by using a green filter on the colposcope. Colposcopy is used not only for diagnosis but to perform directed biopsies [71].

In one study of male partners of infected women, 29% of the men would have been classified as unaffected if this "acetowhite" test had not been performed, and an additional 30% had other lesions discovered in conjunction with their other, easily recognizable disease [102]. Men should soak their penis in 3% acetic acid for 5 minutes before examination, using cotton gauze pads. In women, subclinical infection of the vulva and vagina can be detected using the same 3% to 5% acetic acid, which may sting slightly when applied with large cotton applicators. In the vagina, "acetowhite" flecks against the normal epithelial background (reverse punctation) indicate HPV infection. Colposcopy can aid greatly in the diagnosis [71].

Cervical infection is the most common form of subclinical infection and is usually first discovered by Pap smear. The presence of "koilocytes"—squamous epithelial cells with swollen, raisin-like nuclei surrounded by a halo—is pathognomonic of HPV infection (Fig. 19). Unfortunately, the Pap smear has a relatively poor sensitivity and specificity for determining cervical lesions, with a false-

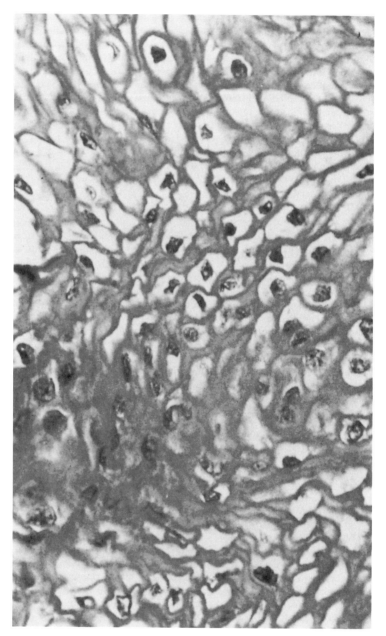

FIG. 19. Koilocytes. Biopsy specimen of a cervical flat condyloma, showing koilocytes in the upper third. Koilocytes are cells with raisin-like nuclei and are suggestive of human papillomavirus infection. (Moscicki B. HPV infections: an old STD revisited. *Contemporary Pediatrics* 1989;6:12; and Meisels A, Morin C. Human papillomavirus and cancer of the uterine cervix. *Gynecol Oncol* 1981;12:S111, with permission.)

negative rate of 20% to 50% [71]. In addition, the terminology can be very confusing (see "The Pap Smear," in the section on Menstrual Disorders). However, Pap smears *can* serve as a useful mass screening tool, determining who should be screened further by colposcopy and directed biopsy (see Table 52). Any of the following terms probably connote HPV infection—"koilocytes," "dysplasia," "carcinoma in situ," "carcinoma," and "reactive atypical cells." Pathologists often use the terms *cervi-*

cal intraepithelial neoplasia (CIN) and *dysplasia* interchangeably, even though the former is a histologic diagnosis and the latter is a cytologic one (see Table 53). HPV infection should be viewed as part of the continuum in the development of cervical cancer, and any dysplasia requires further evaluation and treatment [104].

The natural history of HPV infection varies according to location and subtype. Vulvar or vaginal condylomata often regress within 3 to 5 years, even without treatment [105]. Cervical HPV infection without dysplasia usually regresses (79%), but 8% to 14% of cases progress to CIN within 2 years [106,107]. If dysplasia is initially present, that figure increases to 26%, and an initial diagnosis of "warty atypia" shows a 50% progression rate to either CIN or overt cervical cancer [107]. It is possible that the process of performing a biopsy may alter the normal rate of progression by stimulating the host's immune system [108]. As dysplasia progresses to CIN, the presence of "koilocytes" diminishes. Spontaneous regression is rarer with HPV 16, and 85% of women younger than age 30 years who had CIN were found to have this subtype [108]. Subtypes 16, 18, 31, 33, and 35 are usually associated with subclinical infection but can occasionally be found in exophytic warts [19]. Because they can be associated with moderate or severe dysplasia, young women infected with these subtypes should be considered at relatively high risk [82]. However, in general, there is no way to predict which lesions will progress and which will regress.

With DNA HPV testing has come a new clinical entity, the patient with DNA probe-positive infection who lacks any signs of either clinical disease or dysplasia [109]. Clearly, these patients warrant surveillance, but at present no treatment is considered necessary [71,98]. Indeed, transient infection may be part of the natural history of HPV infection in adolescent women [98].

Treatment

Efforts to treat clinical and subclinical HPV infection have been a bit varied and confusing (Table 76) [72,110,111]. New methods and techniques are constantly evolving. Response rates differ greatly. Nevertheless, the principles of treatment are fairly straightforward: type and duration of treatment are based on location, extent, and clinical expression of the disease. For example, the dense squamous cell epithelium of the vulva can tolerate more chemical treatment than the cervix, and the risk of progression to carcinoma is far less. On the other hand, absorption from the vagina may limit the types of toxins that can be applied. Finally, multicentric disease usually calls for more extreme remedies.

The goal of treatment is removal of visible warts and reduction of the patient's symptoms, *not the elimination of HPV.* No therapy has been shown to eradicate HPV; hence, any treatment that results in scarring should be avoided [19,31,72,111]:

Overt Clinical Disease.   A comprehensive review of the literature found that no one treatment method was superior to another [112] (Fig. 20). Furthermore, all methods had significant recurrence

TABLE 76. *Comparison of therapies for treatment of human papillomavirus infection*

Treatment modality	Average number of treatments required	Success rate	Recurrence rate <6 mo
No treatment	0	20–30%	NA
All treatments	Variable	22–94%	≥25%
Electrocautery	1.4	93%	24%
LEEP	1	93%	29%
CO$_2$ laser	1.3	43–89%	8–95%
Cryotherapy	1.9	63–88%	21–39%
Trichloroacetic acid	4	81%	36%
Fluorouracil	6.6	71%	13%
Podophyllin	4.2	32–79%	27–65%
Podofilox	Variable	45–88%	33–60%
Alpha-interferon	11	44–61%	0–67%

NA, not applicable; LEEP, loop electrosurgical excisional procedure.
Adapted from Centers for Disease Control and Prevention. 1993 Sexually transmitted diseases treatment guidelines. *MMWR Morb Mortal Wkly Rep* 1993;42(no. RR-14):1; and Mayeaux EJ, Harper MB, Barksdale W, et al. Noncervical human papillomavirus genital infections. *Am Fam Physician* 1995;52: 1137.

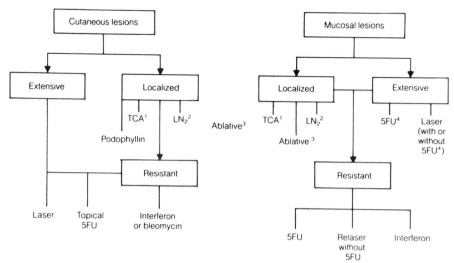

FIG. 20. Treatment of clinical human papillomavirus disease. (Moscicki B. HPV infections: an old STD revisited. *Contemporary Pediatrics* 1989;6:12, with permission.)

rates. Choice of treatment should be determined according to expense, efficacy, convenience, side effects, and patient wishes [112].

Chemical treatment of HPV infections probably should be confined to the use of liquid nitrogen or trichloroacetic acid (TCA). Traditionally, podophyllin has been used widely, but it has a number of drawbacks [113]:

- Variability in potency of solutions
- Severe local irritation
- Need for weekly applications for 4 to 6 weeks
- Major systemic toxicity, including neurologic and bone marrow impairment, if used on mucosal surfaces
- Teratogenicity in pregnant patients

If home trials of weaker solutions of podophyllin are successful, this method may make a comeback. Otherwise, this treatment probably should be limited to external warts, in nonpregnant patients, using the purified preparation of the drug (Podofilox) [113].

Liquid nitrogen and TCA are sometimes combined to treat condylomata and are safe for use on mucosal areas and in pregnant patients. The lesion is first frozen until it and the surrounding 5 mm of tissue turn white. A freeze–thaw–refreeze method may decrease failure rates. Treatments need to be repeated every 7 to 12 days. After liquid nitrogen application, treatment with TCA may also decrease failure rates. TCA is used in an 85% solution and acts as a caustic agent, precipitating proteins. It must be applied carefully to avoid traumatizing nearby normal epithelium, which can be protected using petrolatum or a baking soda paste. After its application, viscous lidocaine can be applied to the same area to minimize discomfort.

Although cervical cryotherapy is inexpensive, does not require anesthesia, and can be performed on outpatients, caution is advised. One report of 67 adolescents undergoing cryotherapy found that PID developed in 9% within 1 month of the procedure (having had negative cultures before treatment), and two patients had cervical stenosis. The authors suggested that the use of prophylactic antibiotics be investigated for adolescents undergoing cervical cryotherapy [110].

Patients with extensive vulvar or vaginal warts may benefit from the use of topical 5-fluorouracil (5-FU), which inhibits DNA and RNA synthesis and stimulates the host immune response. Systemic absorption is usually not significant (<6%); however, it is absolutely contraindicated during pregnancy. Side effects are primarily local: irritation, edema, and an erosive dermatitis. For vaginal disease, one third of an applicator of 5-FU can be inserted once a week for 10 to 12 weeks to avoid the latter complication. In one clinical trial, this regimen resulted in an 85% success rate without any cases of vulvitis from leakage of the cream. However, 40% of the patients showed inflammatory reactions of the vagina [114]. For vulvar disease, a small amount of 5-FU cream can be applied for two consecutive nights once a week for 10 weeks, using petroleum jelly to protect unaffected skin. Idoxuridine, another DNA inhibitor, has also been used with nearly 80% success in one study. A 0.25% ointment is applied to the vulva twice daily for 2 weeks [115]. It may prove useful after further testing.

Other local treatment options include injecting either bleomycin, an antibiotic with antiviral action, or α-2β interferon (Intron A, Schering) [116]. Side effects of interferon injection include a flu-like illness with fever, headaches, myalgia, fatigue, and leukopenia. In addition, no more than five warts can be treated at a time, and treatment requires injections three times a week for 3 weeks [117]. This mode of treatment may be useful in selected patients, but its long-term safety and effectiveness in controlled trials are still unknown; consequently, it is not recommended by the Centers for Disease Control and Prevention (CDC) [19].

One new and still experimental treatment is the use of oral cimetidine for multiple condylomata. A single case report found that a dose of 400 mg qid resulted in the disappearance of all warts within 5 weeks [118]. Cimetidine has been used safely and with considerable success for multiple nongenital warts [119], and this may represent an effective and nontoxic treatment in the future.

Various surgical methods have also been used. Cryotherapy and electrocautery show success rates of 60% to 90% and may be the treatment of choice on keratinized skin (thighs, scrotum), but they also suffer from high morbidity rates. In the late 1980s, the carbon dioxide laser came into vogue [120,121]. Laser treatments may have success rates as high as 95% [81], although a randomized trial puts the rate at 43% [19]. Advantages of laser therapy include 1) ability to treat at one sitting, including external genitalia, perianal area, vagina, and cervix; 2) competitive cure rates; and 3) success in extensive or refractory disease. Disadvantages include 1) high cost of equipment and treatments; 2) need for general or conduction anesthesia; 3) risk of iatrogenic spread if the HPV-containing smoke from the laser is not properly vented; 4) need for specialized training in its use; 5) lack of widespread availability; and 6) occurrence of significant postoperative pain. One controversy in laser therapy is how much to treat the surrounding epithelium, which may look grossly normal but contain HPV. A technique known as "brushing" has been used [121–123] but may be associated with increased morbidity [124]. Patients with a history of anal intercourse or with extensive disease often require anoscopy and uroscopy at the time of laser surgery.

The latest treatment method is LEEP, loop electrosurgical excision procedure, which uses a diathermy wire of varying sizes and configurations to excise tissue by heat destruction. It requires only local anesthesia, and incurs minimal blood loss [125,126]. It is used more as an alternative to cold-knife or laser cone biopsies in cervical dysplasia than in treatment of HPV.

Because laser therapy of urethral condylomata can cause strictures, 5-FU is the treatment of choice for these. In addition, 5-FU is apparently more effective in treating vaginal condylomata. Some surgeons are using 5-FU cream 4 to 6 weeks after laser treatments to prevent reinfection.

Treatment of cervical HPV infection depends on the histologic type of the biopsy specimen. Therefore, *all adolescents with either gross HPV infection of the external genitalia or vagina or cytologic evidence of cervical infection should be referred for colposcopy and directed biopsies* [71]. Treatment options depend on whether the histologic report shows HPV infection with dysplasia or without dysplasia:

- If no dysplasia is present, the options are: 1) observe for 3 months and repeat a Pap smear then, or 2) treat with either cryotherapy or TCA.
- Observation is a viable option because some HPV disease regresses over time, but the Pap is not completely reliable, nor is adolescent compliance.
- Cryotherapy is the most common mode of treatment, with an 85% to 90% success rate, but may constitute a destructive procedure on a young woman with many years of reproductive potential. It also carries potential risks [110].
- Trichloroacetic acid has an 80% cure rate and may be preferable [127].
- Cervical dysplasia (i.e., CIN) requires treatment with either cryotherapy, laser, cone biopsy, or LEEP.

• Young women with HPV infection should urge their sexual partners to have evaluation and treatment and should insist that they use condoms, although the latter do not protect against HPV infection of the external genitalia because the vulvar and scrotal areas remain uncovered. Use of the so-called "female condom" would be completely protective, but it is unlikely that this form of contraception will ever gain any appreciable popularity [128].

Subclinical Disease.   Not only is subclinical disease more difficult to diagnose, it is more difficult to treat (Fig. 21).. However, the benefit of treating patients with subclinical disease has not yet been demonstrated, and the effect of treatment on recurrence or transmission is unknown. Consequently, the CDC recommends no treatment for subclinical disease in the absence of coexistent dysplasia [19]. Failure to appreciate subclinical disease in patients with condylomata or to insist that their partners use condoms may lower their cure rate appreciably. (See the section on Issues for the Male Adolescent for a discussion of male HPV disease.)

Chlamydia trachomatis

C. trachomatis is an obligate intracellular bacteria that causes mucopurulent cervicitis in women and urethritis in men and is the most prevalent bacterial infectious disease in the United States [129,130]. Each year, approximately 4 million new chlamydial infections occur in the United States, with direct and indirect costs exceeding $2.4 billion annually [131]. As many as 14.5% of suburban female adolescents and 35% of urban female adolescents may be infected, although often they are asymptomatic [132–134]. Age is the most powerful predictor of chlamydial infection, and teenagers are at highest risk [135].

The infectious form of the organism, the elementary body, attaches to and is taken into a host cell by the process of endocytosis. After 48 hours, the entire phagosome is extruded, leaving the host cell intact. The organism acts as part-virus, part-parasite, allowing the possibility of prolonged subclinical infection, which is a hallmark of chlamydial disease [136]. This prolonged life cycle has also made it resistant to single-dose treatment regimens until the development of new treatments in the early 1990s [137,138]. In adults with gonorrhea, coinfection with *C. trachomatis* has been reported in 11% to 62% [139].

Besides age, factors associated with an increased risk of chlamydial infection include nonwhite race, use of OCs, nonuse of barrier contraception, multiple sexual partners, recent change in sexual partners, cervical ectopy, smoking, and early age at first intercourse [131,140–144]. Although it is relatively less contagious than gonorrhea, chlamydial infection still occurs in 45% of female partners of infected men, and 50% of male partners of infected women remain asymptomatic [145]. In female adolescents, 33% to 68% can be asymptomatic, constituting an important reservoir of disease [134,135].

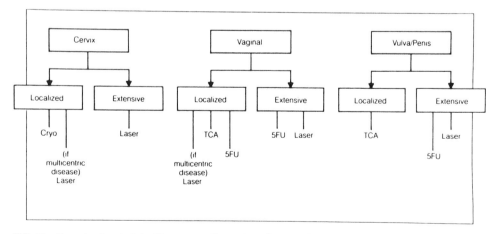

FIG. 21. Flow chart: subclinical human papillomavirus disease. (Moscicki B. HPV infections: an old STD revisited. *Contemporary Pediatrics* 1989;6:12, with permission.)

Newborns are directly infected through an infected birth canal. Many prospective studies have documented that seroconversion occurs in up to two thirds of infants, with conjunctivitis in 50% and pneumonitis in 10% to 20% [146,147].

Signs and Symptoms

Overall, probably 10% to 20% of sexually active female teens harbor chlamydial infections, and up to 70% of the infections are clinically inapparent [148]. In symptomatic patients, cervical inflammation and mucopurulent discharge are the most prominent symptoms. Half of all women with the latter have positive cultures for *C. trachomatis*. Mucopurulent cervicitis can be diagnosed by 1) visualization of yellow "mucopus" in the cervical os, or 2) presence of 10 or more WBCs per high-power field on Gram stain [136,149]. In addition, at least 15 to 20 WBCs/hpf on a saline wet preparation, or a Pap smear that shows severe inflammatory changes, with WBCs present, should alert the clinician to the possibility of chlamydial infection. Often, the cervical os is friable and bleeds easily when wiped with a cotton swab.

The exocervicitis associated with chlamydial infection must be differentiated from gonorrhea and from a more widespread vaginitis caused by either *T. vaginalis* or *C. albicans*. In one study, the presence of exocervicitis alone or a history of a partner with urethritis successfully predicted 80% of all patients with chlamydial infection [150]. In a separate study of over 500 female teens seen for routine gynecologic care, 25% were found to have chlamydial infection. The significant findings on pelvic examination were cervical friability and erythema, endocervical mucopus, and cervical ectopy. By history, those teenagers with more frequent lifetime intercourse or with multiple partners were at highest risk [151].

Patients with the "acute urethral syndrome," caused by chlamydial infection, present with dysuria, frequency, and pyuria with negative urine cultures for conventional pathogens [152]. Chlamydial infection can cause cervicitis, urethritis, or both. In one study of affected women at an STD clinic, half of the patients had both positive cervical and urethral cultures, one fourth had positive cervical cultures, and one fourth had only positive urethral cultures [145]. A more recent study of incarcerated female adolescents had nearly identical results, and the authors suggested that both the cervix and urethra should be cultured [153]. Partners of men with nongonococcal urethritis may have urethral infection only. Chlamydial infection may also be implicated in "honeymoon cystitis."

Diagnosis

A variety of means exist to diagnose chlamydial infection, but each has its own limitations [131,147,154] (Table 77). Part of the problem with the wide range of test results is that sampling techniques can vary greatly. Because *C. trachomatis* is an obligate intracellular pathogen, obtaining a specimen without endocervical cells significantly increases the risk of obtaining a false-negative test [155].

Cell culture remains the gold standard, although it is expensive and requires careful handling of specimens with technical expertise. Sterile cotton or Dacron swabs are used to sample endocervical material, then vigorously swirled into transport medium. This must be sent promptly to the laboratory, held at 4°C or frozen at −70°C. *C. trachomatis* requires cells for growth, and a monolayer of McCoy or HeLa 227 cells is typically used. Organisms are identified in the cell layer by direct immunofluorescence. Cultures are 100% specific, but a single cervical swab may be only 60% to 80% sensitive [156,157].

In adolescent populations, antigen tests have been used most widely during the past decade. Either EIA or direct fluorescent antibody (DFA) tests are cheaper, easier to perform, and have comparable specificity and sensitivity [133,158,159]. EIA tests use chlamydial antibody to combine with antigen in a clinical sample, producing an antigen–antibody sandwich. This can be attached to color-producing enzymes and assayed spectrophotometrically within 4 hours, although the actual turnaround time may be several days because specimens are usually batched. DFA tests use a slide of the clinical material, combined with fluorescein-labeled monoclonal antibodies against outer membrane proteins of the organisms, which are then visualized as apple-green through fluorescence microscopy. The DFA test requires a special microscope and technical expertise, but tests can be done individually and are available within 15 minutes. Neither method should be used as a test of cure because they detect nonviable organisms.

TABLE 77. *Tests for chlamydial infection in women*

Method	Sensitivity	Specificity	Cost	Type
Gold standard				
Culture (1 swab)	85–90%	100%	$40–85	
Specific tests				
Laboratory-based				
Chlamydiazyme (Abbott)	70–100%	97–99%	$40–60	EIA
MicroTrak (Syva)	70–100%	97–99%	$40–60	Direct fluorescent antibody
LCx *Chlamydia trachomatis* (Abbott)	96%	100%	$32	Ligase chain reaction
Pace II (GenProbe)	94%	99%	$35	DNA probe
Amplicor (Roche)	94%	100%	$40	Polymerase chain reaction
Office-based				
TestPack Chlamydia (Abbott)	81%	97%	$8–14	EIA
Surecell (Johnson & Johnson)	85–87%	95–99%	$8–14	EIA
Cleaview (Wampole)	85–94%	98–99%	$8–14	EIA

EIA, enzyme immunoassay.
Adapted from Chernesky MA, Jang D, Lee H, et al. Diagnosis of *Chlamydia trachomatis* infections in men and women by testing first-void urine by ligase chain reaction. *J Clin Microbiol* 1994;32:2682; Skolnik NS. Screening for *Chlamydia trachomatis* infection. *Am Fam Physician* 1995;51:821; Heath CB, Heath JM. *Chlamydia trachomatis* infection update. *Am Fam Physician* 1995;52:1455; and Hsuih TCH, Guichon A, Diaz A, et al. Chlamydial infection in a high-risk population: comparison of Amplicor PCR and Gen-Probe PACE II for diagnosis. *Adolescent and Pediatric Gynecology* 1995;8:71.

Pap smears can be used to detect intracytoplasmic inclusions and are most useful in low-incidence populations. A combination of cervical findings—mucopurulent discharge, cervical ectopy, friability, and presence of more than five polymorphonuclear cells on Gram stain—has been found to be highly specific for chlamydial cervicitis (99%), although not very sensitive (16%) [160]. Complement fixation tests usually are not useful for detecting acute chlamydial infection because, by age 30 years, half of American women show positive antibody titers [161]. Leukocyte esterase testing is a rapid, cheap ($8), and effective way of screening asymptomatic patients who may then require further testing. Because it detects WBCs only in a first-voided urine specimen, a positive test does not rule out other causes of urethritis or urinary tract infection. This technique is particularly useful for screening asymptomatic men (but not women) for urethritis because it is noninvasive and cost effective [156,162,163].

More recently, three variations on DNA probe technology have been tested and show considerable promise, although all are technically demanding:

- *Simple DNA/RNA probes.* These detect the presence of *C. trachomatis* by linking luminescent DNA with ribosomal RNA. PACE 2 (Gen-Probe, San Diego, CA) has been reported to be as sensitive as tissue culture [164]. One advantage of this method is that it tests for both chlamydial infection and gonorrhea using the same sample in the same test tube [165]. Because each organism contains more RNA than DNA, the test's sensitivity is enhanced compared with methods that target only DNA. A study of infected young women found it to be 94% sensitive and 99% specific [166]. It is becoming a popular and widely used test.
- *Polymerase chain reaction.* Amplicor (Roche Diagnostic Systems, Nutley, NJ) combines colorimetric DNA hybridization with PCR in first-voided specimens in men [167]. One study found it to be 100% sensitive and specific [168]. This may represent the new diagnostic method of choice for noninvasive screening of asymptomatic young men. A study of 189 adolescent women also found it to be sensitive (94%) and highly specific (100%) [166].
- *Ligase chain reaction.* LCx *Chlamydia trachomatis* (Abbott Laboratories, North Chicago, IL) is the latest example of noninvasive testing and uses a first-voided urine specimen to test for the presence of chlamydial organisms. One study found it to be superior to culture and rapid tests for screening both men and women, with 96% sensitivity and 100 specificity [169]. In another study, it showed a detection sensitivity that was 30% greater than culture [170]. Ligase chain reaction also may become one of the new diagnostic methods of choice.

Treatment

Antibiotics that interfere with protein synthesis interrupt the chlamydial cell cycle. Therefore, doxycycline has traditionally been the drug of choice (Table 78). More recently, single-dose azithromycin has been found to be an equally acceptable alternative [31,171,172]. Unfortunately, the gain in compliance is offset by the increased cost [154,173]. A single-dose powder formulation costs less, however ($9 vs. $24.50 for four 250-mg capsules) [31,154]. Both doxycycline and azithromycin have similar cure rates (96–98%) and similar side effects (diarrhea, nausea, vomiting, abdominal pain) [138,174]. Both are also effective for treatment of nongonococcal, nonchlamydial urethritis in men [175].

Uncomplicated urethral, cervical, or rectal chlamydial infection in men or nonpregnant women can be treated with doxycycline, 100 mg orally twice a day for 7 days, or azithromycin, 1 g in a single oral dose. Carboxyquinolone antibiotics (e.g., ofloxacin) are active against both chlamydial infection and gonorrhea and are (expensive) alternatives for patients older than 17 years of age. In pregnant women, erythromycin base, 500 mg four times daily for 7 days, 250 mg four times daily for 14 days, or enteric-coated erythromycin, 333 mg three times daily for 7 days may be used. Amoxicillin is also a safe and somewhat less effective but better tolerated alternative [176].

No retesting is necessary after completing treatment with either doxycycline or azithromycin unless symptoms persist or reinfection is suspected, because there is no known resistance. Indeed, false-negative tests can occur because of too few organisms remaining; false-positive nonculture tests can occur because of the continued excretion of dead organisms [19,177]. However, rates of reinfection and repeat infection among adolescents can be high—in one study, which followed 216 female adolescents for 1 to 2 years, 9% had recurrent cervicitis sometime during the follow-up period [178]. Partners need to be identified, evaluated, and treated; unfortunately, only two thirds of female adolescents actually notify their partners [179].

Although the CDC recommends treating all patients with gonorrhea for the possibility of coincident chlamydial infection, the reverse is not yet being advocated in uncomplicated chlamydial disease [19].

Neisseria gonorrhoeae

Gonorrhea was first described by Huang Ti in 2167 BC and named by Galen in 180 AD. It continues to be one of the major STDs in adolescents, but less common than chlamydial infection. Overall, an estimated 1 million new infections with *N. gonorrhoeae* occur each year in the United States [19]. Although the rate of gonorrhea decreased 65% from 1975 to 1993 (from 468 cases per 100,000 people to 166), the United States has the highest rate among Western nations [180].

TABLE 78. *Treatment of chlamydial infection*

Drug	Dose	Cost[a]
Recommended		
Doxycycline	100 mg bid × 7d	$50 (generic, $5)
Azithromycin	1 g, single dose	$24.50
Alternative		
Erythromycin base	500 mg qid × 7d	$11
Erythromycin ethylsuccinate	800 mg qid × 7d	$12.50–15.50
Ofloxacin	300 mg bid × 7d	$48.50
Sulfisoxazole	500 mg qid × 10d	$5
Pregnant patients		
Erythromycin base	500 mg qid × 7d	$11
Amoxicillin	500 mg tid × 7–10d	$7–11.50

[a]Average wholesale cost to pharmacist.
Adapted from Centers for Disease Control and Prevention. 1993 Sexually transmitted diseases treatment guidelines. *MMWR Morb Mortal Wkly Rep* 1993;42(no. RR-14):50; and Heath CB, Heath JM. *Chlamydia trachomatis* infection update. *Am Fam Physician* 1995;52:1455.

Teenagers and young adults have always been at increased risk because of unprotected sex, multiple partners, and poor selection of partners [180]. Young people continue to have some of the highest gonorrhea rates of any age group: 743 cases per 100,000 for boys aged 15 to 19 years, and 936 cases per 100,000 for girls aged 15 to 19 years in 1992 [8]. These rates have actually decreased slightly from 1988, when they peaked at 1,075 cases per 100,000—1% of all teenagers [181]! But most of the decrease occurred only among white and Hispanic teens; rates among black male teenagers continue to rise [182]. Overall, young people 10 to 24 years of age account for nearly two thirds of all cases of gonorrhea [4].

Although there are now 30 drug regimens comprising 21 different antimicrobial drugs for treatment of uncomplicated gonococcal infections [183], increasing drug resistance is always a major concern. One third of *N. gonorrhoeae* isolates are now resistant to penicillin or tetracycline [184], and new strains resistant to fluoroquinolones (ciprofloxacin and ofloxacin) have been reported in Denver and Seattle [185].

In asymptomatic female adolescents, the yield of positive cultures is 7% to 10% [186,187]. In a prospective study of 216 sexually active girls, initial rates for chlamydial infection and gonorrhea were 23.2% and 11.6%, respectively. By the end of the 12- to 24-month follow-up period, 101 episodes of chlamydial infection and 68 episodes of gonococcal infection had been identified [178]. Although the possibility of acquiring gonorrhea from contaminated toilet seats has been widely rumored in some adolescent circles, a scientific study has found no evidence for this mode of transmission [188].

N. gonorrhoeae and *C. trachomatis* can produce remarkably similar clinical pictures, including acute urethral syndrome, Bartholin's gland infection, cervicitis, salpingitis, perihepatitis, and disseminated arthritis–dermatitis [189] (Table 79). Symptoms typically develop within 3 to 5 days after exposure. Urethritis, vaginitis, and a mucopurulent cervicitis are all typically seen. However, asymptomatic disease is also more common in women than men. Cervicitis may be asymptomatic, and a carrier state can last for months or years [190]. In the literature, asymptomatic disease rates in teenagers range from 6% to 12% for girls and 1% to 7% for boys [134]. Men have a one in four chance of acquiring gonorrhea from infected women, but spread from infected men to unaffected women is virtually 100%. Various factors may influence who remains asymptomatic, develops local infection, or suffers from disseminated disease: secretory IgA, serum IgG and complement levels, virulence of the strain, and whether recent intercourse has occurred.

Signs and Symptoms

If symptomatic, young women may have a variety of different vaginal or urinary symptoms, usually 2 to 7 days after intercourse. Classically, a yellowish-green mucopurulent endocervical discharge is observed. Dysfunctional uterine bleeding, dyspareunia, vaginal discharge, and dysuria are also

TABLE 79. *Spectrum of gonococcal and chlamydial disease*

Men
Urethritis
Epididymitis
Proctitis
Conjunctivitis
Disseminated infection (gonococcal arthritis dermatitis syndrome, Reiter's syndrome)
Women
Acute urethral syndrome
Bartholinitis
Cervicitis
Salpingitis
Conjunctivitis
Perihepatitis
Disseminated infection

Adapted from McGregor JA. Chlamydial infection in women. *Obstet Gynecol Clin North Am* 1989; 16:565.

common. Vulvar tissues can be profusely inflamed, with pruritus and burning. The endocervix can also be swollen and intensely inflamed. The clinical spectrum of disease has remained unchanged for several years [191].

Diagnosis

Detecting gonorrhea is straightforward and inexpensive. A cervical culture, plated on Thayer-Martin medium and incubated in a 10% carbon dioxide environment, has become a mandatory part of every pelvic examination in sexually active women. Alternatively, a self-contained culture package with its own source of CO_2 (e.g., Transgrow) is acceptable. Rectal cultures add 5% to the yield of positive cultures, although they may not reflect anal intercourse but rather local spread. If the patient has engaged in oral sex, a throat culture should also be taken and plated on Thayer-Martin medium or Transgrow. Particular care should be taken that the medium is at room temperature when used because *N. gonorrhoeae* is a very fastidious organism that will not grow on chilled plates. Cultures are often available for $10 or less, or free from state laboratories. Although cultures are thought to be the gold standard for this disease, as with chlamydial disease they only detect 65% to 85% of infections in asymptomatic women [192]. This could be due to inadequate sampling, improper transport or preservation of the specimen, or improper media or culturing techniques.

Intracellular gram-negative diplococci in WBCs are diagnostic of gonorrhea. However, extracellular diplococci are *not;* other *Neisseria* species that are not pathogenic can normally inhabit the vagina. A Gram's stain is highly specific for gonorrheal infection but only 50% sensitive, making a culture always necessary. Likewise, the finding of greater than five WBCs on Gram's stain is suggestive of either chlamydial or gonococcal cervicitis, but not diagnostic [160].

Gonozyme (Abbott Laboratories), a rapid test that uses an EIA for gonococcal antigen, has been tested in adolescents and found to be highly sensitive and specific in high-prevalence populations (e.g., 95% predictive), but frequently misleading in low-prevalence populations (e.g., 50% predictive) [187,192]. More recently, PACE-2 (Gee-Probe, Inc.), a DNA probe assay, has been shown to be effective in both diagnosing urogenital gonococcal infection and providing a test of cure [193,194]. In one study, PACE-2 was found to be 50% sensitive but 98% specific for gonococcal infection compared with culture [165]. Its major advantage is enabling testing for chlamydial and gonorrheal infection simultaneously.

Treatment

A number of regimens are used to treat uncomplicated gonorrheal infection [19,31,183]. Intramuscular ceftriaxone, 125 mg intramuscularly (IM) is now the *treatment of choice* for mucosal gonorrhea at any site, according to the CDC (although both authors continue to use the 250-mg IM dose). No ceftriaxone-resistant strains of *N. gonorrhoeae* have been reported, and it may be useful in eradicating incubating syphilis as well [19]. Disadvantages include its expense, the need to administer it by injection, and the discomfort (ameliorated somewhat by using 1% lidocaine as a diluent) [195].

Alternatives include spectinomycin, 2 g IM, or three different choices for one-time oral therapy, cefixime 400 mg, ciprofloxacin 500 mg, or ofloxacin 400 mg. The latter two should not be used in teenagers younger than 18 years of age. *All of these regimens require simultaneous treatment for the possibility of chlamydial coinfection.* Oral treatment should probably be reserved for asymptomatic infection.

If pharyngeal gonorrhea is a concern, either ceftriaxone or ciprofloxacin should be used because studies indicate that either is greater than 90% effective [19]. Pregnant teenagers should be treated with either a cephalosporin or spectinomycin, along with either erythromycin or amoxicillin for chlamydial coinfection, because quinolones (and tetracyclines) are contraindicated.

Partners should be referred immediately for evaluation and treatment. Teenagers treated for gonorrhea (or chlamydial infection) should be considered at high risk for repeat infections in the near future. In a study of nearly 100 adolescents with genital gonorrheal infections, 23% returned within 8 to 14 months with a repeat infection [196]. A similar but larger study of more than 200 sexually active girls found that 11.6% were infected with gonorrhea at the outset, but another 14% of teens initially testing negative became infected during the next 12 to 24 months [178]. Coinfection is also common: a large 1995 Texas study of adults and teenagers with chlamydial infections found that 17% also had gonorrhea, a significant increase from 3 years earlier [197].

Syphilis

In the late 1980s, the United States experienced an epidemic of syphilis, primarily among heterosexuals [198]. In 1990, more than 50,000 cases of primary and secondary syphilis were reported to the CDC, the largest number since 1948. Fortunately, there has been a dramatic decline since then, with only 40% as many cases reported in 1994 as in 1990 (20,627) [199].

Rates for female adolescents are nearly double those for males (35.7 vs. 18.5 per 100,000 in 1991), and although overall rates have decreased for teens since 1990, as they have for the general population, the incidence of the disease among African-American teens is 12 times higher than for white teens [200]. In addition, in New York state, teenagers accounted for 15% of all mothers giving birth to infants with congenital syphilis from 1989 to 1992 [201]. The greatest increases in rates may be coming from rural, not urban, teens [202].

The American Academy of Pediatrics recommends syphilis screening for any sexually active teenager who [3]:

- Lives in an endemic area
- Has had another STD
- Has had more than one sex partner in the past 6 months
- Has exchanged sex for drugs or money
- Is male and is having sex with another man

Particular care should be taken in evaluating any circular or ulcerous lesion of the vulva, vagina, or penis, because the spirochete is present and extremely infectious if the lesion is a chancre. The estimated risk of acquiring syphilis from an infected partner is 30%.

Signs and Symptoms

Primary syphilis is usually heralded by the presence of a chancre—a punched-out, *painless* ulcer with a granular base, rubbery, raised edges, and serous discharge. Associated inguinal adenopathy is usually rubbery and nontender. Incubation period averages 3 weeks but ranges from 10 to 90 days. Occasionally, multiple chancres can occur. Most chancres appear on the lower labia or fourchette, but they can be found on the cervix as well. They heal spontaneously, without scarring, in 3 to 8 weeks. Only about half of cases involve a classic chancre, and an ulcerative genital lesion can sometimes be confused with herpes, chancroid, trauma, or even lymphogranuloma venereum [200].

Within 4 to 10 weeks after the onset of the chancre, untreated patients progress to secondary syphilis, which represents hematogenous spread of the treponeme. The maculopapular or papulosquamous rash of secondary syphilis is best known and is one of the few rashes that occur on the palms and soles [203]. Generalized adenopathy is common, as are constitutional symptoms mimicking a viral illness. The genital lesions can include condylomata lata—whitish-gray, coalescent papules on the labia, and in the perianal area and perineum—and mucous patches—superficial ulcers on the labia minora that may be confused with genital herpes. Like the chancre, these lesions are highly infectious. A few patients (5%) may present with patchy alopecia of the scalp or eyebrows. About one third of patients with secondary syphilis have asymptomatic central nervous system involvement, which can be diagnosed by doing a lumbar puncture. A cell count, protein determination, and a Venereal Disease Research Laboratory (VDRL) test on the spinal fluid show abnormalities that may correlate with the risk for development of later neurosyphilis [204].

After a prolonged latency period, 20% to 30% of untreated patients go on to have tertiary syphilis, which may be due to an exaggerated hyperimmune response to treponemal antigens. Involvement may include granulomatous gummas of the skin, bone, or viscera, aortitis, or neurosyphilis. Fortunately, this is a very rare disease among adolescents and is becoming increasingly rare among adults. However, 53 cases of tertiary syphilis were found in New York State among 10- to 19-year-olds between 1987 and 1993, and most of those had neurosyphilis [200].

Diagnosis

Dark-field testing for *Treponema pallidum* can serve as a rapid test and is the most accurate way to confirm the clinical diagnosis. In a "press preparation,' a slide is used gently to abrade a lesion, then normal saline is added. Nonspecific serologic tests—the rapid plasma reagin and VDRL—can be used as screening tests and to follow therapy. They may not be positive in early primary infection or in patients with HIV infection and secondary syphilis. On the other hand, 1% of normal patients have a biologic false-positive test, usually secondary to febrile illnesses, immunizations, autoimmune diseases, intravenous drug abuse, or laboratory error [205]. These tests usually have low titers. Specific antitreponemal tests are used to confirm infection, such as the fluorescent treponemal antibody absorption test (FTA-ABS) or the microhemagglutination assay—*T. pallidum* test. These tests retain lifelong positivity.

In primary syphilis, the nonspecific serologic tests are reactive in 80% of patients, and the specific treponemal tests in 90%. However, very early in primary disease, just after the appearance of a chancre, nontreponemal tests may be negative in up to 40% of patients [200]. The first test to turn positive is the FTA-ABS, usually 5 to 7 days after appearance of a chancre. Syphilis tests in HIV-infected patients may be either false positive or false negative. In secondary syphilis, nontreponemal tests may be negative because of the prozone phenomenon: patients with a very high titer of antibody do not form antigen–antibody complexes that register as positive tests. The test turns positive if the laboratory is asked to dilute the serum [206].

Because adults with early syphilis often have cerebrospinal fluid abnormalities, yet few go on to have neurosyphilis, a lumbar puncture is not recommended in such patients unless they have neurologic signs and symptoms [19].

Treatment

Standard treatment for primary or secondary syphilis continues to be benzathine penicillin G, 2.4 million units IM [19,31,207]. This long-acting penicillin yields low but constant levels of the drug over several days, compared with the high peak levels required to treat gonorrheal infection. Alternative treatment regimens include doxycycline, 100 mg orally twice daily for 2 weeks, or erythromycin, 500 mg orally four times daily for 2 weeks. Success rates in early syphilis are 98% with penicillin treatment, lower for other drugs. A Jarisch-Herxheimer reaction is common after treatment for secondary syphilis and is manifested by fever, tachycardia, hypotension, headaches, and painful lesions. Considerable controversy now exists about the adequacy of treatment in HIV-infected adults with secondary syphilis [208]. Standard doses of penicillin are sometimes inadequate in preventing serologic and clinical relapses [209].

Posttreatment serology tests at 6 and 12 months are recommended by the CDC [19]. Patients who are adequately treated should have a two-dilution decrease in titer by 3 months in primary infections and by 6 months in secondary infections. Persistently high titers suggest treatment failure or reinfection. Sexual partners must be treated according to their clinical stage.

Pelvic Inflammatory Disease and Other Disseminated Sexually Transmitted Diseases

Pelvic inflammatory disease is one of the most serious and significant diseases of female adolescents. Each year, nearly 1 million episodes of acute PID occur in the United States, at a cost of $4 billion to society [210]. Clinicians need to recognize that *sexually active young women who present with a chief complaint of lower abdominal pain are far more likely to have PID than acute appendicitis or any other abdominal lesion* [100,211]. Sexually active female teens have the highest rate of PID among all women—1 in 8 15- to 19-year-olds, compared with 1 in 80 25-year-olds [212]. By comparison, the *lifetime* incidence of acute appendicitis is 7% to 12% [213]. In 1988, more than 10% of American women reported that they had been treated for PID, and this is undoubtedly an underestimate of the true prevalence of the disease [214,215]. If current rates continue, half of all 15-year-olds in 1970 will have experienced at least one episode of PID by the year 2000 [37].

Risk factors for PID include adolescence, nonwhite race, use of an IUD or nonuse of other barrier contraception, multiple partners, and a previous history of PID. Douching and cigarette smoking may also be linked to the development of PID [216–218]. Cervical ectopy also represents a risk factor unique to adolescents because it predisposes to both chlamydial and gonococcal infections [37,142]. Cervical columnar epithelial cells are less resistant to infection than squamous epithelial cells, and the cervical mucus plug seems to be more permeable [219].

As discussed previously, OCs may play a role in cervical infections and PID [220]. The preponderance of evidence seems to indicate an increased risk of chlamydial cervicitis [221] but a decreased risk of upper tract disease, with 50% less hospitalizations for PID among OC users [222]. Contrary to previous belief, there is only a slightly increased risk of PID among IUD users, which seems to be most strongly related to the insertion process and to the background risk of STDs [223,224].

Etiologic Features

Scientific thinking about PID has changed dramatically since the early 1980s. Previously, the gonococcus was thought to be the primary offender, either exclusively or as the initiator of a mixed superinfection. Then, *C. trachomatis* was suspected as being the most important and prevalent organism. Now, through the use of laparoscopic cultures taken directly from the fallopian tubes, a polymicrobial etiology for PID is suspected [215,218]. Frequently, *N. gonorrhoeae, C. trachomatis,* anaerobic organisms (e.g., *Bacteroides* species and peptostreptococci), facultative bacteria (e.g., *G. vaginalis, E. coli,* enterococci), and genital tract mycoplasmas are found in concert. One theory is that most PID is caused by chlamydial infection or gonorrhea, which sets up an initial infection that alters the oxygen availability and pH of the vaginal environment, enabling overgrowth of other organisms [31,225]. A mixture of organisms then progressively ascends into the upper genital tract [219].

Isolation rates have documented the following rates of infection: *N. gonorrhoeae,* 25% to 50%; *C. trachomatis,* 25% to 43%; and anaerobes and facultative aerobes (i.e., organisms found in bacterial vaginosis), 25% to 84% [226,227]. Gonorrhea is more common among urban teenagers and young adults, chlamydial infection among college students [210]. But the most common organisms recovered from the upper genital tract of women with PID have been anaerobes, although exactly how the organisms involved in bacterial vaginosis become disseminated or increase a woman's susceptibility to upper tract infection is still unknown [215,228]. The role of viruses and of various *Mycoplasma* species also remains unclear. Some experts believe that *M. hominis* and *Ureaplasma urealyticum* are causes of PID as well [19].

Information about dissemination of both gonococcal and chlamydial disease is well known, however. The former disseminates 10% to 17% of the time, and the latter 10% to 30% [1,229]. PID is known to occur during or shortly after menses [227]. Organisms may be refluxed along with blood or transported by sperm [227,229,230]. In addition, the normal vaginal mucosa has a pH-dependent peroxidase system that becomes relatively inactivated during menses, when the pH becomes more alkaline. Blood is also a good culture medium, and the loss of the normal endocervical mucus plug may allow access of both *N. gonorrhoeae* and *C. trachomatis* to the upper genital tract. Once inside the fallopian tubes, organisms are moved along through ciliary action, and the resultant inflammation, scarring, and pitting may result in infertility, ectopic pregnancy, or chronic pelvic pain.

This triad of sequelae is all too common after PID: 18% of women had chronic pelvic pain after PID in one study [231], and ectopic pregnancies were six times more common [232]. Tubal occlusion, however, is the most troublesome result because it often comes after "silent" or atypical disease. In one classic, prospective study, 8% of women were infertile after a single episode of PID, 20% after two episodes, and 40% after three or more episodes [232]. Some studies have found that 30% to 80% of women with infertility and obstructed fallopian tubes have had no clinically recognizable episodes [233], yet most such women have antibodies against *C. trachomatis* [218].

Symptoms

Any female adolescent with acute lower abdominal pain should be suspected of having PID until proven otherwise. This diagnosis should be the first one that comes to the mind of the clinician—ahead of acute appendicitis, urinary tract syndrome, inflammatory bowel disease, and so forth. Because PID is an STD, a reliable negative history of sexual intercourse rules out this disorder (although there *are* a few reported cases of PID in virginal teenagers). In particular, sexually active patients should also be questioned about previous infections, numbers of sexual partners, type of contraception used, and relationship of their symptoms to their last menstrual period. *Onset of lower abdominal pain within a week of the start of menses in a sexually active teenager is very suggestive of PID.*

Classically, girls with PID are said to present with lower abdominal pain, fever, vaginal discharge, and perhaps irregular vaginal bleeding. However, none of these symptoms is specific for PID, and all may be associated with a myriad of other disorders. Therefore, a high index of suspicion must be maintained in evaluating female adolescents with any lower abdominal complaints.

Complicating the situation is the fact that PID can exist within a temporal spectrum of disease: acute, subacute, and chronic. Acute PID most closely mimics acute appendicitis, with ill-appearing patients who are often (but not always) febrile. Subacute PID usually presents as lower abdominal pain or dyspareunia, less acute and more insidious in nature, without constitutional symptoms, or it may be an incidental finding on routine pelvic examination. Typically, no fever is present, and laboratory signs of inflammation are often absent. In chronic PID, pelvic pain of long-standing duration may be the presenting complaint.

Diagnosis

Pelvic inflammatory disease is a *clinical* diagnosis. Unfortunately, no single test or symptom is pathognomonic for the disorder. Cervical cultures may be useful in isolating an organism but do not reflect the pathophysiologic processes ongoing in the fallopian tubes. In addition, the greater the duration of symptoms, the less likely cervical cultures are to be positive.

A classic Swedish study of adult women demonstrated that PID is a disease that probably is underdiagnosed and misdiagnosed frequently, even by astute clinicians: 814 consecutive patients with a diagnosis of acute PID (as made by two independent gynecologists, based on traditional signs and symptoms) underwent laparoscopy. Only 65% actually had PID verified visually. The remaining one third of patients were either normal (23%) or had a different disease process (12%) [234] (Tables 80, 81). Surprisingly, the classic constellation of findings—lower abdominal pain, vaginal discharge, and fever—was found in 20% of the confirmed PID group but also in 14% of the visually normal group. Even adding such findings as adnexal tenderness, an increased erythrocyte sedimentation rate (ESR), and a pelvic mass accounted for only one third of the confirmed PID patients [234].

Clearly, no such study could ever be undertaken in the United States, nor can every teenager suspected of having PID be subjected to a laparoscopy, the diagnostic gold standard [235]. Therefore, clinicians must rely on a high index of suspicion, the clinical history, the findings on pelvic examination, and ancillary laboratory data. Criteria for the diagnosis have been developed and are helpful, but have not been tested clinically (Table 82). For the diagnosis of acute PID, lower abdominal pain and tenderness, cervical motion tenderness, and adnexal tenderness all should be present. Those are three clinical criteria, and they are the minimum criteria necessary to make a diagnosis of PID—that is, fever, elevated WBC count, and elevated ESR are not necessary [19].

The abdominal and adnexal pain is usually bilateral, although it may be more pronounced on one side than the other. This offers the clinician a useful differentiating point from acute appendicitis, which eventually becomes right-sided. Clinicians should be aware that determining cervical motion tenderness requires lateral motion of the cervix (as the examiner faces the patient), which will stretch the broad ligaments, tug on the salpinx, and elicit pain—not up-and-down motion. Depending on the clinical context, any degree of pain elicited may be significant. Therefore, the classic "chandelier's sign" is not a particularly useful or appropriate sign or term. An ultrasonographic evaluation—particularly using a vaginal probe—may provide supporting evidence for the diagnosis, but frequently is not diagnostic [236]. Transvaginal sonograms can provide superior resolution compared with transabdominal studies and can differentiate various stages of PID (pyosalpinx, hydrosalpinx, tuboovarian complex, and tuboovarian abscess [TOA]) [236].

TABLE 80. *Diagnostic accuracy of a clinical diagnosis of pelvic inflammatory disease (PID)*

Prelaparoscopic diagnosis PID = 814 patients
Diagnosis at laparoscopy PID = 532 patients (65%) Normal = 184 patients (23%) Other diagnoses = 98 patients (12%)

Adapted from Jacobson L, Westrom L. Objectivized diagnosis of acute pelvic inflammatory disease. *Am J Obstet Gynecol* 1980;138: 905.

TABLE 81. *If pelvic inflammatory disease is diagnosed clinically but is an erroneous diagnosis, what is the actual diagnosis?*[a]

Diagnosis	No. of patients
Ovarian tumor	20 (22%)
Acute appendicitis	18 (20%)
Ectopic pregnancy	16 (18%)
Chronic salpingitis	10 (11%)
Acute peritonitis	6 (7%)
Miscellaneous	6 (7%)
Endometriosis	5 (5%)
Uterine myoma	5 (5%)
Pelvic pain	5 (5%)
	91 (100%)

[a]*N* =91 patients (all undergoing laparoscopy).
Adapted from Jacobson L, Westrom L. Objectivized diagnosis of acute pelvic inflammatory disease. *Am J Obstet Gynecol* 1980;138: 905.

Interestingly, this is one disorder where the pediatrician or family practitioner may be as experienced as the gynecologist, especially if the latter does not see many adolescent patients. If not, a consultation with an experienced adolescent gynecologist is always appropriate.

Treatment

All patients with PID should be hospitalized [19]. Unfortunately, this does not seem to be the current practice, particularly in pediatric emergency rooms, where the diagnosis is often first made [237]. There is a strong rationale for this rather dogmatic statement:

• Early and intensive intravenous antibiotic treatment may result in increased tubal patency and decreased risk of later infertility [229].
• No matter how astute the clinician is, the diagnosis may be in error (see Tables 80, 81).
• Patients with TOA may require surgical drainage.
• Adolescent compliance is notoriously poor. Compliance with medical regimens may only be as high as 30% to 50% [238,239]. In one study of nearly 400 women with PID given prescriptions for

TABLE 82. *Criteria for the diagnosis of pelvic inflammatory disease (PID)*

Minimum criteria (all three should be present)
• Lower abdominal tenderness
• Cervical motion tenderness
• Adnexal tenderness (can often be unilateral)

Additional criteria that may increase the specificity of the diagnosis
• Oral temperature >38.3°C
• Abnormal cervical or vaginal discharge
• Elevated erythrocyte sedimentation rate
• Elevated C-reactive protein
• Laboratory documentation of cervical infection with *Neisseria gonorrhoeae* or *Chlamydia trachomatis*

Elaborate criteria for making the diagnosis
• Histopathologic evidence of endometritis on endometrial biopsy
• Tubo-ovarian abscess on ultrasonography
• Laparascopic abnormalities consistent with PID

From Centers for Disease Control and Prevention. *1993 Sexually Transmitted Diseases Treatment Guidelines. MMWR Morb Mortal Wkly Rep* 1993;42(RR-14):75.

a standard 10-day regimen of doxycycline, only 31% finished the course of treatment. Nearly one third failed even to fill the prescription, and 41% stopped taking the antibiotic an average of 6 days before completing the course [239].

- Because treatment of PID is empirically based, some patients need close follow-up and some may require a change in antibiotic coverage.
- The patient may be too sick to tolerate oral medications.
- The adolescent's psychosocial needs can be better met by hospitalization.
- Hospitalizing adolescents with PID is the official recommendation of the CDC [19].

Frequently, adolescents with PID are not hospitalized because an adult gynecologist is involved in their care and their "model" is outpatient treatment of affected adults. Adolescent patients have special needs that probably are better served when their uniqueness as patients can be appreciated. However, patients with subacute or chronic PID can be comfortably managed as outpatients (Table 83).

Antibiotic regimens, as recommended by the CDC, were determined empirically and based on organisms' known sensitivities, not on controlled clinical trials [19,240]. Coverage includes an antibiotic active against *N. gonorrhoeae* (e.g., cefoxitin) and one active against *C. trachomatis* (e.g., doxycycline). Patients with a high fever or with a TOA may require three antibiotics, including coverage against anaerobes. Exactly how the new role of anaerobes and bacterial vaginosis will be translated into antibiotic treatment recommendations for PID is unclear.

Current regimens are effective in eradicating gonococci and chlamydiae and producing good clinical responses. However, their efficacy in preventing long-term sequelae is unknown. Some observers have suggested investigation of more aggressive antimicrobial treatment of anaerobes or use of nonsteroidal antiinflammatory agents to try to reduce long-term complications [218].

Ideally, the hospitalized adolescent is treated for 48 to 72 hours intravenously, then switched to oral medications before being sent home. Criteria for switching from intravenous to oral antibiotics are subjective, but amount of fever, pain, and tenderness should be considered. Clinical response to high-dose intravenous antibiotics is usually prompt, within 72 hours. Failure to respond should make the clinician reconsider the primary diagnosis and perhaps ask for a gynecologic or surgical consultation.

Sexual partners must be treated as well. Cervical gonorrhea developed in one fourth of women with gonococcal PID within 3 months after treatment, probably because of untreated male partners [229]. Up to half of these untreated partners are asymptomatic [241]. Outpatient treatment of partners should follow the protocol for treatment of uncomplicated gonococcal infection (see section XX).

TABLE 83. *Management of pelvic inflammatory disease (PID) in adolescents*

Note: Hospitalization of *all* adolescents with acute PID is strongly recommended. Outpatient regimens should be reserved for adolescents with subacute or chronic PID.

Either
Cefoxitin 2 g IV every 6 h *or* cefotetan 2 g IV every 12 h
plus
Doxycycline 100 mg IV or orally every 12 h

- Treat for at least 48 h after the patient clinically improves. After discharge from hospital, continue:
Doxycycline 100 mg orally bid for total of 14 d

or
Clindamycin 900 mg IV every 8 h
plus
Gentamicin 2 mg/kg loading dose IV or IM, followed by a maintenance dose of 1.5 mg/kg every 8 h

- Treat for at least 48 h after the patient clinically improves. After discharge from hospital:
Doxycycline 100 mg orally bid for total of 14 d *or* clindamycin 450 mg orally qid for total of 14 d

For subacute PID
Either: Ceftriaxone 250 mg IM + doxycycline 100 mg orally bid for 14 d
    or: Ofloxacin 400 mg orally bid for 14 d + clindamycin 450 mg orally qid (or metronidazole 500 mg orally bid) for 14 d

---

From Centers for Disease Control and Prevention. 1993 Sexually transmitted diseases treatment guidelines. *MMWR Morb Mortal Wkly Rep* 1993;42(RR-14):75.

Infectious Complications

Tuboovarian Abscess

Tuboovarian abscess is produced by contact between the ovary and purulent material spreading from the fallopian tubes and occurs in up to 15% of patients with PID. A ruptured TOA is a surgical emergency. Ultrasonography of the pelvis can help delineate this complication [236,242]. In one study, adolescents with TOA tended to have less fever but more pain and higher ESRs [243]. Another study found no difference in fever but TOA patients with higher WBC counts and no previous history of PID [244]. In a third and more recent study, teenagers with TOA tended to have had a past history of PID and had lower WBC counts and ESRs. They also usually had their last menstrual period more than 18 days before admission and had a palpable adnexal mass on pelvic examination [245]. Given the inconsistency of these findings and the difficulty of making this diagnosis clinically, transvaginal ultrasonography is worth considering for any teenager hospitalized for PID.

Perihepatitis

Perihepatitis (Fitz-Hugh–Curtis syndrome) presents as right upper quadrant pain and tenderness caused by violin-string adhesions between the anterior capsule of the liver and the peritoneum [246–248]. In 5% to 20% of women with laparascopically verified acute salpingitis, there is acute inflammation of the liver capsule without any parenchymal involvement [37,215]. To date, it has been associated with both gonorrhea and chlamydial infection, but not with organisms found in bacterial vaginosis [249]. Patients with perihepatitis may have findings consistent with PID or no pelvic findings whatsoever [250]. Cervical cultures usually are negative because the pathologic organism is long gone from that site, having passed through the fimbriated end of the fallopian tubes and into the peritoneum. Fitz-Hugh–Curtis syndrome should be suspected in any sexually active young woman with right upper quadrant pain or right-sided chest pain and no signs or symptoms of either hepatitis or gallbladder disease. Serum transaminases are mildly elevated in only one third of cases [251]. Treatment usually requires several days of high-dose parenteral antibiotics (see Table 83).

Disseminated Gonococcal Infection

Disseminated gonococcal infection (DGI) can take the form of arthritis–dermatitis syndrome or, rarely, endocarditis, or meningitis [252–256]. Spread is hematogenous, usually within a week of menses [255]. The risk of PID developing from a local cervicitis is thought to be approximately 15%, and the risk of dissemination of gonorrhea is approximately 0.5% to 3% [255]. Therefore, the overall incidence of DGI is quite low. However, *any female adolescent who presents with septic arthritis should be considered to have DGI until proven otherwise.* DGI is far more common in adolescents than juvenile rheumatoid arthritis (which is a *chronic* illness) or other forms of septic arthritis [257]. By far, the knee is the most commonly affected joint [256]. Most cases of DGI occur in girls, because boys are more often symptomatic with local gonorrheal infection. However, both male and female adolescents are at risk for dissemination from pharyngeal infection, which is often asymptomatic and difficult to eradicate [258].

Disseminated gonococcal infection occurs in two contiguous phases: a bacteremic phase, manifested by fever, chills, skin lesions, and tenosynovitis; and a septic arthritis phase, with involvement of one or more joints:

- In the first phase, blood cultures are positive in 9% to 28% of cases, and skin lesions have a lower yield.
- In the second phase, joint fluid is positive in 18% to 28% of cases and blood cultures are negative.
- Interestingly, cervical cultures may give the highest yield—28% to 90% are positive in DGI [256,259].

Two reasons for the low yield in cultures of synovial fluid are the normal bacteriostatic mechanisms present in such fluid and the fastidiousness of the gonococcus. Skin lesions can be papules, pustules, vesicles, bullae, or necrotic pustules. Initially, joint involvement is manifested by a tenosynovitis of the wrists or ankles. Later, large joints may manifest acute swelling, tenderness, warmth, and pain. Although the knees and ankles are prime targets in the later phase, any joint can be involved, and the process may not necessarily be limited to single joints. Because less virulent strains of the gonococcus remain asymptomatic longer and therefore have a greater opportunity eventually to disseminate, this septicemia is usually extremely sensitive to high doses of parenteral antibiotics (e.g., ceftriaxone 1 g IM or IV every 24 hours, ceftizoxime 1 g IV every 8 hours, or cefotaxime 1 g IV every 8 hours) [260].

Sequelae of Pelvic Inflammatory Disease

Infertility is one of the most feared complications of PID. Tubal damage is the most common known cause of infertility [37,218]. Consequently, an ESR greater than 15 mm/hour and evidence of severe tubal inflammation during PID constitute increased risks [212]. OCs may be relatively protective of post-PID fertility [218,261,262]. Because chlamydial PID is milder clinically (and therefore may go undetected) but is associated with more severe tubal inflammation, *C. trachomatis* probably represents the single greatest infectious threat to adolescents' fertility. Overall, the rate of infertility increases dramatically with each succeeding episode of PID, starting out with a risk of 8% after the initial infection and nearly doubling with each new infection [232]. Obviously, these are statistics only: anyone in the 8% group could be 100% infertile after only one episode of PID. And teenagers are frequently desperately concerned about their future ability to bear children.

Ectopic pregnancy is the other, extremely important complication of PID. It makes this disease a life-threatening one for female adolescents. Chlamydial infection and PID have both been strongly linked to the fourfold increase in ectopic pregnancy noted between 1970 and 1987 [263,264]. The inflammation that occurs in salpingitis forms pits and scars that can potentially trap a fertilized ovum (see Shafer and Sweet [37] for excellent scanning electron micrographs).

Overall, more than one fourth of young women will have permanent or long-standing sequelae from PID, including infertility (21%), ectopic pregnancy (5%), and chronic pelvic pain, dyspareunia, or pelvic adhesions (21%) [37].

Because cervicitis can frequently be asymptomatic, screening for chlamydial disease is imperative, especially among sexually active female adolescents [155]. A study of aggressive screening for cervical infection in women aged 18 to 34 years found a remarkable 56% reduction in the incidence of PID [265]. Clearly, the benefits of widespread screening of all sexually active women exceed the costs [266]. A national prevention campaign could be mounted for $175 million, compared with the overall costs of chlamydial infections of $2.4 billion per year [155].

AIDS and the Human Immunodeficiency Virus

The acquired immunodeficiency syndrome was first reported in the United States in 1981 and now constitutes one of the most urgent public health crises in the history of American public health. According to the World Health Organization, young people aged 15 to 24 years will account for more than 50% of all HIV infection in the next decade [267] (Fig. 22). In 1984, a retrovirus was implicated (HIV-1). This virus has been isolated from semen, cervical secretions, blood, urine, amniotic fluid, breast milk, saliva, and tears in patients with AIDS, although the actual infectivity of these fluids varies significantly. HIV eventually succeeds in crippling the host's immune system, paving the way for opportunistic infections, malignancies, and autoimmune disorders. Although the incubation period averages 7 to 10 years for most patients, some survive 12 years or more without clinical expression of the virus [268]. More recently, another retrovirus, HIV-2, has been found, mainly confined to central Africa, with a much slower progression to full-blown AIDS.

More than 1 million people are infected with HIV in the United States. In 1994, there were 80,689 cases of AIDS reported [269] (Fig. 23). Although only 417 of these were teenagers aged 13 to 19 years, most of the 13,198 patients aged 20 to 29 were probably infected during their adolescence. In 1993, HIV infection became the leading cause of death among people aged 24 to 44 years [270].

Epidemiologic Features

Although less than 1% of AIDS cases occur in 13- to 19-year-olds, there is an increasing realization that most of the young adults were first infected with HIV during adolescence [271,272]. Actual AIDS cases probably represent the "tip of the iceberg": for every case, an estimated 50 to 100 people are infected with HIV but are asymptomatic. If these estimates are correct, the United States could be faced

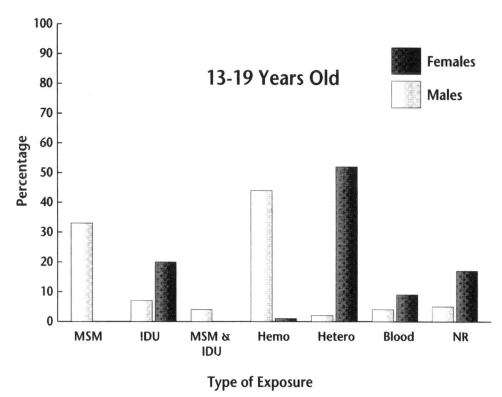

Type of Exposure

FIG. 22. AIDS cases in adolescents, by exposure category and sex, totals through December, 1993, United States. (Centers for Disease Control and Prevention. *HIV/AIDS Surveillance Report* 1994;5:9. Reproduced with permission from *The Contraception Report* 1995;VI[2]:12.) MSM: men having sex with men; IDU: intravenous drug use; HEMO: hemophiliac; HETERO: heterosexual sex; BLOOD: transfusion; NR: not reported.

with 1 to 2 million cases of AIDS in the near future [273]. Although not all clinicians have encountered teenagers with acquired HIV infection or AIDS, endemic areas exist throughout the United States.

Increasing amounts of data are available about the number of HIV-infected adolescents:

- Certain subgroups of adolescents demonstrate high rates of infection—in homeless and runaway youth in New York City, the rate of seropositivity was an astounding 7% in 1,500 teenagers and 16% in 18- to 20-year-olds [274]. Such teenagers may become involved in survival sex (exchanging sex for money, food, or lodging) and in use of crack/cocaine [271].
- Endemic areas (e.g., New York, San Francisco) have the next highest rates: 2.5% in 15- to 19-year-olds attending STD clinics in Baltimore [275]; 5.9% of adolescent women giving birth in the Bronx [276].
- Juvenile offenders also have increased rates of HIV: 1.4% in one study of 37 different correctional facilities [277].
- "Baseline" rates of seroprevalence have been established by 1) anonymous surveillance of blood specimens at hospitals: 1.1% to 3.8% of teenagers were seropositive for HIV in two Northeastern hospitals [278]; 2) surveillance of new military recruits: a 1990 study of over 1 million military recruits younger than 20 years of age found a prevalence rate of 1 in 3,000 infected with HIV [279]; and 3) surveillance of college students: a survey of over 16,000 college students at 19 universities throughout the United States found an overall prevalence of 1 in 50 students infected: all were older than 18 years of age, nearly two thirds were older than 24 years of age, and all but two were men [280].

AIDS annual rates per 100,000 population — United States, January–December 1996

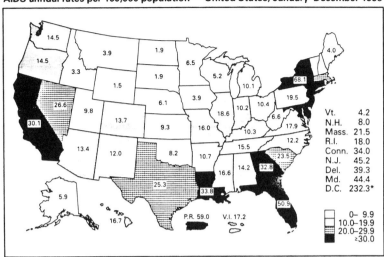

This rate represents only persons residing within the geographic boundaries of the District and differs from the rate for the larger Washington, D.C., metropolitan area (see table).

FIG. 23. AIDS cases per 100,000 population—United States cases reported January–December, 1996. (From *MMWR Morb Mortal Wkly Rep* 1997;46:333.)

- In the most recent review of seroprevalence rates among U.S. teenagers, nearly 80,000 adolescents were screened between 1990 and 1992, with rates ranging as high as 6.8% in correctional facilities, 4.1% in homeless shelters, and 3.5% in STD clinics [281].
- Young people of color, ages 13 to 24, are disproportionately represented among total AIDS cases. African-American youth account for one third of all AIDS cases among men and 55% of all cases among women. Hispanic men and women account for approximately 20% of all cases [4].

Risk factors for teenagers becoming infected with HIV include [282–285] (Table 84):

- Unprotected vaginal or anal receptive intercourse
- Intravenous drug use, or having sex with someone using intravenous drugs
- High rates of oral sex
- Multiple partners
- Having sex under the influence of drugs, especially crack/cocaine

TABLE 84. *Comparison of HIV-positive and HIV-negative adolescents: risk factors*

Risk factor	HIV+ (N = 72)	HIV− (N = 1,142)	P value
Engaged in multiple problem behaviors	72%	30%	$P < 0.01$
Had a sexually transmitted disease	59%	28%	$P < 0.01$
Sex under the influence of drugs	52%	27%	$P < 0.01$
Sexually abused	33%	21%	$P < 0.05$
Anal sex	32%	4%	$P < 0.01$
Survival sex	32%	4%	$P < 0.01$
Used multiple drugs	43%	9%	$P < 0.01$
Unprotected sex with casual partners	42%	23%	$P < 0.05$

HIV, human immunodeficiency virus.
Adapted from Hein K, Dell R, Futterman D. Comparison of HIV+and HIV−adolescents: risk factors and psychosocial determinants. *Pediatrics* 1995;95:96.

- Men having sex with men
- A history of sexual abuse
- A previous history of STDs
- Engaging in survival sex
- Engaging in multiple problem behaviors
- A history of blood transfusions

Among the first 1,200 AIDS cases diagnosed in 13- to 21-year-olds, 70% of noniatrogenic infections were secondary to homosexual or bisexual transmission [280]. However, female adolescents may be at particular risk from heterosexual sex, unlike their male or adult counterparts [286,287] (Table 85). In fact, heterosexual contact is the most rapidly increasing category for women infected with HIV [288].

In New York City, the male-to-female ratio for AIDS cases is 2.9:1 in adolescents, compared with 7:1 for adults [274]. Among the first 50 patients in a New York City adolescent HIV program, 82% of the young women acquired HIV through sexual intercourse [271]. Data from Africa are also extremely worrisome. The male-to-female ratio there is 1:1, with 15- to 19-year-olds in Zaire constituting the highest cohort of seropositive individuals [289]. Female teens in New York and San Francisco also show surprisingly high rates of anal intercourse (18% to 36%), one known high-risk activity [283–285].

Acquired immunodeficiency syndrome is also largely a disease of racial and ethnic minorities. Half of men, three fourths of women, and 84% of children with AIDS are people of color [290]. In seroprevalence studies from U.S. Job Corps entrants, HIV rates were highest among African Americans [291]. However, studies show that the natural history of the disease is not influenced by race or ethnicity but rather by access to and use of health care [292]. Just as teenage pregnancy is sometimes (erroneously) associated with inner-city, minority teenagers, HIV and AIDS funding may suffer because these infections are not viewed as the major public health hazards they really are.

Also alarming is the fact that some HIV-positive adults and adolescents continue to engage in high-risk behavior. In a study of 116 adult men, 34% reported having multiple partners, 28% had vaginal or anal sex without using a condom, and 23% traded sex for drugs or money within the preceding month [293]. In a study of the first 50 HIV-positive adolescents in New York City, many of the teens continued to have intercourse without condoms, particularly those with alcohol or drug dependency [271].

Pathophysiologic Features

Human immunodeficiency virus is a 100-nm RNA retrovirus with a glycoprotein lipid coat, including gp 120, which is capable of recognizing a glycoprotein antigen (CD4) on susceptible host cells. Any activity that can disrupt normal skin, mucous membranes, or blood barriers can lead to infection. This includes intravenous drug use with contaminated needles, transfusion with infected blood products, or contact of vaginal or rectal mucosa with infected bodily fluids. Many host cells are susceptible because of their glycoprotein composition: helper–inducer lymphocytes (T4), macrophages,

TABLE 85. *Acquired immunodeficiency syndrome in adolescents (aged 13–19 years)*

Acquisition profile	Boys	Girls
Hemophilia	43%	0%
Homosexual/bisexual	33%	0%
Heterosexual	3%	50%
Intravenous drug use	6%	33%
Homosexual + drug use	5%	0%
Transfusion	4%	2%
Other	7%	14%

Adapted from Centers for Disease Control and Prevention. HIV/AIDS surveillance report. *MMWR Morb Mortal Wkly Rep* 1995; 7(1):12.

monocytes, B-cell lymphocytes, and neural cells. Infected cell type may determine the type of clinical disease. For example, infected macrophages predispose to systemic *Pneumocystis carinii* infection.

The virus binds to the normal cell surface membrane, fuses with it, and infuses its core into the cell. There, the virus' reverse transcriptase converts its RNA genome into a DNA copy, which is integrated into the host cell genome. Virions are produced and shed by budding from the cell surface. Host cell death occurs at a variable time later [273,294].

Signs and Symptoms

Unfortunately, positive laboratory tests for HIV antibodies may constitute the first and only evidence of initial HIV infection. Antibodies may develop within 2 to 8 weeks after initial exposure, but can also take as long as 35 months in homosexual men at high risk [295]. A brief, flulike illness may signify primary infection, with symptoms similar to infectious mononucleosis, but it is virtually impossible to detect clinically. This is followed by a period of quiescence that can last up to 5 to 7 years, and perhaps longer [268]. Patients in this stage are clinically well but are carriers and transmitters of the virus.

Various factors may contribute to the length of the incubation period, including size and route of the inoculum, number of exposures, past exposure to other viruses, and general health of the host. In adults, it averages 10 years, with a range from a few months to more than 12 years [19]. Unfortunately, there is no sure way of predicting how fast a patient will progress from one stage to another. Elevated levels of neopterin, P-24 antigen, β_2-microglobulin, and HIV RNA may be predictive of a more rapid disease course. Currently, however, the CD4+ T-lymphocyte count is viewed as the best laboratory indicator of clinical progression, and most management schemes use the count to determine the need for intervention. Patients with CD4+ counts greater than 500 cells/μl are usually not clinically immunosuppressed. Patients with intermediate counts, 200 to 500 CD4+ cells/μl, are more likely to have HIV-related symptoms and to require medical treatment. At counts below 200 cells/μl, complicated disease can occur, requiring hospitalization in a specialized facility [19].

Many studies have demonstrated that both ulcerative and nonulcerative genital infections increase the risk of either transmitting or acquiring HIV three- to fivefold [296]. Vaginal candidiasis and genital herpes infections occur more frequently with declining CD4+ counts [297]. In addition, PID, HPV infection, abnormal Pap smears and intraepithelial neoplasia, and syphilis are all either more common or more severe in HIV-infected patients [298].

Teenagers undergoing evaluation for diffuse lymphadenopathy (at two separate sites other than inguinal, for greater than 3 months), fever, weight loss, fatigue, or chronic diarrhea should have HIV testing included in their workup as indicated.

Diagnosis

In 1985, an enzyme-linked immunosorbent assay (ELISA) was developed to detect antibodies to HIV. Although the test is highly sensitive, the incidence of false-positive reactions remains high, especially in screening people at low risk of HIV infection. Therefore, all initially positive tests should be repeated and then must be validated by more specific tests. The Western blot test, which identifies antibodies to specific viral membrane and core proteins, is more specific than the ELISA test and is used to confirm infection [19].

Antibody to HIV is detectable in more than 95% of patients within 6 months of infection. However, antibody tests cannot rule out infection that has occurred within a 6-month period before the test—the so-called "window period." For this reason, there is still a very small risk of HIV associated with receiving a blood transfusion, for example (currently estimated to be 1 case of HIV transmission for every 450,000–660,000 donations of blood) [299]. Finally, a few patients have been described with HIV infection but without detectable HIV-1 antibody even beyond the window period [300].

Ideally, culturing the HIV would confirm infection. The PCR, a selective DNA amplification technique, can now be used to identify a small number of infected monocytes in a patient's peripheral blood, even when antibodies are not detectable. Still a research tool, this test may become the future standard for confirming HIV infection [301].

Who should be screened? Intuitively, it might be thought that careful attention to high-risk factors would be sufficient. Yet, in a large study of 3,520 teenagers in Washington, DC, the 4.1% of "at-risk" teens who were seropositive represented only 38% of all the HIV-positive adolescents discovered

[302]. Clearly, any teenager who is sexually active and who desires HIV testing should be offered it, confidentially. All states allow teenagers to be seen for confidential health visits related to STDs [19], and 12 states expressly allow adolescents older than 12 years of age to consent to HIV testing [303]. However, clinicians need to be absolutely sure that their laboratories are reliable, confidentiality is ensured not only by the laboratory but by the office staff as well, and that they are prepared to handle the emotional and medical aspects of counseling an HIV-positive teenager [303,304].

Treatment and Prevention

There is no cure for AIDS, but early detection does allow for optimal medical and psychological management as well as appropriate immunizations and prophylaxis. An extensive discussion of the evaluation and treatment of the HIV-positive adolescent is beyond the scope of this chapter, but several excellent, detailed reviews are available [272,305,306]. The following preventative measures are recommended by the CDC [19]:

- Preventative therapy for tuberculosis (isoniazid 10 mg/kg daily to a maximum adult dose of 300 mg daily)
- Vaccination against pneumococci, hepatitis B, and influenza
- Prophylaxis against *P. carinii* infection for any patients with CD4+ T-cell counts below 200 cells/µl. Oral trimethoprim–sulfamethoxazole (TMP-SMX) should be given at a dose of one double-strength tablet (800 mg SMX, 160 mg TMP) once a day for the lifetime of the patient. Oral prophylaxis can prevent infection in most patients who take the drug, but side effects (rash, nausea, fever) often result in patients discontinuing the regimen [307].

Increasing numbers of antiretroviral therapeutic agents are being developed, and many researchers have high hopes that HIV infection can be controlled for long periods of time using combination drug therapy [307–310]. Zidovudine (ZDV, AZT) was the first drug of choice, recommended for symptomatic patients with less than 500 CD4+ T cells/µl and for asymptomatic patients with less than 300 CD4+ T cells/µl. Usual dosage is 500 mg/day (100 mg orally every 4 hours while the patient is awake). AZT is a nucleoside analog that inhibits HIV reverse transcriptase, HIV RNA, and can increase levels of CD4+ cells and prolong survival in some patients [19,307]. When given to pregnant women, AZT decreases vertical transmission of HIV from 28% to 8% [311,312]. Side effects include anemia, neutropenia, nausea, vomiting, headache, fatigue, malaise, and hepatitis [307].

However, other, newer drugs to combat HIV have been developed and tested: ddl (dideoxyinosine), ddc (dideoxycytidine), stavudine (d4T), and lamivudine (3TC), all reverse transcriptase inhibitors like AZT, and a variety of potent new protease inhibitors (e.g., indinavir, saquinavir, ritonavir), which prevent HIV replication in vitro [307,308]. Monotherapy with ZDV is no longer recommended because of increased drug resistance. Instead, triple therapy with two nucleoside analogs plus a protease inhibitor, or combinations of protease inhibitors, appears to be the regimen of choice [308,313,314]. Such regimens have been shown to reduce levels of HIV by 99.9%, practically eliminating detectable virus in body tissues [315].

Because AIDS is a fatal disease and no cure exists, prevention is of paramount importance. Among the high-risk populations, homosexual men need to avoid receptive anal intercourse and use condoms. Intravenous drug users must avoid sharing needles. Women whose sexual partners are intravenous drug users or bisexual are also at high risk, and all women should be aware of the fact that male-to-female transmission of the virus appears to be far more efficient than vice versa [316]. Practitioners should counsel their adolescent patients, both male and female, about the component parts of "safe sex" [298,316,317] (Tables 86, 87):

- Reduction in numbers of sexual partners
- Emphasis on permanent mutual monogamy
- Use of condoms
- Avoidance of anal intercourse
- Avoidance of drugs in conjunction with sex

The effectiveness of parental and physician intervention has been demonstrated. Data from a 1989 national sample of over 8,000 high school students demonstrated that students who discussed HIV with their parents were less likely to have had multiple sex partners or unprotected sex [318]. Similarly, teens who discussed AIDS with a physician were more likely to adopt condom use to avoid HIV

TABLE 86. *What sort of HIV-related counseling do adolescents want from their physicians?*[a]

Topic	Want to hear from MD about	Uncomfortable raising issue themselves
HIV	85%	—
Sexually transmitted diseases	82%	—
Safe sex	80%	59%
Condoms	73%	67%
Sex	70%	60%

HIV, human immunodeficiency virus.
[a]N = 845 9th–12th grade students.
Adapted from Rawitscher LA, Saitz R, Friedman LS. Adolescents' preferences regarding human immunodeficiency virus (HIV)-related physician counseling and HIV testing. *Pediatrics* 1995; 96:52.

exposure [319]. Unfortunately, although 80% had seen a physician in the past year, only 13% received counseling about AIDS [319]. Even among high-risk groups like teen runaways or drug users, prevention programs have been effective [320,321].

There is also increasing knowledge about AIDS [322,323], but increases in knowledge and changes in attitude require thoughtful school-based campaigns. In 1994, the CDC conducted a comprehensive review of school health policies in all 50 states and the District of Columbia. Forty states require HIV prevention education. However, only one third of teachers received in-service training on HIV prevention during the previous 2 years. In addition, specific topics like the use of condoms were often neglected [324] (Table 88).

Significant deficits still exist in teenagers' knowledge and attitudes about HIV and AIDS. For example, nearly half of adolescents in one Wisconsin survey reported that homosexuals and intravenous drug users with AIDS were "getting what they deserve" [322]. In another study, only half of adolescent girls knew that heterosexual intercourse placed them at risk for HIV infection [325]. And 70% of nearly 1,000 college students believed that they were unlikely to get AIDS, even though 19% had had sex with a stranger or casual acquaintance recently [326].

And, as discussed previously, the use of condoms remains intermittent at best. Clearly, less than half of sexually active teenagers use condoms correctly, *all the time;* and high-risk teens (i.e., multiple sexual partners or drug users) are the *least likely* to use them [327,328].

Education about AIDS and HIV *can* be effective but should *never* involve so-called "scare tactics." There is no evidence that teenagers can be dissuaded from initiating sexual intercourse by the threat of AIDS, or that scare tactics are successful in dissuading teenagers from engaging in high-risk activities

TABLE 87. *Counseling adolescents about "safe sex"*

Avoid alcohol and drugs. You are more likely to take sexual risks when you are drunk or high.
Never be afraid to say "no" to sex.
Limit the number of your sex partners. Make an agreement to be faithful sexually, and stick to it. The greater the number of your sex partners, the greater your chance of catching an STD.
Remember that you cannot tell that someone has an STD, including AIDS, merely by how they look.
Use a condom every time you have intercourse, even if you are using another method of birth control as well. Condoms help prevent STDs; birth control pills help prevent pregnancies.
Learn the common symptoms of STDs. Seek medical help if any suspect symptoms develop.
Avoid sexual contact with infected people and with those undergoing treatment for STDs. If you're female, having sex with a bisexual male or an intravenous drug user puts you at risk for contracting AIDS.
Avoid receptive anal intercourse.

AIDS, acquired immunodeficiency syndrome; STD, sexually transmitted disease.
Adapted from Brown HP. Recognizing STDs in adolescents. *Contemp Pediatr* 1989;6:17.

TABLE 88. *What do school programs actually teach about HIV and AIDS?*

Topic	Actually being taught[a]
Basic facts about HIV/AIDS	72–87%
How HIV is transmitted	70–84%
Sexual behaviors that transmit HIV	59–78%
Reasons for choosing abstinence	55–78%
Compassion and support for people with HIV/AIDS	42–59%
How well condoms work	33–56%
Information about HIV testing	28–56%
Risk behavior and HIV	28–51%
Correct use of condoms	15–37%

HIV, human immunodeficiency virus; AIDS, acquired immunodeficiency syndrome.

[a]Range results from whether specific topics were taught by health educators (higher figure) or other teachers (lower figure).

From Centers for Disease Control and Prevention. School-based HIV prevention education: United States, 1994. *MMWR Morb Mortal Wkly Rep* 1996;45:760.

[329]. Indeed, normal adolescent psychology would seem to indicate the exact opposite: most teenagers likely think that "it could never happen to me." Therefore, counseling about AIDS should be educational and nonjudgmental, not hysterical or apocalyptic. In addition, health professionals should be prepared for the fact that it may be easier to change teenagers' attitudes than it is to change their behavior. Increasingly, studies are documenting that the so-called "Health Belief Model" ("If I know something is unhealthy, then I won't do it") is not applicable to many adolescents [330]. A study of an Oklahoma AIDS education program documented that such a program could change teens' knowledge and attitudes but *not* their intention to practice good preventative behavior [331].

A number of general recommendations can be made from the now voluminous literature concerning adolescents and HIV [298,317,332]:

* *All* adolescents should receive intensive education about HIV and AIDS. This should include school- and community-based programs and begin with preteenagers.
* Messages about sexuality need to be balanced, open, and reasonable.
* Health care providers need to take a more aggressive role in educating teenagers.
* Condoms need to be made readily available to teenagers. They should be advertised and marketed appropriately.
* Adolescents should have the opportunity to interact with people their age who are HIV positive [333].
* Widespread screening and counseling should be available to all adolescents.

REFERENCES

1. Braverman PK, Strasburger VC. Adolescent sexuality: III. sexually transmitted diseases. *Clin Pediatr* 1994; 33:26.
2. Alan Guttmacher Institute. *Sex and America's teenagers.* New York: Alan Guttmacher Institute; 1994.
3. Committee on Adolescence, American Academy of Pediatrics. Sexually transmitted diseases (policy statement). *Pediatrics* 1994;94:568.
4. Sells CW, Blum RW. Morbidity and mortality among US adolescents: an overview of data and trends. *Am J Public Health* 1996;86:513.
5. Centers for Disease Control and Prevention. Summary of notifiable diseases, United States, 1994. *MMWR Morb Mortal Wkly Rep* 1995;43(Suppl 53):1.
6. Moscicki A-B, Palefsky J, Gonzales J, et al. HPV infection in sexually active adolescent females: prevalence and risk factors. *Pediatr Res* 1990;28:507.
7. Centers for Disease Control and Prevention. Surveillance for gonorrhea and primary and secondary syphilis among adolescents: United States, 1981–1991. *MMWR Morb Mortal Wkly Rep* 1993;42(SS-3):1.

8. Centers for Disease Control and Prevention. *Pregnancy, sexually transmitted diseases, and related risk behaviors among U.S. adolescents.* CDC publication No. 099–4630. Atlanta: Centers for Disease Control and Prevention; 1995.

9. Chacko MR, Taber LH. Epidemiology of sexually transmitted diseases in children and adolescents in the United States. *Seminars in Pediatric Infectious Diseases* 1993;4:71.

10. McGrath JW, Strasburger VC, Cushing AH. Secretory IgA in cervical mucus. *J Adolesc Health* 1994;15:149.

11. Witkin SS, Inglis SR, Polaneczky M. Detection of *Chlamydia trachomatis* and *Trichomonas vaginalis* by polymerase chain reaction in introital specimens from pregnant women. *Am J Obstet Gynecol* 1996;175:165.

12. Chacko M, Kozinetz CA, Hill R, et al. Leukocyte esterase dipstick as a rapid screening test for vaginitis and cervicitis. *Journal of Pediatric and Adolescent Gynecology* 1996;9:185.

13. Demetriou E, Emans SJ, Masland RP. Dysuria in adolescent girls: urinary tract infection or vaginitis? *Pediatrics* 1982;70:299.

14. Johnson J. Sexually transmitted diseases in adolescents. *Prim Care* 1987;14:101.

15. Eckert LO, Loutsky LA, Kiviat NB, et al. The inflammatory Papanicolaou smear: what does it mean? *Obstet Gynecol* 1995;86:360.

16. Braverman P. Literature reviews: adolescent medicine. *Clin Pediatr* 1996;35:541.

17. Jenny C, Hooton TM, Bowers A, et al. Sexually transmitted diseases in victims of rape. *N Engl J Med* 1990;322:713.

18. Reed BD, Eyler A. Vaginal infections: diagnosis and management. *Am Fam Physician* 1993;47:1805.

19. Centers for Disease Control and Prevention. 1993 Sexually transmitted diseases treatment guidelines. *MMWR Morb Mortal Wkly Rep* 1993;42(RR-14):1.

20. Spinillo A, Capuzzo E, Nicola S, et al. The impact of oral contraception on vulvovaginal candidiasis. *Contraception* 1995;51:293.

21. Foxman B. The epidemiology of vulvovaginal candidiasis: risk factors. *Am J Public Health* 1990;80:329.

22. Greydanus DE, Shearin RB. *Adolescent sexuality and gynecology.* Philadelphia: Lea & Febiger; 1990.

23. The Medical Letter. Oral fluconazole for vaginal candidiasis. *The Medical Letter* 1994;36(931):81.

24. Sobel JD, Brooker D, Stein GE, et al. Single oral dose fluconazole compared with conventional clotrimazole topical therapy of *Candida* vaginitis. *Am J Obstet Gynecol* 1995;172:1263.

25. Sobel JD. Pathogenesis and treatment of recurrent vulvo-vaginal candidiasis. *Clin Infect Dis* 1992;14 (Suppl):S148.

26. Reef SE, Levine WC, McNeil MM, et al. Treatment options for vulvovaginal candidiasis, 1993. *Clin Infect Dis* 1995;20:S8O.

27. Paavonen J, Stamm WE. Lower genital tract infections in women. *Infect Dis Clin North Am* 1987;1:179.

28. Judson FN. The importance of coexisting syphilitic, chlamydial, mycoplasmal, and trichomonal infections in the treatment of gonorrhea. *Sex Transm Dis* 1979;6:112.

29. Hammill HA. *Trichomonas vaginalis. Obstet Gynecol Clin North Am* 1989;16:531.

30. Spence M. The clinical and laboratory diagnosis of *T. vaginalis* infection. *Sex Transm Dis* 1980;7:188.

31. The Medical Letter. Drugs for sexually transmitted diseases. *The Medical Letter* 1995;37(964):87.

32. Feingold S. Metronidazole. *Ann Intern Med* 1980;93:585.

33. Eschenbach DA. History and review of bacterial vaginosis. *Am J Obstet Gynecol* 1993;169:441.

34. Gardner HL, Dukes CD. *Haemophilus vaginalis* vaginitis: a newly defined specific infection previously classified as "non-specific vaginitis." *Am J Obstet Gynecol* 1955;69:962.

35. Eschenbach DA. Bacterial vaginosis: emphasis on upper genital tract complications. *Obstet Gynecol Clin North Am* 1989;16:593.

36. Joesoef MR, Schmid GP. Bacterial vaginosis: review of treatment options and potential clinical indications for therapy. *Clin Infect Dis* 1995;20:S72.

37. Shafer M-A, Sweet RL. Pelvic inflammatory disease in adolescent females. *Pediatr Clin North Am* 1989;36:513.

38. Hillier SL, Nugent RP, Eschenbach DA, et al. Association between bacterial vaginosis and preterm delivery of a low-birth-weight infant. *N Engl J Med* 1995;333:1737.

39. Stevens-Simon C, Jamison J, McGregor JA, et al. Racial variation in vaginal pH among healthy sexually active adolescents. *Sex Trans Dis* 1994;21:168.

40. Lugo-Miro VI, Green M, Mazur L. Comparison of different metronidazole therapeutic regiments for bacterial vaginosis: a meta-analysis. *JAMA* 1992;268:92.

41. Hauth JC, Goldenberg RL, Andrews WW, et al. Reduced incidence of preterm delivery with metronidazole and erythromycin in women with bacterial vaginosis. *N Engl J Med* 1995;333:1732.

42. Bump RC, Zuspan FP, Buesching WJ, et al. The prevalence, six-month persistence, and predictive values of laboratory indicators of bacterial vaginosis (nonspecific vaginitis) in asymptomatic women. *Am J Obstet Gynecol* 1984;150:917.

43. Centers for Disease Control and Prevention. 1989 Sexually transmitted diseases treatment guidelines. *MMWR Morb Mortal Wkly Rep* 1989;38(S-8):1.

44. Eschenbach DA, Hillier S, Critchlow C, et al. Diagnosis and clinical manifestation of bacterial vaginosis. *Am J Obstet Gynecol* 1988;158:819.

45. Clark JL, Tatum NO, Noble SL. Management of genital herpes. *Am Fam Physician* 1995;51:175.

46. Huerta K, Berkelhamer S, Klein J, et al. Epidemiology of herpes simplex virus type 2 infections in a high-risk adolescent population. *J Adolesc Health* 1996;18:384.
47. Rauh JL, Brookman RR, Schiff GM. Genital virus surveillance among sexually active adolescent girls. *J Pediatr* 1977;90:844.
48. Bryson I. Genital herpex simplex virus infections. *Adolescent Medicine: State of the Art Reviews* 1990; 1:471.
49. Becker TM, Stone KM, Cates W Jr. Epidemiology of genital herpes infections in the United States: the current situation. *J Reprod Med* 1996;31(Suppl):359.
50. Baker DA. Herpesvirus. *Clin Obstet Gynecol* 1983;26:165.
51. Landy HJ, Grossman JH. Herpes simplex virus. *Obstet Gynecol Clin North Am* 1989;16:495.
52. Adam E, Dreesman GE, Kaufman RH, et al. Asymptomatic virus shedding after herpes genitalis. *Am J Obstet Gynecol* 1980;137:827.
53. Wald A, Zeh J, Selke S, et al. Virologic characteristics of subclinical and symptomatic genital herpes infections. *N Engl J Med* 1995;333:770.
54. Nerurkar LS, West F, May M, et al. Survival of herpes simplex virus in water specimens collected from hot tubs in spa facilities and on plastic surfaces. *JAMA* 1983;250:3081.
55. Nelson CT, Demmier GJ. Superficial HSV infection: How serious is it? What should you do? *Contemporary Pediatrics* 1996;13:96.
56. Corey L, Adams HG, Brown ZA, et al. Genital herpes simplex virus infections: clinical manifestations, course, and complications. *Ann Intern Med* 1983;98:958.
57. Whitley RJ. Neonatal herpes simplex virus infections: presentation and management. *J Reprod Med* 1986;31 (Suppl):426.
58. Kinghorn GR. Genital herpes: natural history and treatment of acute episodes. *J Med Virol* 1993;1(Suppl):33.
59. Guinan ME, MacCalman J, Kern ER, et al. The course of untreated recurrent genital herpes simplex infection in 27 women. *N Engl J Med* 1981;304:759.
60. Harger JH, Pazin GJ, Breinig MC. Current understanding of the natural history of genital herpes simplex infections. *J Reprod Med* 1986.61;31(Suppl):365.
61. Chacko MR, Rosenfeld WD. The uterine cervix: diagnostic opportunities. *Pediatr Ann* 1995;24:317.
62. Verano L, Michalski FJ. Comparison of a direct antigen enzyme immunoassay, Herpchek, with cell culture for detection of herpes simplex virus from clinical specimens. *J Clin Microbiol* 1995;33:1378.
63. Wald A, Zeh J, Barnum G, et al. Suppression of subclinical shedding of herpes simplex virus type 2 with acyclovir. *Ann Intern Med* 1996;124(1 pt. 1):8.
64. Mertz GJ, Jones CC, Mills J, et al. Long-term acyclovir suppression of frequently recurring genital herpes simplex virus infection: a multicenter double-blind trial. *JAMA* 1988;260:201.
65. Kaplowitz LG, Baker D, Gelb L, et al. Prolonged continuous acyclovir treatment of normal adults with frequently recurring genital herpes simplex virus infection: the Acyclovir Study Group. *JAMA* 1991;265:747.
66. Goldberg LH, Kaufman R, Kurtz TO, et al. Long-term suppression of recurrent genital herpes with acyclovir: a 5-year benchmark. *Arch Dermatol* 1993;129:582.
67. Baker DA, Milch PO. Acyclovir for genital herpes simplex virus infections: a review. *J Reprod Med* 1986;31 (Suppl):433.
68. The Medical Letter. Valacyclovir and famciclovir. *The Medical Letter* 1994;36:97.
69. Muckerman DR. Subclinical human papillomavirus infection in a high-risk population. *J Am Osteopath Assoc* 1994;94:545.
70. Vogel LN. Epidemiology of human papilloma virus infection. *Semin Dermatol* 1992;11:226.
71. Craighill MC. Human papillomavirus infection in children and adolescents. *Seminars in Pediatric Infectious Diseases* 1993;4:85.
72. Mayeaux EJ, Harper MB, Barksdale W,, et al. Noncervical human papillomavirus genital infections. *Am Fam Physician* 1995;52:1137.
73. Becker TM, Stone KM, Alexander ER. Genital human papillomavirus infection: a growing concern. *Obstet Gynecol Clin North Am* 1987;14:389.
74. Zaninetti P, Franceschi S, Baccolo M, et al. Characteristics of women under 20 with cervical intraepithelial neoplasia. *Int J Epidemiol* 1986;15:477.
75. Raymond C. Cervical dysplasia upturn worries gynecologists, health officials. *JAMA* 1987;257:2397.
76. Martinez J, Smith R, Farmer M, et al. High prevalence of genital tract papillomavirus infection in female adolescents. *Pediatrics* 1988;82:604.
77. Moscicki AB, Palefsky J, Gonzales J, et al. Human papillomavirus infection in sexually active adolescent females: prevalence and risk factors. *Pediatr Res* 1990;28:507.
78. Bauer HM, Ting YY, Greer CE, et al. Genital human papillomavirus infection in female university students as determined by PCR-based method. *JAMA* 1991;265:472.
79. Figueroa JP, Ward E, Luthi TE, et al. Prevalence of human papillomavirus among STD clinic attenders in Jamaica: association of younger age and increased sexual activity. *Sex Transm Dis* 1995;22:114.
80. Rosenfeld WD, Vermund SH, Wentz SJ. High prevalence rate of human papillomavirus infection and association with abnormal Papanicolaou smears in sexually active adolescents. *American Journal of Diseases of Children* 1989;143:1443.

81. American College of Obstetrics and Gynecology. Genital human papillomavirus infections. *American College of Obstetrics and Gynecology Technical Bulletin* 1987;105:1.
82. Cannistra SA, Niloff JM. Cancer of the uterine cervix. *N Engl J Med* 1996;334:1030.
83. Meisels A, Morin C. Human papillomavirus and cancer of the uterine cervix. *Gynecol Oncol* 1981;12:S111.
84. Moscicki B. HPV infections: an old STD revisited. *Contemporary Pediatrics* 1989;6:12.
85. Brinton LA, Hamman RF, Huggins GR, et al. Sexual and reproductive risk factors for invasive squamous cell cervical cancer. *J Natl Cancer Inst* 1990;79:23.
86. Fisher M, Rosenfeld WD, Burk RD. Cervicovaginal human papillomavirus infection in suburban adolescents and young adults. *J Pediatr* 1991;119:821.
87. Shew ML, Fortenberry JD, Miles P, et al. Interval between menarche and first sexual intercourse, related to risk of human papillomavirus infection. *J Pediatr* 1994;125:661.
88. Kataja V, Syrjanen S, Yliskoski M, et al. Risk factors associated with cervical human papillomavirus infections: a case-control study. *Am J Epidemiol* 1993;138:735.
89. Mitchell H, Drake M, Medley G. Prospective evaluation of risk of cervical cancer after cytological evidence of human papillomavirus infection. *Lancet* 1986;15:573.
90. Reeves WC, Brinton LA, Garcia M, et al. Human papillomavirus infection and cervical cancer in Latin America. *N Engl J Med* 1989;320:1437.
91. Collins JE, Jenkins D, McCance W. Detection of human papillomavirus DNA sequences by in situ DNA-DNA hybridization in cervical intraepithelial neoplasia and invasive carcinoma: a retrospective study. *J Clin Pathol* 1988;41:289.
92. Phelps WC, Yee CL, Munger K, et al. The human papillomavirus type 16 E7 gene encodes transactivation and transformation function similar to those to adenovirus E1A. *Cell* 1988;53:539.
93. Hillard GD, Massey FM, O'Toole FVJ. Vulvar neoplasia in the young. *Am J Obstet Gynecol* 1980;135:185.
94. Johnson TL, Joseph CL, Caison-Sorey TJ, et al. Prevalence of HPV 16 and 18 DNA sequences in CIN III lesions of adults and adolescents. *Diagn Cytopathol* 1994;10:276.
95. Rylander E, Ruusuvaara L, Almstromer MW, et al. The absence of vaginal human papillomavirus 16 DNA in women who have not yet experienced sexual intercourse. *Obstet Gynecol* 1994;83:735.
96. Adimora AA, Quinlivan EG. Papillomavirus infection: recent findings on progression to cervical cancer. *Postgrad Med* 1995;98:109.
97. Bergernon C, Ferencay A, Shah KN, et al. Multicentric human papilloma virus infections of the female genital tract. *Obstet Gynecol* 1987;69:736.
98. Rosenfeld WD, Rose E, Vermund SH, et al. Follow-up evaluation of cervicovaginal human papillomavirus infection in adolescents. *J Pediatr* 1992;121:307.
99. Kellogg ND, Parra JM. The progression of human papillomavirus lesions in sexual assault victims. *Pediatrics* 1995;96:1163.
100. Walker PG, Calley NU, Gruff C et al. Abnormalities of the uterine cervix in women with vulvar warts. *British Journal of Venereal Disease* 1983;59:120.
101. Dyment PG. Human papillomavirus infection. *Adolescent Medicine: State of the Art Reviews* 1996;7:119.
102. Krebs HB, Schneider V. Human papillomavirus-associated lesions of the penis: colposcopy, cytology, and histology. *Obstet Gynecol* 1987;70:299.
103. Moscicki B. Genital human papilloma virus infections. *Adolescent Medicine: State of the Art Reviews* 1990;1:451.
104. Campion MJ. Clinical manifestations and natural history of genital human papillomavirus infection. *Obstet Gynecol Clin North Am* 1987;14:363.
105. Davis A-J, Emans SJ. Human papilloma virus infection in the pediatric and adolescent patient. *J Pediatr* 1989;115:1.
106. Koutsky LA, Wolner-Hanssen P. Genital papillomavirus infections: current knowledge and future prospects. *Obstet Gynecol Clin North Am* 1989;16:541.
107. Drake M, Medley G, Mitchell H. Cytologic detection of human papillomavirus infection. *Obstet Gynecol Clin North Am* 1987;14:431.
108. Campion MJ, McCane DJ, Cuzick J et al. Progressive potential of mild cervical atypia: prospective cytological and virological study. *Lancet* 1986;2:237.
109. Diagnostic and Therapeutic Technology Assessment (DATTA). Human papillomavirus DNA testing in the management of cervical neoplasia. *JAMA* 1993;267:2493–2496.
110. Hillard PA, Biro FM, Wildey L. Complications of cervical cryotherapy in adolescents. *J Reprod Med* 1991;36:711.
111. Miller DM, Brodell RT. Human papillomavirus infection: treatment options for warts. *Am Fam Physician* 1996;53:135.
112. Stone KM. Human papillomavirus infection and genital warts: update on epidemiology and treatment. *Clin Infect Dis* 1995;20(Suppl 1):S91.
113. The Medical Letter. Podofilox for genital warts. *The Medical Letter* 1991;33:117.
114. Krebs H-B. Treatment of vaginal condylomata acuminata by weekly topical application of 5-fluorouracil. *Obstet Gynecol* 1987;70:68.
115. Hasumi K. A trial of topical idoxuridine for vulvar condylomata acuminata. *Br J Obstet Gynaecol* 1987;94:366.

116. Sykes NL Jr. Condyloma acuminatum. *Int J Dermatol* 1995;34:297.
117. The Medical Letter. Interferon for treatment of genital warts. *The Medical Letter* 1988;30:70.
118. Jamieson MA, Hertweck SP, Sanfilippo JS. Successful cimetidine therapy for multiple genital condyloma in an adolescent female. *Journal of Pediatric and Adolescent Gynecology* 1996;9:155.
119. Orlow SJ, Paller A. Cimetidine therapy for multiple viral warts in children. *J Am Acad Dermatol* 1993;28: 794.
120. Ferenczy A, ed. Symposium: treating condylomata. *Contemporary Obstetrics and Gynecology* 1987;32:158.
121. Richart RM, Baggish MS, Ferenczy AM, et al. Using the CO_2 laser for genital surgery. Contemporary Obstetrics and Gynecology 1989;34:106.
122. Gutman LT. Human papillomavirus infections of the genital tract in adolescents. *Adolescent Medicine: State of the Art Reviews* 1995;6:115.
123. Ferenczy A, Mitoo M, Nagar N, et al. Latent papilloma virus and recurring genital warts. *N Engl J Med* 1985; 313:784.
124. Riva JM, Sedlacek TV, Cunnane MF, et al. Extended CO_2 laser vaporization in the treatment of subclinical papillomavirus infection of the lower genital tract. *Obstet Gynecol* 1989;73:25.
125. Krebs HB, Pastore L, Helmkamp BF. Loop electrosurgical excision procedures for cervical dysplasia: experience in a community hospital. *Am J Obstet Gynecol* 1993;169:289.
126. Crane S. Abnormal Pap smears in the adolescent: the role of LEEP. *NASPAG News* 1995;9(1):1.
127. Malviya VK, Deppe G, Pluszczynski R, et al. Tricholoro-acetic acid in the treatment of human papillomavirus infection of the cervix without associated dysplasia. *Obstet Gynecol* 1987;70:72.
128. Kulig JW. Adolescent contraception: nonhormonal methods. *Pediatr Clin North Am* 1989;36:717.
129. Webster LA, Greenspan JR, Nakashima AK, et al. An evaluation of surveillance for *Chlamydia trachomatis* infections in the United States, 1987–1991. *MMWR Morb Mortal Wkly Rep* 1993;42(SS-3):21.
130. Centers for Disease Control and Prevention. Ten leading nationally notifiable infectious diseases: United States, 1995. *MMWR Morb Mortal Wkly Rep* 1996;45:883.
131. Skolnik NS. Screening for *Chlamydia trachomatis* infection. *Am Fam Physician* 1995;51:821.
132. Fisher M, Swenson PD, Risucci D, et al. *Chlamydia trachomatis* in suburban adolescents. *J Pediatr* 1987; 111:617.
133. Soren K, Willis E. *Chlamydia* and the adolescent girl. *American Journal of Diseases of Children* 1989; 143:51.
134. Biro FM, Rosenthal SL, Kiniyalocts M. Gonococcal and chlamydial genitourinary infections in symptomatic and asymptomatic adolescent women. *Clin Pediatr* 1995;34:419.
135. Rettig PJ. Chlamydia trachomatis infection in pediatrics. *Seminars in Pediatric Infectious Diseases* 1993; 4:151.
136. Hammerschlag MR. Chlamydial infections. *J Pediatr* 1989;114:727.
137. Martin DH, Mroczkowski TF, Dalu ZA, et al. A controlled trial of a single dose of azithromycin for the treatment of chlamydial urethritis and cervicitis. *N Engl J Med* 1992;327:921.
138. Hammerschlag MR, Golden NH, Oh MK, et al. Single dose of azithromycin for the treatment of genital chlamydia infections in adolescents. *J Pediatr* 1993;122:961.
139. Schachter J. Chlamydial infections. *West J Med* 1990;153:523.
140. Harrison HR, Costin M, Meder JB, et al. Cervical *Chlamydia trachomatis* infection in university women: relationship to history, contraception, ectopy, and cervicitis. *Am J Obstet Gynecol* 1985;153:244.
141. Shafer MA, Beck A, Blain B, et al. *Chlamydia trachomatis:* important relationships to race, contraception, lower genital tract infection, and Papanicolaou smear. *J Pediatr* 1984;104:141.
142. Moscicki A-B, Winkler B, Irwin CE Jr, et al. Differences in biologic maturation, sexual behavior, and sexually transmitted disease between adolescents with and without cervical intraepithelial neoplasia. *J Pediatr* 1989;115:487.
143. Oh MK, Feinstein RA, Soileau EJ, et al. *Chlamydia trachomatis* cervical infection and oral contraceptive use among adolescent girls. *Journal of Adolescent Health Care* 1989;10:376.
144. Critchlow CW, Wolner-Hanssen P, Eschenbach DA, et al. Determinants of cervical ectopia and of cervicitis: age, oral contraception, specific cervical infection, smoking, and douching. *Am J Obstet Gynecol* 1995;173: 534.
145. McGregor JA. Chlamydial infection in women. *Obstet Gynecol Clin North Am* 1989;16:565.
146. Hammerschlag MR. *Chlamydia trachomatis* in children. *Pediatr Ann* 1994;23:349.
147. Majeroni BA. Chlamydia cervicitis: complications and new treatment options. *Am Fam Physician* 1994;49: 1825.
148. Schacter J. Why we need a program for the control of *Chlamydia trachomatis*. *N Engl J Med* 1989;320:802.
149. Emans SJH, Goldstein DP. *Pediatric and adolescent gynecology.* 4th ed. Philadelphia: Lippincott–Raven Publishers; 1997.
150. Remafedi G, Abdalian SE. Clinical predictors of *Chlamydia trachomatis* endocervicitis in adolescent women. *American Journal of Diseases of Children* 1989;143:1437.
151. Blythe MJ, Katz BP, Orr DP, et al. Historical and clinical factors associated with *Chlamydia trachomatis* genitourinary infection in female adolescents. *J Pediatr* 1988;112:1000.

152. Stamm WE, Wagner KF, Amsel R, et al. Causes of the acute urethral syndrome in women. *N Engl J Med* 1980;303:409.

153. Morris RE, Legault J, Baker C. Prevalence of isolated urethral asymptomatic *Chlamydia trachomatis* infection in the absence of cervical infection in incarcerated adolescent girls. *Sex Transm Dis* 1993;20:198.

154. Heath CB, Heath JM. *Chlamydia trachomatis* infection update. *Am Fam Physician* 1995;52:1455.

155. Hillis SD, Wasserheit JN. Screening for chlamydia: a key to the prevention of pelvic inflammatory disease. *N Engl J Med* 1996;334:1399.

156. Shafer MA, Schachter J, Moncada J, et al. Evaluation of urine-based screening strategies to detect *Chlamydia trachomatis* among sexually active asymptomatic young males. *JAMA* 1993;270:2065.

157. Biro FM, Reising SF, Doughman JA, et al. A comparison of diagnostic methods in adolescent girls with and without symptoms of chlamydia urogenital infection. *Pediatrics* 1994;93:476.

158. Evans EL, Demetriou E, Shalaby H, et al. Detection of *Chlamydia trachomatis* in adolescent females using direct immunofluorescence. *Clin Pediatr* 1988;27:223.

159. Oh MK, Mulchahey KM, Pass MA, et al. Enzyme immunoassay for detection of asymptomatic chlamydia cervical infection in pregnant adolescents. *Adolescent and Pediatric Gynecology* 1989;2:153.

160. Regard MM, Chacko MR, Kozinetz CA, et al. Reliability of cervical findings and endocervical polymorphonuclear cells in detecting chlamydia and gonococcal cervicitis in young women receiving contraceptive services. *Adolescent and Pediatric Gynecology* 1993;6:129.

161. Fraiz J, Jones RB. Chlamydial infections. *Annu Rev Med* 1988;39:357.

162. Werner MJ, Biro FM. Urinary leukocyte esterase screening for asymptomatic sexually transmitted disease in adolescent males. *J Adolesc Health* 1991;12:326.

163. Genc M, Ruusuvaara L, Mardh PA. An economic evaluation of screening for *Chlamydia trachomatis* in adolescent males. *JAMA* 1993;270:2057.

164. Yang LI, Panke ES, Leist PA, et al. Detection of *Chlamydia trachomatis* endocervical infection in asymptomatic and symptomatic women: comparison of deoxyribonucleic acid probe test with tissue culture. *Am J Obstet Gynecol* 1991;165:1444.

165. Bryant DK, Fox AS, Spigland I, et al. Comparison of rapid diagnostic methodologies for chlamydia and gonorrhea in an urban adolescent population: a pilot study. *J Adolesc Health* 1995;16:324.

166. Hsuih TCH, Guichon A, Diaz A, et al. Chlamydial infection in a high-risk population: comparison of Amplicor PCR and Gen-Probe PACE II for diagnosis. *Adolescent and Pediatric Gynecology* 1995;8:71.

167. Jaschek G, Gaydos CA, Welsh LE, et al. Direct detection of *Chlamydia trachomatis* in urine specimens from symptomatic and asymptomatic men by using a rapid polymerase chain reaction assay. *J Clin Microbiol* 1993;31:1209.

168. Domeika M, Bassiri M, Mardh PA. Diagnosis of genital *Chlamydia trachomatis* infections in asymptomatic males by testing urine by PCR. *J Clin Microbiol* 1994;32:2350.

169. Chernesky MA, Jang D, Lee H, et al. Diagnosis of *Chlamydia trachomatis* infections in men and women by testing first-void urine by ligase chain reaction. *J Clin Microbiol* 1994;32:2682.

170. Lee HH, Chernesky MA, Schachter J, et al. Diagnosis of *Chlamydia trachomatis* genitourinary infection in women by ligase chain reaction assay of urine. *Lancet* 1995;345:213.

171. The Medical Letter. Clarithromycin and azithromycin. *The Medical Letter* 1992;34:45.

172. Weber JT, Johnson RE. New treatments for *Chlamydia trachomatis* genital infection. *Clin Infect Dis* 1995; 20(Suppl 1):S66.

173. Nuovo J, Melnikow J, Paliescheskey M, et al. Cost-effectiveness analysis of five different antibiotic regimens for the treatment of uncomplicated *Chlamydia trachomatis* cervicitis. *J Am Board Fam Pract* 1995;8:7.

174. Martin DH, Mroczkowski TF, Dalu ZA, et al. A controlled trial of azithromycin for the treatment of chlamydial urethritis and cervicitis: the Azithromycin for Chlamydial Infections Study Group. *N Engl J Med* 1992; 327:921.

175. Stamm WE, Hicks CB, Martin DH, et al. Azithromycin for empirical treatment of the nongonococcal urethritis syndrome in men: a randomized double-blind study. *JAMA* 1995;274:545.

176. Alary M, Joly JR, Moutquin JM, et al. Randomised comparison of amoxicillin and erythromycin in treatment of genital chlamydial infection in pregnancy. *Lancet* 1994;344:1461.

177. Workowski KA, Lampe MF, Wong KG, et al. Long-term eradication of *Chlamydia trachomatis* genital infection after microbial therapy. *JAMA* 1993;270:2071.

178. Oh MK, Cloud GA, Fleenor M, et al. Risk for gonococcal and chlamydia cervicitis in adolescent females: incidence and recurrence in a prospective cohort study. *J Adolesc Health* 1996;18:270.

179. Rosenthal SL, Baker JG, Biro FM, et al. Secondary prevention of STD transmission during adolescence: Partner notification. *Adolescent and Pediatric Gynecology* 1995;8:183.

180. Centers for Disease Control and Prevention. Increasing incidence of gonorrhea: Minnesota, 1994. *MMWR Morb Mortal Wkly Rep* 1995;44:282.

181. Rosen DS, Xiangdong M, Blum RW. Adolescent health: current trends and critical issues. *Adolescent Medicine: State of the Art Reviews* 1990;1:27.

182. Webster LA, Berman SM, Greenspan JR. Surveillance for gonorrhea and primary and secondary syphilis among adolescents, United States: 1981–1991. *MMWR Morb Mortal Wkly Rep* 1993;42(SS-3):1.

183. Moran JS, Levine WC. Drugs of choice for the treatment of uncomplicated gonococcal infections. *Clin Infect Dis* 1995;20(Suppl 1):S47.

184. Gorwitz RJ, Nakashima AK, Moran JS, et al. Sentinel surveillance for antimicrobial resistance in *Neisseria gonorrhoeae*: United States, 1988–1991. *MMWR Morb Mortal Wkly Rep* 1993;42:29.

185. Centers for Disease Control and Prevention. Fluoroquinolone resistance in *Neisseria gonorrhoeae*: Colorado and Washington, 1995. *MMWR Morb Mortal Wkly Rep* 1995;44:761.

186. Hein K, Marks A, Cohen MI. Asymptomatic gonorrhea: prevalence in a population of urban adolescents. *J Pediatr* 1977;90:634.

187. Demetriou E, Sackett R, Welch DF, et al. Evaluation of an enzyme immunoassay for detection of *Neisseria gonorrhoeae* in an adolescent population. *JAMA* 1984;252:247.

188. Gilbaugh JH Jr, Fuchs PC. The gonococcus and the toilet seat. *N Engl J Med* 1979;301:91.

189. Woods CR Jr. Gonococcal infections in children and adolescents. *Seminars in Pediatric Infectious Diseases* 1993;4:94.

190. Greydanus DE, Sladkin K, Rosenstock R. Vulvovaginitis in the adolescent. In: Strasburger VC, ed. *Basic office gynecology: an office primer.* Baltimore: Urban & Schwarzenberg; 1990:81.

191. Mandegar M, Schaff EA. Is the clinical spectrum of gonorrhea changing? *J Adolesc Health* 1995;17:123.

192. McNeeley SG Jr. Gonococcal infections in women. *Obstet Gynecol Clin North Am* 1989;16:467.

193. Hale YM, Melton ME, Lewis JS, et al. Evaluation of the PACE 2 *Neisseria gonorrhoeae* assay by three public health laboratories. *J Clin Microbiol* 1993;31:451.

194. Hanks JW, Scott CT, Butler CE, et al. Evaluation of a DNA probe assay (Gen-Probe PACE 2) as the test of cure for *Neisseria gonorrhoeae* genital infections. *J Pediatr* 1994;125:161.

195. Schichor A, Bernstein B. Lidocaine as a diluent for ceftriaxone in the treatment of gonorrhea: does it reduce the pain of injection? *Arch Pediatr Adolesc Med* 1994;148:72.

196. Laras L, Craighill M, Woods ER, et al. Epidemiologic observations of adolescents with *Neisseria gonorrhoeae* genital infections treated at a children's hospital. *Adolescent and Pediatric Gynecology* 1994;7:9.

197. Turner BP, Peyton CE, Wisnoski KL, et al. The rate of coinfectivity with *Neisseria gonorrhoeae* from patients infected with *Chlamydia trachomatis.* Presented at the 95th annual meeting of the American Society for Microbiology, Washington, DC, 1995, Abstract No. C-126.

198. Webster LA, Rolfs RT. Surveillance for primary and secondary syphilis: United States, 19@91. *MMWR Morb Mortal Wkly Rep* 1993;42(SS-3):13.

199. Centers for Disease Control and Prevention. Summary of notifiable diseases, United States, 1994. *MMWR Morb Mortal Wkly Rep* 1995;43:1.

200. Coles FB, Hipp SS. Syphilis among adolescents: the hidden epidemic. *Contemporary Pediatrics* 1996;13:47.

201. Coles FB, Hipp SS, Silberstein GS, et al. Congenital syphilis surveillance in upstate New York, 1989–1992: implications for prevention and clinical management. *J Infect Dis* 1995;171:732.

202. Thomas JC, Kulik AL, Schoenback VJ. Syphilis in the South: rural rates surpass urban rates in North Carolina. *Am J Public Health* 1995;85:1119.

203. Goens JL, Janniger CK, De Wolf K. Dermatologic and systemic manifestations of syphilis. *Am Fam Physician* 1994;50:1013.

204. Lukehart SA, Hook EW, Baker-Zander SA, et al. Invasion of the central nervous system by *Treponema pallidum*: implications for diagnosis and treatment. *Ann Intern Med* 1988;109:855.

205. Wendel GD Jr. Early and congenital syphilis. *Obstet Gynecol Clin North Am* 1989;16:479.

206. Jurado RL, Campbell J, Martin PD. Prozone phenomenon in secondary syphilis. *Arch Intern Med* 1993;153:2496.

207. Rolfs RT. Treatment of syphilis, 1993. *Clin Infect Dis* 1995;20(Suppl 1):S23.

208. Berry CD, Hooton TM, Collier AC, et al. Neurologic relapse after benzathine penicillin therapy for secondary syphilis in a patient with HIV infection. *N Engl J Med* 1987;316:1587.

209. Malone JL, Wallace MR, Hendrick BB, et al. Syphilis and neurosyphilis in a human immunodeficiency virus type-1 seropositive population: evidence for frequent serologic relapse after therapy. *Am J Med* 1995;99:55.

210. Augenbraun MH, McCormack WH. Pelvic inflammatory disease: an ongoing epidemic. *Hosp Pract* 1995;30:61.

211. Strasburger VC, Brown RT, eds. Office practice of adolescent medicine. *Pediatr Clin North Am* 1997 (in press).

212. Westrom L. Incidence, prevalence, and trends of acute pelvic inflammatory disease and its consequences in industrialized countries. *Am J Obstet Gynecol* 1980;138:880.

213. Sleisenger MH, Fordtran JS. *Gastrointestinal disease: pathophysiology, diagnosis, and management.* 3rd ed. Philadelphia: WB Saunders; 1983.

214. Aral SO, Mosher WD, Cates W. Self-reported pelvic inflammatory disease in the United States, 1988. *JAMA* 1991;266:2570.

215. Soper DE. Pelvic inflammatory disease. *Infect Dis Clin North Am* 1994;8:821.

216. Washington AE, Aral SO, Wolner-Hanssen P, et al. Assessing risk for pelvic inflammatory disease and its sequelae. *JAMA* 1991;266:2581.

217. Grodstein F, Rothman KJ. Epidemiology of pelvic inflammatory disease. *Epidemiology* 1994;5:234.

218. McCormack WM. Pelvic inflammatory disease. *N Engl J Med* 1994;330:115.

219. Hillis SD. PID prevention: clinical and societal stakes. *Hosp Pract* 1994;29:89.
220. Rosenfeld WD, Swedler JB. Role of hormonal contraceptives in prevention of pregnancy and sexually transmitted diseases. *Adolescent Medicine: State of the Art Reviews* 1992;3:207.
221. Hatcher RA, Trussell J, Stewart F, et al. *Contraceptive technology.* 17th ed. New York: Irvington; 1998.
222. Burkman RT Jr. Oral contraceptives: an update. *Hosp Pract* 1995;30:85.
223. Farley TMM, Rosenberg MJ, Rowe PJ, et al. Intrauterine devices and pelvic inflammatory disease: an international perspective. *Lancet* 1992;339:785.
224. Editorial. Does infection occur with modern intrauterine devices? *Lancet* 1992;339:783.
225. Rice PA, Schachter J. Pathogenesis of pelvic inflammatory disease: what are the questions? *JAMA* 1991;266:2587.
226. Sweet RL. Pelvic inflammatory disease and infertility in women. *Infect Dis Clin North Am* 1987;1:199.
227. Sweet RL, Blankfort-Doyle M, Robbie MO, et al. The occurrence of chlamydial and gonococcal salpingitis during the menstrual cycle. *JAMA* 1986;255:2062.
228. Eschenbach DA, Hillier S, Critchlow C, et al. Diagnosis and clinical manifestations of bacterial vaginosis. *Am J Obstet Gynecol* 1988;155:819.
229. Washington AE, Sweet RL, Shafer MA. Pelvic inflammatory disease in the adolescent female and its sequelae. *Journal of Adolescent Health Care* 1985;6:298.
230. Dan BB. Sex, lives, and chlamydia rates. *JAMA* 1990;263:3191.
231. Westrom L. Effect of acute pelvic inflammatory diseases on fertility. *Am J Obstet Gynecol* 1975;121:707.
232. Westrom L, Joesoef R, Reynolds G, et al. Pelvic inflammatory disease and fertility: a cohort study of 1,844 women with laparoscopically verified disease and 657 control women with normal laparoscopic results. *Sex Transm Dis* 1992;19:185.
233. Wolner-Hansen P, Kiviat NB, Holmes KK. Atypical pelvic inflammatory disease: subacute, chronic, or subclinical upper genital tract infection in women. In: Holmes KK, Mardh PA, Sparling PF, et al, eds. *Sexually transmitted diseases.* 2nd ed. New York: McGraw-Hill; 1990:615.
234. Jacobson L, Westrom L. Objectivized diagnosis of acute pelvic inflammatory disease. *Am J Obstet Gynecol* 1980;138:905.
235. Method MW. Laparoscopy in the diagnosis of pelvic inflammatory disease. *J Reprod Med* 1988;33:901.
236. Bulas DI, Ahlstrom PA, Sivit CJ, et al. Pelvic inflammatory disease in the adolescent: comparison of transabdominal and transvaginal sonographic evaluation. *Radiology* 1992;183:435.
237. Benaim J, Pulaski ME, Coupey SM. Adolescent girls and PID: Treatment in the pediatric emergency room [abstract]. *Journal of Pediatric and Adolescent Gynecology* 1996;9:153.
238. Litt IR, Cuskey WR. Compliance with medical regimens during adolescence. *Pediatr Clin North Am* 1980;27:3.
239. Brookoff D. Compliance with doxycycline therapy for outpatient treatment of pelvic inflammatory disease. *South Med J* 1994;87:1088.
240. Walker CK, Kahn JG, Washington AE, et al. Pelvic inflammatory disease: metaanalysis of antimicrobial regimen efficacy. *J Infect Dis* 1993;168:969.
241. Washington AE, Wiesner PJ. The silent clap. *JAMA* 1981;245:609.
242. Cacciatore B, Leminen A, Ingman-Friberg S, et al. Transvaginal sonographic findings in ambulatory patients with suspected pelvic inflammatory disease. *Obstet Gynecol* 1992;80:912.
243. Cromer BA, Brandstaetter LA, Fischer RA, et al. Tubo-ovarian abscess in adolescents. *Adolescent and Pediatric Gynecology* 1990;3:21.
244. Golden N, Neuhoff S, Cohen H. Pelvic inflammatory disease in adolescents. *J Pediatr* 1989;114:138.
245. Slap GB, Forke CM, Cnaan A, et al. Recognition of tubo-ovarian abscess in adolescents with pelvic inflammatory disease. *J Adolesc Health* 1996;18:397.
246. Fitz-Hugh T Jr. Acute gonococcic peritonitis of right upper quadrant in women. *JAMA* 1934;102:2094.
247. Curtis AH. Cause of adhesions in right upper quadrant. *JAMA* 1930;94:1221.
248. Lopez-Zeno JA, Keith LG, Berger GS. The Fitz-Hugh–Curtis syndrome revisited: changing perspective after half a century. *J Reprod Med* 1985;30:567.
249. Wang S, Eschenbach DA, Holmes KK, et al. *Chlamydia trachomatis* infection in Fitz-Hugh–Curtis syndrome. *Am J Obstet Gynecol* 1980;138:1034.
250. Katzman DK, Friedman JM, McDonald CA, et al. *Chlamydial trachomatis* Fitz-Hugh–Curtis syndrome without salpingitis in female adolescents. *American Journal of Diseases of Children* 1988;142:996.
251. Litt IF, Cohen MI. Perihepatitis associated with salpingitis in adolescents. *JAMA* 1978;240:1253.
252. Hook EW, Holmes KK. Gonococcal infections. *Ann Intern Med* 1985;102:229.
253. Olsen-Noll CG, Convery SR, Bosworth MF, et al. Gonococcal endocarditis. *J Fam Pract* 1989;29:305.
254. Handsfield HH, Pollock PS. Arthritis associated with sexually transmitted diseases. In: Holmes KK, Mardh PA, Sparling PF, et al, eds. *Sexually transmitted diseases.* 2nd ed. New York: McGraw-Hill; 1990:737.
255. Kerle KK, Mascola JR, Miller TA. Disseminated gonococcal infection. *Am Fam Physician* 1992;45:209.
256. Wise CM, Morris CR, Wasilauskas BL, et al. Gonococcal arthritis in an era of increasing penicillin resistance: presentations and outcomes in 41 recent cases (1985–1991). *Arch Intern Med* 1994;154:2690.
257. Strasburger VC. Why adolescent medicine? Four illustrative cases. *Clin Pediatr* 1984;23:12.
258. Brown RT, Lossick JG, Mosure DJ, et al. Pharyngeal gonorrhea screening in adolescents: is it necessary? *Pediatrics* 1989;84:623.

259. Brandt KD, Catheartes ES, Cohen AS. Gonococcal arthritis. *Arthritis Rheum* 1974;17:503.
260. Zenilman J. Gonococcal infections in adolescents. *Adolescent Medicine: State of the Art Reviews* 1990;1:497.
261. Washington AE, Gives S, Schachter J, et al. Oral contraceptives, *Chlamydia trachomatis* infection, and pelvic inflammatory disease: a word of caution about protection. *JAMA* 1985;124:2246.
262. Wolner-Hansen P, Svensson L, Mardh P-A, et al. Laparascopic findings and contraceptive use in women with signs and symptoms suggestive of acute salpingitis. *Obstet Gynecol* 1985;66:233.
263. Centers for Disease Control and Prevention. Ectopic pregnancy: United States, 1987. *MMWR Morb Mortal Wkly Rep* 1990;39:401.
264. Chow JM, Yonekura L, Richwald GA, et al. The association between *Chlamydia trachomatis* and ectopic pregnancy: a matched-pair, case-control study. *JAMA* 1990;263:3164.
265. Scholes D, Stergachis A, Heidrich FE, et al. Prevention of pelvic inflammatory disease by screening for cervical chlamydial infection. *N Engl J Med* 1996;334:1362.
266. Genc M, Mardh PA. A cost-effective analysis of screening and treatment for *Chlamydia trachomatis* infection in asymptomatic women. *Ann Intern Med* 1996;124:1.
267. Advocates for Youth. *Fact sheet: adolescents in peril: The HIV/AIDS pandemic.* Washington, DC: Advocates for Youth; 1996.
268. Cao Y, Qin L, Zhang L, et al. Virologic and immunologic characterization of long-term survivors of human immunodeficiency virus type 1 infection. *N Engl J Med* 1995;332:201.
269. Centers for Disease Control and Prevention. Update: acquired immunodeficiency syndrome: United States, 1994. *MMWR Morb Mortal Wkly Rep* 1995;44:64.
270. Centers for Disease Control and Prevention. Update: mortality attributable to HIV infection among persons aged 25–44 years: United States, 1994. *MMWR Morb Mortal Wkly Rep* 1996;45:121.
271. Futterman D, Hein K, Reuben N. Human immunodeficiency virus-infected adolescents: the first 50 patients in a New York City program. *Pediatrics* 1993;91:730.
272. Hoffman ND, Futterman D. Human immunodeficiency virus infection in adolescents. *Seminars in Pediatric Infectious Diseases* 1993;4:113.
273. Wenstrom KD, Gall SA. HIV infection in women. *Obstet Gynecol Clin North Am* 1989;16:627.
274. Zylke JW. Interest heightens in defining, preventing AIDS in high-risk adolescent population. *JAMA* 1989;262:2197.
275. Quinn T, Glasser D, Cannon R, et al. Human immunodeficiency virus infection among patients attending clinics for sexually transmitted diseases. *N Engl J Med* 1988;318:197.
276. Sperling R, Sacks H, Mayer L,, et al. Umbilical cord blood serosurvey for human immunodeficiency virus in parturient women in a voluntary hospital in New York City. *Obstet Gynecol* 1989;73:179.
277. Centers for Disease Control and Prevention. *National HIV serosurveillance summary: results through 1990.* Atlanta: U.S. Department of Health and Human Services, Public Health Service; 1992.
278. St. Louis ME, Rauch KJ, Peterson LR, et al. Seroprevalence rates of human immunodeficiency virus infection at sentinel hospitals in the United States. *N Engl J Med* 1990;323:213.
279. Burke DS, Brundage JF, Goldenbaum M, et al. Human immunodeficiency virus infections in teenagers: seroprevalence among applicants for US military service. *JAMA* 1990;263:2074.
280. Gayle HD, Keeling RP, Garcia-Tunon M, et al. Prevalence of the human immunodeficiency virus among university students. *N Engl J Med* 1990;323:1538.
281. Sweeney P, Lindegren ML, Buehler JW, et al. Teenagers at risk of human immunodeficiency virus type 1 infection: results from seroprevalence surveys in the United States. *Arch Pediatr Adolesc Med* 1995;149:521.
282. Boyer CB, Kegeles SM. AIDS risk and prevention among adolescents. *Soc Sci Med* 1991;22:11.
283. Moscicki AB, Millstein SG, Broering J, et al. Risks of human immunodeficiency virus infection among adolescents attending three diverse clinics. *J Pediatr* 1993;122:813.
284. Hein K, Dell R, Futterman D, et al. Comparison of HIV+ and HIV− adolescents: risk factors and psychosocial determinants. *Pediatrics* 1995;95:96.
285. Heffernan R, Chiasson MA, Sackoff JE. HIV risk behaviors among adolescents at a sexually transmitted disease clinic in New York City. *J Adolesc Health* 1996;18:429.
286. Vermund SH, Hein K, Gayle HD, et al. Acquired immunodeficiency syndrome among adolescents: case surveillance profiles in New York City and the rest of the United States. *American Journal of Diseases of Children* 1989;143:1220.
287. Centers for Disease Control and Prevention. Update: AIDS among women: United States, 1994. *MMWR Morb Mortal Wkly Rep* 1995;44:81.
288. Centers for Disease Control and Prevention. Heterosexually acquired AIDS: United States, 1993. *MMWR Morb Mortal Wkly Rep* 1994;43:155.
289. Hein K, Hurst M. Human immunodeficiency virus infection in adolescence: a rationale for action. *Adolescent and Pediatric Gynecology* 1988;1:73.
290. Advocates for Youth. *Fact sheet: adolescents, HIV/AIDS and other sexually transmitted diseases (STDs).* Washington, DC: Advocates for Youth; 1995.
291. Conway GA, Epstein MR, Hayman CR, et al. Trends in HIV prevalence among disadvantaged youth: survey results from a national job training program, 1988 through 1992. *JAMA* 1993;269:2887.
292. Chaisson RE, Keruly JC, Moore RD. Race, sex, drug use, and progression of human immunodeficiency virus disease. *N Engl J Med* 1995;333:751.

293. Centers for Disease Control and Prevention. Continued sexual risk behavior among HIV-seropositive drug-using men: Atlanta; Washington, DC; and San Juan, Puerto Rico, 1993. *MMWR Morb Mortal Wkly Rep* 1996;45:151.

294. Weiss RA. How does HIV cause AIDS? *Science* 1993;260:1273.

295. Imagawa DT, Lee MH, Wolinksy SM, et al. Human immunodeficiency virus type I infection in homosexual men who remain seronegative for prolonged periods. *N Engl J Med* 1989;320:1458.

296. Wasserheit JN. Epidemiological synergy: inter-relationship between HIV infection and other STDs. *Sex Transm Dis* 1992;19:61.

297. Carpenter C, Mayer K, Stein M, et al. Human immunodeficiency virus infection in North American women: experience with 200 cases and a review of the literature. *Medicine* 1991;70:307.

298. Anderson JR. Adolescents and human immunodeficiency virus infection. *Curr Opin Obstet Gynecol* 1992;4:849.

299. Lackritz EM, Satten GA, Aberle-Grasse J, et al. Estimated risk of transmission of the human immunodeficiency virus by screened blood in the United States. *N Engl J Med* 1995;333:1721.

300. Centers for Disease Control and Prevention. Persistent lack of detectable HIV-1 antibody in a person with HIV infection: Utah, 1995. *MMWR Morb Mortal Wkly Rep* 1996;45:181.

301. The Medical Letter. Diagnostic tests for AIDS. *The Medical Letter* 1988;30:73.

302. D'Angelo L, Getsan P, Luban N, et al. Human immunodeficiency virus infection in urban adolescents: can we predict who is at risk? *Pediatrics* 1991;88:982.

303. Anderson MM, Morris RE. HIV and adolescents. *Pediatr Ann* 1993;22:436.

304. Futterman D, Hein K, Kunins H. Teens and AIDS: I. identifying testing those at risk. *Contemporary Pediatrics* 1993;10:68.

305. Hein K, Futterman D. Medical management in HIV-infected adolescents. *J Pediatr* 1991;119(Suppl):S18.

306. Futterman D, Hein K, Kunins H. Teens and AIDS: II. treating the HIV-positive adolescent. *Contemporary Pediatrics* 1993;10:55.

307. The Medical Letter. Drugs for AIDS and associated infections. *The Medical Letter* 1995;37(959):87.

308. The Medical Letter. New drugs for HIV infection. *The Medical Letter* 1996;38(972):35.

309. Voelker R. Can researchers use new drugs to push HIV envelope to extinction? *JAMA* 1996;276:435.

310. Goldschmidt RH, Moy A. Antiretroviral drug treatment for HIV/AIDS. *Am Fam Physician* 1996;54:574.

311. Connor EM, Sperling RS, Gelber R, et al. Reduction of maternal–infant transmission of human immunodeficiency virus type I with zidovudine treatment. *N Engl J Med* 1994;331:1173.

312. Sperling RS, Shapiro DE, Coombs RW, et al. Maternal viral load, zidovudine treatment, and the risk of transmission of human immunodeficiency virus type 1 from mother to infant. *N Engl J Med* 1996;325:1621.

313. Corey L, Holmes KK. Therapy for human immunodeficiency virus infection: what have we learned? *N Engl J Med* 1996;335:1142.

314. Deeks SG, Smith MD, Holodniy M, et al. HIV-1 protease inhibitors: a review for clinicians. *JAMA* 1997;277:145.

315. Associated Press. Research: drug mix cut HIV 99 percent. *Albuquerque Journal* November 11, 1996, p. C2.

316. Haverkos HW, Edelman R. The epidemiology of acquired immunodeficiency syndrome among heterosexuals. *JAMA* 1988;260:1922.

317. Rawitscher LA, Satiz R, Friedman LS. Adolescents' preferences regarding human immunodeficiency virus (HIV)-related physician counseling and HIV testing. *Pediatrics* 1995;96:52.

318. Holtzman D, Rubinson R. Parent and peer communication effects on AIDS-related behavior among U.S. high school students. *Fam Plann Perspect* 1995;27:235.

319. Hingson R, Strunin L, Berlin B. Acquired immunodeficiency syndrome transmission: changes in knowledge and behaviors among teenagers, Massachusetts statewide surveys, 1986 to 1988. *Pediatrics* 1990;85:24.

320. Rotheram-Borus MJ, Koopman C, Haignere C, et al. Reducing HIV sexual risk behaviors among runaway adolescents. *JAMA* 1991;266:1237.

321. St. Lawrence JS. Cognitive–behavioral group intervention to assist substance-dependent adolescents in lowering HIV infection risk. *AIDS Educ Prev* 1994;6:425.

322. Steiner JD, Sorokin G, Schiedermayer DL, et al. Are adolescents getting smarter about acquired immunodeficiency syndrome? Changes in knowledge and attitude over the past 5 years. *American Journal of Diseases of Children* 1990;144:302.

323. Holtzman D, Anderson J, Kann L, et al. HIV instruction, HIV knowledge, and drug injection among high school students in the United States. *Am J Public Health* 1991;81:1596.

324. Centers for Disease Control and Prevention. School-based HIV prevention education: United States, 1994. *MMWR Morb Mortal Wkly Rep* 1996;45:760.

325. Slap G, Plotkin S, Khalid N, et al. A human immunodeficiency virus peer education program for adolescent females. *J Adolesc Health* 1991;12:434.

326. Baldwin J, Baldwin J. Factors affecting AIDS-related sexual risk-taking behavior among college students. *J Sex Res* 1989;25:181.

327. Hingson RW, Strunin L, Berlin BM, et al. Beliefs about AIDS, use of alcohol and drugs, and unprotected sex among Massachusetts adolescents. *Am J Public Health* 1990;80:295.

328. Centers for Disease Control and Prevention. Trends in sexual risk behavior among high school students: United States, 1990, 1191, and 1993. *MMWR Morb Mortal Wkly Rep* 1995;44:124.

329. Strasburger VC. Prevention of adolescent drug abuse: why "just say no" just won't work. *J Pediatr* 1989; 114:676.

330. Strunin L, Hingson R. AIDS and adolescents: knowledge, beliefs, attitudes, and behavior. *Pediatrics* 1987; 79:825.

331. Huszti HC, Clopton JR, Mason PJ. Acquired immunodeficiency syndrome educational program: effects on adolescents' knowledge and attitudes. *Pediatrics* 1989;84:986.

332. Futterman D, Hein K, Kunins H. Teens and AIDS: III. reducing AIDS risk in adolescents. *Contemporary Pediatrics* 1993;10:67.

333. Sunwoo J, Brenman A, Escobedo J, et al. School-based AIDS education for adolescents. *J Adolesc Health* 1995; 16:309.

SUGGESTED READING

STDs in Adolescents

American College of Obstetricians and Gynecologists. *Vaginitis.* Technical bulletin No. 226. Washington, DC: ACOG; 1996.

Biro F. *Adolescents and sexually transmitted diseases.* Washington, DC: Maternal and Child Health Bureau; 1992.

Braverman PK, Strasburger VC. Adolescent sexuality: III. sexually transmitted diseases. *Clin Pediatr* 1994;33:26.

Centers for Disease Control and Prevention. 1993 Sexually transmitted diseases treatment guidelines. *MMWR Morb Mortal Wkly Rep* 1993;42(RR-14):1.

Chacko MR, Rosenfeld WD. The uterine cervix: diagnostic opportunities. *Pediatr Ann* 1995;24:317.

Chacko MR, Taber LH, eds. Sexually transmitted diseases and gynecological problems, parts I and II. *Seminars in Pediatric Infectious Diseases* 1993;4(2):69 and 4(3):139.

Committee on Adolescence, American Academy of Pediatrics. Sexually transmitted diseases (policy statement). *Pediatrics* 1994;94:568.

Coupey SM, Klerman LV, eds. Adolescent sexuality: preventing unhealthy consequences. *Adolescent Medicine: State of the Art Reviews* 1992;3:165.

Cromer BA, Brown RT. Update on pregnancy, condom use, and prevalence of selected sexually transmitted diseases in adolescents. *Curr Opinion Obstet Gynecol* 1992;4:855.

Emans SJ, Goldstein DP. *Pediatric and adolescent gynecology.* 4th ed. Philadelphia: Lippincott–Raven Publishers; 1997.

Eng TR, butler WT (eds). *The Hidden Epidemic: Confronting Sexually Transmitted Diseases.* Washington, DC: National Academy Press, 1997

Ford CA, Moscicki AB. Control of sexually transmitted diseases in adolescents: the clinician's role. *Adv Pediatr Infect Dis* 1995;10:263.

Gittes EB, Irwin CE Jr. Sexually transmitted diseases in adolescents. *Pediatr Rev* 1993;14:180.

Hill RB, Hergenroeder AC. Vulvovaginitis and cervicitis in adolescents. *Seminars in Pediatric Infectious Diseases* 1993;4:167.

Jenny C, ed. Sexually transmitted diseases. *Pediatr Ann* 1994;23:327.

Johnson J, Shew ML. Screening and diagnostic tests for sexually transmitted diseases in adolescents. *Seminars in Pediatric Infectious Diseases* 1993;4:142.

Judson FN, Ehret J. Laboratory diagnosis of sexually transmitted diseases. *Pediatr Ann* 1994;23:361.

Mahony JB. Multiplex polymerase chain reaction for the diagnosis of sexually transmitted diseases. *Clin. Lab. Med.* 16:61,1996.

The Medical Letter. Drugs for sexually transmitted diseases. *The Medical Letter* 1995;37(964):117.

Moscicki AB. The pediatrician and the sexually active adolescent: III. an STD primer. *Pediatr Clin North Am* 1997 (in press).

Remafedi G. Sexually transmitted diseases in homosexual youth. *Adolescent Medicine: State of the Art Reviews* 1990;1:565.

Stewart DC. Sexually transmitted diseases in sexually assaulted adolescents. *Seminars in Pediatric Infectious Diseases* 1993;4:191.

Candidiasis

Centers for Disease Control and Prevention. 1993 Sexually transmitted diseases treatment guidelines. *MMWR Morb Mortal Wkly Rep* 1993;42(RR-14):72.

Goode MA, Grauer K, Gums JG. Infectious vaginitis: selecting therapy and preventing recurrence. *Postgrad Med* 1994;96:85.

The Medical Letter. Oral fluconazole for vaginal candidiasis. *The Medical Letter* 1994;36(931):81.

Sobel JD. *Candida* vulvovaginitis. *Clin Obstet Gynecol* 1993;36:153.

Sobel JD, Brooker D, Stein GE, et al. Single oral dose fluconazole compared with conventional clotrimazole topical therapy of *Candida* vaginitis. *Am J Obstet Gynecol* 1995;172:1263.

Spinillo A, Capuzzo E, Nicola S, et al. The impact of oral contraception on vulvovaginal candidiasis. *Contraception* 1995;51:293.
Tobin MJ. Vulvovaginal candidiasis: topical vs. oral therapy. *Am Fam Physician* 1995;51:1715.

Trichomonas

Centers for Disease Control and Prevention. 1993 Sexually transmitted diseases treatment guidelines. *MMWR Morb Mortal Wkly Rep* 1993;42(RR-14):70.
DeCastro FJ. High prevalence of *Trichomonas* infections in adolescents [letter]. *Clin Pediatr* 1989;28:33.
Goode MA, Grauer K, Gums JG. Infectious vaginitis: selecting therapy and preventing recurrence. *Postgrad Med* 1994;96:85.
Hager WD, Rapp RP. Metronidazole. *Obstet Gynecol Clin North Am* 1992;19:497.
Hammill HA. *Trichomonas vaginalis. Obstet Gynecol Clin North Am* 1989;16:531.
Heine P, McGregor JA. *Trichomonas vaginalis*: a reemerging pathogen. *Clin Obstet Gynecol* 1993;36:137.
Wolner-Hanssen P, Krieger JN, Stevens CE, et al. Clinical manifestations of vaginal trichomoniasis. *JAMA* 1989;261:571.

Bacterial Vaginosis

Biswas MK. Bacterial vaginosis. *Clin Obstet Gynecol* 1993;36:166.
Centers for Disease Control and Prevention. 1993 Sexually transmitted diseases treatment guidelines. *MMWR Morb Mortal Wkly Rep* 1993;42(RR-14):68.
Eschenbach DA. History and review of bacterial vaginosis. *Am J Obstet Gynecol* 1993;169:441.
Eschenbach DA. Vaginitis including bacterial vaginosis. *Curr Opin Obstet Gynecol* 1994;6:389.
Hill GB. The microbiology of bacterial vaginosis. *Am J Obstet Gynecol* 1993;169:450.
Joesoef MR, Schmid GP. Bacterial vaginosis: review of treatment options and potential clinical indications for therapy. *Clin Infect Dis* 1995;20(Suppl):S72.
MacDermott RI. Bacterial vaginosis. *Br J Obstet Gynaecol* 1995;102:92.
Mead PB. Epidemiology of bacterial vaginosis. *Am J Obstet Gynecol* 1993;169:446.
Schlicht JR. Treatment of bacterial vaginosis. *Ann Pharmacother* 1994;28:483.
Sweet RL. New approaches for the treatment of bacterial vaginosis. *Am J Obstet Gynecol* 1993;169:479.

Herpes Infections

Centers for Disease Control and Prevention. 1993 Sexually transmitted diseases treatment guidelines. *MMWR Morb Mortal Wkly Rep* 1993;42(RR-14):22.
Chacko MR. Diagnosis and management of genital ulcers. *Seminars in Pediatric Infectious Diseases* 1993;4:182.
Clark JL, Tatum NO, Noble SL. Management of genital herpes. *Am Fam Physician* 1995;51:175.
Corey L. Genital herpes. In: Holmes KK, Mardh P-A, Sparling PF, et al, eds. *Sexually transmitted diseases.* New York: McGraw-Hill; 1990:391.
Ellen JM, Moscicki AB, Shafer MA. Genital herpes simplex virus and human papillomavirus infection. *Adv Pediatr Infect Dis* 1994;9:97.
Frenkel LM. Herpes simplex virus infections in adolescents. *Adolescent Medicine: State of the Art Reviews,* 1995;6:65.
Huerta K, Berkelhamer S, Klein J, et al. Epidemiology of herpes simplex virus type 2 infections in a high-risk adolescent population. *J Adolesc Health* 1996;18:384.
Kinghorn GR. Genital herpes: natural history and treatment of acute episodes. *J Med Virol* 1993;1(Suppl):33.
Nelson CT, Demmier GJ. Superficial HSV infection: how serious is it? What should you do? *Contemporary Pediatrics* 1996;13:96.
Whitley RJ, Gnann JW Jr. Acyclovir: a decade later. *N Engl J Med* 1992;327:782.

Human Papillomavirus

Biro FM, Hillard PA. Genital human papillomavirus infection in adolescents. *Med Clin North Am* 1990;74:1235.
Cannistra SA, Niloff JM. Cancer of the uterine cervix. *N Engl J Med* 1996;334:1030.
Centers for Disease Control and Prevention. 1993 Sexually transmitted diseases treatment guidelines. *MMWR Morb Mortal Wkly Rep* 1993;42(RR-14):83.
Craighill MC. Human papillomavirus infection in children and adolescents. *Seminars in Pediatric Infectious Diseases* 1993;4:85.
Dyment PG. Human papillomovirus infection. *Adolescent Medicine: State of the Art Reviews* 1996;7:119.
Ellen JM, Moscicki AB, Shafer MA. Genital herpes simplex virus and human papillomavirus infection. *Adv Pediatr Infect Dis* 1994;9:97.

Gutman LT. Human papillomavirus infections of the genital tract in adolescents. *Adolescent Medicine: State of the Art Reviews* 1995;6:115.

Krowchuk DP, Anglin TM. Genital human papillomavirus infections in adolescents: implications for evaluation and management. *Semin Dermatol* 1992;11:24.

Mayeaux EJ, Harper MB, Barksdale W, et al. Noncervical human papillomavirus genital infections. *Am Fam Physician* 1995;52:1137.

The Medical Letter. Interferon for treatment of genital warts. *The Medical Letter* 1988;30:70.

The Medical Letter. Podofilox for genital warts. *The Medical Letter* 1991;33:117.

Miller DM, Brodell RT. Human papillomavirus infection: treatment options for warts. *Am Fam Physician* 1996;53:135.

Oriel D. Genital human papillomavirus infection. In: Holmes KK, Mardh P-A, Sparling PF, et al, eds. *Sexually transmitted diseases.* 2nd ed. New York: McGraw-Hill; 1990:433.

Rosenfeld WD. Genital human papillomavirus infection in adolescents. In: Goldfarb AF, ed. *Clinical problems in pediatric and adolescent gynecology.* New York: Chapman & Hall; 1996:89.

Stone KM. Human papillomavirus infection and genital warts: update on epidemiology and treatment. *Clin Infect Dis* 1995;20:S91.

Verdon ME. Issues in the management of human papillomavirus genital disease. *Am. Fam. Physician* 55:1813,1997.

Chlamydial Infection

Biro FM, Rosenthal SL, Kiniyalocts M. Gonococcal and chlamydial genitourinary infections in symptomatic and asymptomatic adolescent women. *Clin Pediatr* 1995;34:419.

Centers for Disease Control and Prevention. 1993 Sexually transmitted diseases treatment guidelines. *MMWR Morb Mortal Wkly Rep* 1993;42(RR-14):50.

Centers for Disease Control. Chlamydia trachomatis genital infections–United States, 1995. *MMWR* 46:193,1997.

Hammerschlag MR. Azithromycin and clarithromycin. *Pediatr Ann* 1993;22:160.

Hammerschlag MR. *Chlamydia trachomatis* in children. *Pediatr Ann* 1994;23:349.

Heath CB, Heath JM. *Chlamydia trachomatis* infection update. *Am Fam Physician* 1995;52:1455.

Hillis SD, Wasserheit JN. Screening for chlamydia: a key to the prevention of pelvic inflammatory disease. *N Engl J Med* 1996;334:1399.

Majeroni BA. Chlamydia cervicitis: complications and new treatment options. *Am Fam Physician* 1994;49:1825.

Reddy SP, Yeturu SR, Slupik R. *Chlamydia trachomatis* in adolescents: a review. *J Pediatr Adolesc Gynecol* 1997; 10:59.

Schachter J. Biology of *Chlamydia trachomatis.* In: Holmes KK, Mardh P-A, Sparling PF, et al, eds. *Sexually transmitted diseases.* 2nd ed. New York: McGraw-Hill; 1990:167.

Schydlower M, Shafer MA. *Chlamydia trachomatis* infections in adolescents. *Adolescent Medicine: State of the Art Reviews* 1990;1:615.

Skolnik NS. Screening for *Chlamydia trachomatis* infection. *Am Fam Physician* 1995;51:821.

Gonorrhea

Biro FM, Rosenthal SL, Kiniyalocts M. Gonococcal and chlamydial genitourinary infections in symptomatic and asymptomatic adolescent women. *Clin Pediatr* 1995;34:419.

Braverman PK. Herpes, syphilis, and other ulcerogenital conditions. *Adolescent Medicine: State of the Art Reviews* 1996;7:93.

Centers for Disease Control and Prevention. 1993 Sexually transmitted diseases treatment guidelines. *MMWR Morb Mortal Wkly Rep* 1993;42(RR-14):56.

Laras L, Craighill M, Woods ER, et al. Epidemiologic observations of adolescents with *Neisseria gonorrhoeae* genital infections treated at a children's hospital. *Adolescent and Pediatric Gynecology* 1994;7:9.

Mardh PA, Danielsson D. *Neisseria gonorrhoeae.* In: Holmes KK, Mardh PA, Sparling PF, et al, eds. *Sexually transmitted diseases.* 2nd ed. New York: McGraw-Hill; 1990:903.

Oh MK, Cloud GA, Fleenor M, et al. Risk for gonococcal and chlamydial cervicitis in adolescent females: incidence and recurrence in a prospective cohort study. *J Adolesc Health* 1996;18:270.

Sparling PR. Biology of *Neisseria gonorrhoeae.* In: Holmes KK, Mardh PA, Sparling PF, et al, eds. *Sexually transmitted diseases.* 2nd ed. New York: McGraw-Hill; 1990:131.

Woods CR Jr. Gonococcal infections in children and adolescents. *Seminars in Pediatric Infectious Diseases* 1993;4:94.

Zenilman J. Gonococcal infections in adolescents. *Adolescent Medicine: State of the Art Reviews* 1990;1:497.

Syphilis

Centers for Disease Control and Prevention. 1993 Sexually transmitted diseases treatment guidelines. *MMWR Morb Mortal Wkly Rep* 1993;42(RR-14):27.

Chacko MR. Diagnosis and management of genital ulcers. *Seminars in Pediatric Infectious Diseases* 1993;4:182.

Coles FB, Hipp SS. Syphilis among adolescents: the hidden epidemic. *Contemporary Pediatrics* 1996;13:47.

Goens JL, Janniger CK, De-Wold K. Dermatologic and systemic manifestations of syphilis. *Am Fam Physician* 1994;50:1013.

Hutchinson CM, Hook EW III. Syphilis in adults. *Med Clin North Am* 1990;74:1389.

Jaffe HW, Musher DM. Management of reactive syphilis serology. In: Holmes KK, Mardh PA, Sparling PF, et al, eds. *Sexually transmitted diseases.* 2nd ed. New York: McGraw-Hill; 1990:935.

Larsen SA, Steiner BM, Rudolph AH. Laboratory diagnosis and interpretation of tests for syphilis. *Clin Microbiol Rev* 1995;8:1.

McCabe E, Jaffe LR, Diaz A. Human immunodeficiency virus sero-positivity in adolescents with syphilis. *Pediatrics* 1993;92:695.

Pandhi RK, Singh N, Ramam M. Secondary syphilis: a clinicopathologic study. *Int J Dermatol* 1995;34:240.

Rolfs RT. Treatment of syphilis, 1993. *Clin Infect Dis* 1995;20(Suppl 1):S23.

Shew ML, Fortenberry JD. Syphilis screening in adolescents. *J Adolesc Health* 1992;13:303.

Sparling PF. Natural history of syphilis. In: Holmes KK, Mardh PA, Sparling PF, et al, eds. *Sexually transmitted diseases.* 2nd ed. New York: McGraw-Hill; 1990:213.

Zenker P. Syphilis. *Adolescent Medicine: State of the Art Reviews* 1990;1:511.

Pelvic Inflammatory Disease and Disseminated Infection

Augenbraun MH, McCormack WH. Pelvic inflammatory disease: an ongoing epidemic. *Hosp Pract* 1995;30:61.

Centers for Disease Control and Prevention. 1993 Sexually transmitted diseases treatment guidelines. *MMWR Morb Mortal Wkly Rep* 1993;42(RR-14):75.

Cromer BA, Brandstaetter LA, Fischer RA, et al. Tubo-ovarian abscess in adolescents. *Adolescent and Pediatric Gynecology* 1990;3:21.

Eschenbach DA, Wolner-Hanssen P. Fitz-Hugh–Curtis syndrome. In: Holmes KK, Mardh PA, Sparling PF, et al, eds. *Sexually Transmitted Diseases.* 2nd ed. New York: McGraw-Hill; 1990:621–626.

Grodstein F, Rothman KJ. Epidemiology of pelvic inflammatory disease. *Epidemiol* 1994;5:234.

Handsfield HH, Pollock PS. Arthritis associated with sexually transmitted diseases. In: Holmes KK, Mardh PA, Sparling PF, et al, eds. *Sexually transmitted diseases.* 2nd ed. New York: McGraw-Hill; 1990:737.

Hillis SD. PID prevention: clinical and societal stakes. *Hosp Pract* 1994;29:89.

Hillis SD, Wasserheit JN. Screening for chlamydia: a key to the prevention of pelvic inflammatory disease. *N Engl J Med* 1996;334:1399.

Huang A, Jay MS, Uhler M. Tuboovarian abscess in the adolescent. *J Pediatr Adolesc Gynecol* 1997;10:73.

Jacobson L, Westrom L. Objectivized diagnosis of acute pelvic inflammatory disease. *Am J Obstet Gynecol* 1980;138:905.

Kapphahn CJ, Moscicki AB. Pelvic inflammatory disease in adolescents. *Seminars in Pediatric Infectious Diseases* 1993;4:102.

Keat A. Sexually transmitted arthritis syndromes. *Med Clin North Am* 1990;74:1617.

Kerle KK, Mascola JR, Miller TA. Disseminated gonococcal infection. *Am Fam Physician* 1992;45:209.

Landers DV, Sweet RL (eds). *Pelvic Inflammatory Disease.* New York: Springer-Verlag, 1997.

Leu RH. Complications of coexisting chlamydia and gonococcal infections. *Postgrad Med* 1991;89:56.

Lopez-Zeno JA, Keith LG, Berger GS. The Fitz-Hugh–Curtis syndrome revisited: changing perspective after half a century. *J Reprod Med* 1985;30:567.

McCormack WM. Pelvic inflammatory disease. *N Engl J Med* 1994;330:115.

Rice PA, Schachter J. Pathogenesis of pelvic inflammatory disease: what are the questions? *JAMA* 1991;266:2587.

Rome ES. Pelvic inflammatory disease in the adolescent. *Curr Opin Pediatr* 1994;6:383.

Scholes D, Stergachis A, Heidrich FE, et al. Prevention of pelvic inflammatory disease by screening for cervical chlamydial infection. *N Engl J Med* 1996;334:1362.

Shafer MA, Sweet RL. Pelvic inflammatory disease in adolescent females. *Adolescent Medicine: State of the Art Reviews* 1990;1:545.

Slap GB, Forke CM, Cnaan A, et al. Recognition of tubo-ovarian abscess in adolescents with pelvic inflammatory disease. *J Adolesc Health* 1996;18:397.

Soper DE. Pelvic inflammatory disease. *Infect Dis Clin North Am* 1994;8:821.

Spence MR, Adler J, McLellan R. Pelvic inflammatory disease in the adolescent. *Journal of Adolescent Health Care* 1990;11:304.

Wolner-Hansen P, Kiviat NB, Holmes KK. Atypical pelvic inflammatory disease: subacute, chronic, or subclinical upper genital tract infection in women. In: Holmes KK, Mardh PA, Sparling PF, et al, eds. *Sexually transmitted diseases.* 2nd ed. New York: McGraw-Hill; 1990:615.

HIV and AIDS

Anderson JR. Adolescents and human immunodeficiency virus infection. *Curr Opin Obstet Gynecol* 1992;4:849.

Anderson MM, Morris RE. HIV and adolescents. *Pediatr Ann* 1993;22:436.

Brown LK, Schultz JR, Gragg RA. HIV-infected adolescents with hemophilia: adaptation and coping. The Hemophilia Behavioral Intervention Evaluation Project. *Pediatrics* 1995;96:459.

Centers for Disease Control and Prevention. 1993 Sexually transmitted diseases treatment guidelines. *MMWR Morb Mortal Wkly Rep* 1993;42(RR-14):11.

Centers for Disease Control and Prevention. Update: Trends in AIDS incidence, deaths, and prevalence—United States, 1996. *MMWR Morb Mortal Wkly Rep* 1997;46:165.

Centers for Disease Control and Prevention. 1997 Sexually transmitted diseases treatment guidelines. *MMWR Morb Mortal Wkly Rep* 1997 (in press).

D'Angelo LJ. Adolescents and HIV infection: a clinician's perspective. *Acta Paediatr* 1994;400(Suppl):88S.

Deeks SG, Smith MD, Holodniy M, et al. HIV-1 protease inhibitors: a review for clinicians. *JAMA* 1997;277:145.

DiLorenzo T, Hein K. Adolescents: the leading edge of the next wave of the HIV epidemic. In: Wallander JL, Siegel LJ, eds. *Adolescent health problems: behavioral perspectives.* New York: Guilford Press; 1995:117.

Futterman D, Hein K, Kunins H. Teens and AIDS: I. identifying testing those at risk. *Contemporary Pediatrics* 1993;10:68.

Futterman D, Hein K, Kunins H. Teens and AIDS: II. treating the HIV-positive adolescent. *Contemporary Pediatrics* 1993;10:55.

Futterman D, Hein K, Kunins H. Teens and AIDS: III. reducing AIDS risk in adolescents. *Contemporary Pediatrics* 1993;10:67.

Hein K, Futterman D. Medical management in HIV-infected adolescents. *J Pediatr* 1991;119(Suppl):S18.

Hoffman ND, Futterman D. Human immunodeficiency virus infection in adolescents. *Seminars in Pediatric Infectious Diseases* 1993;4:113.

Holtzman D, Rubinson R. Parent and peer communication effects on AIDS-related behavior among U.S. high school students. *Fam Plann Perspect* 1995;27:235.

Kipke MD, O'Connor S, Palmer R, et al. Street youth in Los Angeles: profile of a group at high risk for human immunodeficiency virus infection. *Arch Pediatr Adolesc Med* 1995;149:513.

Landesman SH, DeHovitz JA. HIV diagnostic testing: ethical, legal, and clinical considerations. In: Holmes KK, Mardh PA, Sparling PF, et al, eds. *Sexually transmitted diseases.* 2nd ed. New York: McGraw-Hill; 1990:975.

The Medical Letter. Drugs for AIDS and associated infections. *The Medical Letter* 1995;37(959):87.

The Medical Letter. Drugs for sexually transmitted diseases. *The Medical Letter* 1995;37(964):87.

The Medical Letter. New drugs for HIV infection. *The Medical Letter* 1996;38(972):35.

Rawitscher LA, Satiz R, Friedman LS. Adolescents' preferences regarding human immunodeficiency virus (HIV)-related physician counseling and HIV testing. *Pediatrics* 1995;96:52.

Schonberg SK and Hoffman ND. HIV testing in adolescents. *Adolescent Medicine: State of the Art Reviews* 1997;8:463

Society for Adolescent Medicine. HIV infection and AIDS in adolescents (position paper). *Journal of Adolescent Health Care* 1994;15:427.

Stiehm ER, Frenkel LM, eds. AIDS. *Pediatr Ann* 1993;22:399.

Sweeney P, Lindegren ML, Buehler JW, et al. Teenagers at risk of human immunodeficiency virus type 1 infection: results from seroprevalence surveys in the United States. *Arch Pediatr Adolesc Med* 1995;149:521.

Weiss RA. How does HIV cause AIDS? *Science* 1993;260:1273.

ISSUES FOR THE MALE ADOLESCENT

Urethritis

More than 90% of young men presenting with dysuria have a sexually transmitted disease [1,2]. Therefore, a complete sexual history is mandatory. Because estimates of homosexuality among male teens range as high as 10% [3], asking "the sexual question" improperly may alienate a significant number of teenagers. The easiest technique is to link the historical questions to the presenting complaint. For example:

Patient: "I've had this stuff coming out of my penis."

Physician: "I am not trying to pry, but I need to ask you some personal questions so that I can help you get rid of this problem. What you tell me will be kept strictly confidential by me. Are you having sex with anyone?"

Patient: "Yes."

Physician: "With whom, a girl or a guy?"

In this hypothetical example, the nonjudgmental approach of the physician alerts the patient that the topic of homosexuality is permissible to discuss, if necessary. If the teenager is exclusively heterosexual, his reaction will usually be either amusement or vigorous assertion of his sexual taste, but no harm is done.

The 10% of urethritis that is not infectious is related to either trauma or chemical irritation (e.g., desensitizing creams, a female partner's use of spermicides or douches).

Of the infectious causes of urethritis in males, *Neisseria gonorrhoeae* and *Chlamydia trachomatis* far outdistance all other organisms [2,4,5]. Presence of a discharge enables the clinician to differentiate quickly between gonococcal and nongonococcal urethritis (NGU). First, the presence of polymorphonuclear leukocytes (PMNs) on Gram's stain establishes the diagnosis of urethritis; then, gram-negative intracellular diplococci indicate gonorrheal infection. *Ureaplasma urealyticum* is another common cause of urethritis [2,6,7], and may be a useful marker of sexual activity in young men [8]. Other, rarer causes include *Trichomonas vaginalis*, herpes simplex, adenoviruses, *Hemophilus* species, *Staphylococcus saprophyticus*, and coliforms (in homosexual men) [5,7,9].

C. trachomatis is the major cause of NGU—isolated in about 30% to 40% of all cases [7]. However, it can also be isolated in 15% to 25% of men with urethral gonorrhea, and hence the need for simultaneous treatment [10]. Otherwise, patients infected with both organisms but only treated for gonorrhea will contract postgonococcal urethritis. *Ureaplasma urealyticum* accounts for 15% to 25% of NGU [9,11].

Signs and Symptoms

Inflammation of the male urethra may cause dysuria, itching, or a discharge. Typically, gonorrheal urethritis is associated with a more profuse and purulent discharge. NGU has a scantier, more mucoid discharge, if one is present at all. It may be noticed only in the morning or as a stain on underwear [2]. Herpes urethritis is usually severe, with focal urethral ulceration, inguinal lymphadenopathy, and prominent systemic symptoms [5]. Gonorrhea also tends to have a more abrupt onset, within 2 to 6 days of exposure, with a greater incidence of both dysuria and discharge, whereas NGU is more insidious, with onset ranging from 1 to 6 weeks after exposure [10].

However, asymptomatic urethral infection in men is also common [2,12]. Among male partners of women with either gonorrhea or chlamydial infection, one researcher found an infection rate of 78% for *N. gonorrhoeae* and 53% for *C. trachomatis*, but only half of the infected men were symptomatic [13]. Studies of male adolescents have found rates of asymptomatic infection as high as 5% to 10% for chlamydial infection [2,14] and 15% with gonorrhea [15]. Interestingly, men with asymptomatic gonorrhea, particularly pharyngeal, may harbor strains that are more likely to cause disseminated infection. Male partners of women with pelvic inflammatory disease should be treated routinely, even if they are asymptomatic [16].

When urethritis is accompanied by arthritis, conjunctivitis, and mucocutaneous lesions, Reiter's syndrome should be suspected [2,17]. It usually takes the form of an asymmetric oligoarthritis, typically involving the knees, ankles, feet, wrists, and sacroiliac joints, usually within a month of the episode of NGU. Approximately 50% of men with Reiter's syndrome show evidence of *C. trachomatis* infection [18], although cases have been linked to *N. gonorrhoeae* and *U. urealyticum* as well [2,19]. The disease may represent a hyperimmune response in genetically susceptible individuals who possess the HLA-B27 haplotype, and the risk to such patients after NGU is about 20%, compared with 1% to 3% for the general population [2]. Although both gonorrhea and NGU are most common among 20- to 24-year-olds, followed by 15- to 19-year-olds, Reiter's syndrome is most common in the fourth decade of life and relatively rare among adolescents.

Diagnosis

Presence of a urethral discharge, particularly containing five or more PMNs per oil-immersion field, constitutes evidence for urethritis. Gonorrhea is diagnosed through Gram's stain, culture, or rapid test. Absence of gonorrhea constitutes presumptive evidence for NGU. A rapid test for *C. trachomatis* may then differentiate between NGU caused by that organism or other organisms (Table 89). Although traditionally, tissue culture for *C. trachomatis* has been considered the diagnostic gold standard, it is only 70% to 90% sensitive [20]. An array of newer and highly sensitive and specific chlamydial tests are now available (Table 90), including [2,20]:

- *Antigen detection systems.* These use either enzyme immunoassay (EIA) or direct fluorescent antibody techniques to detect *C. trachomatis* antigens. They are sufficiently sensitive for use in symptomatic men, but not in asymptomatic ones. However, EIA can also be used on first-void urine and is sufficiently sensitive and specific for use in asymptomatic patients. Chlamydiazyme (Abbot Laboratories, North Chicago, IL) is a popular EIA test; Syva Micro Trak (Syva Company, San Jose, CA) is a popular direct fluorescent antibody test.
- *DNA probes.* DNA probes use a chemoluminescent probe that is complementary to the RNA of *C. trachomatis* and *N. gonorrhoeae*. It permits testing for both gonorrheal and chlamydial infection us-

TABLE 89. *Strategies for evaluating young men for nongonococcal urethritis*

Patient is symptomatic
- Perform Gram stain of urethral discharge
- Test for *Chlamydia trachomatis* using
  DNA probe[a] *or*
  Polymerase chain reaction *or*
  Antigen test (direct fluorescent antibody or enzyme immunoassay) *or*
  Tissue culture
- Test for *Neisseria gonorrhoeae* using
  DNA probe[a] *or*
  Culture (Thayer-Martin or other medium)

Patient is asymptomatic
- Perform leukocyte esterase test on first-void urine
- If positive, confirm presence of infection as above

Positive test
- If patient is positive for chlamydia infection, treat with either doxycycline, 100 mg bid × 7d, or azithromycin, 1 g single dose. Treat partner(s).
- If patient is positive for gonorrhea, treat with ceftriaxone, 125 mg IM, or cefixime, 400 mg orally in a single dose + treatment for chlamydial infection as above. Treat partner(s).

[a]Offers advantage of testing for both organisms using a single swab.
Adapted from Centers for Disease Control and Prevention. 1993 Sexually transmitted diseases treatment guidelines. *MMWR Morb Mortal Wkly Rep* 1993;42(RR-14):47; and Krowchuck DP. Nongonococcal urethritis: diagnosis, management, and complications. *Adolescent Medicine: State of the Art Reviews* 1996;7:63.

ing a single specimen, and is highly sensitive and specific. The PACE 2 system (Gen-Probe, San Diego, CA) has been tested and found to be as accurate for diagnosing gonorrhea [21] and for documenting test of cure [22] as a standard culture.
- *Polymerase chain reaction (PCR).* PCR uses a technique to amplify DNA sequences to maximize detection, and is also highly sensitive and specific for diagnosing chlamydial infections. Amplicor (Roche Diagnostic Systems, Nutley, NJ) can be used to test urethral or urine specimens.
- *Ligase chain reaction (LCR).* LCR uses an amplification technique to help identify *C. trachomatis* DNA. Like DNA probes and PCR, it is highly sensitive and specific and can be used to test first-void urine specimens.

Testing for gonorrhea is a bit simpler: culture, Gram stain, or DNA probe. Again, although the culture is the gold standard, it affords sensitivity values ranging only from 80% to 96% because of the fastidiousness of the organism and the requirement for incubation in 3% to 10% carbon dioxide and 70% humidity. Use of transport media diminishes the yield of positive cultures as well. Most gono-

TABLE 90. *Diagnosing chlamydial infections in men*

Technique	Specimen	Sensitivity	Specificity
Tissue culture	Urethra	70–90%	100%
Antigen detection			
Enzyme immunoassay	Urethra	83% (70–100%)	97% (85–99%)
	Urine	84% (76–91%)	97% (95–99%)
Direct fluorescent antibody	Urethra	92% (89–100%)	96% (96–100%)
DNA probe	Urethra	95%	100%
Polymerase chain reaction	Urethra	95–98%	99–100%
	Urine	97%	99%
Ligase chain reaction	Urethra	99%	100%
	Urine	96%	100%

Adapted from Krowchuck DP. Nongonococcal urethritis: diagnosis, management, and complications. *Adolescent Medicine: State of the Art Reviews* 1996;7:63.

coccal cultures also require up to 48 hours, and clinicians must remember to warm the modified Thayer-Martin media to room temperature, or even positive specimens will not grow. Cultures are also painful, can result in subsequent dysuria, and do not enhance the prospect of future visits.

A Gram stain is far quicker and is more than 90% accurate if a discharge is present. If the Gram stain is negative for gram-negative intracellular diplococci but PMNs are present (>5 per oil-immersion field), the diagnosis of NGU has been made. Determining the exact organism then requires the use of culture or a rapid detection test for *C. trachomatis* (e.g., Microtrak, Chlamydiazyme) [23].

In the early 1980s, an enzyme immunoassay for gonococcal antigen was developed (Gonozyme; Abbott Laboratories). Sensitivities and specificities have been high (85–100%) in multiple studies, particularly among men in high-risk populations [24,25]. PACE-2 is the more recent DNA probe, now widely used because of its convenience, with sensitivity rates of 97% to 100% and nearly perfect specificity for detecting the gonococcus [21].

What about screening high-risk but asymptomatic teenagers? With asymptomatic rates of chlamydial infection ranging from 1% to 14% and gonorrhea from 1% to 5% [26,27], screening is important, both clinically and from a public health perspective. At the same time, larger numbers of asymptomatic teenagers are not likely to submit willingly to having urethral swabs taken. One solution has been the use of a simple screening procedure, the leukocyte esterase test (LET) to determine the presence of pyuria [28–30]. First-void urine can be tested simply and inexpensively using a commercially available dipstick. An LET of 1+ or 2+ has a sensitivity of 72% to 100% and a specificity of 83% to 96% [2]. However, false-positive results are common; therefore, a positive LET should be followed by a more reliable test for gonorrhea and chlamydial infection, such as EIA, PCR, LCR, or culture. This two-step approach allows for an excellent, sensitive, specific, and cost-effective means of screening men for infection [2,7,29,31]. However, the *absence* of pyuria in asymptomatic men is not a completely reliable indication of the absence of a sexually transmitted disease (STD), especially chlamydial infection [26].

Treatment

Gonococcal Urethritis

Treatment of urethritis in men has changed since the mid-1980s with the development of third-generation cephalosporins, which are active against penicillinase-producing strains of *N. gonorrhoeae*. In adolescents with asymptomatic gonorrhea, an oral regimen of cefixime, 400 mg in a single dose, can be used, but in adults and in adolescents at high risk for contracting resistant strains, ceftriaxone in a single 125-mg injection has become the drug of choice [16]. Although this represents a very low dose of the drug, it reliably eliminates infection in uncomplicated cases [32]. For patients 18 years and older, ciprofloxacin, 500 mg, or ofloxacin, 400 mg, can be given in a single oral dose for asymptomatic cases. All patients treated for gonorrhea should be treated for the possibility of coexisting chlamydial infection with either a 7-day course of doxycycline or a single dose of azithromycin. For pharyngeal gonorrhea, ceftriaxone is also the drug of choice.

If the ceftriaxone and doxycycline regimen is used for gonococcal urethritis, a test of cure is not routinely needed [9]. However, if one is performed, it should ideally be done 3 to 5 days after the oral antibiotic has been finished. Sex partners should be referred immediately for evaluation and treatment.

Nongonococcal Urethritis

Treatment of NGU infections is now easier with the advent of single-dose oral therapy, azithromycin 1 g [33]. This can be considered one of the two treatments of choice, the other being a 7-day course of doxycycline, 100 mg orally twice a day. Alternatives include erythromycin base, 500 mg four times a day for 7 days, or erythromycin ethylsuccinate, 800 mg orally four times a day for 7 days. Both tetracyclines and erythromycins are active against *C. trachomatis* and most strains of *U. urealyticum*. Azithromycin has the advantages of being a single-dose treatment, with assured compliance, and there are no known resistant strains [31]. However, the cost ($25–35) is far greater than for doxycycline ($5) [7]. A new formulation of azithromycin in a single-dose powder is cheaper and may make use of the drug more popular [34]. In a controlled trial of both azithromycin and doxycycline for NGU, the cure rates were similar, 81% for azithromycin and 77% for doxycycline (but 83% and 90%, respectively, in those patients with documented chlamydial infection) [33]. The efficacy of azithromycin may be improved still further by giving 500 mg on day 1, followed by 250 mg on days 2 and 3 [35].

Although the initial response rate in patients is 85% to 95%, up to one third of patients have a recurrence of pyuria, with or without symptoms, 2 to 6 weeks after treatment. However, doxycycline- or azithromycin-resistant strains of *C. trachomatis* have not yet been reported. Longer courses of treatment have not been shown to be any more effective than a 7-day course [9]. Cultures and tests should be repeated, including a renewed search for trichomoniasis or herpes virus infection, because most recurrences are culture-negative for chlamydial or *U. urealyticum* infection [2]. Tetracycline-resistant strains of *U. urealyticum* do exist, however, so that treatment with a 1- to 2-week course of erythromycin may be appropriate. The sexual history should also be reviewed, because heterosexual and homosexual contacts involve exposure to different organisms. Because 30% to 60% of female partners of men with gonorrhea or NGU have documented chlamydial infection, they must be treated aggressively as well.

Nongonococcal urethritis is thought to be a self-limited disease. However, treatment is important for public health reasons and particularly to protect the female partner. In young adults, epididymitis, prostatitis, or Reiter's syndrome may develop in 1% to 3% of patients [2]. The incidence in adolescents is unknown.

Human Papillomavirus Infection

Young men comprise an important and hidden reservoir of human papillomavirus (HPV) disease. They are not eager observers of their own genitalia, nor are they likely to report warts. Detection usually occurs after HPV infection has been found in the sexual partner.

Human papillomavirus infection is now the most common viral STD in the United States. Its prevalence has increased nearly fivefold since the 1960s [36]. A 1988 review estimated the prevalence of HPV infection among American men and women ages 15 to 49 years to be 10% [37]. Not only is identifying men with HPV important as a way of preventing cervical cancer in women, but HPV is an important etiologic agent in penile and anal carcinomas in men. In one study, half of penile carcinomas contained HPV DNA, mostly types 16 and 19 [38]. HPV has also been linked to receptive anal intercourse and genital warts [39].

In one study of male partners of known infected women, 41% had gross lesions but only 16% were aware of them. Use of acetic acid and magnification detected another 29% who would have been considered disease free and 30% with subclinical areas in addition to their gross warts [40]. Lifetime exposure to HPV may be as high as 25% [41]. In another study of nearly 200 male partners of infected women, 50% had macroscopically visible infection, 24% had subclinical infection only, and 27% were negative. However, lesions developed in eight of the negative men (17%) within the following 6 months [41]. Even among the 50% with grossly visible disease, most of the patients were unaware of the lesions or their infectious origin.

Signs and Symptoms

The clinical appearance of overt HPV infection in men can be quite varied, even in the same patient. *Condylomata acuminata* are the easiest to spot, appearing on the frenum, coronal sulcus, glans, and perianal skin. They are fleshy, soft, grapelike growths. Multiple papular warts often appear on the shaft of the penis, 1 to 5 mm in diameter. The urethra may be infected with exophytic condyloma, with 80% in the terminal region, causing complaints of bleeding, discharge, or decreased urinary force. They may be relatively inconspicuous but a significant source of transmission to others [42]. Anal warts are particularly common among homosexual men, but can be seen in heterosexual men as well if vaginal secretions reach the perianal region [36]. Internal warts are present in up to 50% of patients with external lesions [43].

Patients with subclinical HPV infection have no symptoms, however. Frequently, there are flat warts, or keratotic plaques, found on the shaft of the penis and on the scrotum, but they are visible only after application of 3% to 5% acetic acid for 3 to 5 minutes (Table 91). The acetowhite reaction takes longer to develop on keratinized epithelium than on cervical or vaginal mucosa. Visualization is improved by use of a colposcope: this is now called *acetoenhanced androscopy* and is indicated for all men whose partners have been diagnosed with condyloma, squamous intraepithelial lesions, or cervical cancer [36].

TABLE 91. *Subclinical human papillomavirus infection in men[a]*

	No. of patients	Frequency
Penile shaft alone	19	40%
Scrotum alone	8	17%
Shaft and scrotum	20	43%
Total	47	

[a]Detected by acetic acid soaking.
From Rosemberg SK, Greenberg MD, Reid R. Sexually transmitted papillomaviral infection in men. *Obstet Gynecol Clin North Am* 1987;14:495. With permission.

Diagnosis

Over 75% of male partners of infected women show evidence of HPV infection within 6 months. Approximately two thirds of them have grossly visible disease, and one third have subclinical infection only [41]. All such men should have acetic acid applied to their penis, using sterile gauze pads, and to their scrotum and perineal area. An acetowhite reaction is diagnostic for HPV infection; however, not all lesions have a positive reaction. Perianal warts must be distinguished from *condylomata lata*—sheets of whitish, more rounded lesions that contain treponemes and are pathognomonic of secondary syphilis [44]. Other signs and laboratory evidence are usually present as well.

Treatment

Although there is some anecdotal evidence that HPV infection can regress spontaneously, the risk of spread to a partner and the association between HPV and anogenital neoplasia make treatment advisable [36]. This, despite the fact that the Centers for Disease Control and Prevention guidelines suggest that removal is mainly for cosmetic reasons, and the fact that no form of treatment has been shown to eradicate the virus or modify the risk of cervical dysplasia [34]. Successful treatment requires an accurate evaluation of the extent of the infection, simultaneous treatment of the partner, and recognition and treatment of other concomitant STDs. However, success is often elusive because it is difficult to treat all of the lesions.

Conventional Medical Methods

Cryotherapy should probably be the office-based treatment of choice because it is relatively inexpensive, does not require anesthesia, and does not result in scarring [34]. Freezing the wart and a few millimeters of surrounding tissue for 40 seconds is mildly painful but can usually induce remission. Unfortunately, lesions recur in about one third of cases within a year. Transient hypopigmentation may develop, but resolves. A canister of dimethyl ether and propane (Histofreezer) may be more practical than keeping liquid nitrogen in an office [45].

Several chemical approaches have also been widely used. Typically, 20% podophyllin in tincture of benzoin has been applied to gross lesions, allowed to dry, and washed off after 3 to 4 hours. Because podophyllin is not a pure or standardized compound, it can be associated with unacceptably high risks: severe local reactions, or even paralysis and death if applied to highly vascular areas [46]. Also, it has a low success rate, ranging from 22% to 77%, and is ineffective on condylomata on the penile shaft or within the meatus. An 85% solution of trichloroacetic acid may be preferable to podophyllin. It is applied and washed off after 4 hours, and may be effective against small warts. More recently, a self-administered 0.5% solution of podophyllotoxin in ethanol (a standardized podophyllin) has been used with good results [47,48]. Both chemicals, however, are relatively ineffective on keratinized skin.

Intraurethral condylomata have been effectively treated for 20 years with the use of 5% 5-fluorouracil (5-FU) cream (Efudex). Daily instillation of 5-FU cream after voiding for up to a week is highly effective in eradicating warts [49]. Scrotal lesions may also require 5-FU cream because other methods are overly toxic. However, use of the cream elsewhere may be accompanied by unacceptable soreness.

Surgery

In general, surgery should be reserved for extensive or refractory lesions [34]. Electrocautery requires local anesthesia and can be used to treat lesions on the penile shaft or in the perianal area. Its success rate may range as high as 60% [41]. More recently, the CO_2 laser has been used, with an efficacy rate of 43% but recurrences in 95% of patients [34]. Extensive lesions usually require general anesthesia. Adjuvant therapy with 5-FU cream after surgery may also reduce reinfection from surrounding skin containing HPV. Cure rates may be as high as 80% [41].

Interferon

Systemic interferon has been tried but has no advantages over other forms of treatment [34]. Intralesional injection of α-interferon has been shown to be effective and well tolerated in controlled trials, and may be helpful in some patients [50–52].

The Acute Scrotum: Epididymitis Versus Testicular Torsion

Many different scrotal disorders may bring the young male adolescent to the attention of medical personnel [53] (Table 92), but by far the most common and difficult problem is distinguishing testicular torsion from acute epididymitis. Epididymitis and testicular torsion of the testis or appendages account for 95% of all cases of acute scrotal disease [54]. Although "on paper" the distinction is relatively straightforward, in practice it can be exceedingly difficult (Table 93). Whenever there is doubt, a technetium-99m scan (and, if necessary, exploratory surgery) is always indicated [55]. Amazingly, studies indicate that an average patient with testicular torsion has nearly a 25% chance of losing the involved testis when he consults a primary care physician because of the delay in making the proper diagnosis [56].

Testicular Torsion

Testicular torsion actually represents a bilateral congenital defect in the tunica vaginalis, but it usually does not become apparent until adolescence. Twisting of the spermatic cord may compromise testicular and epididymal perfusion, with resulting sudden onset of acute scrotal pain, swelling, and even discoloration. A history of exercise or trauma is common (although it may not represent a precipitat-

---

TABLE 92. *Causes of acute scrotal pain*

Common
Trauma/hematocele
Varicocele
Testicular torsion
Epididymitis

Less common
Orchitis
Inguinal hernia
Torsion of testicular appendages

Rare
Tumor
Idiopathic scrotal edema
Fat necrosis
Cellulitis of the scrotum
Henoch-Schönlein purpura

TABLE 93. *Testicular torsion versus acute epididymitis*

Features	Torsion	Epididymitis
History		
Onset of pain	Acute	Gradual
Nausea and vomiting	50%	Rare
Dysuria	No	50%
Urethral discharge	No	50%
Past history, similar pain	30–50%	Rare
Physical examination		
Epididymal swelling only	10%	Early
Scrotal edema, erythema	Most	Most
Fever	Rare	50%
Laboratory results		
Pyuria	0–30%	20–95%
Urethral Gram stain/culture	Negative	Often positive
Perfusion studies		
Doppler ultrasound	Decreased flow	Nl./increased flow
Tc-99 scan	Decreased flow	Nl./increased flow

From O'Brien WM, Lynch JH. The acute scrotum. *Am Fam Physician* 1988;37:239. Reprinted with permission of the American Academy of Family Physicians.

ing factor). A detailed history often reveals previous episodes of testicular pain that have spontaneously resolved, because intermittent torsion is a well known phenomenon [57]. Frequently, nausea and vomiting accompany the pain. In one large series of nearly 300 patients with testicular torsion, 88% had pain, 42% had vomiting, approximately 10% had a recent history of trauma or exercise, and 8% had urinary symptoms [58].

Clues to the diagnosis may be found on physical examination. With the patient in an upright or standing position, the presence of a tender testis lying in a transverse position high in the scrotum, or a tender epididymis lying in an anterior rather than a posterior position, is suspect. Elevating the testis to produce relief from the pain (Prehn's sign) may *not* represent an accurate sign [56,59]. Both Doppler ultrasound and technetium-99m scanning can provide useful adjuncts to diagnosis, with accuracies as high as 85% to 90%. Torsion results in decreased perfusion in both studies, whereas epididymitis causes increased blood flow [60,61].

Testicular torsion is a surgical emergency, requiring immediate recognition and treatment. Infarction occurs within 5 to 6 hours, although survival of the testis has been reported for up to 24 hours. Approximate salvage rates vary accordingly [56,62]:

- 100% at 3 hours
- 83% to 90% at 5 hours
- 75% at 8 hours
- 50% to 70% at 10 hours
- 10% to 20% at 10 to 24 hours

At surgery, the torsion is reduced and both testes are tacked down (orchiopexy) because contralateral abnormalities are common [63]. Depending on the duration of torsion and the degree of subsequent testicular atrophy, spermatogenesis may be impaired, although endocrine function is usually normal [64,65].

Intermittent torsion has also been well described, and patients benefit from early recognition and surgery [57]. In perhaps 5% of acute scrotal pain, torsion of the testicular appendages is the etiology. Most commonly, either the appendix testis or the appendix epididymis—remnants of the müllerian and wolffian duct systems, respectively—is involved. Pain is typically discrete and localized to the superior aspect of the testis, with no scrotal swelling. Sometimes a "blue dot" can be observed beneath the scrotal skin, which is pathognomonic and represents the cyanotic appendage. Because these represent necrotic remnants that will undergo atrophy on their own, management in such cases consists solely of observation and analgesia [54].

Acute Epididymitis

Acute epididymitis is most often a manifestation of sexually acquired chlamydial or gonococcal infection [2,66]. Other etiologies include infection with coliform or *Pseudomonas* organisms or an association with trauma or exercise. Classically, epididymitis is more insidious in onset, with pain and tenderness localized to the epididymis and sparing the testis. Fever, pyuria, bacteriuria, and leukocytosis are common findings (Fig. 24; see Table 93).

Treatment depends on Gram stain of urethral secretions, testing for chlamydial infection, and a midstream urine specimen for analysis and culture. On Gram stain, the presence of more than four white blood cells per oil-immersion field and gram-negative intracellular diplococci dictates treatment for gonorrhea (and chlamydial infection). However, if azithromycin is used, a 5- to 7-day course should probably be used instead of a single dose. If organisms are not present, treatment should follow the NGU protocol but, again, be extended to 5 to 7 days. If both the Gram stain and chlamydial test are negative but the urine shows white blood cells or organisms, treatment should be aimed against typical urinary tract pathogens (e.g., trimethoprim–sulfamethoxazole) [67].

Other Scrotal Disorders

Varicoceles

Approximately 15% of young men have varicoceles—a dilated, tortuous plexus of veins surrounding the spermatic cord and looking like "a bag of worms" [68,69]. Most teens are unaware of their presence. Occasionally, patients may notice intermittent pain or a feeling of fullness. The veins (part of the pampiniform plexus) are located almost exclusively on the left side of the scrotum because the left internal spermatic vein drains into the renal vein, whereas the right internal spermatic vein enters the vena cava. Consequently, a right-sided mass should be evaluated for the possibility of being a tumor and not be dismissed as a varicocele.

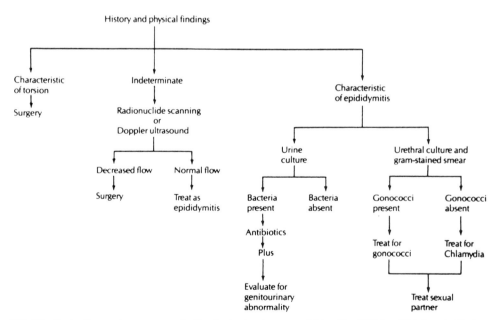

FIG. 24. Evaluation and management of testicular torsion vs. epididymitis. (O'Brien WM, Lynch JH. The acute scrotum. *Am Fam Physician* 1988;37:239. Reprinted with permission of the American Academy of Family Physicians.)

Varicoceles may have important clinical implications. Decreased sperm counts, infertility, and testicular atrophy have all been associated with varicoceles. Among adult men, they represent the leading known cause of male infertility, accounting for about one third of all cases [70,71]. Ligation of the left spermatic vein improves semen characteristics in about two thirds of adult men, and half of these demonstrate fertility [72]. Because this plexus normally functions as a countercurrent heat-exchange unit to keep testicular temperatures down, any anatomic abnormality may result in decreased spermatogenesis and testosterone production [73]. However, many men with varicoceles have normal fertility [71].

To date, only one study [74] has examined testicular function in adolescents with varicoceles: in five patients with normal baseline levels of gonadotropins and normal testicular biopsies, administration of gonadotropin-releasing hormone (GnRH) produced marked elevations in both luteinizing hormone (LH) and follicle-stimulating hormone (FSH)—a picture suggestive of primary testicular insufficiency. After varicocelectomy, the response to GnRH was completely normal. Response of testosterone levels to intramuscular administration of human chorionic gonadotropin (hCG) was also initially abnormal but reversible after surgery. Also, one related study documented that young men with varicoceles did have a significant decrease in left testicular volume, as measured by ultrasound, compared with control subjects [69,75].

The diagnosis of varicoceles is straightforward. In severe or stage III disease, they are noticeable on visual inspection of the scrotum while the patient is standing. Otherwise, having the patient stand upright and perform a Valsalva maneuver may cause greater distention of the pampiniform plexus and accentuate the tortuosity of the varicoceles [69,70].

A few clear indications for varicocelectomy exist: loss of testicular volume on the affected side of more than 20% or 2 ml compared with the normal testis, or infertility in adult life [69,76]. However, what to do with a 14-year-old with equal-sized testes and no symptoms is a dilemma. Short of subjecting them all to sophisticated endocrinologic testing, the best "educated guess" would be to send those young men with large varicoceles for early surgery—to avoid the problems of diminished testis size or function later on.

Hematoceles

The most common traumatic lesion of the scrotum is an accumulation of blood within the tunica vaginalis—a hematocele [61]. Patients complain of scrotal pain, and the involved part of the scrotum is frequently swollen and ecchymotic. The testis does not transilluminate, and ultrasound often demonstrates a lucent area surrounding the testis. Conservative management is indicated for small hematoceles, but larger ones may require surgical drainage. Immediate surgery is also indicated for a suspected ruptured testis, which can usually be visualized using ultrasonography [55]. If there is any doubt, early surgical exploration (within 3 days of injury) avoids compromise of the testis by secondary infection or pressure effect and has a lower subsequent rate of orchiectomy (5–20%), compared with 45% to 55% if exploration is delayed [61].

Orchitis

Viral orchitis, usually caused by mumps, has become uncommon because of widespread immunization efforts. Orchitis develops in 20% to 30% of mumps infections, usually several days after the parotitis [54]. Acute testicular pain and scrotal pain, often unilateral, are accompanied by fever and leukocytosis but not pyuria or bacteriuria. Treatment includes analgesics, bed rest, and scrotal elevation. Both technetium scanning and Doppler studies demonstrate increased blood flow.

Testicular Cancer

Although it is exceedingly rare in adolescents, testicular cancer remains the most common solid tumor in men aged 15 to 34 years and is responsible for 14% of all cancer deaths in this age group [77,78]. Just as young women are taught breast self-examination, many years before their age of peak risk, male adolescents should be taught testicular self-examination [79–81]. Unfortunately, at present, many are not. Curricula to increase awareness about the risk of testicular cancer and to teach self-examination are widely available and have had well documented effectiveness [77,79–83].

Gynecomastia

Gynecomastia represents one of the cruelest "tricks of nature" on boys. It also can represent a significant diagnostic dilemma for the clinician who may not be aware of its prevalence or treatment. In one documented case, an obese 15-year-old with physiologic gynecomastia underwent three computed tomography scans, an arteriogram, and a cisternal puncture as part of the workup for a pituitary tumor that he never had [84].

In most cases, gynecomastia in young men is physiologic and does not require an elaborate neurologic or endocrinologic evaluation. It is most often seen in boys who are between Tanner stages 3 and 4. Indeed, boys who are prepubertal or who have reached Tanner 5 may require a judicious workup, looking for such rare disorders as adrenal or gonadal tumors, liver disease, or Klinefelter's syndrome [85,86]. But even so, the most common cause of gynecomastia that is not physiologic is probably marijuana abuse [87].

In an early study of over 1,800 normal boys in a Boy Scout camp, the overall incidence of gynecomastia was found to be nearly 40%, with a peak incidence of nearly 65% in 14-year-olds. Most often, the breast tissue was bilateral, but in 25% of the boys it was solely unilateral. The condition persisted for up to 2 years in over 25% of the boys and for 3 years in only 7% [88]. In a more recent study of 536 male adolescents, the overall prevalence was 48.5%, with one-sided involvement in 45% [89].

A number of studies have tried to determine the etiology of gynecomastia. Normal levels of LH, FSH, prolactin, testosterone, estrone, and estradiol have been repeatedly documented in such patients [90–93]. Gynecomastia may result from a temporary imbalance in the effects of estrogens versus androgens, or an increased end-organ sensitivity to normal levels of circulating estrogens [88]. In one study, serum estradiol was consistently high in relation to testosterone in adolescent boys with gynecomastia (although absolute levels of both hormones were normal), and the ratio returned to normal as the gynecomastia regressed with age [92]. In the most recent study, lower levels of free testosterone and higher levels of testosterone–estrogen binding globulin (TEBG) were found [89]. Previous studies had not determined levels of free testosterone, and the levels were lower in boys with gynecomastia both at the time of onset and 6 months earlier, as were TEBG levels. Lower levels of the latter could conceivably allow higher levels of unbound estrogen to affect locally sensitive estrogen receptors in male breast tissue [89]. One author postulates the direct testicular secretion of estrogen and the peripheral conversion of prohormones to estrogen as the cause of gynecomastia [94].

Signs and Symptoms

Many young men with gynecomastia are asymptomatic and unaware of the presence of breast tissue. Often they will be forcibly brought in by their mothers, who are concerned about a "tumor." In general, 1.5 to 2 cm of tissue is needed for gynecomastia to be noticed. A small, discoid, subareolar mass can usually be palpated, which is discrete, movable, and associated with varying complaints of tenderness (type I). Occasionally, the amount of male breast development can be quite striking—type II gynecomastia, which may approach the appearance of female Tanner stage 3 breasts.

Diagnosis and Treatment

Clinicians should use tact and common sense in dealing with patients with gynecomastia. Some may prefer to avoid the use of the words "breast tissue" or "breasts" because many male teens may be feeling that their hormones are playing a trick on them, or that they are actually becoming female or having a sexual identity crisis [95]. Others may prefer to describe "some extra tissue" being present without being specific about what kind of tissue it is.

One study has documented that the greater the degree of gynecomastia, the greater the likelihood of adjustment problems, usually involving the patient's self-esteem and concept of his own masculinity [96]. Therefore, the importance of reassurance and counseling should not be underestimated. Patients often respond to the statement that "you are not turning into a girl," whereas their mothers respond to "it is not cancer."

How does the clinician separate out the 99% of boys with physiologic gynecomastia from the 1% who may have underlying disease? Here, a careful history and physical examination are important, as well as judicious restraint. A thorough family, drug, and nutritional history indicates if familial gynecomastia or starvation and refeeding are possibilities, or if the breast tissue could possibly be drug induced (e.g., marijuana, cimetidine, digitalis, tricyclic antidepressants, heroin) [97]. On examination, the body habitus and genitalia should be careful inspected. Careful measurement of the testes is important: testes smaller than 3.5 cm in length may indicate Klinefelter's syndrome, and asymmetric testes may be the only clue to a testicular tumor. Presence of obesity may indicate pseudogynecomastia (fatty tissue rather than true breast tissue). Other endocrine stigmata should also be sought. Most of the time, the male adolescent will be found to be between Tanner stages 2 and 4, and the rest of the history and physical examination will be negative. In such cases, additional laboratory or radiologic workup is neither warranted nor useful. Explicit reassurance should be coupled with sympathetic counseling that in all but 7% of cases, the tissue involutes within 2 to 3 years.

Type II gynecomastia can either be physiologic or pathologic. In either case, corrective surgery may be necessary, especially if the breast development is female Tanner stage 3 or beyond. In such instances, the likelihood of spontaneous resolution is low, and the psychosocial consequences may be severe. Clomiphene citrate and tamoxifen have both been used in medical trials, with limited success, making surgery the treatment of choice ordinarily [85,86]. Workup of gynecomastia that is thought to be pathologic may include a buccal smear, a chromosomal karyotype, measurements of urinary 17-ketosteroids, plasma testosterone, estradiol, LH, thyroid-stimulating hormone, and hCG, and liver function tests [86].

REFERENCES

1. Goldenring JM. Acute urethral syndromes. *Seminars in Adolescent Medicine* 1986;2:125.
2. Krowchuck DP. Nongonococcal urethritis: diagnosis, management, and complications. *Adolescent Medicine: State of the Art Reviews* 1996;7:63.
3. Remafedi G. Male homosexuality: the adolescent's perspective. *Pediatrics* 1987;79:326.
4. Collins KC, Chacko MR. Urethritis and epididymitis in male adolescents. *Seminars in Pediatric Infectious Diseases* 1993;4:176.
5. Braverman PK. Herpes, syphilis, and other ulcerogenital conditions. *Adolescent Medicine: State of the Art Reviews* 1996;7:93.
6. Risi GF Jr, Sanders CV. The genital mycoplasmas. *Obstet Gynecol Clin North Am* 1989;16:611.
7. Schmid GP, Fontanarosa PB. Evolving strategies for management of the nongonococcal urethritis syndrome. *JAMA* 1995;274:577.
8. Chambers CV, Shafer MA, Adger H, et al. Microflora of the urethra in adolescent boys: relationships to sexual activity and nongonococcal urethritis. *J Pediatr* 1987;110:314.
9. Bowie WR. Urethritis in males. In: Holmes KK, Mardh PA, Sparling PF, et al, eds. *Sexually transmitted diseases*. 2nd ed. New York: McGraw-Hill; 1990:627.
10. Kulig J. Gonococcal infection in the adolescent male. *Adolescent Medicine: State of the Art Reviews* 1996;7:63.
11. Bowie WR. Nongonococcal urethritis. *Urol Clin North Am* 1982;11:55.
12. Handsfield HH, Lipman TO, Harnisch JP, et al. Asymptomatic gonorrhea in men: diagnosis, natural course, prevalence, and significance. *N Engl J Med* 1974;290:117.
13. Thelin I, Wennstrom AM, Mardh PA, et al. Contact-tracing in patients with genital chlamydial infection. *British Journal of Venereal Disease* 1980;56:259.
14. Shafer MA, Prager V, Shalwitz J, et al. Prevalence of urethral *Chlamydia trachomatis* and *Neisseria gonorrhoeae* among asymptomatic sexually active adolescent males. *J Infect Dis* 1987;156:223.
15. Smith JA, Linder CW, Jay MS, et al. Isolation of *Neisseria gonorrhoeae* from the urethra of asymptomatic adolescent males. *Clin Pediatr* 1986;25:566.
16. Centers for Disease Control and Prevention. 1993 Sexually transmitted diseases treatment guidelines. *MMWR Morb Mortal Wkly Rep* 1993;42(RR-14):1.
17. Handsfield HH, Pollock PS. Arthritis associated with sexually transmitted diseases. In: Holmes KK, Mardh PA, Sparling PF, et al, eds. *Sexually transmitted diseases*. 2nd ed. New York: McGraw-Hill; 1990:737.
18. Martin DH. Chlamydia trachomatis infections in men with Reiter's syndrome. *Ann Intern Med* 1984;100:207.
19. Horwitz S, Horwitz J, Taylor-Robinson D, et al. *Ureaplasma urealyticum* in Reiter's syndrome. *J Rheumatol* 1994;21:877.
20. Judson FN, Ehret J. Laboratory diagnosis of sexually transmitted infections. *Pediatr Ann* 1994;23:361.
21. Hale YM, Melton ME, Lewis JS, et al. Evaluation of the PACE 2 *Neisseria gonorrhoeae* assay by three public health laboratories. *J Clin Microbiol* 1993;31:451.
22. Hanks JW, Scott CT, Butler CE, et al. Evaluation of a DNA probe assay (Gen-Probe PACE 2) as the test of cure for *Neisseria gonorrhoeae* genital infections. *J Pediatr* 1994;125:161.
23. Stamm WE, Mardh PA. *Chlamydia trachomatis*. In: Holmes KK, Mardh PA, Sparling PF, et al, eds. *Sexually transmitted diseases*. 2nd ed. New York: McGraw-Hill; 1990:917.

24. Mardh PA, Danielsson D. *Neisseria gonorrhoeae*. In: Holmes KK, Mardh PA, Sparling PF, et al, eds. *Sexually transmitted diseases*. 2nd ed. New York: McGraw-Hill; 1990:903.
25. Demetriou E, Sackett R, Welch DF, et al. Evaluation of an enzyme immunoassay for detection of *Neisseria gonorrhoeae* in an adolescent population. *JAMA* 1984;252:247.
26. Braverman PK, Biro FM, Brunner RL, et al. Screening asymptomatic adolescent males for chlamydia. *Journal of Adolescent Health Care* 1990;11:141.
27. Shafer MA. Sexually transmitted diseases in adolescents: prevention, diagnosis and treatment in pediatric practice. *Adolescent Health Update* 1994;6:1.
28. Werner MJ, Biro FM. Urinary leukocyte esterase screening for asymptomatic sexually transmitted disease in adolescent males. *J Adolesc Health* 1991;12:326.
29. Shafer MA, Schachter J, Moncada J, et al. Evaluation of urine-based screening strategies to detect *Chlamydia trachomatis* among sexually active asymptomatic young males. *JAMA* 1993;270:2065.
30. Woods CR Jr. Gonococcal infections in children and adolescents. *Seminars in Pediatric Infectious Diseases* 1993;4:94.
31. Genc M, Ruusuvaara L, Mardh PA. An economic evaluation of screening for *Chlamydia trachomatis* in adolescent males. *JAMA* 1993;270:2057.
32. Judson FN. Treatment of uncomplicated gonorrhea with ceftriaxone: a review. *Sex Transm Dis* 1986;13:199.
33. Stamm WE, Hicks CB, Martin DH, et al. Azithromycin for empirical treatment of the nongonococcal urethritis syndrome in men: a randomized double-blind study. *JAMA* 1995;274:545.
34. The Medical Letter. Drugs for sexually transmitted diseases. *The Medical Letter* 1995;37(964):117.
35. Whatley JD, Thin RN, Mumtaz G, et al. Azithromycin vs doxycycline in the treatment of nongonococcal urethritis. *Int J STD AIDS* 1991;2:248.
36. Dyment PG. Human papillomavirus infection. *Adolescent Medicine: State of the Art Reviews* 1996;7:119.
37. Koutsky LA, Galloway DA, Holmes KK. Epidemiology of human papillomavirus infection. *Epidemiol Rev* 1988;10:122.
38. McCance DJ, Kalache A, Ashdown K, et al. Human papillomavirus types 16 and 18 in carcinomas of the penis from Brazil. *Int J Cancer* 1986;37:55.
39. Daling JR, Weiss NS, Hislop TG, et al. Sexual partners, sexually transmitted diseases, and the incidence of anal cancer. *N Engl J Med* 1987;317:973.
40. Krebs HB, Schneider V. Human papilloma virus-associated lesions of the penis: colposcopy, cytology, and histology. *Obstet Gynecol* 1987;70:299.
41. Rosemberg SK, Greenberg MD, Reid R. Sexually transmitted papillomaviral infection in men. *Obstet Gynecol Clin North Am* 1987;14:495.
42. Levine RU, Crum CP, Herman E, et al. Cervical papillomavirus infection and intraepithelial neoplasia: a study of male sex partners. *Obstet Gynecol* 1984;64:16.
43. Schlappner OLA, Shaffer EA. Anorectal condylomata acuminata: a missed part of the condylomata spectrum. *Can Med Assoc J* 1978;118:172.
44. Braverman PK. Herpes, syphilis, and other ulcerogenital conditions. *Adolescent Medicine: State of the Art Reviews* 1996;7:93.
45. Dyment PG. Cryosurgery with dimethyl ether and propane for condylomata in male college students. *Pediatr Res* 1995;37(Suppl):4A-9.
46. Slater GE, Rumack BH, Peterson RG. Podophyllin poisoning: systemic toxicity following cutaneous application. *Obstet Gynecol* 1978;52:94.
47. von Krog G. Topical self-treatment of penile warts with 0.5% podophyllotoxin in ethanol for four or five days. *Sex Transm Dis* 1987;14:135.
48. The Medical Letter. Podofilox. *The Medical Letter* 1991;33:117.
49. Dretler SP, Klein LA. The eradication of intraurethral condylomata acuminata with 5 per cent 5-fluorouracil cream. *J Urol* 1975;113:195.
50. Eron LJ, Judson F, Tucker S, et al. Interferon therapy for condylomata acuminata. *N Engl J Med* 1986;315:1059.
51. The Medical Letter. Interferon for treatment of genital warts. *The Medical Letter* 1988;30:70.
52. Sykes NL Jr. Condyloma acuminatum. *Int J Dermatol* 1995;34:297.
53. Dyment PG, ed. Male reproductive health. *Adolescent Medicine: State of the Art Reviews* 1996;7:1.
54. O'Brien WM, Lynch JH. The acute scrotum. *Am Fam Physician* 1988;37:239.
55. Witherington R. The "acute" scrotum: lesions that require immediate attention. *Postgrad Med* 1987;82:207.
56. Prater JM, Overdorf BS. Testicular torsion: a surgical emergency. *Am Fam Physician* 1991;44:834.
57. Stillwell TJ, Kramer SA. Intermittent testicular torsion. *Pediatrics* 1986;77:908.
58. Williamson RCN. Torsion of the testis and allied conditions. *Br J Surg* 1976;63:465.
59. Haynes BE, Bessen HA, Haynes VE. The diagnosis of testicular torsion. *JAMA* 1983;249:2522.
60. Barloon TJ, Weissman AM, Kahn D. Diagnostic imaging of patients with acute scrotal pain. *Am Fam Physician* 1996;53:1734.
61. Monga M, Hellstrom WJG. Testicular trauma. *Adolescent Medicine: State of the Art Reviews* 1996;7:141.
62. Sonda LP, Want S. Evaluation of male external genital diseases in the emergency room setting. *Emerg Med Clin North Am* 1988;6:473.

63. Laor E, Fisch H, Tennenbaum S, et al. Unilateral testicular torsion: abnormal histological findings in the contralateral testis—cause or effect? *Br J Urol* 1990;65:520.

64. Krarup T. The testes after torsion. *Br J Urol* 1978;40:43.

65. Thomas WE, Cooper MJ, Crane GA, et al. Testicular exocrine malfunction after torsion. *Lancet* 1984;2:1357.

66. Ireton RC, Berger RE. Prostatitis and epididymitis. *Urol Clin North Am* 1984;11:83.

67. Bowie WR. Approach to men with urethritis and urologic complications of sexually transmitted diseases. *Med Clin North Am* 1990;74:1543.

68. Kass EJ, Reitelman C. Adolescent varicocele. *Urol Clin North Am* 1995;22:151.

69. Monga M, Sofkitis N, Hellstrom WJG. Benign scrotal masses in the adolescent male: varicoceles, spermatoceles, and hydroceles. *Adolescent Medicine: State of the Art Reviews* 1996;7:131.

70. Boyd AS. Varicoceles and male infertility. *Am Fam Physician* 1988;37:252.

71. Trantham P. The infertile couple. *Am Fam Physician* 1996;54:1001.

72. Berger OG. Varicocele in adolescents. *Clin Pediatr* 1980;19:810.

73. Pryor JL, Howards SS. Varicocele. *Urol Clin North Am* 1987;14:499.

74. Castro-Magana M, Angulo MA, Canas JA, et al. Improvement of of Leydig cell function in male adolescents after varicocelectomy. *J Pediatr* 1989;115:809.

75. Sayfan J, Soffer Y, Manor H, et al. Varicocele in youth: a therapeutic dilemma. *Ann Surg* 1988;207:223.

76. Kass EJ, Belman AB. Reversal of testicular growth failure by varicocele ligation. *J Urol* 1990;137:475.

77. Vaz RM, Best DL, Davis SW, et al. Evaluation of a testicular cancer curriculum for adolescents. *J Pediatr* 1989;114:150.

78. Thomas R. Testicular tumors. *Adolescent Medicine: State of the Art Reviews* 1996;7:149.

79. Goldenring JM. A lifesaving exam for young men. *Contemporary Pediatrics* 1992;9:63.

80. Kapphahn C, Schlossberger N. Male reproductive health: I. painful scrotal masses. *Adolescent Health Update* 1991;4(3):1.

81. Kapphahn C, Schlossberger N. Male reproductive health: II. painless scrotal masses. *Adolescent Health Update* 1992;5(1):1.

82. Goldenring JM. Teaching testicular self-examination to young men. *Contemporary Pediatrics* 1985;3:73.

83. Sayger SA, Fortenberry JD, Beckman RJ. Practice patterns of teaching testicular self-examination to adolescent patients. *Journal of Adolescent Health Care* 1988;9:441.

84. Strasburger VC. Why adolescent medicine? Four illustrative cases. *Clin Pediatr* 1984;23:12.

85. Braunstein GD. Gynecomastia. *N Engl J Med* 1993;328:490.

86. Braunstein GD. Diagnosis and treatment of gynecomastia. *Hosp Pract* 1993;28:37.

87. Harmon J, Aliapoulios MA. Gynecomastia in marijuana users. *N Engl J Med* 1972;287:936.

88. Nydick M, Bustos J, Dales JH Jr, et al. Gynecomastia in adolescent boys. *JAMA* 1961;178:449.

89. Biro FM, Lucky AW, Huster GA, et al. Hormonal studies and physical maturation in adolescent gynecomastia. *J Pediatr* 1990;116:450.

90. Editorial. *Br Med J* 1964;2:1548.

91. Lee PA. The relationship of concentrations of serum hormones to pubertal gynecomastia. *J Pediatr* 1975;86:212.

92. Knorr K., Bidlingmaier F. Gynaecomastia in male adolescents. *Clin Endocrinol Metab* 1975;4:157.

93. Biro FM, Lucky AW, Huster GA. Hormonal studies and physical maturation in adolescent gynecomastia. *J Pediatr* 1990;116:450.

94. Kulin HE, Muller J. The biological aspects of puberty. *Pediatr Rev* 1996;17:75.

95. Greydanus DE, Shearin RB. *Adolescent sexuality and gynecology*. Philadelphia: Lea and Febiger; 1990.

96. Schonfield WA. Gynecomastia in adolescence: effects on body image and personality adaptation. *Psychosom Med* 1962;24:379.

97. Thompson DF, Carter JR. Drug-inducted gynecomastia. *Pharmacotherapy* 1993;13:37.

SUGGESTED READING

Urethritis

Bowie WR. Approach to men with urethritis and urologic complications of sexually transmitted diseases. *Med Clin North Am* 1990;74:1543.

Braverman PK. Herpes, syphilis, and other ulcerogenital conditions. *Adolescent Medicine: State of the Art Reviews* 1996;7:93.

Collins KC, Chacko MR. Urethritis and epididymitis in male adolescents. *Seminars in Pediatric Infectious Diseases* 1993;4:176.

Krowchuck DP. Nongonococcal urethritis: diagnosis, management, and complications. *Adolescent Medicine: State of the Art Reviews* 1996;7:63.

Kulig J. Gonococcal infection in the adolescent male. *Adolescent Medicine: State of the Art Reviews* 1996;7:63.

Roberts JA. Management of urinary tract infections in the adolescent male. *Adolescent Medicine: State of the Art Reviews* 1996;7:1.

Shafer MA. Sexually transmitted diseases in adolescents: prevention, diagnosis and treatment in pediatric practice. *Adolescent Health Update* 1994;6:1.

Schmid GP, Fontanarosa PB. Evolving strategies for management of the nongonococcal urethritis syndrome. *JAMA* 1995;274:577.

Zenilman J. Sexually transmitted diseases in homosexual adolescents. *Journal of Adolescent Health Care* 1988;9:129.

HPV Infection

Brown DR, Fife KA. Human papillomavirus infections of the genital tract. *Med Clin North Am* 1990;74:1455.

Dyment PG. Human papillomavirus infection. *Adolescent Medicine: State of the Art Reviews* 1996;7:119.

Kraus SJ, Stone SM. Management of genital infection caused by human papillomavirus. *Rev Infect Dis* 1990;12(Suppl):S620.

Krebs HB, Schneider V. Human papilloma virus-associated lesions of the penis: colposcopy, cytology, and histology. *Obstet Gynecol* 1987;70:299.

Oriel D. Genital human papillomavirus infection. In: Holmes KK, Mardh PA, Sparling PF, et al, eds. *Sexually transmitted diseases*. 2nd ed. New York: McGraw-Hill; 1990:433.

Shah KV. Biology of genitral tract human papillomaviruses. *Urol Clin North Am* 1992;19:63.

Scrotal Disorders

Barloon TJ, Weissman AM, Kahn D. Diagnostic imaging of patients with acute scrotal pain. *Am Fam Physician* 1996;53:1734.

Dyment PG, ed. Male reproductive health. *Adolescent Medicine: State of the Art Reviews* 1996;7:1.

Goldenring JM. A lifesaving exam for young men. *Contemporary Pediatrics* 1992;9:63.

Kapphahn C, Schlossberger N. Male reproductive health: I. painful scrotal masses. *Adolescent Health Update* 1991;4(3):1.

Kapphahn C, Schlossberger N. Male reproductive health: II. painless scrotal masses. *Adolescent Health Update* 1992;5(1):1.

Kass EJ, Reitelman C. Adolescent varicocele. *Urol Clin North Am* 1995;22:151.

Monga M, Hellstrom WJG. Testicular trauma. *Adolescent Medicine: State of the Art Reviews* 1996;7:141.

Monga M, Sofkitis N, Hellstrom WJG. Benign scrotal masses in the adolescent male: varicoceles, spermatoceles, and hydroceles. *Adolescent Medicine: State of the Art Reviews* 1996;7:131.

O'Brien WM, Lynch JH. The acute scrotum. *Am Fam Physician* 1988;37:239.

Prater JM, Overdorf BS. Testicular torsion: a surgical emergency. *Am Fam Physician* 1991;44:834.

Skoog SJ, Roberts KP, Goldstein M et al. The adolescent varicocele: what's new with an old problem in young patients? *Pediatr* 1997;100:112.

Thomas R. Testicular tumors. *Adolescent Medicine: State of the Art Reviews* 1996;7:149.

Gynecomastia

Braunstein GD. Gynecomastia. *N Engl J Med* 1993;328:490.

Braunstein GD. Diagnosis and treatment of gynecomastia. *Hosp Pract* 1993;28:37.

Greydanus DE, Parks DS, Farrell EG. Breast disorders in children and adolescents. *Pediatr Clin North Am* 1989;36:601.

Kulin HE, Muller J. The biological aspects of puberty. *Pediatr Rev* 1996;17:75.

Lee PA. The relationship of concentrations of serum hormones to pubertal gynecomastia. *J Pediatr* 1975;86:212.

Neuman JF. Evaluation and treatment of gynecomastia. *Am Fam Physician* 1997;55:1835.

Nydick M, Bustos J, Dale JH Jr, et al. Gynecomastia in adolescent boys. *JAMA* 1961;178:449.

Thompson DF, Carter JR. Drug-inducted gynecomastia. *Pharmacotherapy* 1993;13:37.

HEALTH CARE FOR GAY, LESBIAN, AND BISEXUAL YOUTH

Written with Gary Remafedi

During the 1980s, the impact of sexual orientation on adolescent health became an important new topic. Bisexual and homosexual youth are disproportionately affected by serious medical, mental

Gary Remafedi, M.D., M.P.H., is Associate Professor of Pediatrics and Director, Youth and AIDS Projects, Department of Pediatrics, University of Minnesota School of Medicine.

health, social, and public health problems. For example, multiple studies have found consistently high rates of attempted suicide, in the range of 20% to 42%, in volunteer samples of gay and lesbian youths [1]. It has been estimated that gays and lesbians may account for up to 30% of completed suicides among U.S. adolescents each year [2]. Currently, 38% of reported U.S. acquired immunodeficiency syndrome (AIDS) cases in 13- to 19-year-olds and 74% in 20- to 24-year-olds have involved men who have sex with men [3]. Bisexual and homosexual youths may comprise a large share of runaways, the homeless, and youth adolescent prostitutes [4]. In addition, surveys of bisexual and gay male adolescents have uncovered high rates of dropping out of school, victimization by sexual assault, substance abuse, sexually transmitted diseases (STDs), and arrests for misconduct [5].

Despite the need, few health professionals have received instruction about the special issues involved in caring for homosexual youth. Disapproval of homosexuality is widespread, among professionals and lay persons alike. As a result of misinformation, lack of information, and cultural taboos, the health problems of gay and lesbian youth have been largely untended. This is reflected in the problems of inadequate immunization against hepatitides [5], lack of specific human immunodeficiency virus (HIV) prevention programming for gay and lesbian youth, and underutilization of STD screening and HIV antibody counseling and testing [6].

This section focuses on the practical aspect of working with gay and lesbian youth, with special attention devoted to questions most often asked by professionals: How do I know if my patient is gay? What are the best ways to discuss homosexuality with youths and their families? How should I counsel an adolescent who is confused about his or her sexuality? What kinds of interventions might be useful?

This discussion is based on an understanding of the following principles [7–10]:

1. The term "sexual orientation" indicates an individual's pattern of attraction toward men, women, or both [7]. It may involve sexual fantasies, emotional attachments, sexual behavior, or group affiliation. "Homosexuality" encompasses a spectrum of sexual orientations, generally characterized by a persistent pattern of homosexual attraction and absent or weak heterosexual attraction.

2. "Homophobia" is a pervasive and irrational fear of homosexuality, which can affect homosexual or heterosexual individuals [8]. Bisexual and homosexual youth may experience "internalized" homophobia as lowered self-esteem, shame, and self-compromising behaviors. Such adolescents may also encounter homophobia from others in the form of verbal abuse, physical violence, parental rejection, and discrimination.

3. Homosexuality is not pathologic [9]. Although the stigma of homosexuality may be destructive—especially for adolescents—adverse medical and psychosocial sequelae are not inevitable. Therapies that purport to change sexual orientation are not only unsuccessful but exacerbate the damaging effects of homophobia as well.

4. Sexual orientation appears to be established early in childhood and, perhaps, even before birth [10]. There is no evidence that homosexuality is "caused" by harmful life experiences.

Psychosexual Development

Acquisition of a homosexual identity is not a sudden event but a gradual unfolding of identity that spans the life cycle [11]. This process often begins in childhood with a vague sense of "being different." Atypical gender interests or behavior may be displayed. At puberty, homosexually oriented adolescents often become aware of an attraction to people of the same gender. Such a realization may lead to severe distress or confusion. During middle or late adolescence, or adulthood, the individual may resolve this confusion and adopt a homosexual or bisexual identity, although ambivalence may persist. Gay teenagers may discuss homosexuality with others—usually trusted friends rather than parents. Assumption of a homosexual identity usually precedes sexual activity with partners of the same gender. Given the stigma of homosexuality, adolescents do not often identify themselves as gay or lesbian without considerable forethought.

Acceptance of one's homosexuality is characterized by the absence of distress, unwillingness to change sexual orientation, and the development of intimate relationships. Often, full acceptance is not attained before adulthood.

Presenting Issues

Homosexual youth do not usually come to the attention of physicians during childhood or early adolescence. A notable exception is the severely gender-atypical child. In this case, parents may be distressed by the child's mannerisms, gender-inappropriate play, or identification with people of the opposite gender. They may express worries about the child's physical constitution, social adaptation, or sexual identity.

Adolescents seeking a professional's assistance are likely to be at a point of identity confusion or assumption. Often, they turn to trusted school nurses or counselors for help. Such teens may present with anxiety, depression, attempted suicide, STDs, family conflict, deteriorating school performance, substance abuse, or school misconduct. If the underlying concerns about sexual orientation can be detected, effective counseling is possible. Some youth seek help with "coming out," changing sexual orientation, managing peer and family relationships, making independent living arrangements, and locating information and social support.

Adolescents who are struggling with their sexual identities may not clearly articulate their concerns. Fearing disapproval, even the most self-confident individuals may appear confused. Many homosexual adults report prior consultation with mental health professionals, yet important sexual concerns are often not discussed.

Older adolescents and adults have often reached the point of acceptance and present to physicians for detection and treatment of STDs or other health-related issues. They may seek counseling for relationship problems, HIV-related issues, chemical dependence, or sequelae of social stigmatization.

Contrary to popular stereotypes, homosexual youth are indistinguishable from their heterosexual peers in appearance or mannerisms. The only reliable indicator of sexual orientation is the patient's own self-report. However, adolescents with the most urgent concerns about their sexual orientation are often the least likely to initiate such a discussion. Health professions can ease the process by taking a sensitive and comprehensive sexual history.

Sexual History

Physicians need to explore their own attitudes toward homosexuality and other controversial sexual issues. Thinking about such topics in advance improves the quality of the interview and helps to control verbal and nonverbal cues to the patient.

The context of the sexual history may be as important as the content. Adolescents are more apt to discuss their sexual orientation if waiting rooms and offices contain posters, brochures, and periodicals about gay and lesbian issues. Health history intake forms should begin with an acknowledgment of confidentiality and should not assume the respondents' heterosexuality.

Given their sensitive nature, questions about sexuality should be prefaced with an explanation of their purpose and the limits of confidentiality. For example, the interview might begin: "In order to offer you the best care possible, I first need to ask you some personal questions about sex. I ask all of my patients these questions. With the exception of my having to report abuse, all of your answers will remain completely confidential." From this point, questions should follow a logical progression from general to more specific information: "Have you had any sexual experiences? Have your sexual experiences been with males, females, or both? How many partners have you had during the past year? What kinds of sexual experiences have you had—oral sex? vaginal intercourse? anal intercourse?"

Questions about sexual behavior might lead to additional discussion about sexual orientation: "Do you consider yourself to be gay/lesbian, bisexual, or heterosexual? Have you discussed your feelings with other people? Are you currently in a steady relationship?" Ideally, the conversation should lead to an accurate depiction of the patient's psychosexual development and ideas for constructive interventions.

Sometimes the sexual history reveals inconsistencies in orientation. For example, a patient might report predominantly homosexual fantasies, experiences, and emotional attractions but assumes a heterosexual identity. If identity confusion is suspected, the hypothesis might be tested further: "What do you think about homosexuality? Have you known any gay/lesbian people? What do you think it would be like to be gay? How does a person know if he is gay?"

The goal of the sexual history is to assist the patient, not to assign him or her a sexual orientation. Gay adolescents may be distressed by their sexual feelings and unable to cope with a homosexual identity. In such situations, clinicians should offer information, support, and reassurance that the teenager will eventually resolve their identity in a healthy and normal way, whether heterosexual or homosexual.

Occasionally, adolescents are labeled as homosexual by others, before they have considered this as a possibility. This is a common predicament for gender-atypical boys and girls who are taunted by their classmates for being different. In other cases, physicians might suspect that sexual orientation confusion underlies serious problems such as depression, attempted suicide, or substance abuse. Professional counseling may be warranted in these situations.

Epidemiology and Clinical Presentation of Sexually Transmitted Diseases

Various anatomic, physiologic, and psychosocial risk factors contribute to the spread of sexually transmitted disease among young men who have unprotected sex with men [12]. Pathogens in semen are efficiently transmitted during anal intercourse, both locally in the rectum and parenterally across damaged epithelial surfaces. Among all sexual behaviors, unprotected anal intercourse poses the greatest risk of spreading HIV, hepatitis B, and cytomegalovirus (CMV). Other common sexual practices, such as oral–genital and oral–anal contact, can transmit hepatitis A and enteric infections. Ulcerative diseases, like syphilis and herpes, compound the risk of HIV transmission during intercourse by creating a portal of entry or exit for the virus or possibly increasing the host's susceptibility to infection. Finally, psychosocial comorbidities, such as substance abuse in sexual situations, promote the spread of STDs by their deleterious effects on safer sex precautions.

Although gay adults have demonstrated one of the most rapid and profound responses to a health threat that has ever been documented [13], ongoing HIV risk among gay and bisexual adolescents continues to be problematic. A study of gay and bisexual adolescents enrolled in an HIV prevention program found that 64% were at extreme risk for HIV infection based on reports of unprotected anal intercourse or injecting drug use [14]. Perceived likelihood of HIV acquisition, substance use, relationship status, noncommunication with partners about risk reduction, and frequent intercourse were found to be significantly associated with unprotected anal intercourse in the previous year [15].

Seroprevalence of HIV among young men who have sex with men has been found to be 4.2% in a New York City runaway/homeless shelter [16], 13% to 17% in a national sample of adolescent clinics [17], 26% in a Maryland college clinic [18], and 30% in a national sample of STD clinics [19]. A longitudinal, household survey of young gay and bisexual men (median age, 25 years) found the HIV seroincidence to be 2.6% annually; at the observed infection rate, seroprevalence was projected to reach 35% in 9 years, approaching levels observed among gay adults at the height of the epidemic [20].

Gay adolescents with STDs can experience symptoms related to any organ system, but the most common clinical syndromes are pharyngitis, urethritis, dermatologic conditions, gastrointestinal infections, hepatitis, and mononucleosis-like illnesses [13]. Gonococcal infections of the throat, urethra, or rectum and ectoparasitic infections (pediculosis pubis and scabies) are among the most common problems. Studies of gay men in STD clinics have found a peak incidence of gonorrhea and chlamydial infections in the 15- to 20-year-old group [21]. In addition to ectoparasitic infections, other common dermatologic problems include ulcerative lesions caused by syphilis or herpes and genital or perianal condylomata acuminata.

Sexually transmitted gastrointestinal and rectoanal infections [12] may present with proctitis (commonly caused by gonorrhea, herpes simplex virus, human papillomavirus, syphilis, or lymphogranuloma venereum), *proctocolitis* (caused by enteric parasites or bacteria such as *Shigella, Campylobacter,* and *Salmonella* species), *enteritis* (commonly caused by *Giardia lamblia* or opportunistic infections), or *esophagitis* (especially in immunocompromised individuals, due to *Candida albicans,* herpes simplex virus, or CMV).

Hepatitis B virus is one of the most common and serious sexually transmitted pathogens in homosexual men. During the 18-month vaccine trials, 35% of unvaccinated men showed serologic evidence of infection. Among the more than 1,000 participants, 52 non-B hepatitis events were recorded. Of these, 27 were caused by hepatitis A virus, 8 by CMV, and 2 by Epstein-Barr virus [22]. More recently, there have been reports of a marked increase in hepatitis A in homosexual men from cities in the United States, Canada, and Australia [23].

Physical Examination and Laboratory Testing

In general, the medical care of gay, lesbian, and bisexual youth should be determined by their sexual behavior, not their sexual orientation [7]. The sexual history should elicit specific information about the frequency of sexual activity, gender and numbers of partners, specific sexual behaviors, condom use, and the use of alcohol or other drugs in sexual situations. Lesbian and gay youth may still engage in heterosexual as well as homosexual intercourse. Others may be sexually inexperienced. Like other teenagers, many homosexual youth are poorly informed about reproductive health, contraceptive use, STDs, and AIDS.

Women who have sex only with women are at lower risk for STDs than are women who have intercourse with men. However, symptoms or signs of an STD should be investigated with appropriate testing [24]. Although the incidence of cancers among lesbians has not been well studied, nulliparity may increase their risk for breast, ovarian, and endometrial lesions [24]. Like women who have sex with men, young women who limit their sexual activity to female partners need regular gynecologic examinations and Pap tests. The need for family planning services should be individually determined by the sexual history.

Male adolescents who have sex with other men require periodic testing for syphilis and gonorrhea (oral, rectal, or urethral) at intervals suggested by the sexual history. In addition, hepatitis A and B serologies should be obtained, and vaccination is recommended.

The risks and benefits of HIV antibody testing should be discussed with all sexually active teens, regardless of gender or sexual orientation. Recommendations should take into account the potential educational or diagnostic value for the individual patient as well as his or her maturity, emotional state, suicide risk, social vulnerability, and expected response to the results. Testing should be voluntary. Individual state reporting and contact notification requirements and handling of laboratory results should be discussed. Pretest and posttest counseling should be conducted in accordance with suggested national guidelines [25].

Special Services

Most gay and lesbian youth can benefit from educational information about homosexuality. Such topics include etiology and normality of homosexuality, gay and lesbian life-styles, "coming out" to parents and friends, developing intimate relationships, legal protections, and STDs. A thorough understanding of AIDS prevention is especially urgent.

Referrals for special services should be guided by the individual's needs, but most youth benefit from social support groups. Youth groups that exist in many cities offer opportunities for learning, friendship, positive role models, and safe entertainment. Their goal is to prevent the medical and psychosocial problems that arise from stigma and isolation. Parents and family members should be encouraged to obtain information and support from local chapters of the Federation of Parents and Friends of Lesbians and Gays (PFLAG) [26]. More intensive psychotherapy usually is reserved for patients who are experiencing severe distress or serious psychiatric symptomatology unrelieved by educational and supportive measures.

REFERENCES

1. Remafedi G, ed. *Death by denial: studies of suicide in gay and lesbian teenagers*. Boston: Alyson Publications; 1994:7–14.
2. U.S. Department of Health and Human Services. *Report of the Secretary's Task Force on Youth Suicide, Volume 3: Prevention and interventions in youth suicide*. Rockville, MD: 1989.
3. Centers for Disease Control and Prevention. *HIV/AIDS Surveillance Report* 1995;7:12.
4. Deisher R, Robinson G, Boyer D. The adolescent female and male prostitute. *Pediatr Ann* 1982;11:819.
5. Remafedi G. Adolescent homosexuality: psychosocial and medical implications. *Pediatrics* 1987;79:331.
6. Povinelli M, Remafedi G, Tao G. Trends and predictors of human immunodeficiency virus antibody testing by homosexual and bisexual adolescent males, 1989–1994. *Arch Pediatr Adolesc Med* 1996;150:33.
7. West J, Remafedi G. Caring for lesbian and gay youth. *Contemporary Pediatrics* 1989;6:125.
8. Smith KT. Homophobia: a tentative profile. *Psychol Rep* 1971;29:1091.
9. Gonsiorek JC. Mental health issues of gay and lesbian adolescents. *Journal of Adolescent Health Care* 1988; 8:114.
10. Savin-Williams RC. Theoretical perspectives accounting for adolescent homosexuality. *Journal of Adolescent Health Care* 1988;8:95.
11. Troiden RR. Homosexual identity development. *Journal of Adolescent Health Care* 1988;8:105.
12. Remafedi G. Sexually transmitted diseases in homosexual youth. *Adolescent Medicine: State of the Art Reviews* 1990;1:565.
13. Becker MH, Joseph JG. AIDS and behavioral change to reduce risk: a review. *Am J Public Health* 1988; 78:394.
14. Remafedi G. Predictors of unprotected intercourse among gay and bisexual adolescents: knowledge, beliefs, and behavior. *Pediatrics* 1994;94:163.
15. Remafedi G. Cognitive and behavioral adaptations to HIV/AIDS among gay and bisexual adolescents. *J Adolesc Health* 1994;15:142.
16. Stricof RL, Kennedy JT, Nattell TC, Weisfuse IB, Novick LF. HIV seroprevalence in a facility for runaway and homeless adolescents. *Am J Public Health* 1991;81(Suppl):50.
17. Wendell DA, Onorato IM, McCray E, Allen DM, Sweeney PA. Youth at risk: sex, drugs, and human immunodeficiency virus. *American Journal of Diseases of Children* 1992;146:76.

18. Kotloff KL, Tachet CO, Clemens JD, et al. Assessment of the prevalence and risk factors for human immuno-deficiency virus type 1 infection among college students using three survey methods. *Am J Epidemiol* 1991;133:2.

19. Sweeney P, Lindegren M, Buehler JW, Onorato IM, Janssen RS. Teenagers at risk of human immunodeficiency virus type 1 infection. *Arch Pediatr Adolesc Med* 1995;149:521.

20. Osmond DH, Page K, Wiley J, et al. HIV infection in homosexual and bisexual men 18 to 29 years of age: the San Francisco Young Men's Health Study. *Am J Public Health* 1994;84:1933.

21. Rompalo AM, Roberts PL. Potential value of rectal screening cultures for *Chlamydia trachomatis* in homosexual men. *J Infect Dis* 1986;153:888.

22. Hadler SC, Francis DPL, Maynard JE, et al. Long-term immunogenicity and efficacy of hepatitis B vaccine in homosexual men. *N Engl J Med* 1986;315:209.

23. Centers for Disease Control and Prevention. Hepatitis A among homosexual men: United States, Canada, and Australia. *MMWR Morb Mortal Wkly Rep* 1992;41:161.

24. Council on Scientific Affairs, American Medical Association. Health care needs of gay men and lesbians in the United States. *JAMA* 1996;275:1354.

25. English A. AIDS testing and epidemiology for youth: recommendations of the work group. *Journal of Adolescent Health Care* 1989;10(Suppl):52S.

26. Borhek MV. Helping gay and lesbian adolescents and their families: a mother's perspective. *Journal of Adolescent Health Care* 1988;8:123.

SUGGESTED READING

Alter MJ, Margolis HS. The emergence of hepatitis B as a sexually transmitted disease. *Med Clin North Am;* 1990;74:1529.

Borhek MV. Helping gay and lesbian adolescents and their families: a mother's perspective. *Journal of Adolescent Health Care* 1988;8:123.

Council on Scientific Affairs, American Medical Association. Health care needs of gay men and lesbians in the United States. *JAMA* 1996;275:1354.

Gonsiorek JC. Mental health issues of gay and lesbian adolescents. *Journal of Adolescent Health Care* 1988;8:114.

Friedman RC, Downey JI. Homosexuality. N Engl J Med 1994;331:923.

Povinelli M, Remafedi G, Tao G. Trends and predictors of human immunodeficiency virus antibody testing by homosexual and bisexual adolescent males, 1989–1994. *Arch Pediatr Adolesc Med* 1996;150:33.

Rompalo A. Sexually transmitted causes of gastrointestinal symptoms in homosexual men. *Med Clin North Am* 1990;74:1633.

Remafedi G. Male homosexuality: the adolescent's perspective. *Pediatrics* 1987;79:326.

Remafedi G. Adolescent homosexuality: psychosocial and medical implications. *Pediatrics* 1987;79:331.

Remafedi G. Sexually transmitted diseases in homosexual youth. *Adolescent Medicine: State of the Art Reviews* 1990;1:565.

Remafedi G. Predictors of unprotected intercourse among gay and bisexual adolescents: knowledge, beliefs, and behavior. *Pediatrics* 1994;94:163.

Remafedi G. Cognitive and behavioral adaptations to HIV/AIDS among gay and bisexual adolescents. *J Adolesc Health* 1994;15:142.

Ryan C, Futterman D, eds. Lesbian and gay youth: care and counseling. *Adolesc Medicine: State of the Art Reviews* 1997;8:207.

Savin-Williams RC. Theoretical perspectives accounting for adolescent homosexuality. *Journal of Adolescent Health Care* 1988;8:95.

Troiden RR. Homosexual identity development. *Journal of Adolescent Health Care* 1988;8:105.

6

Adolescent Sports Medicine

More than 20 million children and adolescents between the ages of 8 and 16 years participate in youth sports (i.e., nonscholastic, organized sports activities), and more than 3.5 million boys and 2 million girls are involved in a wide variety of high school sports [1,2]. Clearly, our nation's youth are predominantly a physically active population. This chapter attempts to give the reader a comprehensive overview of the place of sports in the lives of adolescents and a set of guidelines for helping teenagers participate in sports activities in the most healthful manner possible. Why do adolescents participate in sports activities? Six primary reasons can be identified:

1. *To attain self-confidence and a feeling of personal satisfaction.* Adolescence is a time of life when personal doubts can be pervasive and feelings of confidence and self-control can be low. Achievement in sports activities may be the sole way, or one of several ways, in which adolescents can overcome these feelings of inadequacy.
2. *To combat boredom.* Young adolescents, in particular, cannot yet participate in more adult activities, such as driving a car or going out by themselves with friends. Sports activities can fill this gap.
3. *To socialize.* Venues in which sports activities occur are generally viewed by adults as conducive to wholesome entertainment for youngsters. Here, they can be safe from the dangers of the streets, such as involvement with drugs and other risk-taking behaviors. With some exceptions (which are discussed later), this is true. Sports can help adolescents further life goals both in general terms (e.g., becoming personally competent and learning to work with a group) and in personal terms (e.g., gaining self-control and individual achievement).
4. *To satisfy peer and parental pressure.*
5. *To participate in socially acceptable risk-taking behavior.*
6. *To have fun.* Participation in sports and other physical activities just plain feels good, and many adolescents feel better when they are fit.

How, then, can clinicians help adolescents to participate in sports and fitness activities successfully? First, we must provide the adolescent with a proper preparticipation evaluation. Then we should help him or her select an effective conditioning program and advise the patient about injury prevention. Next, we must advise the adolescent to participate in activities in which he or she can participate for life. Finally, we should become involved as consultants, educators, and team physicians. With so many adolescents active in scholastic and nonschool sports, and with the understanding that those who are not physically active should be, there is a large component of the primary care clinician's practice that can be directly or indirectly involved with sports health. Mastering the facts and becoming comfortable with the principles of sports health for adolescents is obligatory for any physician who cares for adolescents.

Preparticipation Evaluation

Much has been written about the preparticipation evaluation for sports [2–8]. This evaluation is accepted universally for youths who wish to participate in scholastic sports and is highly recommended for youngsters who wish to become involved in nonscholastic sports and fitness activities. The goals of the preparticipation evaluation include assessing the overall health of the adolescent, detecting conditions that might eliminate the teenager from participation, taking anthropometric measurements, determining the adolescent's fitness for the specific sport in question (which includes an assessment of maturation), and providing an opportunity for counseling and education. In adolescents, who may see a physician only when a sports examination is needed, this evaluation can also serve as an entryway into other areas of the adolescent's health [9].

The preparticipation examination has a variable rate of detecting conditions that may disqualify a youth from participation. The rates of various studies are listed in Table 1. Almost as important as detecting potentially disqualifying conditions is the detection of other conditions that need medical attention but that are not serious enough to disqualify a youth from participation. Three studies have shown rates of detection of such conditions in 17% to 62% adolescents being evaluated [10–12].

Three basic types of evaluation have been described: an examination by the personal physician, the "station" (or multiple examiner) type of evaluation, and the "locker room" evaluation. The latter type is the least desirable because it can be cursory, with little done except screening for obvious conditions that would disqualify a youth from participation. A preparticipation evaluation by the youth's personal physician has the benefit of being performed by a practitioner who presumably knows the youth well; therefore, the evaluation can be part of the ongoing health care of the adolescent. However, the personal physician may not be well versed in the essentials of a sports evaluation, such as risks associated with certain types of sports and the factors that might predispose a youth to certain types of injury. Consequently, certain parts of the preparticipation evaluation may be inadequately performed.

The multiple examiner, or station, evaluation has been shown to be the best way to detect conditions that either need further evaluation or will disqualify a youth from participating in a certain sport [2,8]. In this type of evaluation, athletes are examined in a single setting by several examiners. The evaluation is sports oriented and is performed by evaluators who are interested in sports medicine and who are aware of the risks of athletic participation. The station examination may also use examiners who are subspecialists and who might not participate in another type of evaluation.

Medical History

In the station evaluation, the first station should be one where the medical history is reviewed. The medical history is the most important part of the screening process. Obtaining the history can be facilitated by using preprinted check-off forms that can be sent to the youths before the evaluation. The adolescent brings the form to the evaluation, and the information on it is reviewed with the youth by the examiner. If records from the personal physician would be needed for clarification of an historic item, the youth would have been directed to bring them along as well. Important points that need to be covered include conditions that might limit the youth's ability to participate, such as asthma or a

TABLE 1. *Effectiveness of athletic examinations in identifying athletes who should be disqualified from participation*

Study	N	True-positive rate	False-positive rate
Goldberg et al	701	12.8/1,000	79.5/1,000[a]
Linder et al	1,268	1.6/1,000	50.5/1,000
Tennant et al	2,719	Unknown	11.8/1,000[b]
Thompson et al	2,670	Unknown	11.6/1,000[b]
McKeag	989	11/1,000	89/1,000
DuRant et al			
Station examination	752	4.0/1,000	59.8/1,000
Single-provider	170	0/1,000	23.5/1,000
Risser et al	2,114	2.8/1,000	30.7/1,000

[a]These exclude a number of adolescents who had asymptomatic bacteriuria.

[b]In these two studies, the numbers of athletes referred for further evaluation and subsequently disqualified were not given. The false-positive rates, therefore, represent a maximum possible figure.

From American Medical Association. Athletic preparticipation examinations for adolescents. From the Group on Science and Technology. Report of the Board of Trustees. *Arch Pediatr Adolesc Med* 1994;148:93. Used with permission, "copyright 1994–95, American Medical Association."

seizure disorder. Here, factors that could indicate a risk for sudden death, such as a history of syncope with exercise or a family history of sudden death, can be reviewed. A history of previous injuries and subsequent rehabilitation is elicited as well.

Anthropometric Assessment

The next station can be the one in which anthropometric measurements are taken. Here, height, weight, triceps skinfold thickness, and blood pressure are measured. Tanner stage can be assessed here as well. If it is not possible to assess Tanner stage directly, pictures of various stages should be available for the youth to look at so that he or she can perform a self-assessment. Such self-assessments have been shown to be fairly accurate, although they are less desirable than direct observation by a clinician [13]. The value of measuring height and weight is obvious. These measurements should be plotted on a growth chart.

Maturation assessment is especially important in sports in which heavy contact and collision is common (Table 2). It is also important for counseling purposes, such as when a girl is interested in gymnastics, a sport in which less mature participants seem to have a competitive advantage, and when a less than fully mature boy is interested in baseball but is at risk for elbow problems if he is allowed to throw curve balls. In New York State, there is a Selection Classification Age Maturity Program in the public schools in which physical maturity is used to match athletes for competition. When the five criteria used for matching—type of sport selected; level of competition; degree of agility, endurance, strength and speed; proficiency in the sport; and a physical examination, including level of physical maturity—are used to match athletes, the number of injuries is reduced significantly [14].

Measurement of skinfold thickness is crucial in evaluating a youth's percentage of body fat as well as in providing a baseline for youths who wish to lose weight for competition. Blood pressure is of obvious importance for detection of hypertension. Clinicians should be cautioned to have blood pressure cuffs of various sizes available, whether the examination is done in stations or at a private physician's office.

TABLE 2. *Classification of sports*

Contact/ collision	Contact/impact	Noncontact		
		Strenuous	Moderately strenuous	Nonstrenuous
Boxing	Baseball	Aerobic dancing	Badminton	Archery
Field hockey	Basketball	Crew	Curling	Golf
Football	Bicycling	Fencing	Table tennis	Riflery
Ice hockey	Diving	Field events		
Lacrosse	Field events	Discus		
Martial arts	High jump	Javelin		
Rodeo	Pole vault	Shot put		
Soccer	Gymnastics	Running		
Wrestling	Horseback riding	Swimming		
	Skating	Tennis		
	Ice	Track		
	Roller	Weight lifting		
	Skiing			
	Cross-country			
	Downhill			
	Water			
	Softball			
	Squash, handball			
	Volleyball			

Reproduced with permission from the Committee on Sports Medicine. Recommendations for participation in competitive sports. *Pediatrics* 1988;81:737.

Limited Physical Examination

The next station usually is the one for physical examination of paired organs, the cardiovascular system, and the musculoskeletal system. *A complete physical examination is not indicated at a sports preparticipation evaluation.* Particular attention should be paid to the detection of heart murmurs, clicks, or arrhythmias. Heart murmurs are especially important if they worsen with mild exercise. Therefore, any young athlete who has either a murmur, a history of syncope or dyspnea with exercise, or a family history of sudden death in a close relative younger than 40 years of age should be examined after exercising. Having the youngster do jumping jacks, run in place, or step up and down one step for 10 minutes to raise the heart rate to 120 beats per minute is sufficient to accentuate a murmur due to hypertrophic cardiomyopathy [15], the most common cause of sudden death in young athletes when such a murmur is present [16]. Auscultating adolescents while they squat also is valuable to accentuate a mitral regurgitation murmur, which may be indicative of hypertrophic cardiomyopathy. Although sudden death is decidedly uncommon in this group [17], it is the catastrophe that clinicians should attempt to avoid above all others. Figure 1 shows the causes of sudden cardiac arrest in young competitive athletes. Other causes of sudden death in athletes, all considerably less common than even hypertrophic cardiomyopathy, include cystic medial necrosis of the aorta leading to rupture of the aorta (Marfan's syndrome), congenital anomalous coronary arteries, and prolonged QT syndrome and other arrhythmias [18]. Of these disorders, cystic medial necrosis is worth mentioning because of its association with Marfan's syndrome.

The diagnosis of Marfan's syndrome in adolescents is, for several reasons, more difficult than one might suspect. First, the final bodily proportions that characterize Marfan's syndrome may not be readily apparent until the end of physical development. Second, all tall and thin athletes do not have Marfan's syndrome. The at-risk athletes whom the evaluating clinician should be seeking are those who are tall and hyperextensible and who have lower body segments that are disproportionately long compared

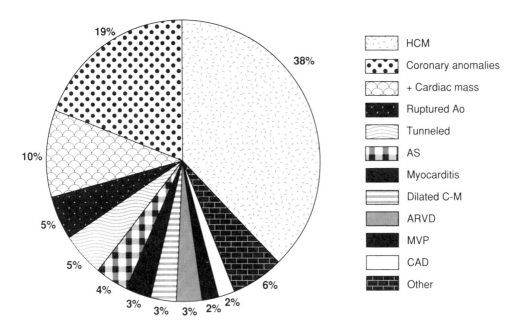

FIG. 1. Causes of sudden cardiac death in young competitive athletes (median age, 17 years), based on systematic tracking of 158 athletes in the United States, primarily from 1985 to 1995. Ao, aorta; LAD, left anterior descending coronary artery; AS, aortic ventricular dysplasia; MVP, mitral valve prolapse; CAD, coronary artery disease; HCM, hypertrophic cardiomyopathy; ↑, increased. (Maron BJ, Thompson PD, Puffer JC, et al. Cardiovascular preparticipation screening of competitive athletes. *Circulation* 1996;94:850, with permission.)

with the upper body segments. If there is a family history suggestive of the condition or other stigmata such as a history of ocular lens dislocation, then referral for genetic and cardiac evaluation is indicated [19]. Table 3 gives another classification of sports more oriented to cardiovascular risk.

Problems with paired organs are unusual. When they are identified, referral is necessary only if this is a new finding; if there is a long-established and fixed deficiency, only counseling about which sports may cause the least risk of further damage may be needed.

In terms of prevention of the most common health problems of young athletes, evaluation of the musculoskeletal system is the most important part of the physical examination. No other system is subjected to more injuries in young athletes [20–22]. Boys incur most of these injuries, primarily in football [2,23,24]. When contact sports are eliminated from consideration, injuries are comparable among boys and girls (Table 4).

Assessment of physical maturation may not be as important as was once believed for identifying youths at higher risk for epiphyseal injury. There are no conclusive data that open epiphyses lead to increased risk of skeletal injury [25]. In fact, there are data to the contrary [26]. Screening for Tanner stage *is* important, however, because there is evidence that, during the period of peak height velocity (the growth spurt) and immediately thereafter, the young athlete is at increased risk for strains, sprains, and overuse injuries [27]. This may be a consequence of stretching of the musculotendinous unit by rapid growth of the long bones, which may lead to decreased flexibility.

TABLE 3. *Classification of sports (based on peak dynamic and static components during competition)*

	A. Low dynamic	B. Moderate dynamic	C. High dynamic
I. Low static	Billiards Bowling Cricket Curling Golf Riflery	Baseball Softball Table tennis Tennis (doubles) Volleyball	Badminton Cross-country skiing (classic technique) Field hockey[a] Orienteering Race walking Racquetball Running (long distance) Soccer[a] Squash Tennis (singles)
II. Moderate static	Archery Auto racing[a,b] Diving[a,b] Equestrian[a,b] Motorcycling[a,b]	Fencing Field events (jumping) Figure skating[a] Football (American)[a] Rodeoing[a,b] Rugby[a] Running (sprint) Surfing[a,b] Synchronized swimming[b]	Basketball[a] Ice hockey[a] Cross-country skiing (skating technique) Football (Australian rules)[a] Lacrosse[a] Running (middle distance) Swimming Team handball
III. High static	Bobsledding[a,b] Field events (throwing) Gymnastics[a,b] Karate/judo[a] Luge[a,b] Sailing Rock climbing[a,b] Waterskiing[a,b] Weight lifting[a,b] Windsurfing[a,b]	Body building[a,b] Downhill skiing[a,b] Wrestling[a]	Boxing[a] Canoeing/kayaking Cycling[a,b] Decathlon Rowing Speed skating

[a]Danger of bodily collision.
[b]Increased risk if syncope occurs.
From Mitchell JH, Haskell WL, Raven PB. Classification of sports. *J Am Coll Cardiol* 1994;24:864, with permission.

TABLE 4. *Injuries in boys' and girls' sports*

Sport	Boys		Girls	
	No. of participants	Injury rate/ 1,000	No. of participants	Injury rate/ 1,000
Track	1,682	16.6	1,141	7.0
Cross-country running	389	23.1	187	0.0
Swimming	233	4.2	165	30.3
Tennis	430	0.0	457	6.6
Volleyball	19	0.0	429	4.0
Soccer	118	8.5	50	20.0
Basketball	1,638	59.8	1,605	65.4
Baseball, softball	1,969	14.2	773	11.6
Total	6,478	25.4	4,807	27.7

From Shively RA, Hodgson JL, Kwiterovich PO, et al. High school sports injuries. *Phys Sports Med* 1981;9:46.

The risk factors for musculoskeletal injuries for which a youth may be screened include body type, ligamentous laxity or flexibility, muscle strength, inadequate rehabilitation from previous injury, and skeletal anomalies and malalignment [28] (Table 5). Heavier adolescents experience more injuries in youth football [29]. Certain body builds seem to be at greater risk for injury in gymnastics.

Flexibility is another significant factor in assessing risk of injury in the young athlete. Stretching tight musculotendinous units before exercise can prevent injuries [30,31]. On the other hand, total body laxity can also lead to increased incidence of injury [30]. It may be that injury does not depend on flexibility, although this might be a reflection of which sports are considered and how well conditioned, in general, the particular athletes are.

Muscle strength is also important in discerning those athletes at increased risk for injury. Increasing neck muscle strength decreases risk of injury in football players [32]. Weak and dysplastic quadriceps muscles, especially the vastus medialis, can lead to increased incidence of patellofemoral disorders [33], which can be alleviated, to some degree, by strengthening the extensor muscles of the legs.

TABLE 5. *The 90-second orthopedic screening examination*

Instruction to athlete	Area to observe
Stand facing examiner	Acromioclavicular joints; general habitus
Look at ceiling, floor, over both shoulders; touch shoulder to ears	Cervical spine motion
Shrug shoulders (examiner provides resistance)	Trapezius muscle strength
Abduct shoulders 90°(examiner provides resistance at 90°)	Deltoid muscle strength
Fully rotate arms externally	Shoulder motion
Flex and extend elbows	Elbow motion
With arms at sides and elbows flexed 90°, pronate and supinate wrists	Elbow and wrist motion
Spread fingers; make fist	Hand and finger motion and deformity
Tighten and relax quadriceps muscles	Symmetry and knee effusion; ankle effusion
"Duck walk" (buttocks on heels) four steps away from examiner	Hip, knee, and ankle motion
Duck walk back to examiner	Shoulder symmetry; scoliosis
With knees straight, touch toes	Scoliosis, hip motion, hamstring tightness
Raise up on toes, raise heels	Calf symmetry, leg strength

Adapted, with permission, from American Academy of Pediatrics Committee on Sports Medicine. Preparticipation health evaluation. In: Smith NJ, ed. *Sports medicine: health care for young athletes.* Evanston, IL: American Academy of Pediatrics; 1983:75–92.

Bratton RL, Agerter DC. Preparticipation sports examinations: efficient risk assessment in children and adolescents. *Postgrad Med* 1995;98:123.

Inadequate rehabilitation from previous injury is a major cause of reinjury, and evidence for it should be sought assiduously in the preparticipation evaluation. During the Junior Olympics of 1985, 26% of all injuries occurred at sites of previous injury [34]. A study of 84 basketball players showed that 70% had a history of ankle sprains, and 80% of these had had multiple sprains [35]. In addition to a propensity to reinjure an inadequately rehabilitated site, athletes may also be at risk for injury at a distant site. For example, a pitcher with an inadequately healed leg injury may be at greater risk of an arm injury owing to an alteration in throwing mechanics.

Skeletal malalignment and anomalies are the last category to consider in the preparticipation musculoskeletal evaluation of the young athlete. Anomalies such as a cervical rib can lead to arm pain and wasting of the hand muscles due to thoracic outlet syndrome. Scoliosis is not an indication for decreased sports participation, but other spinal problems can cause trouble in the young athlete. Atlantoaxial subluxation is present in 10% to 20% of children with Down's syndrome [36–39]. Although no Down's syndrome athlete has had a significant injury related to atlantoaxial subluxation during Special Olympics training or competition [40], the Special Olympics rules include statements restricting those so affected from activities that result in "hyperextension, radical flexion, or direct pressure on the neck and upper spine" [41]. In addition, athletes with a 50% spondylolisthesis (forward displacement of a vertebra) should not participate in vigorous sports because of the risk of further slippage [42]. In ballet dancing, decreased external fibular rotation can lead to overuse syndromes, but foot pronation and increased external tibial torsion can compensate for this somewhat [43]. Patellar problems have been associated with a multitude of malalignment factors (see section on Types of Injuries).

Various sports categories are listed according to intensity, contact, and disqualifying conditions in Tables 2 and 6.

Counseling

The last station in the multiple examiner evaluation (or the last part of the private physician's examination) should be a counseling session with the young athlete and, ideally, with his or her parents. All the findings of the evaluation should be reviewed and put into perspective. Findings that call for further evaluation should be discussed, and reassurance that most findings do not preclude participation should be given. As stated previously, the station examination is the most efficient and productive type of preparticipation evaluation, primarily because private physicians have been found not to do an adequate job. When the private practitioner performs a correct and thorough evaluation, then the optimum is reached, because completeness is combined with continuity of care under the guidance of a clinician who has a personal relationship with the youth and the family. The effectiveness of the preparticipation physical assessment depends to a degree on whether its main purpose is detection of conditions that might disqualify a youth from sports, or to find health problems in adolescents who happen to be athletes. The station examination in better at the former, and the private clinician's examination is better at the latter [2].

Nutrition in Sports

One area with which pediatricians and other clinicians who deal with adolescents should be familiar is nutrition. Proper nutrition is critical in all adolescents and even more so in adolescent athletes. Fortunately, in the United States, nearly all adolescents get adequate amounts of protein, carbohydrates, and fats. By doing so, they also ingest adequate amounts of vitamins. The nutrients that may not be taken in adequate amounts are minerals, especially iron and calcium in young women.

The basics of good nutrition for athletes are the essentials for all adolescents. The food pyramid (Fig. 2) includes a base of cereals and grains augmented by fruits and vegetables, with adequate amounts of animal protein, including dairy products, and a small amount of sweets. The other major item that is critical for athletes is fluids, particularly water.

Water

Water performs three main functions pertinent to exercise: 1) it helps regulate body temperature; 2) it is the transport medium for nutrients, oxygen, and waste in the plasma; and 3) it is a necessary component of biochemical reactions in energy production. Water is lost from the body through urination, evaporation from the respiratory tract during breathing, and perspiration. The greater the intensity and

TABLE 6. *Advisability of participation in competitive sports for children and adolescents with various medical conditions*

Condition	Contact sports		Strenuous	Noncontact sports	
	Significant contact or collision	Limited contact or collision		Moderately strenuous	Nonstrenuous
Acute illness	Depends on specific problem (e.g., contagiosity, risk of worsening disease).				
Asthma	Yes	Yes	Yes	Yes	Yes
Atlantoaxial instability	No	No	Yes, except for butterfly or breast-stroke or diving stars in swimming	Yes	Yes
Carditis	No	No	No	No	No
Congenital heart disease	Patients with mild forms may participate in all sports; those with severe forms or who have undergone recent surgery need individual evaluation.				
Convulsive disorder					
Well controlled	Yes	Yes	Yes	Yes	Yes
Poorly controlled	No	No	Yes; no swimming or weight lifting	Yes	Yes; no archery or riflery
Detached retina	Before any sports activities, consult an ophthalmologist.				
Enlarged liver	No	No	Yes	Yes	Yes
Enlarged spleen	No	No	No	No	No
Function in one eye only	Participation is usually allowed with use of eye guards approved by American Society for Testing materials; individual evaluation is required.				
History of serious head or spine trauma, repeated concussions, or craniotomy	IA	IA	Yes	Yes	Yes
Hypertension					
Mild	Yes	Yes	Yes	Yes	Yes
Moderate/severe	IA	IA	IA	IA	IA
Inguinal hernia	Yes	Yes	Yes	Yes	Yes
Musculoskeletal disorder	IA	IA	IA	IA	IA
Pulmonary insufficiency	Participate if oxygenation remains satisfactory during graded stress test.				
Sickle cell trait	Yes	Yes	Yes	Yes	Yes
Skin disease (boils, herpes, impetigo, scabies)	No gymnastics on mats, martial arts, wrestling, or contact sports if contagious.			Yes	Yes
Solitary kidney	No	Yes	Yes	Yes	Yes
Solitary ovary	Yes	Yes	Yes	Yes	Yes
Testis undescended/absent	Use of protective cup recommended in certain sports.		Yes	Yes	Yes

IA, individual assessment needed.

Adapted from American Academy of Pediatrics Committee on Sports Medicine. Recommendations for participation in competitive sports. *Pediatrics* 1988;81:737.

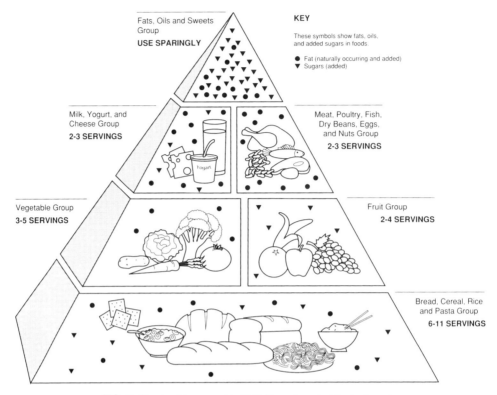

FIG. 2. Food guide pyramid. (U.S. Department of Agriculture.)

duration of the exercise and the higher the environmental temperature, the more water is lost. As much as 1.0 L/m²/hour may be lost through sweating in hot and humid weather with intense exercise [44]. Body weight is the most sensitive indication of water lost and, therefore, of water requirements. For each kilogram of weight lost through exercise, 1 L of water needs to be taken in (or approximately 16 oz for each pound lost). Because athletes are not weighed during competition or practice, water must be supplied prophylactically throughout the activity. The hotter and more humid the conditions in which the activity is performed, the more water is needed. The risk of heat injury increases with the increase in the wet bulb thermometer index, or WBGT index. This calculation takes into account the environmental temperature, the ambient humidity, and the solar radiant energy factor. The formulas and criteria for activities at various levels of the WBGT index are listed in Table 7.

TABLE 7. *WBGT index for outdoor activities*

Range (°F)	Signal flag	Activity
Below 64	None	Unlimited
64–76	Green	Alert for possible increase in index and for symptoms of heat stress
73–81	Yellow	Curtail active exercise for people not acclimatized to heat
82–85.9	Red	Curtail active exercise for all but the well-acclimatized
86+	Black	Stop all training

Note: Runners who are not accustomed to running in the heat must proceed with caution at any temperature.

From Raven PB. Heat stress and athletic performance: medical concerns. *Sports Medicine Digest* 1995;17:1.

Thirst is not a good indicator of water loss, so water should be provided regardless of whether the athlete is thirsty. A loss of 2% to 3% of body weight should dictate cessation of activity until the fluid deficit is restored, because this amount of loss can stress the circulatory system and impair thermoregulation and endurance [45]. It has been argued that rehydration fluids should not be plain water [46,47]. Rather, they should contain less than 2.5 g sugar per 100 ml and should be hypotonic, with an osmolality of 200 mmol/L or less [48]. Most sports drinks (e.g., Gatorade) have excessive carbohydrate concentrations and should be diluted with one to two parts water. Cold fluids are emptied by the stomach more quickly than warm ones [49], and glucose and sodium may enhance fluid absorption by the small intestine [50]. If one has to choose a fluid to be on hand during practice or competition, however, water is as good as anything else and is considerably less expensive. A good prophylactic regimen is to have athletes drink an 8-oz glass of water or dilute fluid every 15 to 20 minutes during activities.

One final caution with respect to water concerns the use of dehydration by athletes who have to meet weight restrictions for a competition such as a wrestling match. Trying to lose a few pounds by losing water is an activity that should be condemned by all clinicians and coaches. The resultant dehydration can be extremely dangerous and will, in fact, reduce performance.

Minerals and Electrolytes

Sodium in the form of salt should not be provided during competition except as part of dilute hydration fluids. The old practice of giving athletes salt tablets is unnecessary and even potentially harmful. Athletes who eat an adequate diet ingest enough sodium to replace any losses from exercise. The only role for extra potassium for athletes may be to limit muscle cramping.

One mineral that may be inadequately supplied in an athlete's typical diet is iron. The U.S. Food and Drug Administration's recommended dietary allowance (RDA) for iron for menstruating girls is 18 mg/day. One study found that female track athletes ingest an average of only 10 mg/day if they are not on iron supplements [51]. That same study showed that female high school athletes are at greater risk for iron deficiency than are nonathletes, particularly if the athletes are black. Athletes who are involved in intense exercise can have impaired iron absorption [52]. Iron deficiency is particularly common in athletes involved in regular, strenuous endurance exercise [53–55]. Menstruating girls are at increased risk for iron deficiency with or without anemia compared with boys. Iron-deficiency anemia can reduce endurance performance [56], and iron deficiency without anemia seems to be related to a reduction in physical work capacity [57,58].

No expert has ever advocated routine iron supplementation in all adolescent female athletes. Nonetheless, given the high prevalence of iron deficiency in teenage girls, as well as their inadequate iron intake, such supplementation with ferrous sulfate and ascorbic acid in a single tablet daily may prevent iron deficiency in female adolescent athletes [59]. No such supplementation is necessary for the typical male athlete.

One added caution is that iron deficiency, with or without anemia, should be expected in any girl who has excessively heavy menstrual periods. Whether laboratory tests such as serum iron, iron-binding capacity, or serum ferritin levels should be drawn in these circumstances is problematic, given the cost of such tests. Hemoglobin and hematocrit determinations are probably cost effective and, therefore, should be obtained routinely for all female athletes.

In general, vitamins are not needed as a supplement because the average American teenager's diet provides all the necessary vitamins.

Proteins, Carbohydrates, and Fats

Proteins, carbohydrates, and fats are, of course, the primary constituents of our diet. Any adolescent eating a well balanced diet with foods from all four major food groups should need no further adjustments or supplementations for any athletic endeavor. A typical athlete's diet should consist of 15% to 20% protein, 55% to 75% carbohydrate, and 10% to 30% fat. The main sources of energy for competition are carbohydrates and fats. Protein is used only at times of caloric deprivation. Normally, fat is the source of energy for activities while at relative rest. Carbohydrate in the form of stored glycogen is used for intense exercise of relatively short duration (primarily anaerobic), whereas fat is used for energy production in lower-intensity exercise of longer duration (aerobic). Prior aerobic training increases the ability of muscle to bring oxygen to energy metabolism, thereby increasing the body's ability to use fat as an energy source [60]. This use of fat is good because it spares carbohydrate resources, and glycogen (the form carbohydrate assumes to be used by muscle) is in limited supply. Therefore, in preparation for endurance events, some athletes resort to glycogen loading in an effort to extend their endurance ability. Glycogen loading involves the depletion of muscle glycogen followed by the consumption of excessive amounts of complex carbohydrates in the few days preceding an athletic competition. This can almost double the amount of glycogen available to muscle [61], but it can be deleterious as well. It can create a feeling of sluggishness, especially considering that it enhances retention of water. Diarrhea has been associated with excessive carbohydrate intake, and this is clearly not a good thing in an endurance event. Physicians should not encourage glycogen loading in adolescent athletes unless the latter are elite athletes who regularly engage in endurance activities of longer than 1 hour's duration.

Protein in the average diet of an adolescent is usually adequate for any athletic endeavor. Protein or amino acid supplements are a waste of money and are potentially harmful. Fats should be ingested in the suggested amounts, but probably should be limited in the pregame meal because they can delay gastric emptying and give a feeling of sluggishness that can last for several hours. A light meal of pasta, vegetables, and fruit is much more advisable just before strenuous activity.

The guiding light of sports nutrition in adolescents should be common sense. A helpful list of Do's and Don'ts as suggested by Primos and Landry [62] is found in Table 8.

TABLE 8. *Do's and don'ts of sports nutrition*

Do's

Do eat a well balanced diet consisting of elements of the four basic food groups. Your diet should include dairy products, cereals and grains, meats and animal products, fruits and vegetables.

Do drink water at regular intervals during exercise.

Do monitor your weight before and after exercise to prevent dehydration.

Do drink 16 oz. of water for each pound of fluid lost through exercise.

Do drink water or beverages with small amounts of simple sugars or glucose polymers and no or small amounts of electrolytes. If you choose a sports drink, such as Gatorade, be sure to dilute it with one or two parts water, as it contains high levels of carbohydrates.

Do follow a goal of achieving a certain percentage of body fat when trying to lose weight. You want to lose body fat, not lean body tissue or water.

Do reduce caloric intake to not less than 1,200 calories for women and 1,500 calories for men per day if you're trying to lose weight.

Do combine increased calories with muscle work (such as weight training) to gain weight.

Do eat a pregame meal at least 2½ hours before competition. The meal should be mostly carbohydrates. You should avoid slowly digested foods such as fats and desserts and those with a great deal of sugar.

Don'ts

Don't return to exercise activity if you've lost more than 3% of your body weight (through fluid loss). Return only after the fluid is restored.

Don't take salt tablets. They are rarely needed and may actually be harmful and increase dehydration.

Don't engage in glycogen loading by consuming large amounts of foods high in carbohydrates (such as breads, cereals, and pasta) unless you are engaging in long endurance exercise that takes more than an hour (marathons, cross-country ski racing).

Don't take amino acids or protein supplements. They are potentially harmful.

Don't take vitamin supplements. They are usually unnecessary and a waste of money, and excessive doses can be harmful. One daily multivitamin is not harmful and would be helpful if you are not eating a well balanced diet.

Don't take mineral supplements unless you have developed a specific deficiency, such as iron.

Don't lose more weight than 1–2 lb per week. Any more weight loss could be water or lean body tissue.

Don't gain more than 1–2 lb per week. Any more weight gain could be body fat.

From Primos WA Jr, Landry GL. Fighting the fads in sports nutrition. *Contemporary Pediatrics* 1989; 6:14.

Issues for Female Athletes

The mass participation of girls in sports is a relatively recent phenomenon that has brought to the forefront the need for physicians and others involved in sports health to be knowledgeable about issues particularly relevant to female athletes. In 1970 and 1971, 294,000 girls were on high school athletic teams; in 1983 and 1984, the number had risen to more than 1,800,000, an increase of more than 600% [63]! Intercollegiate sports were no different. Youth sports (nonscholastic, organized sports activities), once the domain of male Little Leagues, had similar increases in female participation. Instrumental in this explosive increase was Title IX of the Federal Education Act of 1972, which mandated equal athletic facilities for boys and girls. Concomitant societal changes that have enhanced the opportunities for female participation in all areas of life have further facilitated female involvement in sports activities.

Prepubertal boys and girls who are in comparable physical condition are equally capable of participating in all sports activities. The differences that develop with physical maturation can be ascribed to the larger muscle mass of male adolescents and adults. Differences attributable to different physiques (i.e., women having narrower shoulder girdles and wider hips) also limit female participation in certain sports compared with men. Given those differences, however, there are no true limits to the sports activities to which girls can devote themselves successfully. All team sports can also be the purview of teenage girls, with the possible exception of heavy collision sports, and those can be played successfully by girls if proper equipment is used, if participants are matched for strength, and if societal norms are altered.

A study of teenage girls going through preparticipation evaluations showed that girls had fewer physical problems than did boys in the same study [64]. The types of problems that were encountered suggested that girls might benefit from more aerobic and strength training before the sports season. Studies of injury rates among female athletes and their male counterparts showed no greater rate nor seriousness of injury among the girls except for basketball participants. Female basketball players had higher rates of major knee injuries [65,66], which might be attributable to a greater degree of genu valgum (knock knees) in girls and an increased Q angle (Fig. 3). The latter can be produced by a wide pelvis, external tibial torsion, or laterally placed tibial tubercles. This increased Q angle causes the patella to slide laterally with flexion at the knee, increasing the risk of acute and chronic injury [59]. (See further discussion under Injuries to Specific Sites.)

Major concerns for adolescent female athletes are summarized in the concept of the female athlete triad: amenorrhea, osteoporosis, and disordered eating (see also Menstrual Disorders, Chap. 5). All women should adhere to recommended levels of calcium intake (1,200 mg/day). Adolescent female athletes may need that amount of calcium—or more—if they are to mineralize their skeletons effectively and avoid problems in the future. The major portion of the bone mass is acquired by the time a girl reaches 20 years of age [67–69]. Minimal increases of bone mineral density occur later than 2 years postmenarche [70]. Female athletes involved in endurance training who are amenorrheic or oligomenorrheic have inadequate estrogen levels, resulting in decreased calcium absorption and increased calcium excretion [71]. This leads to decreased bone density [72] and an increased risk of skeletal injury. Therefore, female adolescent athletes should be encouraged to consume between 1,200 and 1,500 mg of calcium per day through diet or supplement [73–76].

Another concern vis-à-vis female adolescent athletes is aberrations in menstrual pattern. Several studies have documented that highly conditioned athletes can have delayed menarche and an increase in secondary amenorrhea and oligomenorrhea [77–79]. Reduction in training intensity usually leads to a rapid return to normal menstrual function. Several factors may account for this phenomenon. A decrease in the pulsatility of luteinizing hormone release in heavily training athletes causes an increase in anovulation [80,81]. This may be mediated by elevated levels of enkephalins produced by intense physical activity [59]. Another factor that may predispose young female athletes to delayed menarche is the body habitus of those girls who successfully pursue this intense level of activity. Success comes to those girls in sports in which a thin, willowy, flexible physique is desirable, such as running, gymnastics, or ballet. It may be that girls who are successful and are then urged to excel further in these activities are predisposed to being late maturers, with consequent physiologic delay in achieving menarche. It is known that the later a girl matures, the longer it takes her to achieve regular ovulation.

A good rule of thumb is to evaluate a female adolescent athlete with menstrual dysfunction if no menses have appeared by her 16th birthday. Additional clues for concern are as follows:

- More than 4 years have passed since the first sign of puberty occurred.
- There is no sign of puberty by 13½ years old.

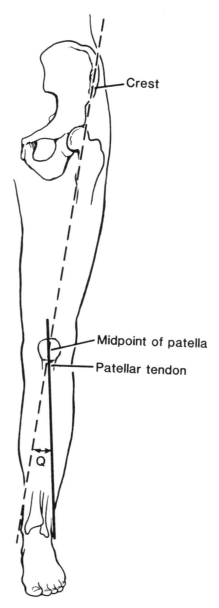

FIG. 3. Q angle. (Adapted from Squire DL. Female athletes. *Pediatr Rev* 1987;9:183.)

- There is oligomenorrhea interspersed with rare but heavy menstrual bleeding.
- Secondary amenorrhea has persisted longer than 6 months.

If relatively simple evaluations are negative, a trial of rest from the girl's activity should be tried to see whether puberty swiftly progresses or regular menstruation rapidly ensues.

A final area of concern that is more prevalent in female adolescents is that of eating disorders, particularly anorexia nervosa. It is well known that girls with anorexia nervosa exercise vigorously in an attempt to get rid of fat that only they perceive. In sports, where vigorous activity is the norm, it should be no surprise to find an increased prevalence of girls with anorectic tendencies. Therefore, weight loss in highly trained athletes should cause as much concern as it does in less active young women.

With attention to these issues, a physician or other clinician should be able to provide adequate nutritional support and guidance to young female athletes.

Types of Injuries

Incidence of Various Injuries

Along with the maintenance and improvement of health, prevention and treatment of injury and rehabilitation after injury are the reasons for the participation of health professionals in sports medicine for children and adolescents. The assessment for injury potential was discussed earlier in this chapter.

Many adolescents are injured in athletic activities each year. The annual estimated number of injuries from sports and recreation in the United States in 1988 was 4,379,000, with over 1.3 million being from serious injuries [82]. From emergency department data, it is estimated that 1.5 million injuries occurred to participants in basketball, football, gymnastics, soccer, volleyball, and wrestling in 1991 [83]. Sports and recreational injuries accounted for significantly more of all the serious injury episodes in the 10- to 13-year-old age group than in other age groups. Boys had more injuries from sports and recreation than did girls [82]. Figure 4 shows the rates of injury by age and gender. Figure 5 shows the types of injuries by age. A study at a large high school showed that 22% of the school's

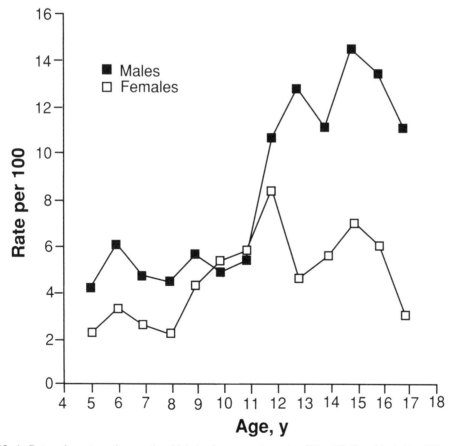

FIG. 4. Rates of sports and recreational injuries by age and gender. (Bijur PE, Trumble A, Harel Y, et al. Sports and recreation injuries in US children and adolescents. *Arch Pediatr Adolesc Med* 1995;149:1009, with permission.)

athletes suffered an injury in 1 year [84]. Football had the highest injury rate (61%), followed by girls' and boys' gymnastics, wrestling, and boys' basketball. In five sports, there were no injuries: boys' tennis, golf, boys' and girls' swimming, and girls' water polo. Girls' track had the greatest number of days lost per injury (320), followed by girls' basketball, girls' cross-country, boys' track, and boys' wrestling. Sprains and strains accounted for 57% of all injuries. Only five athletes required surgery. In a study of Seattle high school athletes, the types and frequency of injuries were comparable when contact sports were eliminated [25]. In a review of injuries from Oklahoma high schools, girls and boys had similar rates of injury [85], but girls experienced a significantly greater number of major injuries. Most injuries were to the lower extremities, with girls having a greater number of knee injuries. Sprains and strains were the most common type of injury [82], the ankle being the area most frequently sprained. Girls suffered more major ankle injuries than boys.

Strains and Sprains

Before specific body regions are considered, we discuss the most common types of injuries: strains and sprains. A muscle *strain* is a partial or complete tear of the musculotendinous unit [86]. Strains are divided into first-, second-, and third-degree strains (Table 9). This type of injury occurs when the muscle undergoes an eccentric lengthening type of contraction (intrinsic pace) to counteract the excessive stretching force applied to the point of injury. Several factors that contribute to the possibility of a muscle strain include inadequate flexibility, inadequate strength or endurance, insufficient warm-up, inadequate rehabilitation from a previous injury, and out-of-phase muscle contractions [87,88]. The weakest structural element and the most likely place for a strain to occur is at the muscle–tendon junction [87,89,90].

Sprains are partial or complete tears of ligamentous tissue. They are graded in the same manner as strains. Evaluation of sprains and strains should take place immediately after the injury, because swelling can obscure the degree of injury. The most common ligaments sprained are those of the ankle.

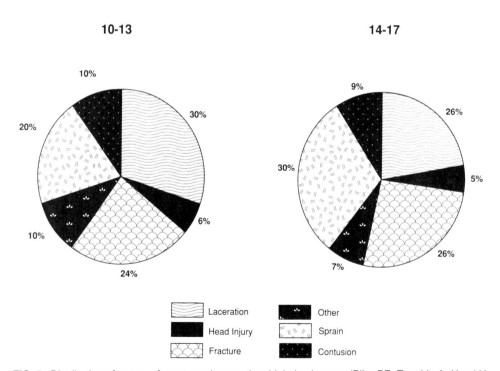

FIG. 5. Distribution of nature of sports and recreational injuries by age. (Bijur PE, Trumble A, Harel Y, et al. Sports and recreation injuries in US children and adolescents. *Arch Pediatr Adolesc Med* 1995; 149:1009, with permission.)

TABLE 9. *Severity of strains and sprains*

Grade	Description
1	Mild: little tissue disruption with minimal loss of function
2	Moderate: moderate tissue disruption with partial loss of function
3	Severe: complete or nearly complete tissue disruption with marked or complete loss of function

Adapted from Dyment PG. Athletic injuries. *Pediatr Rev* 1989;10:291.

Assigning a Degree of Injury

All sprains and strains should be considered serious until they are fully evaluated and a degree of injury is assigned. A first-degree sprain can be treated acutely with ice and compression and, if no decrease in function is apparent, the participant can soon return to play [7]. If swelling occurs immediately and if there is apparent decrease in function, a second-degree injury must be assumed, and participation must be forbidden until painless function with preinjury strength has returned. An abnormal increase in the range of motion at the site of a ligament or musculotendinous junction signals a third-degree sprain or strain (i.e., a complete rupture), and evaluation by an orthopedist is mandatory. When stressing the injury site to assess degree of injury, care should be taken not to apply too much force because of the possibility of exacerbating a growth plate injury at that site.

Treatment

The classic treatment regimen for strains and sprains is *rest, ice, compression*, and *elevation* (RICE) [91]. Because athletes may ignore the simple suggestion to rest the affected area, it may be necessary to insist, in the case of leg injuries, that the athlete use crutches to avoid weight bearing. It also is useful to use the concept of "relative rest" when prescribing return-to-play guidelines [92]. Relative rest is described in Table 10. During the rehabilitative period, and athlete is permitted to resume activities of daily living unless pain or swelling occur or worsen during the activity or within the ensuing 24 hours. *Rest should be mandatory* for first- and second-degree injuries for 2 or 3 days. If, after this period, there is residual pain, swelling, or tenderness, rehabilitative exercises should be prescribed, because prolonged disuse produces atrophy and consequent weakening of the muscles that help stabilize the joint, or of the affected muscles themselves, which sets the stage for reinjury [93]. For specific rehabilitation regimens, the primary care clinician should consult with an orthopedist or an athletic

TABLE 10. *Relative rest and return to play*

Skeletally immature (prepubertal and early pubertal) adolescent athletes should not play or exercise if there is pain or swelling during or after activity.
- Discuss pain thresholds and pain-free movement as they apply to rehabilitation.
- Explain that normal activities are allowed if they cause no pain at any time within the next 24 hours.
- Address pain-free alternatives to maintain strength and improve flexibility.

When an athlete fails to improve in a rehabilitative program, one of the three explanations is likely:
- The diagnosis is incorrect
- The patient is not compliant with the rehabilitation or is not practicing relative rest
- The rehabilitation program is not appropriate

In rare instances, a mature, older adolescent at an advanced level of competition may be permitted to practice and return to play during rehabilitation. This is an exception to the rule, and assumes that the following conditions have been met:
- The diagnosis is correct
- The athlete has complied with an appropriate rehabilitative program, and shown progress toward recovery
- A sports medicine or orthopedic specialist has been consulted, if possible

From Hergenroeder AC. Acute shoulder, knee, and ankle injuries: Part 2. rehabilitation. *Adolescent Health Update* 1996;8:1, with permission.

trainer for details, depending on the site and severity of the injury. General principles of rehabilitation of musculoskeletal injuries are listed in Table 11.

The second treatment method is the application of *cold* to the injured site. Effective use of cryotherapy has been shown to decrease the recovery time for injuries such as sprains [94]. Chipped ice is the most effective source of cold, and this can be applied in disposable plastic bags. The cold packs should be applied intermittently for the first 48 hours after injury for 20 to 30 minutes per session, three to four times daily.

Compression by an elastic bandage should be used because it assists in minimizing the amount of edema. The bandage should be worn for a minimum of several days. Edema is deleterious for at least

---

TABLE 11. *General principles in rehabilitation of musculoskeletal trauma*

Phase I: Limit further injury; control pain and swelling
    The first priorities are protection, rest, and support for the injured area. Wraps, splints, crutches, and slings are commonly used for this purpose. An initial treatment regimen that follows the RICE protocol should limit further damage.

• Icing begins immediately postinjury. The ice (crushed ice is preferable) should be put in a plastic bag and applied directly to the skin for 20 minutes at a time.
• More frequent applications are more effective. The injury should be iced three to four times daily while swelling persists.
• Some discomfort is to be expected in the first 3 to 4 minutes after ice is applied. Numbness will follow.
• Effective cooling will occur over the next 10 to 15 minutes *if the ice is kept in place.* Effective cooling will not occur if the ice is removed when discomfort occurs, then replaced in a minute or two.

    For injuries with rapid swelling and moderate to severe pain, consider modalities such as transcutaneous electrical nerve stimulation. This is ordinarily applied by a physical therapist or athletic trainer.

Phase II: Measures to improve strength and range of motion
    Immediate postinjury rehabilitation exercises are designed to improve both strength and flexibility without causing further damage. These exercises can begin as early as the day of the injury, if they are not associated with increased pain.
    Instruct the athlete to maneuver the injured structures within the pain-free range of motion. Pain and swelling may severely limit flexibility in the first days after injury. Isometric muscle contractions, which generate force but do not move the joint, can help to maintain strength in the injured area.
    It is important to provide adequate analgesia in appropriate dosages. Pain inhibits full muscular contraction and delays recovery. For oral analgesia, start with acetaminophen or nonsteroidal antiinflammatory drugs. Maintenance of strength, flexibility, and endurance will be compromised if persistent pain inhibits muscle use over days to weeks.
    As pain and swelling are reduced, and rehabilitation exercises are begun, strength and range of motion improve. Protective devices can be removed when the patient's strength and flexibility improve sufficiently.

Phase III: Achieve near-normal strength and range of motion
    The third phase focuses on a return to near-normal strength and range of motion. This applies to the injured extremity, and the rest of the body as well. Encourage the athlete to maintain cardiovascular fitness and other-extremity strength and flexibility while the injured joint is rehabilitated. Swimming, water jogging, and cycling on a stationary bike can increase cardiovascular fitness without disturbing the injured extremity, which can be rested or exercised, as comfort allows.

Phase IV: Return to the preinjury level of activity without pain, swelling, or compromised range of motion
    In the final phase, the athlete transitions from exercises intended to improve strength and range of motion to functional rehabilitation. The athlete can begin sports-specific activities once near-normal strength and flexibility have returned. Full range of motion and strength do not imply a safe return to play without some transition into the sport.

RICE, rest, ice, compression, and elevation.
From Hergenroeder AC. Acute shoulder, knee, and ankle injuries: Part 2. rehabilitation. *Adolescent Health Update* 1996;8:1, with permission.

three reasons: 1) it may act as an insulator, keeping cold therapy from reaching deeper tissues; 2) it can mechanically decrease range of motion, thereby decreasing the effectiveness of rehabilitation exercises; and 3) it can keep ruptured ligament fibers apart, thereby promoting fibrous scarring rather than ligament-to-ligament regrowth [93]. Consistent compression is most difficult to apply around the ankle. This can be accomplished by padding the hollow between the malleoli and the Achilles tendon with felt pads or layered disposable diapers, cut into horseshoe shape and placed around and inferior to the malleolus. This is then covered with an elastic bandage.

Elevation can reduce edema, especially if the injured part can be raised at least to the level of the heart.

Alleviation of pain is a consistent goal of injury treatment. Acetaminophen or nonsteroidal antiinflammatory drugs (NSAIDs) are the analgesics of choice.

Injuries to Specific Sites

Our discussion now turns to injuries to specific anatomic sites, their assessment, and treatment. This description of injuries is not exhaustive, but emphasizes the most common injuries.

Knee Injuries

As stated earlier, injuries to the knee occur very frequently in athletic activities. They are most common in football. During each week of the football season, it is estimated that 6,000 high school and college players injure their knees, and 10% of these injuries require surgery [93]. The most frequent injuries of significance are ligamentous injuries, meniscal (cartilage) injuries, and injuries involving the patellofemoral structures.

Ligamentous Injuries

Ligamentous injuries occur when there is excessive rotatory, medial, or lateral force applied to the knee. The most common ligaments affected are the medial collateral and anterior cruciate ligaments (Fig. 6). The medial collateral ligament is usually injured when there is a direct blow to the lateral aspect of the knee. The resulting medial stress can cause a first-, second-, or third-degree sprain. Because medial knee pain is felt at the time of injury, the knee may feel unstable when the player gets up and walks. Pain over the ligament or separation of the medial aspect of the joint when the abductor stress test is performed indicates a high probability that this structure is injured. A medial opening of more than 1 cm with the abductor stress test indicates possible damage to the anterior and posterior cruciate ligaments as well. If the knee is stable in extension but opens in 30° of flexion, rotatory instability should also be considered [95].

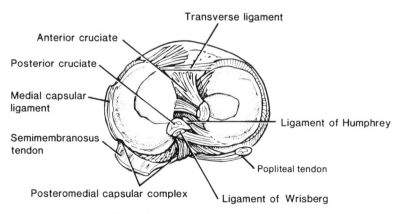

FIG. 6. Anatomic structures of the knee.

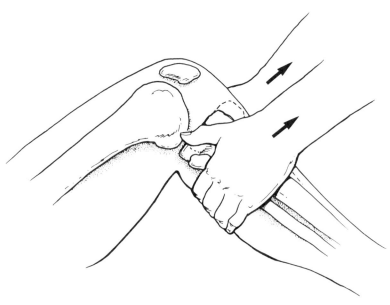

FIG. 7. The anterior drawer test.

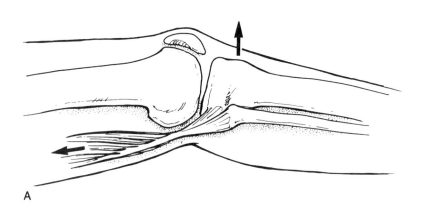

A

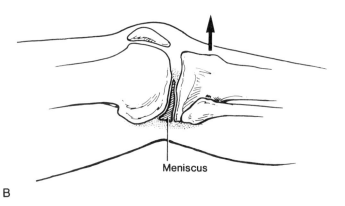

Meniscus

B

FIG. 8. False-negative anterior drawer tests due to hamstring muscles opposing pull on tibia **(A)** or restriction by meniscus **(B)**.

The anterior cruciate ligament is the most common site of severe injury to the knee [93]. The injury usually occurs when the athlete is running and changes direction. A pop may be felt and the player falls and is unable to continue playing. An anterior drawer test with the knee in 90° of flexion and with the knee in 15° to 30° of flexion—the Lachman test—should be performed as soon after the injury as possible because a bloody effusion will accumulate over the next 24 hours, making it difficult to assess the type or degree of injury. If the tibia moves anteriorly on the femur, an anterior cruciate tear has occurred. Lateral collateral and posterior cruciate ligament injuries do occur, but they are decidedly less common than those just mentioned. Various tests for assessment of ligamentous integrity are illustrated in Figures 7 through 14.

Meniscal Injuries

Injuries to the cartilage in the knee may occur after a twisting impact, hyperflexion, or hyperextension. The medial meniscus is attached to the medial collateral ligament and is frequently damaged along with that ligament when a tackle hits the lateral side of the knee and produces external rotation of the tibia, stretching the medial collateral ligament and rupturing the medial meniscus. Examination reveals tenderness over the medial or lateral joint line, pain at the medial or lateral joint line with hyperextension or hyperflexion of the knee, and pain with external tibial rotation when the knee is flexed to 90°. Internal rotation produces pain with a lateral meniscus injury. Often, the examiner can feel a grating or crunch with fingers at the joint line when rotating the tibia in these maneuvers.

For either ligamentous or meniscal injuries, when it appears that significant rupture has occurred, the primary practitioner should refer to orthopedic colleagues. RICE should be used until such consultation can be obtained.

Patellofemoral Disorders

The third most frequent knee problems are patellofemoral disorders. These are more often due to abnormal anatomy and overuse than to injuries [96]. A 1981 study looked at athletes who complained

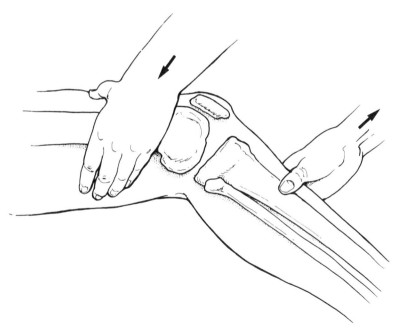

FIG. 9. The Lachman test.

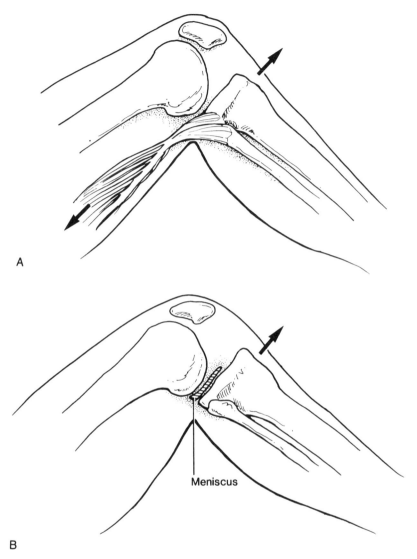

FIG. 10. Slight flexion of knee relieves resistance by hamstrings **(A)** or meniscus **(B)**.

of anterior knee pain or patellar instability [32]. The athletes could be classified into three fairly distinct groups:

1. Those who complained of frank dislocation. These athletes exhibited vastus medialis deficiency and infrapatellar fat pad enlargement and had increased general ligamentous laxity, increased patellar mobility, and out-facing patellae with subsequent decreased Q angles in chronic cases.
2. Patients who complained of classic knee pain consistent with chondromalacia patellae and who had no swelling. These patients had normal ligamentous laxity and patellar mobility, more in-facing patellae, and normal Q angles.
3. Patients with pain and swelling who had findings somewhere between the other two groups. They generally fit into the group with what is commonly called *subluxation of the patella*. They had

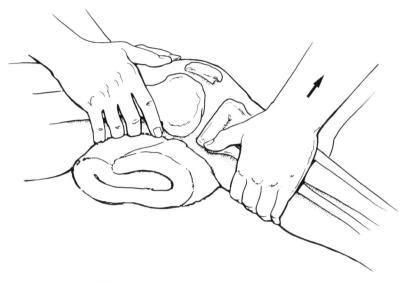

FIG. 11. Modified Lachman test (patient supine).

normal ligamentous tone, increased patellar mobility, and normal Q angle, but more in-facing patellae and fat pad enlargement.

Most adolescents with these syndromes fall into the first group, known better as patellofemoral pain syndrome, or PFS [96]. The symptoms of the primary pathologic process result in relative disuse with secondary loss of quadriceps muscle strength. From a practical viewpoint, PFS can be viewed as a tracking disorder of the patella that often occurs secondary to a weakness of the vastus medialis, which is incapable of maintaining normal patellar alignment through the whole range of motion [97].

Symptoms of PFS are usually vague and start insidiously. Actually, the vagueness of the pain is a good differentiating clue from the acute pain of a meniscal tear. The pain is usually related to activity, and aching usually occurs from prolonged sitting with the knees flexed. It is difficult for patients with this problem to pinpoint exactly the location of their pain. The consequent swelling, decreased range of motion, and feeling of instability usually occurs fairly late in the course of the condition. Although patients complain frequently of their knees "locking," this is not true total immobility but actually a stiffening or "gelling" from prolonged flexion that resolves slowly with repeated flexion and extension.

Depending on the length of time that symptoms have been present, the most dramatic finding on physical examination may be relative atrophy of the vastus medialis. Contracting the muscle may reveal what appears to be a normal muscle mass, but palpation reveals a soft, ineffective muscle. The presence of an effusion is relatively common and is of little diagnostic value. Patellofemoral crepitation is also innocuous, occurring as it does in affected and unaffected knees alike. Obviously, a complete knee examination should be performed. Radiographs are of little assistance and should not be performed unless there is a high index of suspicion of other pathologic processes. The different characteristics of the three causes of anterior knee pain mentioned previously are listed in Table 12.

To correct this chronic problem, the patient must be actively involved. He or she must not only be taught to do the therapeutic exercises but must be convinced of their value. Controlling the symptoms and strengthening the vastus, the primary objectives of treatment, can often be accomplished without major intrusion into the patient's athletic activities. These patients know that total rest will alleviate their symptoms, but they want relief while still remaining active. The object is to maintain the highest level of activity without pain. To that end, the clinician may prescribe a Neoprene sleeve with a lateral pad. Patients who cannot perform their activity without pain can be put in a knee immobilizer for a week at the commencement of their quadriceps-strengthening regimen.

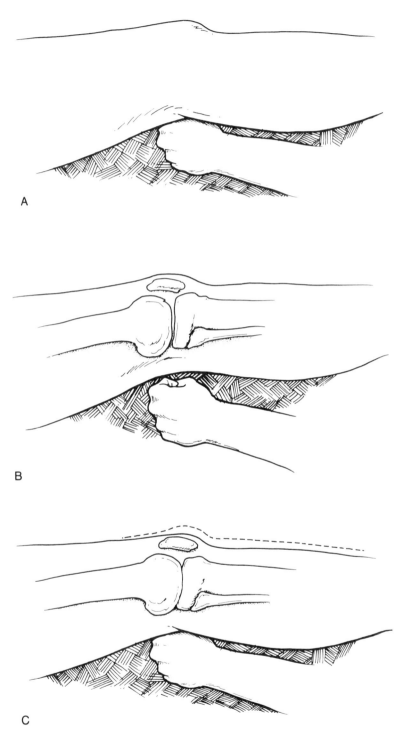

FIG. 12. Dynamic extension test.

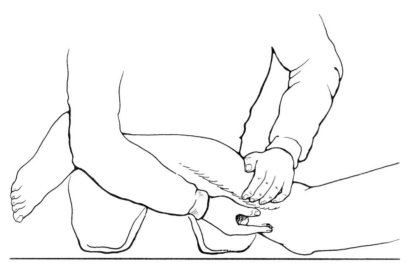

FIG. 13. Alternate Lachman test.

It is primarily the vastus medialis that must be strengthened. Isometric exercises (quad settings) work best [97]. For these, the legs are fully extended and the patient is instructed to pull the kneecap toward the waist as hard as possible, hold it for 5 to 6 seconds, and then relax. Four contractions are done 15 to 20 times daily. It is best to associate these with some other activity, such as at the end of each television commercial when viewing, or after each period at school. The patient should be told to feel the vastus medialis while performing this exercise to ensure that he or she is contracting the correct muscle. Straight leg raises and terminal arc extensions also are recommended [96]. Once this strengthening regimen is well under way, rehabilitation for any hamstring weakness or tightness or quadriceps tightness should begin. As the symptoms decrease, the patient should slowly increase the level of activity until it reaches optimum. Setting up a specific timetable for return to full activity is

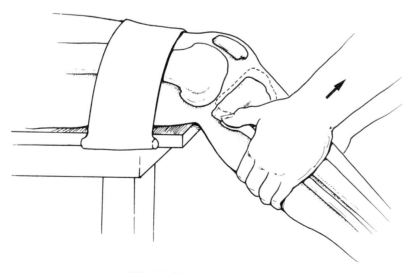

FIG. 14. Femur stabilization test.

TABLE 12. *Differential diagnosis of patellofemoral pain syndrome*

Disorder	Presentation	Physical examination	Radiographs	Pathophysiology
Patellofemoral pain syndrome	Younger patients Related to overuse Insidious onset Retropatellar or peripatellar knee pain	Pain at patellar facets or retinacula Malalignment may be present Pain with compression of the patella against the femoral condyles	Usually normal	Repetitive trauma of the subchondreal bone of the patella against the femur Retinacular strain and inflammation
Chondromalacia patellae	Older patients Chronic anterior knee pain Pain worse on walking up or down stairs	Pain at patellar facets Malalignment usually present Crepitation Recurrent effusions common	Early radiographs are normal[a] Late radiographs show patellar thinning or lateral displacement of the patella	Softening, then fissures, then erosion of the articular cartilage of the patella
Patellar subluxation	Initial episode usually traumatic Subsequent episodes result in acute exacerbation Instability with pivoting ("giving way")	Severe knee pain and effusion after initial injury or subsequent exacerbation Patient becomes apprehensive when lateral displacement of the patella is attempted	Axial radiographs show lateral displacement of the patella	Laxity of medial retinaculum Lateral patellar trauma against femoral condyles

[a]Patellar pathology visible only on direct visualization (e.g., via arthroscopy).
From Davidson K. Patellofemoral pain syndrome. *Am Fam Physician* 1993;48:1254, with permission.

important to give the patient concrete goals at which to aim. Failure to improve after 2 or 3 months should prompt an investigation into other possible etiologies.

Another common cause of knee pain in the adolescent, especially a boy who is at Tanner stage 3 or 4, is *Osgood-Schlatter disease* (OSD). Pain, tenderness, and swelling at the anterior tibial tubercle (which is an apophysis, a prominent site where tendon unites with bone) where the patellar tendon inserts are diagnostic. Activity invariably exacerbates the symptoms, as does local trauma to the tubercle. The cause of OSD probably relates to the lengthening of the long bones during the pubertal growth spurt without immediate lengthening of the muscle–tendon unit, with consequent stress on the cartilaginous growth center of the bone to which the tendon attaches. Affected people have avulsion lesions in small areas of the developing ossification center in the anterior part of the tibial tuberosity [98–100].

Physical examination is diagnostic. A swollen anterior tibial tubercle is noted with tenderness on direct palpation in a Tanner stage 3 or 4 youth. No other knee or bony pathologic finding is noted on examination. Radiographs usually are not necessary. If done, irregularity of the tuberosity ossification center as well as anterior soft tissue swelling would be seen.

Initial treatment is RICE. Stretching of the quadriceps is initiated twice daily, followed by a 20-minute application of ice. When the patient can easily touch the buttock with the heel of the offending leg without difficulty while lying prone, quadriceps-strengthening exercises are added to the regimen and resumption of activity is allowed [101].

Consequences of OSD are usually limited to a permanently enlarged anterior tibial tuberosity once ossification has been completed, although fracture of the tubercle is possible.

Ankle Injuries

The lateral ligament complex of the ankle is the most commonly injured site in interscholastic and intercollegiate sports [102,103]. Nearly 85% of all ankle injuries are sprains, of which 80% occur to the lateral ligament complex [35,104]. The ankle is the most common site of injury in basketball players and soccer players [105]. Knowledge of the bones and ligaments of the ankle is necessary for proper diagnosis of ankle injuries [106] (Fig. 15).

The ankle joint has been described as a mortise and tenon. The mortise is formed by the inferior surface of the tibia, the medial or tibial malleolus, and the lateral or fibular malleolus. The lateral malleolus is longer than the medial and prevents excessive eversion of the ankle, the result being infrequent injury to the deltoid ligament on the medial side of the joint. The tenon of the joint is the cartilaginous surface of the dome of the talus.

The three major groups of ankle ligaments are the medial collateral, lateral collateral, and tibiofibular groups. Of the three lateral collateral ligaments, the anterior talofibular ligament, which links the anterior border of the lateral malleolus and the lateral surface of the talar neck, is the weakest and most frequently injured [104,107]. The strongest of the three is the calcaneofibular ligament, and the other is the posterior talofibular. The three lateral ligaments can be palpated at 4, 6, and 8 o'clock distal to the bony prominence of the lateral malleolus.

The ankle joint was, in the past, assumed to be uniaxial in movement, but orientation of the joint axis actually changes position and direction as the ankle moves. The movement of the foot in the joint has been likened to a badly mounted wheel [108]. The normal ankle can move approximately 18° from horizontal in dorsiflexion and approximately 50° in plantar flexion; it can invert to almost 33° and evert to nearly 18° [107].

Most ankle injuries occur when the foot is slightly plantarflexed and inverted with internal rotation, damaging the anterior talofibular ligament [106,107]. The injury is usually abrupt. An attempt should be made to ascertain the mechanism of injury, and an examination should be performed as soon as possible before the swelling that is imminent. Common scenarios for injury include a poorly executed cutting move enhanced by inadvertent foot fixation, landing on an irregular playing surface, and uncontrolled landing from jumps. One can picture this occurring most frequently in basketball.

It is prudent first to examine the normal ankle to get a good idea of the patient's normal anatomy and range of motion. Then the bony structures should be examined for evidence of fracture. The ligaments should be palpated for point tenderness, and the stability of the ankle should be determined. This is done by stabilizing the leg and pulling the ankle forward with the foot in neutral position. A positive anterior drawer sign is produced when the talus slides forward more than 4 mm. An anterior talofibular ligament tear can result in an anterior drawer sign of 4 to 16 mm [109]. Gradation of

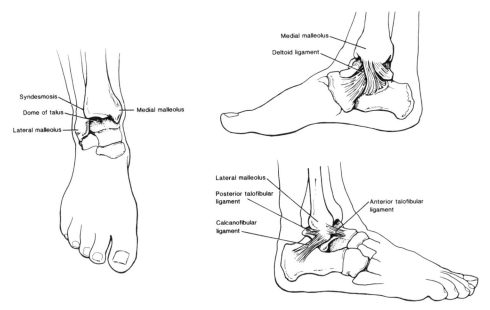

FIG. 15. Ankle ligaments. (Adapted from Harvey J. Ankle injuries in children and adolescents. *Pediatr Rev* 1981;2:217.)

sprains is as in other anatomic sites: first-degree sprains consist of stretching of ligaments; second-degree sprains show tearing of some fibers and stretching of others; and third-degree sprains tear the whole ligament. Differentiation between grades 2 and 3 is most critical because many grade 3 injuries require surgical intervention. Radiographic evaluation can be used to determine *talar tilt*, which is the angle formed by the opposing articular surfaces of the tibia and talus when an inverting force is applied to the ankle. A significant difference in the amount of separation between the lateral tibiotalar surfaces or a significant difference between the two legs indicates instability [110,111]. Whether radiographs should be obtained in the first place is determined by the Ottawa Ankle Rules, which state that a radiograph is needed if there is pain near the malleoli and one or more of the following exists: age 55 years or older; unable to bear weight; and bone tenderness at the posterior edge or tip of either malleolus [112,113]. Functional tests to allow decisions about returning to play at the time of injury are listed in Table 13.

Proper treatment and rehabilitation are critical. Eighty percent of high school varsity basketball players with ankle sprains have multiple episodes. Forty percent of patients with previous injuries to the lateral ligaments complain of chronic instability [114]. The most common cause of chronic ankle pain after an ankle sprain is incomplete rehabilitation [115].

Immediate treatment for grade 3 sprains and for probable fractures is immobilization and referral to an orthopedist. For grade 1 and 2 sprains, RICE is the initial treatment. Avoidance of weight bearing should be reinforced, especially with impulsive adolescents, by having the patient use crutches for a few days. Pain is a good guide for what the patient may or may not do. Pain-free activities should be encouraged.

Rehabilitation should be begun within a few days of injury. The principles of rehabilitation are listed in Table 14.

Lower Leg Pain

Most causes of lower leg pain in athletes can be ascribed to overuse syndromes. Overuse injuries of this area are frequently called *shin splints*, but more properly should be described by the severity of injury and site of involvement. Injury can range from simple transient pain after activity (due to minor inflammation or overdoing an activity) to stress fractures of the tibia. The site of involvement can be the tibia, the various muscle compartments in the lower leg, the periosteum, or the Achilles tendon and its attachments. The authors recommend the following system of assessing and treating such injuries [116].

Pain that is transient usually is of no major concern and is easily treated with ice and mild analgesia. It can be prevented by wearing proper shoes and by conditioning. Pain that begins late in an activity, lasts for an hour or two, and recurs for more than 2 weeks is usually due to mild musculotendinous inflammation. Examination reveals no point tenderness. Ice, decreased activity, and adherence to proper techniques along with proper equipment usually suffice for treatment.

Pain that has recurred for more than 3 to 4 weeks and that begins earlier in an activity is of more concern. If there is evidence of inflammation and point tenderness with pain at that site when pressure is applied to other sites in the leg, the cause is major inflammation of the musculotendinous unit, pe-

TABLE 13. *Functional tests for sideline decisions on return to play after ankle injury*

No evidence of fracture or grade 2 or 3 sprain
Can walk without a limp or undue pain
Can job in straight line without limp or undue pain
Can run figure-eights and cut, stop quickly, and jump
Can hop freely on injured leg without undue pain
Tape ankle and return to play[a]

[a]Observe athlete closely during remainder of game and remove from play if athlete's performance deteriorates or is hampered by pain or limp.

From Harvey J. Ankle injuries in children and adolescents. *Pediatr Rev* 1981;2:217. Reproduced with permission from *Pediatrics*.

TABLE 14. *Ankle sprain rehabilitation: a walk/run program for transition from crutches to running*

Patients recovering from ankle sprain can begin a rehabilitative walk/run program as soon as they can bear weight with minimal discomfort. Walk/run rehabilitation enables the athlete to build strength over a period of 2 to 3 weeks. Instruct the patient as follows:

- **Avoid weight-bearing on the ankle until you can step down with minimal discomfort.**
- **Start a walking routine, beginning with 5 minutes per day, and increasing up to 20 minutes at a time, until you can walk for the full 20 minutes.**
- Begin to substitute 5 minutes of jogging for 5 minutes of walking at a time, until you are jogging for the full 20 minutes without pain.
- Begin straight-ahead sprints, then figure-eight sprints. Start with 20-yard figure-eights (e.g., figure-eights that are 20 yards long from top to bottom), and gradually restrict your running path to a 10-yard figure-eight.
- Once you are sprinting figure-eights without pain and swelling, it should be safe to return to play with ankle support.
- If pain or swelling occurs at any time, stop the regimen for a day or two, ice frequently, then resume your routine at the last comfortable level.

Athletes with grade 3 sprains who follow this regimen (*as tolerated*) can expect to return to play in about 3 weeks.

From Hergenroeder AC. Acute shoulder, knee, and ankle injuries: Part 2. rehabilitation. *Adolescent Health Update* 1996;8:1, with permission.

riostitis, or bone microtrauma. Radiographs and a bone scan are indicated. A bone scan may be positive in 75% of these cases. RICE is indicated for treatment initially with use of NSAIDs. Slow return to activity is prescribed after pain resolves, and attention should be paid to proper equipment and techniques.

The most severe symptom is pain that has lasted longer than 4 weeks and occurs early in activity, preventing or affecting performance. Findings are the same as in the previous category, with further disturbance in function, decreased range of motion, and possible muscle atrophy. This type of injury is usually due to breakdown in soft tissue, stress fracture, or a compartment syndrome (especially if swelling is marked). Radiographs and a bone scan should be performed. The bone scan is positive in up to 95% of cases. Initially, treatment consists of RICE and NSAIDs followed by a gradual return to activity when pain resolves. Again, attention should be paid to proper equipment and techniques.

Common sites and types of lower leg injuries are highlighted next. There are several other, more obscure causes of lower limb pain in adolescent athletes, including foot problems and the like, but most fit into the categories described here.

Anterior Tibial Strain

Anterior tibial strain produces pain along the anterior lateral tibia. It is especially common among beginning runners, athletes who run repetitively on hard surfaces, and those who indulge in too much activity too soon. Ice, relative rest, resistive dorsiflexion Achilles tendon stretching, well cushioned shoes, and running on softer surfaces all aid in alleviating this syndrome.

Medial Tibial Stress Syndrome

Medial tibial stress syndrome produces pain along the distal third of the medial border of the tibia. Pain comes from the soft tissues, not the bone. Hyperpronation of the foot is part of this syndrome. It results from several causes, including malalignment of the Achilles tendon, hypermobility of the subtalar joints, or pes planus. In the toe-off phase of gait, the soleus and posterior tibial muscles are forced into a position of mechanical inefficiency. Also, as the foot pronates, the lower leg rotates internally, and in runners with hyperpronation, the transmission of force up the leg is exaggerated [116]. This problem is common among long-term runners. Methods used to treat this problem include ice, relative rest, correction of biomechanical problems with proper shoes or orthoses, resistive plantar flexion, and stretching of the Achilles tendon.

Compartment Syndromes

Compartment syndromes are another source of chronic leg pain in athletes. There are four compartments in the lower leg (Fig. 16). Symptoms that are characteristic of a compartment syndrome include consistent onset of pain early in an activity, weakness of the involved muscles, tenseness on palpation, and paresthesias in the areas supplied by the nerves in that compartment [116]. The symptoms occur only with exercise and are relieved shortly thereafter, especially if ice is applied. Rest and treatment for inflammation are usually successful, but occasionally the fascia is tight, producing high intracompartmental pressures. Surgery (fasciotomy) is then required.

Achilles Tendinitis

Achilles tendinitis presents with pain just above the insertion of the Achilles tendon into the calcaneus. There is tenderness at that site along with crepitation and thickening of the tendon. Causes include a tight Achilles tendon, uphill running, and hyperpronation. Treatment consists of relative rest, ice, use of a temporary heel pad, stretching, and correction of biomechanical problems. Included in the differential diagnosis of this problem in young athletes is a condition similar to OSD, *Sever's disease* or *traction apophysitis* at the insertion of the Achilles tendon into the calcaneus. Various apophyseal injuries are listed in Table 15.

Stress Fracture

The final syndrome is stress fracture, which is particularly troublesome in adolescents, especially girls. Girls who are athletic and are amenorrheic are more prone to this type of injury secondary to relative decreased bone density. The most common site of stress fracture in young athletes is the proximal tibial metaphysis [117]. Stress fractures can be viewed as the body's inability to heal microfractures because of repeated stress and trauma to the site. The problem is augered by pain that begins relatively early in a workout and persists throughout the day, pain that prevents exercise, erythema, warmth, and point tenderness on palpation. Radiographs do not detect this type of fracture early in its course; a bone scan is necessary for its diagnosis. Some bony deformities, such as tibia vara and anterior tibial bowing, can predispose to this type of injury. Frequently, the problem is preceded by a significant increase in training intensity. Treatment with relative rest, ice, NSAIDs, and prescription of alternative exercise until the pain is gone usually is adequate.

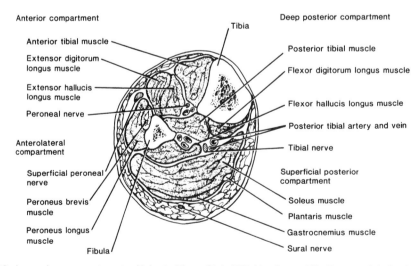

FIG. 16. Lower leg compartments. (Adapted from Clain MR, Hershman EB. Overuse injuries in children and adolescents. *Phys Sports Med* 1989;17:111.)

TABLE 15. *Apophyseal injuries*

Injury	Age (y)	Site	Presentation	Differential diagnosis	Treatment
Sever's disease	8–13	Posterior calcaneus	Heel pain with activity	Achilles tendinitis, stress fracture	Heel cups, RICE < decrease activity, NSAIDs
Osgood-Schlatter disease	Boys: 10–15 Girls: 8–13	Tibial tuberosity	Anterior knee pain	PFD, OCD, stress fracture	RICE, activity modification, knee strap, NSAIDs
Sindig-Larsen-Johannson syndrome	10–13	Inferior pole of patella	Anterior knee pain	PFD < OCD, stress fracture	RICE, activity modification, NSAIDs
Apophysitis of the hip	9–13	ASIS, AIIS, iliac crest, ischial tuberosity	Dull ache around the hip	Muscle strain, stress fracture	RICE, stretching program, NSAIDs
Medial epicondylitis	9–13	Humeral medial epicondyle	Medial elbow pain with activity	Flexor tendinitis, UCL sprain	RICE, activity modification, NSAIDs

NSAIDs, nonsteroidal antiinflammatory drugs; PFD, patellofemoral dysfunction; OCD, osteochondritis dessicans; RICE, rest, ice, compression, and elevation; ASIS, anterior superior iliac spine; AIIS, anterior inferior iliac spine; UCL, ulnar collateral ligament.
From Peck DM. Apophyseal injuries in the young athlete. *Am Fam Physician* 1995;51:1891, with permission.

Shoulder and Arm Problems

Upper extremity problems frequently seen in adolescent athletes are Little League elbow, swimmer's shoulder, hand injuries such as sprains and finger dislocations, navicular fractures, and shoulder injuries such as dislocations.

Hand and Wrist Disorders

Common hand injuries include finger sprains and dislocations. Sprains should be evaluated for degree of injury, if they are not third degree, splinting for 7 to 10 days, with ice and analgesia as necessary, is usually sufficient. Dislocations of fingers should be assessed on the scene for functional impairment and for direction of the dislocation. The direction in which the finger is dislocated can suggest possible ligament tears. Once evaluation is complete, simple longitudinal traction with or without nerve block is sufficient to reduce the problem. Splinting for a week or two and rehabilitation to return to previous flexibility is usually all that is required for treatment [118].

A fracture of the navicular bone in the wrist easily can be overlooked because the symptoms can mimic a sprain and radiographs may be negative for several days after the injury. Untreated navicular fractures can lead to nonunion and may require secondary surgery [118]. This type of fracture is associated with tenderness in the anatomic snuffbox and pain at extremes of wrist motion. Standard treatment consists of using a long thumb spica cast for as long as 4 months until the fracture has healed.

Elbow Disorders

Elbow problems, particularly in pitchers, are frequently encountered. Most of these can be grouped under the rubric of *Little League elbow*, a group of disorders resulting from repetitive valgus stress of the elbow as a consequence of throwing. Most such disorders are a direct result of repetitive pitching and poor throwing mechanics in an immature elbow. Valgus forces applied to the elbow create compression forces across the lateral structures (radial head and capitellum) and tension on the medial structures (medial epicondyle, medial collateral ligaments; Figs. 17, 18). In immature arms, the ten-

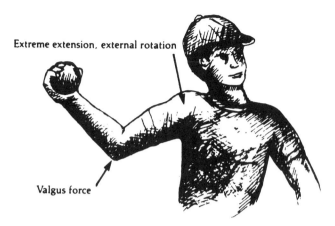

Extreme extension, external rotation

Valgus force

FIG. 17. Forces on the elbow and shoulder with throwing. (Reprinted with permission from Emans JB. Upper extremity injuries in sports. In: Micheli LJ, ed. *Pediatric and adolescent sports medicine.* Boston: Little, Brown; 1984:71.)

sion forces can create chronic medial epicondylitis with overgrowth of the medial epicondyle from chronic traction [119,120]. Occasionally, an avulsion fracture of the medial epicondyle can occur.

The most common presenting symptom is medial elbow pain. Locking or catching may also be present. Tenderness is produced with palpation over the medial ligaments or the epicondyle. Radiographs can help, but more extensive imaging studies may be necessary to evaluate fully the damage to the joint structures. In general, the hallmark of treatment is rest until symptoms are gone. A slow return to throwing may be allowed when pain has subsided and full range of motion is achieved. Prohibiting immature athletes from throwing curve balls, throwing sidearm, and from pitching an excessive number of innings is mandatory. If the young pitcher does not abide by the therapeutic dictates of the physician or trainer, chronic elbow problems may ensue.

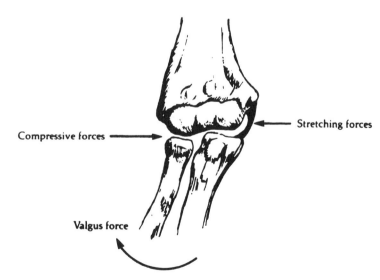

Compressive forces

Stretching forces

Valgus force

FIG. 18. At the elbow, lateral compression forces and medial distraction forces result from throwing. (Reprinted with permission from Emans JB. Upper extremity injuries in sports. In: Micheli LJ, ed. *Pediatric and adolescent sports medicine.* Boston: Little, Brown; 1984:71.)

Shoulder Disorders

The most common upper arm injury in sports that requires a physician's attention probably is the dislocated shoulder [118]. Anterior and inferior dislocations are most common, although posterior ones do occur. The usual mechanism for the injury is a fall on the abducted or extended arm. Initial dislocations generate much pain and swelling and the appearance of a hollow on the lateral aspect of the shoulder. There are several methods for reduction of the dislocation. These include the Aronen method, in which the injured person grasps the ipsilateral knee and slowly extends the knee while continuing to hold the knee. This is a self-reduction technique that should be taught to anyone with recurrent dislocations. The Rockwood technique uses countertraction with a cloth around the body and under the affected shoulder while the clinician pulls the arm in line with the countertraction (Fig. 19). Most shoulders are immobilized after manipulative reduction for approximately 6 weeks, followed by a rehabilitative program.

Recurrent dislocations need surgical correction to stabilize the joint. Swimmer's shoulder is characterized by pain in the anterior and lateral aspects of the shoulder and is commonly associated with impingement of the structures in the subacromial space [121]. The tendons of the supraspinatus and biceps muscles are most often involved. The problem is almost exclusively due to faulty stroke mechanics with either faulty technique or deterioration of technique as muscles fatigue. Relative rest, ice, and NSAIDs are used for the immediate symptoms, followed by a rehabilitation period in which proper stroke mechanics are emphasized [121].

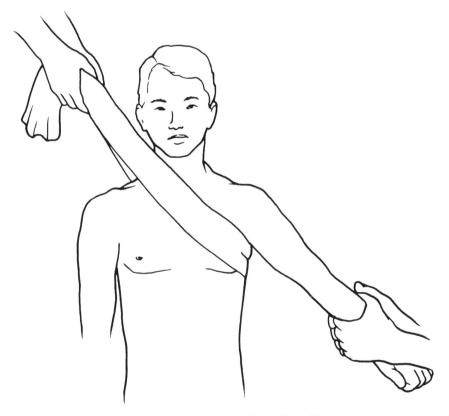

FIG. 19. Rockwood technique for closed reduction of left shoulder with traction against counteraction. (Adapted from Rockwood CA, Green DP, eds. *Fractures in adults.* vol. 1. 2nd ed. Philadelphia: JB Lippincott; 1984.)

Acromioclavicular separation is more common in older adolescents and adults. It usually results from a fall directly on the point of the shoulder. There is discrete tenderness at the acromioclavicular joint. With a grade 1 acromioclavicular separation, there is tenderness over the joint, and with grades 2 and 3, there is also a gap appreciated between the acromion and clavicle because of tearing of ligaments. Length of rehabilitation depends on the degree of separation, but the process is the same: RICE, range-of-motion exercises, and slow return to function with strengthening exercises as the separation heals [92].

Back Injuries

Any acute injury to the back with possible neurologic consequences should be evaluated immediately at the time of injury. The neck should be immobilized, a neurologic assessment should be performed, and appropriate radiographs should be obtained. Lower back pain from muscle spasm is also commonly encountered. This can be diagnosed by finding no neurologic deficiencies and no point tenderness over the spine with meticulous palpation of the vertebrae. Tenderness and firmness of the paraspinal muscles and exacerbation of the pain with hyperextension at the hip on the affected side while the victim is lying prone are typical findings. Treatment is rest on a hard surface, application of wet heat, and NSAIDs until pain is gone. Flexion exercises should be prescribed before any further physical activity.

A significant cause of back pain in the young athlete is *spondylolysis*, which is defined as a defect or cleft in the pars interarticularis of a vertebra without displacement of the vertebral body. It is most common at L5. The vertebral body can also move anteriorly on the one below it, which is called *spondylolisthesis*.

Spondylolysis appears to be an acquired, stress-induced fracture of the pars interarticularis [122,123]. It is probably due to repetitive hyperextension of the spine or to a single significant trauma. It may occur in as many as 11% of female gymnasts compared with 2% to 4% of the general population of similar adolescents who are not gymnasts or dancers [124]. It has also been described in 15% to 20% of dancers with back symptoms [125]. The pain is usually generalized lower back pain that is not necessarily consonant with the degree of objective injury but is more likely due to associated soft tissue changes [126]. Usually unilateral, the pain is exacerbated by hyperextension activities such as back walkovers in gymnastics and by arabesques in ballet. The only objective signs may be tenderness over the affected area due to soft tissue reaction. A radiograph may reveal the classic broken neck of the Scotty dog in the oblique view. If the radiograph is negative, a bone scan frequently reveals increased uptake characteristic of fracture. Early detection may prevent progression of the problem and permit eventual return to activity. Rest until the patient is free of pain and analgesia are usually adequate treatment. Antilordotic bracing also can be of benefit [123]. Resolution of findings on bone scan is a good indicator of the time to return to activity, although this may take as long as 8 months.

Concussion

A concussion has been defined as a clinical syndrome characterized by immediate and transient posttraumatic impairment of neural functions [127]. Each year, approximately 20% of high school football players sustain a concussion [128]. Concussion also can be a serious problem in sports such as boxing, ice hockey, and horseback riding [129]. These can be graded from 1 to 3 in severity [130]. Table 16 describes the levels of concussion with recommended rules for return to competition. For grade 2 concussion, radiographs and full neurologic evaluation must be performed to rule out a cervical spine injury. Return to competition is delayed until at least 7 days after all symptoms have resolved. For a grade 3 concussion, immediate neurologic consultation should be obtained. No youth should return to activity until all concussive symptoms have resolved to avoid the chance of second-impact syndrome. This condition occurs when an athlete returns to activity before fully recovering from the initial head trauma and sustains a seemingly minor head injury. A rapid neurologic deterioration ensues, and the patient can die [131]. More than two concussions should exclude the adolescent from further hard collision sports. Neuroimaging tests such as magnetic resonance imaging and computed tomography should be considered when symptoms worsen or persist for more than a few days. Finally, the clinician should be aware that sudden death in young athletes can occur after blunt trauma to the chest [132,133].

TABLE 16. *Grading scale for concussion in sport*

Grade 1. Confusion without amnesia, no loss of consciousness
Grade 2. Confusion with amnesia, no loss of consciousness
Grade 3. Loss of consciousness

Guidelines for return to competition

Grade 1. Remove from contest. Examine immediately and every 5 minutes for the development of amnesia or postconcussive symptoms at rest and with exertion. May return to contest if amnesia does not appear and no symptoms appear for at least 20 minutes.
Grade 2. Remove from contest and disallow return. Examine frequently for signs of evolving intracranial pathology. Reexamine the next day. May return to practice only after 1 full week without symptoms.
Grade 3. Transport from field by ambulance (with cervical spine immobilization if indicated) to nearest hospital. Thorough neurologic evaluation emergency. Hospital confinement if signs of pathology are detected. If findings are normal, instructions to family for overnight observation. May return to practice only after 2 full weeks without symptoms.
Prolonged unconsciousness, persistent mental status alterations, worsening postconcussion symptoms or abnormalities on neurologic examination require urgent neurosurgical consultation or transfer to a trauma center.

From Feinstein RA, Owen C, Guralnick D. Sports medicine: clinical update. *International Pediatrics* 1995;10:292, with permission.

Steroids

Adolescent athletes and adolescents in general who feel insecure about their bodies are particularly susceptible to any solicitations that hold out the illusory promise of better body build and improved performance in many arenas of life. Adolescents are susceptible to these blandishments because of their self-perceived physical inadequacies and because of the feeling that enhanced physical appearance compensates for perceived personal inadequacies.

Adolescent athletes are particularly prone to looking for quick fixes for their performance deficiencies. When faced with a choice between hard work and long hours versus taking a few pills or even a few injections to improve performance, some teenagers may succumb to the easy way out. That may mean using anabolic steroids to produce large muscles and increase strength quickly.

Anabolic steroids are derivatives of the natural male hormone testosterone. Their use in human performance enhancement was described during World War II, when they were allegedly supplied to German soldiers to make them more ferocious during battle [134]. Athletes who needed lots of muscle size and definition, such as body builders, or who needed lots of muscle power, such as power lifters, shot putters, and the like, seized the opportunity to use these substances [135,136]. Despite anecdotal reports about the high prevalence of steroid use, few data exist. Over a million Americans are estimated to be using anabolic steroids, and approximately half of them are high school students [137,138]. The use among adolescent male athletes has been stated to be between 2% and 3% [139], and another study reported a 6.6% use rate among male high school seniors [140]. A survey in a suburban Chicago high school revealed a similar use rate [141].

Anabolic steroid use has significant side effects. These include liver tumors and disease, acne, a decrease in high-density lipoprotein cholesterol, an increase in low-density lipoprotein cholesterol, hypertension, gynecomastia, baldness, and decreased testicular size with oligospermia or azoospermia. There is also an increase in aggressive behavior as well as occasional psychotic symptoms. In addition, use of anabolic steroids accelerates closure of bony epiphyses in the prepubertal and pubertal adolescent, thereby decreasing ultimate height. In girls, these drugs cause acne, baldness, and other signs of masculinization. Although the combination of steroids and intensive weight training combined with a high-calorie, high-protein diet increases muscle size and strength [142,143], the side effects of long-term use can greatly outweigh any transient benefits.

In addition to the risks incurred by use of these drugs, adolescents who use anabolic steroids also are at increased risk for use of other illicit, harmful drugs and of participating in other high-risk behaviors [144,145]. Other drugs also may be used by adolescents to enhance athletic performance. These include those listed in Table 17. Physicians must be aware of the use of these drugs and include

TABLE 17. *Commonly abused ergogenic drugs*

Drug	Desired effect	Activity	Bans
Amphetamines	Euphoria Masked fatigue	Endurance and strength sports	USOC NCAA
Anabolic steroids	Increased muscle Increased strength	Strength sports Body building	USOC NCAA
Beta-blockers	Decreased tremor Decreased heart rate	Shooting Music Archery	USOC NCAA (selected sports)[a]
Caffeine	Stimulation Increased free fatty acids	Sprint and distance running	Restricted use by NCAA and USOC[b]
Cyproheptadine (Periactin)	Appetite stimulation Weight gain	Size sports Body building	USOC
Diuretics	Weight loss Masked urine	Wrestling Banned drug use	USOC NCAA
Erythropoietin	Increased hematocrit	Endurance sports	USOC NCAA
Growth hormone	Increased muscle mass Enhanced healing	Strength sports Body building	USOC NCAA

USOC, United States Olympic Committee; NCAA, National Collegiate Athletic Association.

[a]Banned in riflery by NCAA; USOC tests 14 sports, including gymnastics, figure skating, fencing, and diving.

[b]Urine concentrations allowed up to 12 μg/ml by USOC and 15 μg/ml by NCAA.

From Foley JD, Schydlower M. Anabolic steroid and ergogenic drug use by adolescents. *Adolescent Medicine: State of the Art Reviews* 1993;4:341, with permission.

counseling against their use by adolescents in their health supervision visits. History of steroid use also should be sought in adolescents who abuse other drugs.

Being a Team Physician

Pediatricians and other primary care practitioners are ideally suited to be the physicians responsible for athletic teams at secondary schools and even at the college level. Although orthopedists garner the most headlines as team doctors for professional and large college sports programs, their role with scholastic sports is primarily as consultants.

Years ago, being a team physician meant showing up at varsity games and treating injuries. Today, this role encompasses much more. The team "doc" must play an active role in all aspects of the sports program. Frequently, groups of physicians share the role of team physician for a whole scholastic sports program, supported by an employed or volunteer athletic trainer and trained members of the school health staff. The team physician must have expertise in many more areas than just sports traumatology. He or she must have competence in the sports aspects of cardiovascular, respiratory, dermatologic, gynecologic, infectious, metabolic, nutritional, and psychological problems. Along with this goes the need for a comprehensive understanding of principles of preventive health in sports and of the preparticipation evaluation, conditioning, rehabilitation, and the effective use of consultants. With this kind of expertise and support, the physician can ensure that the coaches and school administration are well educated about sports issues and that the school views her or him as an integral part of the program.

Specific Job Responsibilities

The team physician's specific job responsibilities should include the following [130]:

- Being present at all athletic events where the chance of injury is high
- Treating and making appropriate referral for those injuries that occur at athletic contests
- Assisting in rehabilitation and determining the return to action for athletes
- Educating coaches and officials associated with the school

- Working with the athletic directors and trainers in establishing an ongoing program for student trainers at the high school level
- Assisting the athletic trainers of the school or system in determining the appropriate protocol for management of specific injuries
- Establishing, with the assistance of the athletic trainers and directors, the authority to restrict or release injured athletes from practice and games

Team physicians should be aware that in some states any actions they take for assessment or treatment of injuries on the field of play will not expose them to liability as long as they do not take compensation for their services.

General Roles of the Team Physician

There are several roles that the team physician can play in the school's athletic program and in the medical life of his or her community [146]. As *acute care provider*, the physician provides on-site care for game injuries and is available for assessment of practice injuries at his or her office. To provide *ongoing care*, the team doctor can hold a weekly clinic at the school to assess athletes who have recently been injured and those who are in the midst of a rehabilitation program.

Educating coaches and (para)medical personnel at the school is an important aspect of the team physician's role. The lessons to be taught are not only those of what to do if someone is injured. They also include instruction on nutrition, preventive health issues, and conditioning. Frequently, the physician can also be an educator for the athletes themselves and for their parents. He can bring a caring but unbiased perspective to the athletic arena in a secondary school setting. The education of other physicians, medical students, and residents in the area can be a rewarding aspect of the team doctor's educational activities.

The physician's *administrative duties* should include ensuring that all medical equipment is appropriate and usable. He or she should also review all preparticipation evaluation forms and consultant instructions and all rehabilitation plans. Proper maintenance of records falls under the doctor's purview as well. Also, the team doctor should be responsible for ensuring that emergency medical services are appropriately on call whenever a game is being played.

Being a team physician is a demanding but very rewarding activity in which the clinician can directly contribute to one aspect of adolescent development.

REFERENCES

1. McKeag DB. Adolescents and exercise. *Journal of Adolescent Health Care* 1986;7:121S.
2. American Medical Association Board of Trustees. Athletic preparticipation examinations for adolescents. *Arch Pediatr Adolesc Med* 1994;148:93.
3. Kemper HCG. Longitudinal studies on the development of health and fitness and the interaction with physical activity of teenagers. *Pediatrician* 1986;13:52.
4. Fripp RR, Hodgson JL, Kwiterovich PO, et al. Aerobic capacity, obesity, and atherosclerotic risk factors in male adolescents. *Pediatrics* 1985;75:813.
5. Hulse E, Strong WB. Preparticipation evaluation for athletes. *Pediatr Rev* 1987;9:173.
6. DuRant RH, Seymore C, Linder CW, et al. The preparticipation examination of athletes. *American Journal of Diseases of Children* 1985;139:657.
7. Micheli LJ, Yost JG. Preparticipation evaluation and first aid for sports. In: Micheli LJ, ed. *Pediatric and adolescent sports medicine*. Boston: Little, Brown; 1984:30.
8. Bratton RL, Agerter DC. Preparticipation sports examinations: efficient risk assessment in children and adolescents. *Postgrad Med* 1995;98:123.
9. Krowchuk DP, Krowchuk HV, Hunter DM, et al. Parents' knowledge of the purposes and content of preparticipation physical examinations. *Arch Pediatr Adolesc Med* 1995;149:653.
10. Linder CW, DuRant RH, Seklecki RM, et al. Preparticipation health screening of young athletes: results of 1268 examinations. *Am J Sports Med* 1981;9:187.
11. Risser WL, Hoffman HM, Bellah GG, et al. A cost–benefit analysis of preparticipation sports examinations of adolescent athletes. *J Sch Health* 1985;55:270.
12. DuRant RH, Seymore C, Linder CW, et al. The preparticipation examination of athletes: comparison of single and multiple examiners. *American Journal of Diseases of Children* 1985;139:657.
13. Duke PM, Litt IF, Gross RT. Adolescent's self-assessment of sexual maturation. Pediatrics 1980;66:918.
14. Hafner J. Problems in matching athletes: baby fat, peach fuzz, muscle and moustache. *Sports Med* 1975;3:96.

15. Tomassoni TL, Galioto FM Jr. Cardiologic aspects of adolescent sports medicine. *Seminars in Adolescent Medicine* 1987;3:185.
16. Maron BJ, Roberts WC, McAllister HA, et al. Sudden death in young athletes. *Circulation* 1980;62:218.
17. Epstein SE, Maron BJ. Sudden death and the competitive athlete: perspectives on preparticipation screening studies. *J Am Coll Cardiol* 1986;7:220.
18. Maron BJ, Thompson PD, Puffer JC, et al. Cardiovascular preparticipation screening of competitive athletes: a statement for health professionals from the Sudden Death Committee (Clinical Cardiology) and Congenital Cardiac Defects Committee (Cardiovascular Disease in the Young), American Heart Association. *Circulation* 1996;94:850.
19. Bracer MD, Jones KL, Moore BS. Suspected Marfan syndrome in a female basketball player. *Phys Sports Med* 1988;16:69.
20. Guyer B, Gallegher SS. An approach to the epidemiology of childhood injuries. *Pediatr Clin North Am* 1985;32:5.
21. Garrick JG, Requa RK. Girls sports injuries in high school athletics. *JAMA* 1978;239:2245.
22. Garrick JG. Characterization of the patient population in a sports medicine facility. *Phys Sports Med* 1985;13:73.
23. Tursz A, Crost M. Sports-related injuries in children: a study of their characteristics, frequency, and severity, with comparison to other types of accidental injuries. *Am J Sports Med* 1986;14:294.
24. DeHaven KE, Lintner DM. Athletic injuries: comparison by age, sport, and gender. *Am J Sports Med* 1986;14:218.
25. Rowland TW. Preparticipation sports examination of the child and adolescent athlete: changing views of an old ritual. *Pediatrician* 1986;13:3.
26. Garrick JG, Requa RK. Injury patterns in children and adolescent skiers. *Am J Sports Med* 1979;8:377.
27. Micheli LJ. Pediatric and adolescent sports injuries: recent trends. *Exerc Sport Sci Rev* 1986;14:359.
28. Moskwa CA Jr, Nicholas JA. Musculoskeletal risk factors in the young athlete. *Phys Sports Med* 1989;17:49.
29. Goldberg B, Rosenthal PP, Nicholas JA. Injuries in youth football. *Phys Sports Med* 1984;12:122.
30. Nicholas JA. Risk factors, sports medicine and the orthopedic system: an overview. *Sports Med* 1976;3:243.
31. Miller AP. Strains of the posterior calf musculature ("tennis leg"). *Am J Sports Med* 1979;7:172.
32. Brooks WH, Young AB. High school football injuries: prevention of injury to the central nervous system. *South Med J* 1976;69:1258.
33. Reider B, Marshall JL, Warren RF. Clinical characteristics of patellar disorders in young athletes. *Am J Sports Med* 1981;9:270.
34. Martin RK, Yesalis CE, Foster D, et al. Sports injuries at the 1985 Junior Olympics: an epidemiologic analysis. *Am J Sports Med* 1987;15:603.
35. Smith RW, Reischl SF. Treatment of ankle sprains in young athletes. *Am J Sports Med* 1986;14:465.
36. Diamond LS, Lynne D, Sigman B. Orthopedic disorders in patients with Down's syndrome. *Orthop Clin North Am* 1981;12:57.
37. Committee on Sports Medicine. Atlanto-axial instability in Down syndrome. *Pediatrics* 1984;74:152.
38. Pueschel SM. Atlanto-axial subluxation in Down's syndrome [Letter]. *Lancet* 1983;1:980.
39. Hreidarsson S, Magram G, Singer H. Symptomatic atlantoaxial dislocation in Down syndrome. *Pediatrics* 1982;69:568.
40. Hudson PB. Preparticipation screening of Special Olympics athletes. *Phys Sports Med* 1988;16:97.
41. Special Olympics Bulletin. *Participation by individuals with Down syndrome who suffer from the atlantoaxial dislocation condition*. Washington, DC: Special Olympics Committee; 1983.
42. Micheli LJ. Low back pain in the adolescent: differential diagnosis. *Am J Sports Med* 1979;7:3652.
43. Staheli LT. Medial femoral torsion. *Orthop Clin North Am* 1980;11:39.
44. Costill DL, Kammer WF, Fisher A. Fluid ingestion during distance running. *Arch Environ Health* 1970;21:520.
45. McArdle WD, Katch FI, Datch VL. *Exercise physiology: energy, nutrition, and human performance*. Philadelphia: Lea & Febiger; 1986.
46. Lamb DR, Brodowicz GR. Optimal use of fluids of varying formulations to minimize exercise-induced disturbances in homeostasis. *Sports Med* 1986;3:247.
47. Murray R. The effects of consuming carbohydrate–electrolyte beverages on gastric emptying and fluid absorption during and following exercise. *Sports Med* 1987;4:322.
48. Costill DL. Water and electrolyte requirements during exercise. *Clin Sports Med* 1984;3:639.
49. Costill DL, Saltin B. Factors limiting gastric emptying during rest and exercise. *J Appl Physiol* 1974;37:679.
50. Davis JM, Lamb DR, Burgess WA, Bartoli WP. Accumulation of deuterium oxide in body fluids after ingestion of D20 labeled beverages. *J Appl Physiol* 1987;63:2060.
51. Brown RT, McIntosh SM, Seabolt VR, Daniel WA Jr. Iron status of adolescent female athletes. *Journal of Adolescent Health Care* 1985;6:349.
52. Ehn L, Carlmark B, Hoglund S. Iron status in athletes involved in intense physical activity. *Med Sci Sports Exerc* 1980;12:61.
53. Clement DB, Sawchuck LL. Iron status and sports performance. *Sports Med* 1984;1:65.

54. Rowland TW, Black SA, Kelleher JF. Iron deficiency in adolescent endurance athletes. *Journal of Adolescent Health Care* 8:322, 1987;.
55. Wishnitzer R, Vorst E, Berrebi A. Bone marrow iron depression in competitive distance runners. *Int J Sports Med* 1983;4:27.
56. Gardner GW, Edgerton VR, Senerwiratne B, et al. Physical work capacity and metabolic stress in subjects with iron deficiency anemia. *Am J Clin Nutr* 1977;30:970.
57. Dallman PR, Beutler E, Finch CA. Effects of iron deficiency exclusive of anemia. *Br J Haematol* 1978;40:179.
58. Finch CA, Miller LR, Inamdar AR, et al. Iron deficiency in the rat: physiological and biochemical studies of muscle dysfunction. *J Clin Invest* 1976;58:447.
59. Squire DL. Female athletes. *Pediatr Rev* 1987;9:183.
60. Holloszy JO. Muscle metabolism during exercise. *Arch Phys Med Rehabil* 1982;63:231.
61. Bergstrom J, Hultman E. Muscle glycogen synthesis after exercise: an enhancing factor localized to the muscle cells in man. *Nature* 1966;210:309.
62. Primos WA Jr, Landry GL. Fighting the fads in sports nutrition. *Contemporary Pediatrics* 1989;6:14.
63. Primos WA Jr, Landry GL. Five-on-one: should men coach women's sports? *Journal of Physical Education and Recreational Dance* 1986;57:62.
64. DuRant RH, Linder CW, Sanders JM, et al. Adolescent females' readiness to participate in sports. *Journal of Adolescent Health Care* 1988;9:310.
65. Shively RA, Hodgson JL, Kwiterovich PO, et al. High school sports injuries. *Phys Sports Med* 1981;9:46.
66. Chandy TA, Grana WA. Secondary school athletic injury in boys and girls: a three year study. *Phys Sports Med* 1985;13:106.
67. Gilsanz V, Gibbens DT, Roe TF, et al. Vertebral bone density in children: effect of puberty. *Radiology* 1988;166:847.
68. White CM, Hergenroeder AC, Klish WJ. Bone mineral density in eumenorrheic and amenorrheic, 15–21 year old females. *American Journal of Diseases of Children* 1992;146:31.
69. Theintz G, Buchs D, Rizzoli R, et al. Longitudinal monitoring of bone mass accumulation in healthy adolescents: evidence for marked reduction after 16 years of age at the levels of lumbar spine and femoral neck in female subjects. *J Clin Endocrinol Metab* 1992;75:1060.
70. Hergenroeder AC. Bone mineralization, hypothalamic amenorrhea, and sex steroid therapy in female adolescents and young adults. *J Pediatr* 1995;126:683.
71. Heaney RP. Nutritional factors and estrogen in age-related bone loss. *Clin Invest Med* 1982;5:147.
72. Drinkwater BL, Nilson K, Chesnut CH III, et al. Bone mineral content of amenorrheic and eumenorrheic athletes. *N Engl J Med* 1984;311:277.
73. Slemenda CW, Reister TK, Hui SL, et al. Influences on skeletal mineralization in children and adolescents evidence for varying effects of sexual maturation and physical activity. *J Pediatr* 1994;125:201.
74. Johnston CC, Miller JZ, Slemenda CW, et al. Calcium supplementation and increases in bone mineral density in children. *N Engl J Med* 1992;327:82.
75. Shangold M, Rebar RW, Wentz AC, et al. Evaluation and management of menstrual dysfunction in athletes. *JAMA* 1990;263:165.
76. Matkovic V, Ilich J. Calcium requirements for growth: are current requirements adequate? *Nutr Rev* 1993;51:171.
77. Frisch RE, Getz-Welbergen AV, McArthur JW, et al. Delayed menarche and amenorrhea of college athletes in relation to age of onset of training. *JAMA* 1981;246:1559.
78. Malina RM, Spirduso WW, Tate C, et al. Age at menarche and selected menstrual characteristics in athletes at different competitive levels and in different sports. *Medicine and Science in Sports* 1978;10:218.
79. Warren MP. The effects of exercise on pubertal progression and reproductive function in girls. *J Clin Endocrinol Metab* 1980;51:1150.
80. Bullen BA, Skrinar GS, Beitens IZ, et al. Induction of menstrual disorders by strenuous exercise in untrained women. *N Engl J Med* 1985;312:1349.
81. Bonen A, Keizer HA. Athletic menstrual cycle irregularity: endocrine response to exercise and training. *Phys Sports Med* 1984;12:78.
82. Bijur PE, Trumble A, Harel Y, et al. Sports and recreation injuries in US children and adolescents. *Arch Pediatr Adolesc Med* 1995;149:1009.
83. *Accident facts 1992 edition*. Itasca, IL: National Safety Council; 1992.
84. McLain LG, Reynolds S. Sports injuries in a high school. *Pediatrics* 1989;84:446.
85. Shively RA, Grana WA, Ellis D. High school sports injuries. *Phys Sports Med* 1981;9:46.
86. Burkett LN. Causative factors in hamstring strains. *Medicine and Science in Sports* 1970;2:39.
87. Garrett WE, Safran MR, Seaber AV, et al. Biomechanical comparison of stimulated and nonstimulated skeletal muscle pulled to failure. *Am J Sports Med* 1987;15:448.
88. Agre JC. Hamstring injuries: proposed etiological factors, prevention and treatment. *Sports Med* 1985;2:21.
89. Nicholaou PK, MacDonald BL, Bilsson RR, et al. Biomechanical and histological evaluation of muscle after controlled strain injury. *Am J Sports Med* 1987;15:9.

90. Garrett WE, Almekinders LC, Seaber AV. Biomechanics of muscle tears in stretching injuries. *Transactions of the Orthopedic Research Society* 1984;9:384.
91. Hergenroeder AC. Acute shoulder, knee, and ankle injuries: part 1. diagnosis and management. *Adolescent Health Update* 1996;8:1.
92. Hergenroeder AC. Acute shoulder, knee, and ankle injuries: part 2. rehabilitation. *Adolescent Health Update* 1996;8:1.
93. Dyment PG. Athletic injuries. *Pediatr Rev* 1989;10:291.
94. Hocutt JE, Jaffe R, Rylander CR, et al. Cryotherapy in ankle sprains. *Am J Sports Med* 1982;10:316.
95. Kennedy JC. Ligamentous injuries in the adolescent. In: Kennedy JC, ed. *The injured adolescent knee*. Baltimore: Williams & Wilkins; 1979:1.
96. Davidson K. Patellofemoral pain syndrome. *Am Fam Physician* 1993;48:1254.
97. Ogden JA, Tross RB, Murphy MJ. Fractures of the tibial tuberosity in adolescents. *J Bone Joint Surg [Am]* 1980;62:205.
98. Ogden JA, Southwick WO. Osgood-Schlatter's disease and tibial tuberosity development. *Clin Orthop* 1976; 116:180.
99. Clain MR, Hershman EB. Overuse injuries in children and adolescents. *Phys Sports Med* 1989;17:111.
100. Peck DM. Apophyseal injuries in the young athlete. *Am Fam Physician* 1995;51:1891.
101. Toney JM, Requa RK, Garrick JG. Antifriction devices and injury in skiing. *Am J Sports Med* 1977;5:241.
102. Saunders EA. Ligamentous injuries of the ankle. *Am Fam Pract* 1980;22:132.
103. Brostrom L. Sprained ankles: 1.anatomic lesions in recent sprains. *Acta Chirurgica Scandinavica* 1964;128: 483.
104. Brostrom L. Sprained ankles: 3. clinical observations in recent ligament ruptures. *Acta Chirurgica Scandinavica* 1965;130:560.
105. Harvey J. Ankle injuries in children and adolescents. *Pediatr Rev* 1981;2:217.
106. Attarian DE, McCrackin JH, DeVito DP, et al. Biomechanical characteristics of human ankle ligaments. *Foot Ankle* 1985;6:54.
107. Nike, Inc. Lateral ankle sprains. *Sport Research Review* 1989;July/August.
108. Wyller T. The axis of the ankle joint and its importance in subtalar arthrodesis. *Acta Orthop Scand* 1968; 33:320.
109. Klein SN, et al. Functional and surgical anatomy of the lateral ankle. *J Foot Surg* 1981;20:170.
110. Johannsen A. Radiological diagnosis of lateral ligament lesion of the ankle: a comparison between talar tilt and anterior drawer sign. *Acta Orthop Scand* 1978;49:295.
111. Freeman MA. Instability of the foot after injuries to the lateral ligament of the ankle. *J Bone Joint Surg [Br]* 1965;47:669.
112. Stiell IG, Green berg GH, McKnight RD, et al. A study to develop clinical decision rules for the use of radiography in acute ankle injuries. *Ann Emerg Med* 1992;21:384.
113. Chande VT. Decision rules for roentgenography of children with acute ankle injuries. *Arch Pediatr Adolesc Med* 1995;149:255.
114. Bosien WR, Staples OS, Russell SW. Residual disability following acute ankle sprains. *J Bone Joint Surg [Am]* 1955;37:1237.
115. Grana WA. Chronic pain after ankle sprain: consider differential diagnosis. *Phys Sports Med* 1995;23:67.
116. McKeag DB, Dolan C. Overuse syndromes of the lower extremity. *Phys Sports Med* 1989;17:108.
117. Walter M, Wolf M. Stress fractures in young athletes. *Am J Sports Med* 1977;5:165.
118. Emans JB. Upper extremity injuries in sports. In: Micheli LJ, ed. *Pediatric and adolescent sports medicine*. Boston: Little, Brown; 1984:49.
119. Fox GM, Jebson PJ, Orwin JF. Overuse injuries of the elbow. *Phys Sports Med* 1995;23:58.
120. Nirschl RP, Kraushaar BS. Assessment and treatment guidelines for elbow injuries. *Phys Sports Med* 1996;24:43.
121. Murphy TC, Riester JN. Managing the young swimmer. *Student Athlete* 1988;1:4.
122. Pennel RG, et al. Stress injuries of the pars interarticularis: radiologic classification and indication for scintigraphy. *American Journal of Radiology* 1985;145:763.
123. Micheli LJ, Fehlandt AF Jr. Overuse injuries to tendons and apophyses in children and adolescents. *Clin Sports Med* 1992;11:713.
124. Gelfand MJ, Strife JL, Kereiakes JG. Radionuclide bone imaging in spondylolysis of the lumbar spine in children. *Radiology* 1985;140:191.
125. Hamilton WG. Paper presented at the Third Annual Dance Medicine Symposium, Cincinnati, Ohio, 1981.
126. Epstein BS. *The spine: a radiological text and atlas*. 4th ed. Philadelphia: Lea & Febiger; 1976.
127. Report of the Ad Hoc Committee to study head injury nomenclature: proceedings of the Congress of Neurological Surgeons in 1964. *Clin Neurosurg* 1964;12:386.
128. Meuller PO, Cantu RC. Catastrophic injuries and fatalities in high school and college sports, fall 1982–spring 1988. *Med Sci Sports Exerc* 1990;22:737.
129. Bond GR, Christoph RA, Rodgers BM. Pediatric equestrian injuries: assessing the impact of helmet use. *Pediatrics* 1995;95:487.
130. Jackson DW, Wiltse LL, Cirincione RJ. Spondylolysis in the female gymnast. *Clin Orthop* 1976;117:68.

131. Cantu RC, Voyu R. Second impact syndrome: a risk in any contact sport. *Phys Sports Med* 1995;23:27.
132. Maron BJ, Poliac LC, Kaplan JA, et al. Blunt impact to the chest leading to sudden death from cardiac arrest during sports activities. *N Engl J Med* 1995;333:337.
133. Estes NAM III. Sudden death in young athletes [Editorial]. *N Engl J Med* 1995;333:380.
134. *Roles and responsibilities of the team physician.* Columbus, OH: Academy of Medicine of Columbus and Franklin County; 1989.
135. AAP Committee on Sports Medicine. Steroids. In: *Sports medicine: health care for young athletes.* Evanston, IL: American Academy of Pediatrics; 1983:181.
136. Strauss RH. Anabolic steroids. In: Strauss RH, ed. *Drugs and performance in sports.* Philadelphia: WB Saunders; 1987:59.
137. Brower KJ, Blow FC, Eliopulos GA, et al. Anabolic-androgenic steroids and suicide. *Am J Psychiatry* 1989; 146:1075.
138. Yesalis CE, Kennedy NJ, Kopstein AN, et al. Anabolic-androgenic steroid use in the United States. *JAMA* 1993;270:1217.
139. Dyment PG. The adolescent athlete and ergogenic acids. *Journal of Adolescent Health Care* 1987;8:68.
140. Pope HG, Katz DL, Champoux R. Anabolic-androgenic steroid use among 1,010 college men. *Phys Sports Med* 1988;16:75.
141. Terney R, McLain LG. The use of anabolic steroids in high school students. *American Journal of Diseases of Children* 1990;144:99.
142. Johnson MD, Jay MS, Shoup B, Rickert VI. Anabolic steroid use by male adolescents. *Pediatrics* 1989;83: 921.
143. Bhasin S, Storer TW, Berman N, et al. The effects of supraphysiologic doses of testosterone on muscle size and strength in normal men. *N Engl J Med* 1996;335:1.
144. DuRant RH, Escobedo LG, Heath GW. Anabolic-steroid use, strength training, and multiple drug use among adolescents in the United States. *Pediatrics* 1995;96:23.
145. Middleman AB, Faulkner AH, Woods ER, et al. High-risk behaviors among high school students in Massachusetts who use anabolic steroids. *Pediatrics* 1995;96:268.
146. American College of Sports Medicine. Position statement on anabolic/androgenic steroids. *Sports Medicine Bulletin* 1984;19:8.

SUGGESTED READING

American Academy of Family Physicians, American Academy of Pediatrics, American Medical Society for Sports Medicine, American Orthopaedic Society for Sports Medicine, American Osteopathic Academy of Sports Medicine. *Preparticipation physical evaluation.* 2nd ed. Minneapolis, MN: The Physician and Sportsmedicine, Division of McGraw-Hill; 1992.

American College of Sports Medicine. Position statement on anabolic/androgenic steroids. *Sports Medicine Bulletin* 1984;19:8.

Bonen A, Keizer HA. Athletic menstrual cycle irregularity: endocrine response to exercise and training. *Phys Sports Med* 1984;12:78.

Chandy TA, Grana WA. Secondary school athletic injury in boys and girls: a three year study. *Phys Sports Med* 1985;13:106.

Council on Scientific Affairs. Medical and nonmedical uses of anabolic-androgenic steroids. *JAMA* 1990; 264:2923.

Donahue P. Preparticipation exams: how to detect a teenage crisis. *Phys Sports Med* 1990;18:53.

DuRant RH, Linder CW, Sanders JM, et al. Adolescent females readiness to participate in sports. *Journal of Adolescent Health Care* 1988;9:310.

Dyment PG. The adolescent athlete and ergogenic acids. *Journal of Adolescent Health Care* 1987;8:68.

Dyment PG. Athletic injuries. *Pediatr Rev* 1989;10:291.

Dyment PG. Steroids: breakfast of champions. *Pediatr Rev* 1990;12:103.

Dyment PG, ed. Sports and the adolescent. *Adolescent Medicine: State of the Art Reviews* 1991;2:1.

Emans JB. Upper extremity injuries in sports. In: Micheli LJ, ed. *Pediatric and adolescent sports medicine.* Boston: Little, Brown; 1984:49.

Garrick JG. Anterior knee pain (chondromalacia patellae). *Phys Sports Med* 1989;17:75.

Hergenroeder AC, Garrick JG. Sports medicine. *Pediatr Clin North Am* 1990;37:1021.

Hudson PB. Preparticipation screening of Special Olympics athletes. *Phys Sports Med* 1988;16:97.

Hulse E, Strong WB. Preparticipation evaluation for athletes. *Pediatr Rev* 1987;9:173.

Lane SE. Severe ankle sprains. *Phys Sports Med* 1990;18:43.

McKeag DB. Adolescents and exercise. *Journal of Adolescent Health Care* 1986;7:121S.

McKeag DB, Dolan C. Overuse syndromes of the lower extremity. *Phys Sports Med* 1989;17:108.

Metcalf TS, Bernhardt DT. Evaluating and managing shoulder injury in young athletes. *Contemporary Pediatrics* 1996;13:94.

Moskwa CA Jr, Nicholas JA. Musculoskeletal risk factors in the young athlete. *Phys Sports Med* 1989;17:49.

Murray R. The effects of consuming carbohydrate–electrolyte beverages on gastric emptying and fluid absorption during and following exercise. *Sports Med* 1987;4:322.

Risser WL, Risser JMH. Iron deficiency in adolescents and young adults. *Phys Sports Med* 1990;18:87.

Sullivan JA, Grana WA. *The pediatric athlete.* Park Ridge, IL: American Academy of Orthopedic Surgeons; 1990.

Tomassoni TL, Galioto FM Jr. Cardiologic aspects of adolescent sports medicine. *Seminars in Adolescent Medicine* 1987;3:185.

Tursz A, Crost M. Sports-related injuries in children: a study of their characteristics, frequency, and severity, with comparison to other types of accidental injuries. *Am J Sports Med* 1986;14:294.

7

Practical Adolescent Psychology

It is normal for an adolescent to behave in an inconsistent and unpredictable manner; to deny his impulses and to accept them; to love his parents and to hate them; to be deeply ashamed to acknowledge his mother before others and, unexpectedly, to desire heart to heart talks with her; to thrive on imitation of and identification with others while searching unceasingly for his own identity; to be more idealistic, artistic, generous, and unselfish than he will ever be again, but also the opposite: self-centered, egoistic, calculating. Such fluctuations between extreme opposites would be deemed highly abnormal at any other time of life. At this time they may signify no more than that an adult structure of personality takes a long time to emerge, that the ego of the individual in question does not cease to experiment and is in no hurry to close down on possibilities.

- Anna Freud [1]

NORMAL ADOLESCENCE

Teenagers are the kids that adults love to hate. The history of Western civilization is replete with a litany of complaints about teenagers: from Hesiod's comment that they disrespect their elders to Aristotle's criticism of their lack of "sexual restraint" to Shakespeare's suggestion that they be put into suspended animation until age 23. Adulthood comes approximately 5 years later than most adolescents claim and 5 years before most parents will admit. In some ways, we see our own flaws come to life in our adolescents. As the writer James Baldwin once commented, "Children have never been very good at listening to elders, but they have never failed to imitate them."

Yet we sometimes forget how adolescents have changed the world. Many of the signers of the Declaration of Independence were still in their teens. In the 1960s, it was the student unrest on college campuses that catalyzed public opinion against the Vietnam War. Today, many adults spend literally hours of their day watching adolescents on television, competing in the Olympics or playing college football, basketball, and professional tennis.

What Is Adolescence?

Is adolescence necessary? The short answer to this somewhat facetious question is "no." Adolescence is not a result of raging hormonal tides, nor is it necessarily a time of great turmoil and angst. Adolescence is a *cultural phenomenon* and, as such, must be recognized as an inevitable by-product of adult, Western civilization. Many non-Western societies have no such equivalent (and, therefore, no problem with adolescent acting-out behavior). In these societies, the transition from childhood to adulthood is a rapid and smooth one, usually marked by a *rite of passage*. This could include fasting on a mountain, being tattooed, or even having a circumcision or clitorectomy. But whatever the initiation ceremony, the transition is quickly accomplished and adult obligations are gradually imposed.

By contrast, Western society has no single rite of passage. American teenagers can drive at age 16 but not vote, vote at age 18 but not drink, and drink at age 21 but not necessarily have achieved complete self-sufficiency. These incomplete rites of passage are confusing and may lead teenagers to believe that they have achieved adult status when they have not. Furthermore, we use a sliding scale to determine when one becomes an adult—for example, in the 1930s, Youth Groups were formed to keep adolescents out of the labor market, but in World War II, recruiters looked the other way when underage youngsters wanted to enlist.

With time, American society is giving adolescents less help in making the transition easier. The divorce rate among adults in the United States is the highest among all Western countries. Consequently, an adolescent's friends and peers assume more important roles in their lives, as do adult role models viewed on television [2]. Moreover, despite much data to the contrary, many American adults still believe that sex education in schools and availability of contraceptives make teenagers more likely to engage in early sexual intercourse. Just Say No clubs are far more popular than substantive efforts to educate teenagers about the dangers of early experimentation with sex or drugs [3]. The adolescent suicide rate—which has risen 300% since the 1960s to nearly 13 suicides a day in the United States—may serve as a crude index of adolescent stress in contemporary American society.

Universal Characteristics of Adolescents

Even if contemporary adolescence is considered prolonged (to 15 or 20 years in some cases, compared with colonial times), there is a great deal that must be accomplished in a very short time span. During adolescence, youngsters must strive to:

- Establish independence from parents
- Learn to establish relationships with one's peers and with the opposite sex
- Finish one's formal schooling
- Begin to assess one's place in modern society and formulate plans for a career or job

Given this complicated and difficult set of tasks, certain dynamics of adolescence become more understandable. These dynamics include the following:

- The peer group relationship is prized over all other associations.
- Discontinuity with other generations is nurtured and links with tradition are severed.
- Symbols or hallmarks of the group gain universal acceptance (e.g., music, language, dress).
- A critical, rebellious posture is developed toward established social systems and convention.

Certainly, if the primary goal of adolescence is to define an identity that is independent of one's parents, then many former ties must be broken. Parents may suddenly wonder why their children no longer want to be seen in public with them, let alone spend time with them. Along with this parents-as-lepers syndrome comes a new-found criticism of virtually anything that the parents say or think [4]. As young Anne Frank wrote in her diary [5]: "Why do grown ups quarrel so easily, so much, and over the most idiotic things? . . . I'm simply amazed again and again over their awful manners and especially their stupidity." And Mark Twain wryly observed [6], "When I was 14 I was amazed at how ignorant my father was, but when I reached the age of 21 I was surprised how much he had learned in seven years."

Need for Privacy

Among the nearly universal characteristics of adolescents is the need for privacy. If an identity is to be created and perfected, it requires molding, shaping, and practice. Different identities must be tried out—hence, the resemblance of the stereotypical teenager to a patient with a multiple personalities. At any one time, you may be addressing the child, the teenager, or the adult—all contained within the same rapidly changing body. In private, adolescents can perfect the social masks that they wear. Giving teenagers privacy acknowledges respect for this process and lets them know that they do have a life of their own, apart from their parents.

Peer Group

If the average teenager is to be successful at breaking away from his parents, he will need a new superego figure. The peer group fills the void. Young teenagers with fragile, emerging identities cannot be satisfied with what they think about themselves; they need external validation. In addition, the need for popularity has already been learned from one's parents. Indeed, parents are usually just as anxious about their teenagers' popularity as the teens themselves, although parents are likely to regard nearly every other adolescent as a potentially bad influence. Although peer pressure is a real phenomenon, particularly among early adolescents (ages 12–14 years), it may be overrated. First, there are a variety of peer groups with which a young adolescent can identify. To a great extent, their choice of peer group is predetermined by how much self-reliance and self-esteem they have been endowed with during their preteen years [4]. Contrary to many parents' fears, there is not merely one Adolescent Peer Group, comprised of sex-crazed, beer-swilling juvenile delinquents, that begins circling one's house after dark once the children reach adolescence.

Fads

Fads are a necessary but paradoxical component of adolescence. It does seem odd that a teenager who wishes to assert his or her individuality does so by conforming to whatever ridiculous fad is prevalent at the time (e.g., torn jeans, earrings, a particular brand of sneakers). However, fads enable adolescents to distinguish themselves from their parents. Thus, if Mom and Dad frequently watched Music Television (MTV) and were particularly enamored of Smashing Pumpkins and Pearl Jam, it is likely that their teenage offspring would prefer "Masterpiece Theatre" and Chopin. In fact, one reason for the increased popularity of heavy metal music in the past decade may be that this formerly fringe type of rock 'n' roll music is all that's left to the children of parents who grew up listening to The Beatles and The Rolling Stones.

Idealism and Narcissism

Adolescence is simultaneously a time of intense idealism and extreme narcissism. When teenagers complain about being misunderstood, they frequently mean that adults are failing to see their idealistic side. Groucho Marx once quipped that he would never want to join a club that would have him as a member. Teenagers, too, are investigating the club that they will soon join—adult society—and they do not always like what they see. In literature, such classic characters as Huckleberry Finn and Holden Caulfield have demonstrated this *weltschmerz* or "world pain." At the same time, teenagers must be extremely narcissistic if they are to succeed in creating a coherent identity for themselves. For example, such egocentrism will lead a teenage daughter to complain to her mother, "Oh, Mom, you just don't know how it feels to be in love!"

Idiosyncratic Thinking

By age 16 years, 70% of teenagers are capable of sequential logical thinking (the last, adult stage of cognitive operational thought, according to Piaget) [7]. Without formal operational thinking, a girl would not be able to conceive of the possibility of becoming pregnant, for example, if she were to engage in sexual intercourse. Yet teenagers still suffer from idiosyncratic thought processes that may interfere with optimal health care. According to Elkind [8], they frequently demonstrate "pseudostupidity": "The capacity to conceive many different alternatives is not immediately coupled with the ability to assign priorities and to decide which choice is more or less appropriate than others." In a sense, young adolescents may appear stupid because they are too bright, but certainly they should not be blamed for failing at something of which they are psychologically incapable (e.g., using contraception at a young age).

Already preoccupied with their rapidly changing bodies, teenagers may also become obsessed with their newly acquired logical abilities. Consequently, they begin to believe that everyone is thinking about what they are thinking about—themselves! This belief constitutes the *imaginary audience* and explains much adolescent behavior [9]. The need to play to the "imaginary audience" helps to explain the extreme self-consciousness of the adolescent. At the same time, teenagers want to be looked at and thought about because that confirms their sense of self-worth [10]. They see themselves as actors in their own *personal fable*, and their lives assume heroic proportions. As The Girl in *The Fantasticks* sings: "I am special. I am special. Please, God, *please*: Don't let me be normal" [11]. Such egocentricity explains how a 16-year-old girl can counsel her best friend to use birth control if she has intercourse yet not use it herself: the 16-year-old believes "it can't happen to me."

Teenagers with chronic illnesses may feel that they do not have to take their medicines. In deference to the imaginary audience, they do not want to appear different, but, at the same time, they think that they are different and can cope quite well without treatment (although others with the same disease should, of course, be compliant with treatment). In the same fashion, risk-taking behavior appears much less risky if teens believe that they are invulnerable. These behaviors infuriate adults, who think that teenagers are acting irresponsibly; in fact, the real issue involved is cognitive processing and maturation, not willfulness.

Ambivalence About Growing Up

Many teens have a real ambivalence about growing up and becoming an adult. On the one hand, they desperately want all of the rights and privileges of being an adult (e.g., using the car, no curfew). On the other hand, they loathe the responsibilities attached to the privileges. Whereas parents view the ability to bear responsibility as a mark of maturity, their teenagers view responsibility as something that is imposed by adults and therefore a degrading token of their inferior status. Often, grandparents have greater success in dealing with teenagers than parents simply because they are more ready to acknowledge that the child is growing up.

Physical Characteristics

As if all of these psychological idiosyncrasies were not enough, there is also the physical side of adolescence for young people to contend with. Both boys and girls are maturing faster in the 20th century than ever before: American girls menstruate at an average age of 12.6 years, and English boys' voices change at an average age of 13.3 years (compared with 18 years in Bach's 18th-century choirs) [12–14]. This produces the difficult situation of young people who are marginally able to cope with the world intellectually and experientially but who nevertheless possess the biologic ability to reproduce at a very young age—"babies having babies," as it has been labeled in the mass media. Yet what most adults fail to understand is teens do not mature early by choice: the accelerated rate of sexual maturation in the past century is correlated directly with better nutrition and medical care and higher socioeconomic standards in Western nations. In other words, earlier maturation is a by-product of Western civilization and technology.

Adolescents sometimes display remarkable *asynchrony* in their own growth. Arms, legs, noses, and breasts seem to sprout up with total disregard for overall proportions or symmetry. In addition, although there is a wide age range over which normal development takes place, where one fits in the spectrum may be crucially important. A unique longitudinal research project, the Oakland Growth Study, followed the 16 most and least advanced (by bone age) young men and women in a public school far into their adulthood [15]. They found that early-maturing males were more poised, relaxed, popular, and self-confident than late maturers, who tended to be more restless, impulsive, and have childish social techniques. In fact, the single best predictor of adult male social success was the rate of skeletal development during adolescence. For women, the early maturers suffered and were below average in prestige, popularity, cheerfulness, and leadership. Such work confirmed what many high school educators already knew: the early-maturing young men become the successful athletes and school leaders, but the early-maturing young women are frequently ridiculed. The significance of such research extends beyond the obvious findings: The study demonstrates that even normal physiologic adolescence may have extremely important and lifelong psychological consequences. Clinicians need to appreciate this *variability* in normal growth and assess the potential repercussions.

Is Adolescent Turmoil Normal?

Research has disputed the notion that teenagers must experience a difficult adolescence. Some psychologists have gone so far as to claim that the notion of adolescent turmoil as being normative is "a myth" [16]. In particular, Offer et al. examined psychological questionnaire data across three decades (1960s through 1980s) and found that the rate of behavioral disturbance among adolescents is the same as among people at other parts of the life cycle [17]. Nonetheless, even Offer et al. caution that clinicians should not underestimate the severity of adolescent problems.

The national Youth Risk Behavior Survey adds even more fuel to the controversy. Using a representative sample of more than 10,000 9th- through 12th-grade students nationwide, this survey revealed remarkable threats to the health and well-being of American teenagers [18]:

- More than 21% of students rarely if ever use a seat belt when they ride in a car driven by someone else. In the 30 days before being surveyed, more than one third reported riding with a driver who had been drinking alcohol.
- Nearly 40% of the students had been in a physical fight during the previous 12 months, for a prevalence rate of 127 fighting incidents per 100 students per year. Male students were far more likely to have been in a fight (46.1%) than female students (30.6%).
- More than one third (37.9%) of the students had had sexual intercourse during the 3 months before the survey. Eighteen percent had had four or more sexual partners. In an earlier version of this survey, 25% of the girls reported that someone had tried to force them to have sexual relations during the past year [19].
- During the previous 30 days, one fifth of students (20%) nationwide had carried a weapon to school; 8% had carried a gun. One student in 22 reported missing at least 1 day of school in the previous 30 days because they either felt unsafe at school or traveling to or from school.
- Suicidal ideation and behavior were common. Nearly one fourth of students (24%) had seriously considered attempting suicide in the previous year, 17% had actually made a plan, and 8.7% had made an attempt.
- Nearly 60% of the girls were currently dieting at the time of the survey, and one third of all students felt that they were overweight. Nearly 9% of girls reported using diet pills, and 7% had tried either self-induced vomiting or laxatives.
- Nationwide, 86% of students had been taught about AIDS or human immunodeficiency virus (HIV) infection in their schools. An earlier survey had found that nearly half of all the students thought that donating blood increases the likelihood of becoming infected with HIV, and over half were unsure or believed that "washing after having sex" decreases the likelihood of infection [18].

Despite these noticeable threats to adolescent health, an average of only one third to one half of teenagers had received any instruction in school about these major health areas (Fig. 1). The notable exception was for alcohol and drugs, where nearly 90% of students reported school programs. Clearly, the "just say no" mentality is alive and well in the United States, and just as clearly, it will not protect teenagers against the most significant threats to their health and well-being [3]. Whether teenagers have to suffer through adolescence is still a matter of controversy and debate, but the threats to their health are probably unparalleled in the history of the Western world [20] (Table 1).

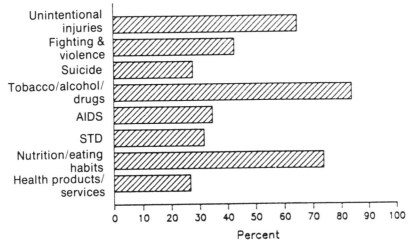

FIG. 1. Percentage of students participating in the National Adolescent Student Health Survey who reported having received school instruction in major health areas. More than 11,000 8th- and 10th-grade students in 20 states were surveyed. AIDS, acquired immunodeficiency syndrome; STD, sexually transmitted disease. (From Centers for Disease Control and Prevention. Results from the National Adolescent Student Health Survey. *MMWR Morb Mortal Wkly Rep* 1989;38:147.)

TABLE 1. *Leading causes of death for men, aged 15 to 34 years: United States, 1991*

Cause	Number	Percentage
Unintentional injury	23,108	32%
Homicide	13,122	18%
Suicide	9,434	13%
AIDS	8,661	12%
Cancer	3,699	5%
Other	13,234	19%

From Centers for Disease Control and Prevention. Homicides among 15–19-year-old males: United States, 1963–1991. *MMWR Morb Mortal Wkly Rep* 1994;43:725.

Counseling Parents

Adolescence is an age of paradoxes, "the best of times and the worst of times." Yet few parents exist who actually look forward to their children's adolescence with great enthusiasm [4,21]. Clinicians can make an important contribution to their patients' health by helping to anticipate some of the problems associated with normal adolescence and counseling parents prophylactically [22].

Psychiatric research demonstrates that most (80%) teenagers survive adolescence with little or no difficulty; only 20% of adolescents suffer from a significant mental or emotional disorder [17]. Interestingly, the notion that adolescence is a period of turmoil is *conditional*: one researcher reviewed 100 years of articles and found that in times of economic depression, adolescents were viewed as immature and in need of more education, whereas during wartime, their psychological competence was suddenly recognized [23]. Another researcher's "baby-boom-baby-bust" theory states that the greater the number of adolescents in proportion to the general population in the United States, the more problems adolescents will have [24]. What the latest research [17] demonstrates, rather, is that people's *opinions* of adolescents probably deteriorate as the number of adolescents increases.

Many important principles need to be conveyed to parents of preteenagers and teenagers, but the most crucial is that only about 15% of teens and their parents experience a disruption in their relationship; most teenagers survive adolescence healthy and intact [17,25]:

* Much of what happens during adolescence is probably already preordained by what has occurred during childhood [4]. In other words, a child who has been taught to be self-reliant and independent and who carries a strong sense of self-esteem is unlikely to suffer a disastrous adolescence. The years between ages 5 to 10 may be absolutely crucial to determining how much turmoil an adolescent will have to experience.
* Similarly, when their children turn 12 or 13 years, parents cannot suddenly "immunize" them against all of the threats they are likely to begin encountering. Sex education, drug education, and discussions about morality and responsibility all should have begun well before adolescence begins. Parents often forget that their youngster has been exposed to over a decade of parental guidance and influence. Although at times it may appear that they have lost control over them, this anxiety is more illusory than real.
* Because parents will no longer be with the teenager at all times or be able to anticipate all of the problems she may encounter, they need to focus their efforts on helping her develop the critical thinking and independent judgment that will permit her to cope with any new situation.

There are four factors that lead to the production of independent, mature young adults rather than adolescent rebels [26,27]: 1) good family communication, 2) enhancing the teenager's self-image, 3) teaching effective decision making, and 4) implementing effective discipline.

There are striking parallels between these basic tenets and the principles elucidated in the pediatric resiliency literature [28,29]. *Mahskroosbarn* is Swedish for "dandelion child," a child who can grow and thrive anywhere. Given the complexities of modern society, parents need to understand how to raise their children to be "unbreakable." In numerous studies examining how children survive international tragedies (war, poverty, famine), researchers have found that those who were successful in overcoming the stresses of their environment had easy, responsive temperaments, experienced considerable social support from friends and relatives, and had an individual sense of purpose and identity. According to Boyce et al. [29], this all adds up to the child or teenager being able to answer four important questions:

- Who am I?
- Am I loved?
- Whom can I count on?
- What am I here for?

Good Family Communication

Family therapy emphasizes good family communication. Good relationships between parents and teenagers result in positive emotional growth and healthy self-esteem [30]. Young teens who feel secure in their relationships with their parents tend to report good relationships with teachers at school and have positive attitudes about learning [31]. Conversely, teens with poor rapport with their parents are more likely to have school problems, drug and alcohol use, delinquent acts, and early sexual activity [32–34].

Whether a family is functional or dysfunctional may depend on the *clarity*, *completeness*, and *congruence* of the communications among its members. The mother who tells her daughter to be home before dark and then is angry when the daughter returns home in the evening, although the daughter insists that it was still light when she left her friend's house and, in fact, it is not quite dark yet, has not exhibited *clarity*. If the mother had changed her message to "Please be home by 5 o'clock," the entire conflict would have been avoided. An example of *incomplete communication* is the father who criticizes his son for not trimming the hedges after cutting the lawn—not that he had specifically asked his son to do it, but the father assumes the youngster should have known anyway. *Congruence* is the extent to which verbal communication matches nonverbal communication. The mother with a repressive upbringing who tries to tell her teenage daughter how wonderful marital sex is will probably fail because her daughter may spot the tension in her voice or her signs of embarrassment—incongruent communication. She can succeed by prefacing her talk with admitting how uncomfortable she is with the topic and explaining how she does not want her daughter to have the same anxieties about sex that she had.

Enhancing the Teenager's Self-Image

Self-esteem, unfortunately, has become the catchword of the 1990s. Educators and health professionals talk about it as if it were contained in a vial and could be administered to children like a vaccine. One's self-image begins forming long before adolescence. In fact, its formation could be said to begin before the child's conception, as reflected in his or her parents' own self-perceptions, their attitude toward themselves and their future, and their temperament. Freud [35] asserted that the ego is based in the body and therefore is most completely shaped in the first year of life. Erickson [36] agreed that the development of self-image begins early, but emphasized that it accelerates during adolescence and represents the most crucial developmental task during those years.

Parents can enhance a child's self-esteem by knowing themselves and their feelings, by serving as role models for their children, and by finding a positive niche for each child. Every child has some area in which he or she is talented or unique [4,22].

An important corollary to this is to learn how to criticize or to be angry. Parents are entitled to be angry and should express their feelings, taking heed of one major caveat—*never attack*! Anger without insult is crucial to the preservation of a teenager's self-esteem. When things go wrong, that is not the ideal time to tell a teenager anything negative about his personality or character. Dealing with the situation at hand is far more important and rewarding. Likewise, learning how to praise a child is extremely important. Remember that praise represents an evaluation by someone sitting in judgment. Consequently, parents should praise efforts and accomplishments, not personality or character [26].

Decision Making

How parents balance the goals of allowing adolescents autonomy in decision making while, at the same time, maintaining control and setting appropriate limits is a particularly difficult part of raising adolescents. Parents must decide what is negotiable and what is not. If something is nonnegotiable, it should be clearly stated to the adolescent as a rule of the house. As long as the number of such rules is not too large and they are not grossly different from other parents' rules in the community, reluctant compliance can be expected. For example, there should probably be a rule in every American household that television viewing does not begin until all homework is completed [2].

The negotiable areas provide the best learning ground for honing decision-making skills. Parents still control the final decision, but "we value your input" can be a very effective phrase, especially if parents do give the teenager's opinion serious consideration and weight. Such traditionally controversial areas as chores, allowances, and curfews can be negotiated and compromises can be made, rather than being handled in a dictatorial fashion. Giving teenagers choices within choices is extremely important [26]: it is far easier to foster cooperation by giving someone a set of possible choices than to announce a single option and insist on its being carried out. No one likes to be presented with a *fait accompli* over which he or she has no control. Giving teens a set of alternatives from which they can choose—a "corral"—allows them the freedom they desire but enables the parents to set the crucial boundaries.

A democratic family allows teenagers choices that stimulate their decision-making skills and help avoid angry confrontations. For example, in many households chores are done in a "prison warden–prison convict" fashion, if at all. Much more can be accomplished by telling teenagers what needs to be done and setting appropriate deadlines, but allowing the teen to do it in any order he or she chooses.

Discipline

Discipline represents another much-maligned and misused area of parenting. Although parents usually associate discipline with punishment, in fact positive reinforcement is a far more effective mode of disciplining than negative reinforcement. Still, parents frequently reject the notion of having to "bribe" their children [37]. Therefore, punishment becomes an important topic. One must remember that not all punishments are created equal, and the goal of punishment is to modify future behavior, not to hurt the child.

When is punishment appropriately used? When children have some sense that they have done wrong, when they have respect for the punisher, and *when the punishment fits the crime*, punishment may be effective. In the case of a child who fails to do his homework and is grounded for a month, the punishment represents an unpleasant experience but it also has no logical or timely connection to the undesired behavior. On the other hand, establishing a new rule of the house that homework must be completed before watching television or using the telephone, especially if these are major reasons why she had not been doing her homework, may make more sense to (and have a greater impact on) the teenager. Likewise, preventing a star athlete from competing because he or she talks back to a parent or comes in after a curfew may serve only to eliminate one of the prime sources of that teenager's self-esteem and increase resentment of the parents without teaching any lesson. Important rules of punishing include the following:

- Never punish in anger.
- Effective punishment is administered as quickly as possible.
- The punishment should be no worse and no longer than necessary to eliminate the probability that the undesired behavior will recur.
- If possible, the teenager should be able to express his or her opinion about types of punishment.
- Punishment should be consistently applied.
- Only the teenager should be punished, not the rest of the family.
- The punishment should focus on the misbehavior itself and not on the perpetrator. Punishments that denigrate young people tend to become self-fulfilling prophecies.

There are many other important lessons that many parents may not recognize or understand [4,21,22,26,27,38,39]:

1. Parents must learn to acknowledge the inevitable: their children are growing up. The sooner parents accept the teenager's impending adulthood, the sooner he or she will assume the role. Therefore, acknowledgments of maturity cannot be coupled with reproaches such as, "I'm surprised at you" or "When I was your age . . ..." Such phrases bring instant deafness to teenage ears.
2. There is no way to win a war with one's children.

3. Parents need to learn how to listen to their teenagers, always conveying respect and trying to preserve their self-esteem. Acknowledging feelings can be a tremendously powerful tool. On the other hand, denying a teen's perceptions can be counterproductive, even if the parent knows better. Experience is not something that can be gift-wrapped and given to teenagers, like a Christmas present. Parents know that the end of the world is not imminent simply because their teenager did not make the basketball squad or the cheerleading team, but to the teenager it *feels* that way. Telling a disappointed teen "You'll have many more chances in life" is not effective or empathetic, despite the fact that it may be true.

4. When it comes to their teenagers' behavior, parents need to learn to tolerate much but sanction little. Teenagers in the 1990s have tremendous freedom. Parents can use that freedom to their advantage by trusting their children to do the right thing. They should not rescind a privilege because it is abused the first time it is used: mistakes are to be expected. The average teenager is going to try things that the parents do not know about in advance or would judge too risky; parents must simply trust in the 10 or 15 years they have already invested in their children and hope for the best.

   One common example of tolerating but not sanctioning certain behavior is the mother who brings her teenage daughter to the doctor's office because the latter has begun having sexual intercourse with her boyfriend. The mother may give a strong message of disapproval of premarital or early sex but, at the same time, she acknowledges the daughter's ability to conduct her own life and wants to protect her by having her examined and placed on appropriate birth control.

5. In their apparent disregard for any adult's opinion (especially their parents'), adolescents sometimes resemble catatonic schizophrenics. They act as if they are not listening to what is being said, yet they can often repeat it word for word. Parents need to realize that if they take the time to explain their own philosophy to their teenagers, the teens will inevitably have to deal with what is being said and incorporate it into their own lives. Nonetheless, the teenager's philosophy and future behavior may not exactly match the parent's.

Office Practice and Counseling

Incorporating Adolescent Patients in an Office Practice

Adolescents make rewarding patients [40–43], but attention must be paid to their unique physical and psychological needs. Clinicians who understand the basics of caring for teenage patients can go far in improving the health care of their adolescent patients [44]. However, to use pediatricians as an example, those who are currently practicing did not always receive adequate training in adolescent medicine during their residencies. A 1992 study surveyed 3,000 pediatricians who had completed their residency training since the American Academy of Pediatrics' Task Force on Pediatric Education Report in 1978 [45]. Among the more recent graduates (completing training since 1984), the following percentages of pediatricians found their residency training experiences to be insufficient in the listed areas:

Care of adolescents 51%
Psychosocial problems 50%
Interviewing and counseling 33%
School health 61%
Child advocacy 44%

Sadly, if the pediatric experience holds true for other primary care physicians, studies show that the next generation of physicians also is not gaining enough training in adolescent medicine, nor is it very fond of teenagers as patients. A recent national survey of 715 pediatric house officers in 65 different programs found that only 20% had had a structured experience in adolescent medicine during medical school, compared with 70% in neonatology. Although half of the respondents expected to enter practice, 77% identified adolescents and young adults as the age group they least enjoyed working with. Only 12% identified teens as the group they most enjoyed [46]. Similarly, a 1995 survey of 277 incoming pediatric residents found that 11% believe that making birth control available to teens condones their sexual activity, 24% would not include abortion counseling when seeing a pregnant teen, and 31% believe that homosexuality is abnormal [47]. Until academic medicine gets serious about adolescent medicine, the situation likely will continue [48].

Office Environment

Although it is not mandatory, a separate waiting area goes a long way to assuring the adolescent patient that he or she has a separate identity and the practitioner he or she is about to see is no longer "just a baby doctor." Office walls that are plastered with Disney and *Sesame Street* characters do not inspire the confidence of the average adolescent patient; nor does waiting room literature consisting solely of *Ladies Home Journal* or *Curious George*.

More important than the office surroundings is the attitude of office personnel. Many receptionists and nurses do not like adolescents, and they communicate their feelings very quickly and effectively to prospective patients. When office personnel smile at cute babies but groan when they see a teenage girl who needs a pelvic examination, good reviews from the patient are not likely. Although they may not personally approve of premarital sexual activity, for example, office personnel need to understand that they are providing a vital health service and should be tolerant of adolescent patients who may be engaging in activities that the staff, as parents, might not condone.

Patient–Practitioner Rapport

Of paramount importance is the need to guarantee the confidentiality of health care visits, unless the teenager is actively suicidal or homicidal. Telling a teenager that "what you tell me will stay in this room, between us, unless you are about to harm yourself or someone else" is a powerful and important tool in dealing with adolescent problems. Just as parents must learn to respect their teenager's newfound sense of privacy, physicians must respect confidentiality.

Several studies demonstrate that confidentiality is the single most crucial issue for teenagers, yet physicians frequently fail to discuss it with their patients [49–51]. A 1993 survey of nearly 1,300 9th through 12th graders found that 58% reported having health concerns that they wished to keep private from their parents, and 25% reported that they would forego health care in some situations if it meant that their parents might find out [49]. Although physicians' assurances of confidentiality do increase adolescents' willingness to disclose sensitive information about sex, substance abuse, and mental health issues [50], only 56% of 1,210 primary care physicians in California reported discussing it with their patients [51].

Another key issue for practitioners is compliance. Because adolescents at differing levels of maturity cannot be expected to act similarly, compliance can vary greatly. Failures should be expected and should be accepted philosophically. By their very nature, teenagers sometimes engage in risk-taking behaviors that are not in their own best interests, even after a physician has counseled them appropriately.

In eliciting the history, how questions are phrased can determine what sort of answers are received. Young adolescents tend to be very concrete in their thinking, so questions must be phrased at their level (Table 2). In addition, many clinicians prefer to question their patients directly, rather than using impersonal questionnaires [52].

TABLE 2. *The importance of phrasing questions properly*

Bad: How do you get along with your parents?
Expected answer: Okay
Good: Who lives at home with you? Do you like them?
Reason: More specific. Elicits more environmental history. Parents may be divorced or deceased.

Bad: How are you doing at school?
Expected answer: Fine.
Good: What grades do you get at school? Do you like school? What is your best subject?
Reason: More specific. Acknowledges the teenager as an individual, with his or her own preferences.

Bad: Are you sexually active?
Expected (comic) answer: No, I just lie there.
Good: Are you having sex with anyone?
Reason: Unclear what "sexually active" means. Good question does not discriminate between homosexual and heterosexual activity.

Adapted from Goldenring JM, Cohen E. Getting into adolescent heads. *Contemporary Pediatrics* 1988;5:75.

Other important aspects of the clinician's interaction with adolescents include [44]:

- Ensuring the shortest possible delay in the patients' being seen. Teenagers have high anxiety levels and low tolerance for frustration.
- Seeing the patient alone first, or with the parents and then alone. If both are being seen together, it is important for the physician to introduce himself or herself to the adolescent *first*; after all, the adolescent is the patient, not the parent.
- Making the teenager feel that the clinician has a genuine interest in him or her as a person. Asking questions about the teenager's social environment (using the the HEADDS inventory or the West Virginia University Adolescent Risk Score) [52,53] facilitates this.
- Avoiding the twin pitfalls of being overly judgmental or too authoritarian. This does not mean, however, that the clinician should be shy about pointing out potentially harmful health behaviors to the teen, but such discussions should be confined to the realm of medicine, not philosophy or morality.
- Being honest with the adolescent.
- Speaking to the adolescent patient in the physician's own (normal) language, rather than trying to mimic whatever adolescent lingo the physician thinks is current.

Ideally, physicians and nurses can be strong advocates for adolescent patients and can be important sources of guidance in their lives. Adolescents make enjoyable patients and, unlike infants, are able to communicate their feelings to the practitioner. Appropriate and well timed interventions can preserve the health of many adolescents and provide great satisfaction to physicians who incorporate adolescents into their practice. But clinicians must understand and be sensitive to the basic principles of adolescent medicine and adolescent psychology to be successful in treating such patients [54,55].

The Primary Care Practitioner as Counselor

Primary care clinicians are ideally suited for counseling, as long as they understand the basic principles of adolescent psychology and can recognize their own prejudices and limitations [56,57]. With a good child or adolescent psychiatrist or psychologist available for consultation and liaison [58], the practitioner can undertake brief intervention and counseling with teenagers who have minor mental health disorders. Many adolescents resist referral to psychiatrists or psychologists for fear that their imaginary audience will label them as "mental cases" [10]. In addition, in many communities, only adult psychiatrists are available to see adolescent patients and, like other practitioners who specialize in adult patients, they may vary widely in their interest and skill with teenagers.

If the practitioner decides to undertake counseling in his or her office practice, a few principles should be observed. First, *counseling is not psychotherapy*. Although the prime issues of transference and countertransference are inevitably present in a counseling relationship, they are not used in the explicit way that they are in more formal psychotherapy. Teenagers benefit from counseling because they see an interested and attractive adult role model spending time with them and listening to their problems and concerns. Although the amount of actual insight generated in counseling may vary according to the baseline intelligence of the patient, self-esteem is generated according to the therapeutic bond that develops between counselor and patient.

Counseling for psychological problems should be distinguished from routine health counseling. The latter exists squarely within the purview of all primary care practitioners, although they often choose not to do it [59] (Table 3).

Patients should be carefully selected and screened for counseling, and treatment should be brief (less than 6 months in duration, no more than once a week in frequency). If clinicians have any doubts about their ability to deal with a particular patient, consultation with a child or adolescent psychiatrist, psychologist, or social worker should be sought. The ideal patient is one with an adjustment reaction of adolescence, rather than a teenager with a severe depression, borderline personality, or psychosis. However, at times, despite a clinician's self-doubts, a supportive mental health specialist may still want the clinician to serve as the primary caregiver, while the mental health specialist provides the necessary supervision.

Counseling time should be sacred. Phone calls and other interruptions should not be allowed. Many practitioners find that they can accomplish this only at the end of the day or on Saturdays, but counseling sessions interspersed throughout the day may also serve to vary the clinician's practice and enliven the day.

TABLE 3. *Are physicians counseling teenagers about their health concerns?*

Topic	Percentage of students reporting no counseling	
	Male	Female
Suicide	91	89
Breast/testicular self-examination	**90**	**53**
Seat belt use	89	91
Contraception	**89**	**70**
Eating disorders	**88**	**75**
Cigarette smoking	81	70
Alcohol use	83	76
Sexually transmitted diseases	80	78
Weight control	**71**	**54**

Survey of 362 college freshman.
Boldface indicates statistically significant differences.
Adapted from Joffe A, Radius S, Gall M. Health counseling for adolescents: what they want, what they get, and who gives it. *Pediatrics* 1988;82:481.

Practitioners who do office counseling should bill for their services according to the amount of time spent [40]. Typically, counseling sessions may last 30 to 45 minutes. Although pediatricians should not expect to realize the same income as psychiatrists, for example, they should still be able to bill according to their usual cost per unit time.

Counseling is an active, not a passive process. The stereotypical "How-does-that-make-you-feel?" passive psychiatric approach is doomed to failure with most adolescents, who cannot tolerate much uncertainty or silence in such a session. Good counseling requires efforts actively to engage the adolescent in discussion and reflection: ventilation, problem definition and exploration, definition and exploration of options, and provision of ongoing support all are key aspects of the process [60].

Case 1

A 15-year-old girl is brought in by her parents: they dislike her new boyfriend, they are worried about her declining school performance, and family arguments have increased to the point that she is threatening to run away. The teenager, seen separately, reports that her parents do not trust her and that she is angry and depressed about living at home. Weekly counseling sessions are set up, with the teenager being seen first for 30 minutes, followed by a session with the parents for 30 minutes. Because the teenager is sexually active, she is referred to an office colleague for a pelvic examination and confidential birth control counseling. After 6 weeks, the parents and teenager are seen together for four more sessions. After 10 counseling sessions, the teenager is able to accept that some of her behavior has been provocative, and the parents are willing to set more appropriate limits. Everyone has had a chance to ventilate his or her feelings, both in private and to each other. The teenager's grades begin to improve in school, but she continues to see her boyfriend and have intercourse. However, she does take her birth control pills as prescribed.

Case 2

A 14-year-old boy is referred from school for vandalism. He is extremely bright but repeatedly gets into trouble. His grades vary from A's to D's, depending on whether the teachers penalize him for his behavior. His parents report that he "hangs around with the wrong crowd," and indeed he reports that some of his friends indulge in drinking, drugs, and street fights. He denies suicidal ideation. Weekly counseling sessions are established, and he gradually begins to trust his counselor. His parents are having increasing marital difficulties, he feels that he is overweight and not developing according to plan, and he dislikes school because it is "boring." He does, however, have a number of hobbies, including electronics and model cars, and the counselor encourages him to bring in some of his favorite items. His parents are encouraged to provide more structure in his environment, and they talk to school officials about giving him more vocational training. They are also referred for marriage counseling. He is seen weekly for 6 weeks, then once a month for 6 months, with gradual improvement in his school behavior, although the parents do eventually get a divorce.

Case 3

A 13-year-old girl is referred from adolescent clinic because her mother complains that she is "lying all the time and seems depressed." The teenager is well developed for her age and is extremely provocative, although she does not yet have a boyfriend and is not sexually active. She is intelligent and verbal and says that she "hates her parents." Her mother is a busy real estate agent and rarely has time for her. Her father is an electrical engineer and is dominated by his wife. Weekly counseling sessions are established, and the teenager seems to be relating well to her counselor. After six sessions, however, she informs her counselor that she is going to kill herself. Asked about a plan, she informs him that she has a bottle of her father's sleeping pills and is going to swallow them all that evening. The clinician explains that he is going to have to breach her confidentiality and tell the mother (although this does not seem to disturb the teenager). She is referred to a child psychiatrist and is hospitalized on an adolescent unit for a week-long stay, after which the child psychiatrist and counselor continue treatment as cotherapists with her.

Other Considerations

Office counseling can be extremely rewarding and challenging. Although there are virtually no legal risks involved in counseling a "mature minor" without parental consent [61], it stands to reason that the clinician will want parental involvement, not only for billing purposes but because many adolescent problems have their roots in the parent–child relationship. Techniques can be learned from the adolescent medicine literature, as well as at national meetings or by participating as a cotherapist with a psychiatrist or psychologist. On both an intellectual and an emotional level, counseling can rejuvenate clinicians suffering from burnout, but, as in all aspects of medicine, the clinician needs to be careful not to exceed his or her own ability.

REFERENCES

1. Freud A. Adolescence. *Psychoanal Study Child* 1958;13:255.
2. Strasburger VC. *Adolescents and the media: medical and psychological impact.* Thousand Oaks, CA: Sage; 1995.
3. Strasburger VC. Prevention of adolescent drug abuse: Why "Just Say No" just won't work. *J Pediatr* 1989;114:676.
4. Strasburger VC. *Getting your kids to say no in the '90s when you said yes in the '60s.* New York: Fireside/Simon & Schuster; 1993.
5. Frank A. *The diary of Anne Frank.* New York: Doubleday; 1989.
6. Zall PM, ed. *Mark Twain laughing: humorous anecdotes by and about Samuel L. Clemens.* Knoxville, TN: University of Tennessee Press; 1987.
7. Piaget J. Intellectual evolution from adolescence to adulthood. *Human Development* 1972;15:1.
8. Elkind D. Understanding the young adolescent. *Adolescence* 1978;13:127.
9. Elkind D. Egocentrism in adolescence. *Child Dev* 1967;38:1025.
10. Elkind D. Teenage thinking: implications for health care. *Pediatric Nursing* 1984;1:383.
11. Jones H, Schmidt H. *The fantasticks.* New York: Avon; 1968.
12. Zacharias L, Wurtman RJ. Age at menarche: genetics and environment. *N Engl J Med* 1969;280:868.
13. Wyshak G, Frisch RE. Evidence for a secular trend in age of menarche. *N Engl J Med* 1982;306:1033.
14. Berger KS. *The developing person.* New York: Worth Publishers; 1980.
15. Gross RT, Duke PM. The effect of early versus late physical maturation on adolescent behavior. *Pediatr Clin North Am* 1980;27:71.
16. Zylke JW. Characterizing health adolescent development: distinguishing it from possible disturbances. *JAMA* 1989;262:880.
17. Offer D, Ostrov E, Howard KI. Adolescence: what is normal? *American Journal of Diseases of Children* 1989;143:731.
18. Centers for Disease Control and Prevention. Youth risk behavior surveillance: United States, 1995. *MMWR Morb Mortal Wkly Rep* 1996;45(SS-4):1.

19. Centers for Disease Control and Prevention. Results from the national adolescent student health survey. *MMWR Morb Mortal Wkly Rep* 1989;38:147.
20. Sells CW, Blum RW. Morbidity and mortality among US adolescents: an overview of data and trends. *Am J Public Health* 1996;86:513.
21. Elkind D. *Parenting your teenager in the 90's.* Rosemont, NJ: Modern Learning Press; 1993.
22. Comerci GD, Daniel WA Jr, eds. Parenting the adolescent. *Adolescent Medicine: State of the Art Reviews* 1991;2:251.
23. Enright RD, Levy VM Jr, Harris D, et al. Do economic conditions influence how theorists view adolescents? *Journal of Youth and Adolescence* 1987;16:541.
24. Easterlin RA. *Birth and fortune.* New York: Basic Books; 1980.
25. Peterson AC, Leffert N. What is special about adolescence? In: Rutter M, ed. *Psychosocial disturbances in young people: challenges for prevention.* Cambridge, England: Cambridge University Press; 1994.
26. Leiman AH, Strasburger VC. Counseling parents of adolescents. *Pediatrics* 1985;76(Suppl):664.
27. Ginott HG. *Between parent and teenager.* New York: Macmillan; 1965.
28. Garmezy N. Resilience in children's adaptation to negative life events and stressed environments. *Pediatr Ann* 1991;20:459.
29. Boyce WT, Barr RG, Zeltzer LK, eds. Collection of papers from the William T. Grant Foundation Research Consortium on the Developmental Psychobiology of Stress. *Pediatrics* 1992;90(Suppl):483.
30. Flannery DJ, Torquati JC, Lindemeier L. The method and meaning of emotional expression and experience during adolescence. *Journal of Adolescent Research* 1994;9:8.
31. Ryan RM, Stiller JD, Lynch JH. Representations of relationships to teachers, parents and friends as predictors of academic motivation and self-esteem. *Journal of Early Adolescence* 1994;14:226.
32. Whitbeck LB, Hoyt DR, Miller M, et al. Parental support, depressed affect and sexual experience among adolescents. *Youth and Society* 1992;24:166.
33. Licitra-Kleckler DM, Waas GA. Perceived social support among high-stress adolescents: the role of peers and family. *Journal of Adolescent Research* 1993;8:381.
34. Yancy WS. Juvenile delinquency: considerations for pediatricians. *Pediatr Rev* 1995;16:12.
35. Freud S. *The ego and the id* (1923). London: Hogarth Press; 1947.
36. Erikson EH. *Childhood and society.* 2nd ed. New York: WW Norton; 1963.
37. Patterson GR, Gullion ME. *Living with children.* Chicago: Research Press; 1968.
38. Ginott HG. *Between parent and teenager.* New York: Avon; 1971.
39. Hofmann A. Managing adolescents and their parents: avoiding pitfalls and traps. *Adolescent Medicine: State of the Art Reviews* 1992;3:1.
40. Tolmas HC, Long WA Jr, Grace E. Solutions: the role of the private practitioner. *Adolescent Medicine: State of the Art Reviews* 1990;1:145.
41. Williams RL. The office setting for adolescent care: concerns of physicians, patients and parents. *Adolescent Medicine: State of the Art Reviews* 1992;2:381.
42. Shapiro E. Obstacles to adolescent care in general practice. *Adolescent Medicine: State of the Art Reviews* 1992;2:389.
43. Lopez RI. Obstacles to adolescent care: economic issues. *Adolescent Medicine: State of the Art Reviews* 1992;2:415.
44. Braverman PK, Strasburger VC. Office practice of adolescent medicine. *Adolescent Medicine: State of the Art Reviews* 1997;8(1):1.
45. Wender EH, Bijur PE, Boyce WT. Pediatric residency training: ten years after the Task Force report. *Pediatrics* 1992;90:876.
46. Rosen DS. Expectations of entering pediatric residents toward the care of adolescents [Abstract]. *J Adolesc Health* 1996;18:118.
47. Hornberger LL, Lynch DA. Results of a national survey of life experiences, beliefs, and attitudes of incoming pediatric residents [Abstract]. *J Adolesc Health* 1996;18:119.
48. Strasburger VC. Adolescent medicine in the 1990s: no more excuses. *Clin Pediatr* 1997;36:87.
49. Cheng TL, Savageau JA, Sattler AL, et al. Confidentiality in health care: a survey of knowledge, perceptions, and attitudes among high school students. *JAMA* 1993;269:1404.
50. Ford CA, Millstein SG, Halpern-Feisher B, et al. Confidentiality and adolescents' disclosure of sensitive information [Abstract]. *J Adolesc Health* 1996;18:111.
51. Ford CA, Millstein SG. Delivery of confidentiality assurances to adolescents by primary care physicians [Abstract]. *J Adolesc Health* 1996;18:112.
52. Goldenring JM, Cohen E. Getting into adolescent heads. *Contemporary Pediatrics* 1988;5:75.
53. Perkins K, Ferrari N, Rosas A, et al. You won't know unless you ask: the biopsychosocial interview for adolescents. *Clin Pediatr* 1997;36:79.
54. Strasburger VC. Why adolescent medicine? Four illustrative cases. *Clin Pediatr* 1984;23:12.
55. Strasburger VC. Why adolescent medicine? More illustrative cases. *Conn Med* 1985;49:501.
56. Lopez RI. Role of the primary care pediatrician in adolescent psychosocial assessment and intervention. *Adolescent Medicine: State of the Art Reviews* 1992;3:147.
57. Pratt HD, Greydanus DE. Social learning theory as a basis for office counseling: a tool for the primary care physician of the 1990s. *Adolescent Medicine: State of the Art Reviews* 1994;5:451.

58. Davis G, Hendren RL. What pediatricians should know about adolescent psychiatry. *Adolescent Medicine: State of the Art Reviews* 1992;3:131.
59. Joffe A, Radius S, Gall M. Health counseling for adolescents: what they want, what they get, and who gives it. *Pediatrics* 1988;82:481.
60. Hofmann AD, Greydanus DE. Principles of psychosocial evaluation and counseling. In: Hofmann AD, Greydanus DE. *Adolescent medicine.* 2nd ed. Norwalk, CT: Appleton & Lange; 1989:533.
61. Holder AR. *Legal issues in pediatrics and adolescent medicine.* 2nd ed. New Haven: Yale University Press; 1985.

SUGGESTED READING

For Physicians

Alderman EM, Friedman SB. Behavioral problems of affluent youth. *Pediatr Ann* 1995;24:186.

Braverman PK, Strasburger VC. Office practice of adolescent medicine. *Adolescent Medicine: State of the Art Rev* 1997;8(1):1.

Comerci GD. Parents and society: how much the problem; how much the solution? *Adolescent Medicine: State of the Art Reviews* 1991;2:251.

Comerci GD, Daniel WA Jr, eds. Parenting the adolescent. *Adolescent Medicine: State of the Art Reviews* 1991;2:251.

DiClemente RJ, Hansen WB, Ponton LE. *Handbook of adolescent health risk behavior.* New York: Plenum Press; 1996.

Elkind D. Understanding the young adolescent. *Adolescence* 1978;13:127.

Elkind D. *All grown up and no place to go.* Reading, MA: Addison-Wesley; 1984.

Emery RE, Coiro MJ. Divorce: consequences for children. *Pediatr Rev* 1995;16:306.

Freud A. Adolescence. *Psychoanal Study Child* 1958;13:255.

Hofmann A. Managing adolescents and their parents: avoiding pitfalls and traps. *Adolescent Medicine: State of the Art Reviews* 1992;3:1.

Hutter MJ. Office evaluation and management of family dysfunction. *Adolescent Medicine: State of the Art Reviews* 1991;2:303.

Kaufman KL, Brown RT, Graves K, et al. What, me worry? A survey of adolescents' concerns. *Clin Pediatr* 1993;32:8.

Kreipe RE. Principles of office counseling: the healthy adolescent. *Adolescent Medicine: State of the Art Reviews* 1991;2:277.

Litt IF. Pubertal and psychosocial development. *Pediatr Rev* 1995;16:243.

MacKenzie RG, Peel JL. Principles of office counseling: the high-risk or troubled adolescent. *Adolescent Medicine: State of the Art Reviews* 1991;2:291.

Meuer JR, Meurer LN, Holloway RL. Clinical problems and counseling for single-parent families. *Am Fam Physician* 1996;54:864.

Tolmas HC, Long WA Jr, Grace E. Solutions: the role of the private practitioner. *Adolescent Medicine: State of the Art Reviews* 1990;1:145.

Wallander JL, Siegel LJ, eds. *Adolescent health problems: behavioral perspectives.* New York: Guilford Press, 1995.

Yancy WS. Juvenile delinquency: considerations for pediatricians. *Pediatr Rev* 1995;16:12.

For Physicians and Parents

American Medical Association. *"Teen talk": a guide to understanding your body and your self.* Chicago: American Medical Association; 1996.

Elkind D. *Parenting your teenager in the 90's.* Rosemont, NJ: Modern Learning Press; 1993.

Faber A, Mazlish E. *How to talk so kids will listen and listen so kids will talk.* New York: Avon; 1989.

Ginott HG. *Between parent and teenager.* New York: Avon; 1971.

Greydanus DE, ed. *Caring for your adolescent, ages 12 to 21.* New York: Bantam; 1991.

Orvin GH. *Understanding the adolescent.* Washington, DC: American Psychiatric Press; 1995.

Pipher M. *Reviving Ophelia: saving the selves of adolescent girls.* New York: Ballantine, 1994.

Schmitt BD. Parents' guide to behavior problems: dealing with normal adolescent rebellion. *Contemporary Pediatrics* 1990;7:55.

Steinberg L, Levine A. *You and your adolescent: a parent's guide for ages 10–20.* New York: Harper & Row; 1990.

Strasburger VC. *Getting your kids to say no in the '90s when you said yes in the '60s.* New York: Fireside/Simon & Schuster; 1993.

Winn M. *Children without childhood.* New York: Penguin; 1984.

VIOLENCE

Today's children and adolescents are experiencing one of the most violent cultures in the history of the United States [1–3]. However, they are not just experiencing it; sometimes they are perpetrating it as well [4,5]. For any primary care practitioner interested in the health and welfare of teenagers, the data are chilling:

- In 1991, nearly half of the 26,513 homicide victims in the United States were boys and men, aged 15 to 34 years [6] (Table 4). Expressed differently, 22 young people are murdered every day in the United States, almost 1 every hour [4]. In California alone, the homicide rate for 15- to 19-year-olds has increased fourfold between 1970 and 1993 [7].
- Students report high levels of victimization, especially boys at large-city schools. As many as 44% report being hit at school, 22% have been mugged in their own neighborhood, and 33% have been shot at [1].
- Students report even higher levels of witnessing violence (see Table 4), and exposure to violence correlated with depression, anxiety, and posttraumatic stress [1]. One study of 246 inner-city adolescents found that 42% had seen someone shot or knifed, and 22% witnessed a killing [8].

Guns play a key role in this cascade of violence, particularly handguns; the modern practitioner needs to know how to address this issue with his or her patients, their parents, and their communities as well:

- Firearms are involved in 68% to 75% of all homicides, mostly handguns [4]. In California, among 15- to 19-year-olds, guns now account for 90% of all homicides [7].
- The United States has the highest homicide rate among 21 industrialized countries [9].
- The United States is also the most heavily armed nation on earth, with as many guns as households (200 million) [10].
- Firearm injuries are the third or fourth leading cause of accidental death among children (depending on age and region) [11].
- In one survey of 29 different practices in 7 different states, 37% of families with children reported owning guns (26% rifles, 17% handguns). Of the handguns, 13% were kept loaded and not locked up [11].
- The National Adolescent Student Health Survey studied 5,560 10th graders and found that 41% of boys and 24% of girls reported that they could get a gun easily if they so desired [12]. Nearly 8% of

TABLE 4. *Adolescents' exposure to violence*

Type of violence	Cleveland central city (N = 1,228)		Small Ohio city (N = 862)	
	M	F	M	F
Students victimized by violence				
Threatened at home	24%	25%	29%	32%
Threatened at school	35%	31%	48%	39%
Beaten at home	9%	10%	6%	9%
Sexually abused/assaulted	7%	16%	4%	17%
Knife attack	16%	9%	15%	4%
Shot at or shot	33%	10%	19%	4%
Students witnessing violence				
Threat at home	39%	47%	35%	42%
Threat at school	82%	79%	89%	88%
Beating at home	23%	31%	16%	19%
Beating at school	75%	75%	82%	82%
Sexual assault	21%	20%	16%	19%
Knife attack	46%	44%	35%	28%
Shooting	62%	49%	36%	25%

Adapted from Singer MI, Anglin TM, Song LY, et al. Adolescents' exposure to violence and associated symptoms of psychological trauma. *JAMA* 1995;273:477.

students had carried a gun to school during the 30 days before the 1995 Youth Risk Behavior Survey [13].

From a public health perspective, these data are remarkable and alarming, but what practitioners need to realize and counsel their patients about are the following findings:

- Although Americans say that they are purchasing handguns for protection, guns in the home are 43 times more likely to kill a family member than an intruder [14].
- Adolescents and handguns at home do not mix well; the presence of a handgun at home makes a successful adolescent suicide nearly 10 times more likely. Handguns at home are a particularly significant risk factor for suicide in teenagers without any apparent psychiatric disorder [15].
- The Second Amendment of the U.S. Constitution links the "right" to bear arms closely to the preservation of state militias. It also poses no obstacle to broad gun control legislation, based on several Supreme Court rulings [16].

Guns are not the sole cause of the increasing level of violence in society, however. American media are among the most violent in the world [17], and nearly 1,000 studies demonstrate a significant link between media violence and real-life violence [18,19]. The most recent content analysis of American television, which examined 2,500 hours of programming, found that violence is ubiquitous (57% of programs contained it), negative consequences are rarely portrayed (16% of incidents), and few programs (4%) have an antiviolence theme [20]. Although media violence is estimated to cause perhaps only 15% to 20% of real-life violence in society [21], changing the nature of programming would be far easier than eliminating poverty, racism, or the family and individual factors that probably play a greater role in fostering violence [22].

Much has been written about what the primary care practitioner can do to decrease violence among young people [23–27]. Office-based efforts can include identifying high-risk youth, counseling parents to avoid exposing their young children to media violence, identifying violence-prone families, counseling adolescents who may feel victimized by incidents at school or home, and having preventative discussions concerning guns and gun storage. Practitioners may also want to align themselves with local schools and community efforts to encourage the adoption of violence prevention programs, which have been shown to be effective [6,28–32]. Other strategies suggested by the Centers for Disease Control, the American Academy of Pediatrics, and other groups include:

- Strengthening the scientific base for prevention efforts
- Establishing primary prevention programs
- Targeting youths of all ages
- Involving adults (e.g., parents and other role models)
- Presenting messages in multiple settings
- Addressing societal and personal factors

REFERENCES

1. Singer MI, Anglin TM, Song L, et al. Adolescents' exposure to violence and associated symptoms of psychological trauma. *JAMA* 1995;273:477.
2. Zuckerman B, Augustyn M, Groves BM, et al. Silent victims revisited: the special case of domestic violence. *Pediatrics* 1995;96:511.
3. Bain JE, Brown RT. Adolescents as witnesses to violence. *J Adolesc Health* 1996;19:83.
4. Cohall AT, Cohall RM. "Number one with a bullet": epidemiology and prevention of homicide among adolescents and young adults. *Adolescent Medicine: State of the Art Reviews* 1995;6:183.
5. Rachuba L, Stanton B, Howard D. Violent crime in the United States: an epidemiologic profile. *Arch Pediatr Adolesc Med* 1995;149:953.
6. Centers for Disease Control and Prevention. Homicides among 15–19-year-old males: United States, 1963–1991. *MMWR Morb Mortal Wkly Rep* 1994;43:725.
7. Chu LD, Sorenson SB. Trends in California homicide, 1970 to 1993. *West J Med* 1996;165:119.
8. Schubiner H, Scott R, Tzelepis A. Exposure to violence among inner-city youth. *J Adolesc Health* 1993;14:214.
9. Fingerhut LA, Kleinman JC. International and interstate comparisons of homicide among young males. *JAMA* 1990;263:3292.
10. Davidson OG. *Under fire: the NRA and the battle for gun control.* New York: Holt; 1993.
11. Senturia YD, Christoffel KK, Donovan M. Children's household exposure to guns: a pediatric practice-based survey. *Pediatrics* 1994;93:469.

12. Centers for Disease Control and Prevention. Results from the national adolescent student health survey. *MMWR Morb Mortal Wkly Rep* 1989;38:147.

13. Centers for Disease Control and Prevention. Youth risk behavior surveillance: United States, 1995.*MMWR Morb Mortal Wkly Rep* 1996;44(SS-4):1.

14. Kellerman AL, Reay DT. Protection or peril? An analysis of firearm-related deaths in the home. *N Engl J Med* 1986;314:1557.

15. Brent DA. Depression and suicide in children and adolescents. *Pediatr Rev* 1993;14:380.

16. Vernick JS, Teret SP. Firearms and health: the right to be armed with accurate information about the Second Amendment. *Am J Public Health* 1993;83:1773.

17. Strasburger VC. *Adolescents and the media: medical and psychological impact.* Thousand Oaks, CA: Sage; 1995.

18. Sege R, Dietz W. Television viewing and violence in children: the pediatrician as agent for change. *Pediatrics* 1994;94:600.

19. Committee on Communications, American Academy of Pediatrics. Media violence. *Pediatrics* 1995;95:949.

20. Mediascope. *National television violence study, executive summary, 1994–1995.* Studio City, CA: Mediascope; 1996.

21. Comstock GC, Strasburger VC. Media violence: Q & A. *Adolescent Medicine: State of the Art Reviews* 1993; 4:495.

22. Strasburger VC. "Sex, drugs, Rock 'n' Roll" and the media - are the media responsible for adolescent behavior? *Adolescent Medicine: State of the Art Reviews* 1997; 8(3):403.

23. Deutsch M, Brickman E. Conflict resolution. *Pediatr Rev* 1994;15:16.

24. Spivak H, Harvey B, eds. The role of the pediatrician in violence prevention. *Pediatrics* 1994;94(Suppl):577.

25. Grossman DC, Mang K, Rivara FP. Firearm injury prevention counseling by pediatricians and family physicians: practices and beliefs. *Arch Pediatr Adolesc Med* 1995;149:973.

26. Camosy PA. Incorporating gun safety into clinical practice. *Am Fam Physician* 1996;54:971.

27. Garrity C, Baris MA. Bullies and victims: a guide for pediatricians. *Contemporary Pediatrics* 1996;13:90.

28. Slaby RG, Stringham P. Prevention of peer and community violence: the pediatrician's role. *Pediatrics* 1994; 94:608.

29. Orpinas P, Parcel GS, McAlister A, et al. Violence prevention in middle schools: a pilot evaluation. *J Adolesc Health* 1995;17:360.

30. Wilson-Brewer R. Peer violence prevention programs in middle and high schools. *Adolescent Medicine: State of the Art Reviews* 1995;6:233.

31. DuRant RH, Treiber F, Getts A, et al. Comparison of two violence prevention curricula for middle school adolescents. *J Adolesc Health* 1996;19:111.

32. Hausman A, Pierce G, Briggs L. Evaluation of comprehensive violence prevention education: effects on student behavior. *J Adolesc Health* 1996;19:104.

SUGGESTED READING

Amaya-Jackson L, March JS. Post-traumatic stress disorder in adolescents: risk factors, diagnosis, and intervention. *Adolescent Medicine: State of the Art Reviews* 1995;6:251.

American Medical Association. *Physician guide to media violence.* Chicago: American Medical Association; 1996.

Anglin T. The medical clinician's role in preventing adolescent involvement in violence. *Adolescent Medicine: State of the Art Reviews* 1997;8(3):501.

Bain JE, Brown RT. Adolescents as witnesses to violence. *J Adolesc Health* 1996;19:83.

Centerwall BS. Television and violence: the scale of the problem and where to go from here. *JAMA* 1992;267:3059.

Christoffel KK, Naureckas SM. Firearm injuries in children and adolescents: epidemiology and preventive approaches. *Curr Opin Pediatr* 1994;6:519.

Cohall AT, Cohall RM. "Number one with a bullet": epidemiology and prevention of homicide among adolescents and young adults. *Adolescent Medicine: State of the Art Reviews* 1995;6:183.

Committee on Communications, American Academy of Pediatrics. Media violence (policy statement). *Pediatrics* 1995;95:949.

Comstock GC, Strasburger VC. Media violence: Q & A. *Adolescent Medicine: State of the Art Reviews* 1993;4:495.

Derksen DJ, Strasburger VC. Media and television violence: effects on violence, aggression, and antisocial behaviors in children. In: Hoffman AM, ed. *Schools, violence, and society.* Westport, CT: Praeger; 1996:61.

Deutsch M, Brickman E. Conflict resolution. *Pediatr Rev* 1994;15:16.

Donnerstein E, Linz D. Sexual violence in the mass media. In: Costanzo M, Oskamp S, eds. *Violence and the law.* Newbury Park, CA: Sage; 1994:9.

Donnerstein E, Linz D. The mass media: a role in injury causation and prevention. *Adolescent Medicine: State of the Art Reviews* 1995;6:271.

Garrity C, Baris MA. Bullies and victims: a guide for pediatricians. *Contemporary Pediatrics* 1996;13:90.

Haggerty RJ, Sherrod LS, Garmezy N, et al, eds. *Stress, risk, and resilience in children and adolescents.* New York: Cambridge University Press; 1994.

Harrington D, Dubowitz H. Family violence and development during adolescence. *Adolescent Medicine: State of the Art Reviews* 1995;6:199.

Hoffman AM, ed. *Schools, violence, and society.* Westport, CT: Praeger; 1996.

Jenkins EJ, Bell CC. Adolescent violence: can it be curbed? *Adolescent Medicine: State of the Art Reviews* 1992; 3:71.

Mediascope. *National television violence study, executive summary, 1994–1995.* Studio City, CA: Mediascope; 1996.

Prothrow-Stith D. *Deadly consequences: how violence is destroying our teenage population and a plan to begin solving the problem.* New York: HarperCollins; 1991.

Prothrow-Stith DB. The epidemic of youth violence in America: using public health prevention strategies to prevent violence. *J Health Care Poor Underserved* 1995;6:95.

Rachuba L, Stanton B, Howard D. Violent crime in the United States: an epidemiologic profile. *Arch Pediatr Adolesc Med* 1995;149:953.

Rodriguez LJ. *Always running: la vida loca—gang days in L.A.* Willamantic, CT: Curbstone Press; 1993.

Saner H, Ellickson P. Concurrent risk factors for adolescent violence. *J Adolesc Health* 19:94, 1996;.

Sells CW, Blum RW. Morbidity and mortality among US adolescents: an overview of data and trends. *Am J Public Health* 1996;86:513.

Singer MI, Anglin TM, Song L, et al. Adolescents' exposure to violence and associated symptoms of psychological trauma. *JAMA* 1995;273:477.

Slaby RG, Stringham P. Prevention of peer and community violence: the pediatrician's role. *Pediatrics* 1994; 94:608.

Spivak H, Harvey B, eds. The role of the pediatrician in violence prevention. *Pediatrics* 1994;94(Suppl):577.

Strasburger VC. *Adolescents and the media: medical and psychological impact.* Thousand Oaks, CA: Sage; 1995.

Vernick JS, Teret SP. Firearms and health: the right to be armed with accurate information about the Second Amendment. *Am J Public Health* 1993;83:1773.

Webster DW, Wilson MEH. Gun violence among youth and the pediatrician's role in primary prevention. *Pediatrics* 1994;94(Suppl):617.

Wilson-Brewer R. Peer violence prevention programs in middle and high schools. *Adolescent Medicine: State of the Art Reviews* 1995;6:233.

Yancy WS. Juvenile delinquency: considerations for pediatricians. *Pediatr Rev* 1995;16:12.

Zuckerman DM. Media violence, gun control, and public policy. *Am J Orthopsychiatry* 1996;66:378.

School Curricula

Center for Media Literacy. *Beyond blame: challenging violence in the media.* Five units (high school level), $249.95. Elementary and middle school curriculum, $149.95. Available from: Center for Media Literacy, 4727 Wilshire Blvd., Suite 403, Los Angeles, CA 90010; (213) 931-4177.

SUICIDE

I hope I die before I get old.
—Lyrics from "My Generation," The Who

Many people, including physicians, would be surprised to know that adolescent suicide is relatively uncommon and that teenagers have lower rates of completed suicides than adults [1,2]. Yet teenage suicide is considered (rightfully) a serious and important health problem. Why does this discrepancy exist?

First, any loss of life during childhood or adolescence is considered tragic, given the potential for a full and productive life span of perhaps 70 or 80 years. Second, teenage suicide represents the third leading cause of death among adolescents aged 15 to 19 years (after accidents and homicides) and the second leading cause of death among young people aged 15 to 34 years [3,4]. It alone accounts for 12% of overall mortality during adolescence [5]. A total of about 2,000 teenagers aged 15 to 19 years and 3,500 young adults aged 20 to 24 years commit suicide each year [6]. And, as with accidents and homicides, many suicides appear to be preventable by society in general, or parents and health professionals in particular. Third, the number of completed suicides represents a "tip of the iceberg" phenomenon. Statistically, attempts outnumber completions by an estimated 100 to 200:1 [7]. In addition, many studies have documented that suicidal ideation is common among adolescents [7–11] (Table 5). In the most recent Youth Risk Behavior Survey, nearly one fourth (24.1%) of more than 10,000 high

TABLE 5. *How common are suicide attempts or suicidal ideation among adolescents?*

	Suicidal ideation	Ideation with a plan	At least one suicide attempt	Suicide attempt requiring treatment
Females	34%	20%	10%	3%
Males	21%	12%	6%	2%

Adapted from Centers for Disease Control and Prevention. Attempted suicide among high school students: United States, 1990. *MMWR Morb Mortal Wkly Rep* 1991;40:633.

school students nationwide reported seriously considering suicide during the preceding year, and 8.7% had actually attempted it [12].

Adolescent suicide is not only a tragedy, it angers many adults. They want to know how teenagers can "throw away their lives when they have so much to live for." Again, the idiosyncrasies of normal adolescent psychology play a major role here: teenagers frequently do not have an adult concept of death. The concepts of the "imaginary audience" and the "personal fable" lead most teenagers to have a more immature view of death. In a classic study of nearly 600 13- to 16-year-olds, researchers found that 20% thought that they would still be cognizant after death, 60% envisioned some form of spiritual continuation, and only 20% viewed death as total cessation [13]. It may be useful to ask teenagers who have made suicide attempts what they think would have happened if they had succeeded; such a question may tap into some substantial fantasies.

One important clinical and research problem has always been how to distinguish and categorize successful completors from attempters. Unfortunately, the term *suicide gesture* has been increasingly used to designate a suicide attempt of high impulsivity and low lethality (i.e., one that, ostensibly, need not be taken seriously by the health professionals involved). The authors contend that the use of the term *gesture* in this minimalistic fashion has no place in the medical literature. *All suicide attempts are serious and are meant to be taken seriously. The term "suicidal gesture" is misleading, inappropriate, and should be avoided.* Ideally, teenagers who attempt suicide—even if they swallow only a handful of aspirin—deserve hospitalization on an adolescent medical unit at least overnight [14,15]. Although managed care organizations may not like or accept this recommendation, hospitalization accomplishes a number of important things:

- It removes the teenager from his or her previously stressful environment.
- It also ensures that a reattempt will not be made immediately.
- It alerts the parents that a serious threat to the teenager's health and well-being exists.
- It allows the primary clinician and the psychiatrist or psychologist to make a joint assessment of the teenager's behavior and stressors and to determine whether he or she needs inpatient hospitalization on a psychiatric unit.
- Finally, it enables the mental health specialist to make an initial contact and bond with the teenager so that compliance with outpatient treatment can be maximized.

Hospitalization can be deferred only if an unusually supportive family situation exists, if therapy can be started immediately, or, if the patient is already in therapy, the therapist is contacted and can see the patient no later than the following day.

Epidemiologic Features

Rates

The number of adolescent suicides has tripled from 1952 to 1992 [3] (Fig. 2). In 1992, 1,847 young people aged 15 to 19 years committed suicide [15]. The overall rate for 15- to 19-year-olds is now approximately 10.9 per 100,000 [3]. Although rare, suicides among adolescents younger than 15 years are increasing as well. In 1992, 314 committed suicide, a 100% increase between 1980 and 1992 [15]. In addition, such figures probably represent underestimates of the true incidence, given that suicide

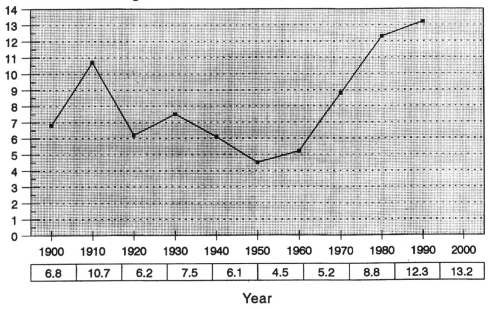

Suicide Rate, Ages 15-24 Years

	1900	1910	1920	1930	1940	1950	1960	1970	1980	1990
	6.8	10.7	6.2	7.5	6.1	4.5	5.2	8.8	12.3	13.2

Year

FIG. 2. Age-specific suicide rates for 15- to 24-year-olds, 1900 to 1990. Rates are given as deaths per 100,000 population per year. (From NCHS mortality files. Kachur SP, Potter LB, Powell KE, et al. Suicide; epidemiology, prevention, treatment. *Adolescent Medicine: State of the Art Reviews* 1995;6:171, with permission.)

has religious, social, and financial implications and is therefore underreported [2]. Many single-vehicle traffic fatalities are thought to be suicides masquerading as accidents as well [16].

Several reasons have been suggested for these significant increases in the teen suicide rate, including:

1. An increase in the rates of suicide for all age groups
2. Wider availability of more lethal means of suicide, especially handguns [17–22]
3. Increased use of alcohol and other drugs among the post-World War II generation [2,23–25]
4. Increased divorce rate among adolescents' parents
5. Increased number of adolescents in the overall population
6. Greater role of the mass media in adolescents' lives [26]
7. Greater stress in adolescents' lives, especially when compared with the "golden age" of the 1950s [27–29]

The increase does appear to be genuine and not merely a result of coroners' changes in how they certify adolescent deaths [30].

As might be expected, the number of suicide attempts is increasing as well. Self-poisoning suicide attempts in Oxford, England have ranged as high as 343 per 100,000 for 16- to 20-year-olds [31]. Oregon is the only state that has a mandatory report form for suicide attempts; between 1988 and 1993, 3,773 attempts and 123 completed suicides occurred (a ratio of 30:1). In addition, more than 40% of the attempters had made at least one previous suicide attempt during the preceding years [25]. Some studies estimate a lifetime prevalence of adolescent attempts as high as 8% [14].

Gender

In general, three to nine times as many female adolescents attempt suicide, but three to five times as many male adolescents succeed [14,30,31]. Primarily this is because boys choose more lethal ways of attempting suicide—guns and hanging—rather than ingestion [2,15]. In addition, antisocial and aggressive behavior is highly correlated with suicidal behavior [32].

Race

White teenagers have higher rates of suicide attempts than all other teens. A few Native American tribes (e.g., Arapahoe and Shoshone) have rates that are up to 20 times the national average [33–36]. However, some Native American tribes also have lower rates than the national average [36]. Rates

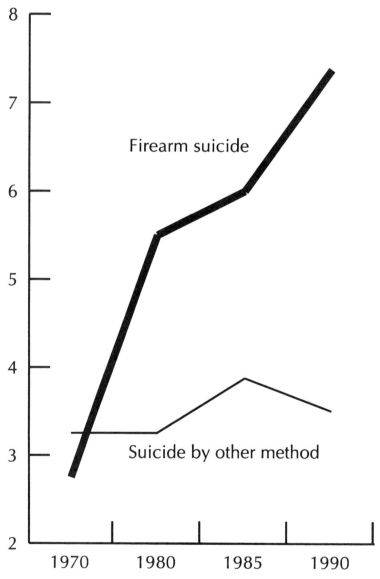

FIG. 3. Firearm suicide among adolescents. Suicides among 15- to 19-year-olds, by method, 1970 to 1990. (From Fingerhut, unpublished data, NCHS. From Youth, suicide, and guns. *FL Educator,* 1996;14(3):10, with permission.)

TABLE 6. *Adolescent suicide rates by method, race, and gender, 1991*[a]

Gender/Race	All Methods	Firearms	Hanging	Poisoning	Cutting	Other
Total	10.8	7.3	1.9	1.1	0.04	0.4
Male						
White	18.3	12.8	3.4	1.4	0.1	0.7
Black	14.8	12.6	1.7	0.2	0.0	0.3
Other	17.4	11.0	4.8	1.2	0.00	0.5
Female						
White	3.7	1.7	0.6	1.1	0.0	0.2
Black	1.9	1.3	0.1	0.4	0.0	0.1
Other	5.0	1.3	1.8	2.0	0.0	0.0

[a]Adolescents ages 15–19 years. All rates are per 100,000 population per year.
From Kachur SP, Potter LB, Powell KE, et al. Suicide: epidemiology, prevention, treatment. *Adolescent Medicine: State of the Art Reviews* 1995;6:171, with permission.

among whites peaked in 1988, but have since stabilized; rates for black and other minority males are continuing to increase [37].

Method

Firearms have revolutionized teenage suicide. For both sexes, firearms are the most common method of completed suicide, particularly when alcohol is also involved, and the suicide rate by firearms is rising faster than any other method [38] (Fig. 3). By far, the problem is handguns, not rifles. *There is ample evidence that the suicide rate is directly correlated with the production, sales, and ownership of handguns and inversely proportional to the restrictiveness of handgun control laws* [17,23,20,39–41] (Tables 6, 7). Relatively recent increases in completed suicides among young teenagers (aged 10–14 years) without concomitant increases in suicide attempts indicate that more lethal means are being used [3].

In North Carolina, one study documented that half of male adolescents own a gun [42]. In addition, studies show that although guns are usually purchased by adults as a defense against intruders, they are far more likely to be used by or against a family member [43]. In fact, in one study, nearly one fourth of attempters reported that their families continued to have a firearm in the home, even after their attempt [44]. Among high-risk adolescents, as many as 20% report playing Russian roulette, usually in conjunction with using alcohol or other drugs [45].

After firearms, hanging is the next most common method for male adolescents and jumping from a height for female adolescents. Although toxic ingestion accounts for the most attempts by girls, it re-

TABLE 7. *Handguns and American children*

- Firearms rank as the second leading cause of fatal injuries in the United States (33,000 deaths annually). Other countries have relatively few such deaths.
- Each year, the United States has over 10,000 handgun homicides, compared to 52 or fewer in other developed countries.
- In addition, there are over 150,000 nonfatal firearm injuries per year.
- The proportion of gun owners in different regions of the United States parallels the percentage of homicides involving firearms and the suicide rate.
- Guns are six times more likely to kill or injure a member of the owner's household than an intruding criminal.
- Toy guns cause over 1,500 injuries per year.
- The sale of toy guns represents a nearly $100 million industry.
- Weapons appear an average of nine times per hour in prime-time programs.

Data from Christoffel KK, Christoffel T. Handguns as a pediatric problem. *Pediatr Emerg Care* 1986;2:343; and Schetky D. Children and handguns: a public health concern. *American Journal of Diseases of Children* 1985;139:229. Reprinted from Strasburger VC. Television and adolescents: sex, drugs, rock 'n' roll. *Adolescent Medicine: State of the Art Reviews* 1990;1:161, with permission.

sults in few completed suicides by either gender [2]. Wrist slashing is the second most common means of attempt in the United States [46].

Diagnostic Impressions

Many experts believe that as many as 90% of all adolescents who committed suicide had previous psychiatric symptoms [2,14,47]. Researchers use a technique called the *psychological autopsy* to piece together full psychological profiles of victims. Symptoms have existed for months or even years in most teenagers, although the diagnosis was not apparent until too late in many cases [15]. At least half of all teenagers committing suicide have had contact with a mental health professional [1]. Of attempters, 40% make a repeat attempt, and 14% eventually succeed [2].

Some researchers believe that adolescents who commit suicide can be divided into four broad categories:

1. Teenagers with a long history of school and behavior problems, school problems, fighting at school and with parents, and impulsiveness (50%)
2. Anxious, perfectionist, rigid teenagers—"model children," performing well at school (20–25%)
3. Depressed girls (20–25%)
4. Psychotic adolescents (1–2%)

Of course, it is the second category of adolescents—those who have never been any trouble to their parents and who are often admired as ideal adolescents—that parents and educators find most troubling [47]. Compared with community controls, these victims show greater evidence of psychiatric risk factors but have not yet come to the attention of any mental health personnel. Unfortunately, there is a higher prevalence of loaded handguns at home, and often these are teenagers who are confronting legal or serious disciplinary crises for the first time [47].

Precipitants

Adolescent suicide is a complex and multifactorial disorder (Fig. 4), but loss, especially a humiliating loss, is a key feature in most cases. The loss can be the break-up of a personal relationship, parents' divorcing, the loss of self-esteem after being ridiculed by friends, the impending loss of self-esteem after being arrested and having to face one's parents, the loss of a good grade on a test, or the death of a close friend, family member, or pet [2]. Many teenagers commit suicide in the interval be-

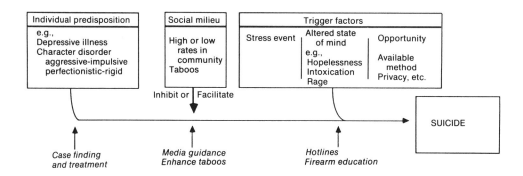

FIG. 4. One model for adolescent suicide causation. (Reprinted with permission from Shaffer D, Garland A, Gould M, et al. Preventing teenage suicide: a critical review. *J Am Acad Child Adolesc Psychiatry* 1988;27:675. Copyright 1988, the American Academy of Child and Adolescent Psychiatry.)

tween the loss and the impending humiliation or disciplinary action, and the stress–suicide interval can be brief [48]. Alcohol or other drugs are a frequent accompaniment to the attempt and may be at least partially responsible for the increase in suicide rates since the 1960s [6,17]. Adolescents who have been sexually abused also are at threefold greater risk of attempting suicide [49]. Among a group of teenagers in Oregon, the reasons given most often for attempting suicide were [25]:

- Rape or sexual abuse (61%)
- Substance abuse (57%)
- Physical abuse (54%)

For completors, psychological autopsies demonstrate that the incidence of psychopathology is extremely high [50,51]. Unipolar and bipolar affective disorders or antisocial disorders can be found in two thirds to three fourths of suicide victims [50–52]. The family history is also frequently positive for similar disorders. Many adolescents have made suicide threats or attempts in the past. They demonstrate a strong desire to die, as manifested by timing the suicide so they will avoid discovery, choosing a lethal method, leaving a suicide note, and proclaiming their intent to die ahead of time. In one study, nearly 85% of teenagers who committed suicide had informed others of their intent before their deaths [50]. Of teen suicide victims, young women are more likely to have made a previous attempt, been diagnosed as having a major depression, or actually been under psychiatric care previously than young men [53].

Attempters manifest similar precipitants for their behavior, although *conflict* may be the operative condition rather than *loss*. This can include interpersonal conflict with a parent or significant other, family conflict, and physical or sexual abuse [54]. When teenagers are surveyed about stressors in their lives, a number of negative events are reported [55] (Tables 8, 9). In addition to not having the coping skills of adults, teenagers also may find certain setbacks stressful that adults would easily shrug off (e.g., receiving a B on an examination instead of an A, or not making the junior varsity swim team). An estimated two thirds of attempters *do not want to die*. Rather, they make impulsive attempts, seeking to communicate anger, escape a difficult situation, or influence others [31]. This may be the derivation of the concept of a gesture, or *cry for help*. Certainly, if these attempts do represent a cry for help, it is in the best interests of both the patient and the practitioner to listen to it and make a significant intervention. Hospitalization on an adolescent medical service accomplishes this without

TABLE 8. *What, me worry?*
The 10 most frequent worries of adolescents

Men
1. Terrorism
2. Feelings that I'm a bad person
3. Having sex or thoughts about having sex
4. Eating too little or too much
5. My parents' physical or mental health
6. Too much free time
7. Getting special recognition at school
8. Going out on a date
9. Popularity with friends and classmates
10. Trouble with the law

Women
1. Terrorism
2. My parents' physical or mental health
3. My periods
4. Feelings that I'm a bad person
5. Getting bad grades
6. Having sex or thoughts about having sex
7. Death or illness of a friend or family member
8. People being afraid of me
9. Going out on a date
10. Getting special recognition at school

From Kaufman KL, Brown RT, Graves K, et al. What, me worry? A survey of adolescents' concerns. *Clin Pediatr* 1993;32:8.

TABLE 9. *Common Adolescent Stresses*[a]

Stress	Reported incidence
Failing grades on report card	34%
Increased arguments between parents	28%
Serious family illness	28%
Broke up with boy/girlfriend	24%
Death in family	22%
Problem with siblings	21%
Teacher problems	14%
Parents divorced	13%
Death of a close friend	11%

[a]Survey of 172 11-19-year-olds in a general adolescent clinic.
Adapted from Greene JW, Walker LS, Hickson G, et al. Stressful life events and somatic complaints in adolescents. *Pediatrics* 1985; 75:19

stigmatizing or scaring the teenager by admitting him or her to a psychiatric ward (particularly an adult ward).

Psychological and Social Risk Factors

Clinicians need to familiarize themselves with the risk factors for attempts or repeated attempts adequately to evaluate adolescents in trouble (Fig. 5). By far, the most significant risk factor is a *history of prior attempts* (Tables 10, 11). Once a teenager makes a suicide attempt, he or she has a 1% to 14% chance of eventually succeeding in future attempts [2,48]. In general, however, there is a fine line between those adolescents at risk and those who actually attempt suicide [56].

This is another area in which exposure to violence takes its toll. One study found that students who knew someone who was murdered were twice as likely to report having suicidal ideation and four times as likely to make a suicide attempt [57]. Likewise, in examining suicides of teenagers with no apparent psychopathology, researchers found that these adolescents had a greater prevalence of loaded firearms at home compared with either normal control subjects or other suicide victims with known psychiatric disturbances [47].

Other major risks for teen suicide include exposure to suicide in family members or friends, major depression, substance abuse, homosexuality, antisocial behavior, and availability of firearms at home [44,58–61]. In one study, 40% of attempters had used drugs within 8 hours of their attempt [44]. A study of 137 gay and bisexual young men, aged 14 to 21 years, found that 29% had made at least one suicide attempt, with nearly one third of the attempts coming in the same year that they identified themselves as being bisexual or homosexual [62]. Of course, the biggest problem is that although risk factors are useful to discuss from an epidemiologic viewpoint, they are not very accurate or useful in individual cases; many false positives will be identified [2].

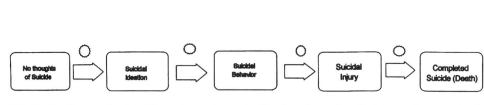

FIG. 5. Continuum of suicidal behavior and opportunities for intervention. O, intervention opportunity. (From Kachur SP, Potter KE, Powell KE, et al. Suicide: epidemiology, prevention, treatment. *Adolescent Medicine: State of the Art Reviews* 1995;6:171, with permission.)

TABLE 10. *Risk factors associated with adolescent suicide*

Category of risk	Risk factor
Demographic	
Age	Older adolescents and young adults
Gender	Male
Race	Whites, certain Native Americans
Psychiatric	
Affective disorders	Depression, bipolar disorder
Substance abuse	Alcohol, drug abuse
Other	Prior suicide attempt; anxiety; conduct or personality disorder
Biologic	
Genetic	Family history of suicide
Neurobiologic	Altered serotonin metabolism
Social/environmental	
Geographic	Western states, rural areas
Exposure	Media exposure; suicide of friend or peer
Predisposing circumstances	Discipline, relationship problems
Availability of means	Firearm in the home

Adapted from Kachur SP, Potter LB, Powell KE, et al. Suicide: epidemiology, prevention, treatment. *Adolescent Medicine: State of the Art Reviews* 1995;6:171.

One researcher has produced a screening model for rapid identification of suicidal adolescents: a history of previous attempts, previous mental health care, poor school performance, marijuana use, and dependence on the emergency room for primary health care accounted for 84% of the 58 suicide attempters [63].

Hopelessness—a major feature in completed adult suicides—is unusual for adolescent attempters but characteristic of teens who commit suicide. It also correlates with severity of the attempt and is predictive of future attempts [64].

TABLE 11. *Risk factors for completed teenage suicide*

Risk factor	Odds ratio	Suicide rate/100,000 affected by risk factor
Male adolescents		
General population	—	14
Prior attempt	23 : 1	270
Major depression	9 : 1	100
Substance abuse	7 : 1	70
Antisocial behavior	4 : 1	40
Family history of suicide	3 : 1	35
Female adolescents		
General population	—	4
Prior attempt	9 : 1	20
Major depression	49 : 1	80
Substance abuse	1 : 1	3
Antisocial behavior	3 : 1	8
Family history of suicide	3 : 1	6

Adapted from Shaffer D. The epidemiology of teen suicide: an examination of risk factors. *J Clin Psychiatry* 1988;49:36.

One interesting risk factor more recently added to the list is media exposure [26]. Numerous studies, both in the United States and Europe, have documented a link between television programming or news reports and an increase in teenage suicide [1,65–68]. A key factor may be the extent to which a susceptible teenager identifies with the suicide victim [69]. On the other hand, it is impossible to know *which* media reports may affect which *particular* teenagers because, again, epidemiologic studies cannot pinpoint individuals at risk. One excellent study examined the effect of four made-for-TV movies about suicide and subsequent rates of attempts and completions. There was a consistent increase, even when all other known variables were controlled [65]. Rock music has also been implicated as a possible catalytic factor [70]. Two teenagers in the United States have committed suicide while listening to Ozzy Osbourne's song, "Suicide Solution" [26]. Overall, these studies and incidents point to an increased risk of imitative behavior probably only in certain susceptible teenagers.

Biologic Risk Factors

Ongoing research is beginning to establish a link between serotonin metabolism and risk of depression and suicide. For example, alcohol abuse, a known concomitant of suicide attempts, is also associated with depletion of serotonin reserves [71]. In adult studies, suicide victims have had low levels of 5-hydroxyindoleacetic acid (5-HIAA), a serotonin metabolite, in their cerebrospinal fluid and in prefrontal cortical tissue [72–74]. In one study that looked at cerebrospinal fluid 5-HIAA levels in adult suicide attempters, researchers found a 10-fold increased risk of completed suicide within a year if levels were below 90 nmoles/L [75]. Studies have also identified a peripheral marker of impaired serotonin metabolism (increased platelet serotonin-2 receptor binding sites) in depressed or suicidal individuals [76]. Although this is still experimental and no studies have yet been conducted in adolescents, it is possible that a lumbar puncture or venous blood sample for serotonin metabolites will become part of the routine evaluation of adolescent suicide attempters in the future.

Suicide Clusters

Epidemics of suicide have occurred throughout recorded history—from the young women of Miletus in ancient Greece, to 665 AD, when English people jumped from seaside cliffs to avoid catching the plague, to imitators of Goethe's *The Sorrows of Young Werther* in 1774, to present-day outbreaks in New Jersey and New Mexico [34,77]. Teenagers are unique in being susceptible to this suicide "contagion" [67]; even so, relatively few suicides (5%) occur in clusters [15].

Controlled studies have documented that adolescent suicide victims are more likely to have been exposed to a suicide than their best friends [51]. Case–control studies also demonstrate increased rates of depression and suicidal ideation among surviving friends and siblings of adolescent suicide victims [78,79]. Such exposure, whether in real-life or fictional media accounts, probably serves as a catalyst for someone who is already susceptible to making an attempt, based on the factors enumerated earlier. Even normal teenagers are susceptible to modeling influences, especially when the model is prominent and attractive, and the outcome is viewed as being desirable. But imitation, alone, does not directly cause suicidal behavior [34].

Evaluation of the Suicidal Adolescent

Suicide prevention begins in the office, with accurate psychological assessment of adolescents. Yet, most studies show that pediatricians avoid the issue entirely [80]. A few key questions can make the difference between spotting an adolescent in trouble and missing a potential suicide victim:

- Have you thought about harming or killing yourself? If so, how would you do it?
- Have you made previous suicide attempts?
- Is there anyone in your family who has committed suicide or had a serious mental illness or depression? Has anyone you know or heard about committed suicide recently?
- Do you use alcohol, marijuana, or other drugs?
- Do you have access to a gun?
- Have you had any major difficulties with parents, peers, school, or the police?
- Has anything bad happened to you recently (e.g., a loss of any kind)?

Contrary to popular belief, asking teens about the possibility of suicide does not "give them ideas," any more than asking about a history of sexual activity gives them ideas about sex. Because many people think about suicide at one time or another, asking about a specific plan helps the clinician to gauge the seriousness and immediate threat of the situation. For example, responses to the question about a plan might range from "Sometimes I think about running in front of a bus, but I know it would be too painful" (low intent, no immediate danger) to "My father keeps a bottle of heart pills in the medicine cabinet, and I think tonight I'll go home and swallow all of them" (high intent, immediate danger).

Once the physician discovers that a patient is potentially suicidal, he or she needs to try to obtain a no-suicide agreement from the teenager [81]. In addition, immediate consultation with a psychiatrist or psychologist is indicated. If a consultation is *readily obtainable*, then the physician, psychiatrist or psychologist, and parents can decide on the best therapeutic intervention: hospitalization, outpatient psychotherapy, family therapy, or outpatient counseling (by the physician). *Physicians must remember that simply referring a patient to a mental health specialist is no guarantee that the patient will actually be seen* [82].

If possible, a teenager who has already made a suicide attempt—no matter how seemingly trivial—merits at least a 24- to 48-hour hospitalization on an adolescent medical unit [14,15,31]. A study of first-time suicide attempters seen in an emergency room who were given outpatient mental health appointments found that only 33% of patients actually complied with the referral [82]. The medical and legal implications of allowing two thirds of suicide attempters to receive no therapy at all are frightening: therefore, *when in doubt, hospitalize*. This communicates to the family the seriousness of the situation, allows further testing to ensure that the patient is out of danger medically, permits immediate mobilization of psychiatric services, and removes the teenager from a stressful environment. Studies have shown that once hospitalized on an adolescent medicine unit, 90% of teenagers do well and only 10% require transfer to a psychiatric facility [83]. Unless strong mental health and social work services (with outreach) are readily obtainable, treating attempters as outpatients is doomed to failure because the teenagers return home to the same stressful environment, and there is no guarantee of appropriate follow-up.

Suicide Prevention Efforts

Based on a thorough review of programs throughout the United States, the Centers for Disease Control and Prevention has identified a number of strategies for preventing adolescent suicides [3,84]:

- Training school and community leaders to identify high-risk youth
- Educating young people about suicide, risk factors, and intervention strategies
- Establishing screening and referral programs
- Developing peer-support programs
- Establishing suicide crisis centers and hotlines
- Limiting access to highly lethal means of suicide
- Intervening after a suicide to prevent copycatting
- Continuing rigorous research into what prevention programs are most effective

Restricting Access to Firearms

Because firearms are highly lethal and represent the most common mode of committing suicide, it is entirely possible that restricting access to them would decrease the suicide rate—especially among impulsive adolescents [1,47,85,86]. Studies have demonstrated reduced suicide rates in some communities that have implemented strong antihandgun restrictions [40,87,88]. Analogously, in Britain, where self-asphyxiation with domestic cooking gas (carbon monoxide poisoning) accounted for 40% of all suicides, switching to natural gas resulted in a steady decrease in both carbon monoxide asphyxiation and total suicide rate [1]. Clearly, removal of a lethal means of death results in fewer deaths and possibly forces suicidal individuals to choose a less lethal means such as self-poisoning.

School-Based Educational Programs

Clustering of suicides among adolescents frequently leads to the creation of intensive educational efforts to discourage such behavior. In a review of 300 prevention programs, researchers concluded that the most effective ones were based on a sound foundation of empirical knowledge (i.e., understanding the risks and problems of adolescents and compiling data to evaluate efficacy) [89]. Unfortunately, few programs do so. For example, most programs present adolescent suicide as a reaction to extreme stress, not as a sign of underlying mental illness. Because such programs are created to increase awareness of the problems, they sometimes exaggerate the incidence of teen suicide [2].

Only a few studies have examined the effectiveness of school-based suicide prevention programs, and the results are not extremely encouraging [2,15]. A 1987 study examined whether such school programs are effective by evaluating 1,000 high school students exposed to a program and a similar number of control subjects. Between 5% and 20% of the students in both groups had high-risk views about suicide, and the educational program did not alter those views. However, nearly 3% of the students in the programs identified themselves as being suicidal or troubled and wanting professional help [1]. Another large, well controlled study in New Jersey [90] found few positive effects of three different programs and one negative effect: students who were at greatest risk for suicide (those who had attempted previously) found the programs unsettling [91].

According to one group of experts, the following concepts are important for any school-based curriculum [34]:

- Suicide is a permanent solution to a temporary problem that can be improved.
- Death is permanent and final and does not allow the teenager any satisfaction from whatever ensues after his or her death.
- Suicidal thoughts are common, but if they persist, help should be sought.
- People who commit suicide are dysfunctional and, sadly, lack the ability to find help for problems that are usually solvable.

Hotlines

One traditional and popular strategy to prevent suicide has been the creation of hotlines. Here, too, few data exist concerning their actual efficacy, and the evidence seems to indicate that suicide hotlines are only minimally effective in reducing suicidal behavior [2,91,92]. One report that examined suicide rates in counties with and without hotlines, and before and after their establishment, found a potential reduction of 1.75 suicides/100,000 young white women (who are the most frequent hotline callers) [93]. However, in another study, one third of the men and one fifth of the women reported that the hotline advice had made their problem worse [94].

Media

Suicide stories seem to beget more suicides. Although much more research is needed, teenagers seem particularly vulnerable to media portrayals of suicide, both fictional and nonfictional [26,95]. Reducing the publicity surrounding actual suicides would be useful but might not be viewed as a recommendation that is compatible with the First Amendment. Certainly, television executives and Hollywood producers should take note that their well meaning attempts to publicize this issue may, in fact, be backfiring. Finally, clinicians who are aware of publicity surrounding suicides in their community or upcoming made-for-TV movies should be particularly vigilant for signs of depression or suicidal behavior in their patients.

REFERENCES

1. Shaffer D, Garland A, Gould M, et al. Preventing teenage suicide: a critical review. *J Am Acad Child Adolesc Psychiatry* 1988;27:675.
2. Garland AF, Zigler E. Adolescent suicide prevention: current research and social policy implications. *Am Psychol* 1993;48:169.
3. Centers for Disease Control and Prevention. Suicide among children, adolescents, and young adults: United States, 1980–1992.*MMWR Morb Mortal Wkly Rep* 1995;44:289.
4. Centers for Disease Control and Prevention. Homicides among 15–19-year-old males: United States, 1963–1991. *MMWR Morb Mortal Wkly Rep* 1994;43:725.
5. Shaffer D, Fisher P. The epidemiology of suicide in children and young adolescents. *Journal of the American Academy of Child Psychiatry* 1981;20:545.

6. Elster AB, Kuznets NJ. *AMA guidelines for adolescent preventive services (GAPS): recommendations and rationale.* Baltimore: Williams & Wilkins, 1994.

7. Centers for Disease Control and Prevention. Attempted suicide among high school students: United States, 1990. *MMWR Morb Mortal Wkly Rep* 1991;40:633.

8. Smith K, Crawford S. Suicidal behavior among "normal" high school students. *Suicide Life Threat Behav* 1986;16:313.

9. Hibbard RA, Brack CJ, Rauch S, et al. Abuse, feelings, and health behaviors in a student population. *American Journal of Diseases of Children* 1988;142:326.

10. Centers for Disease Control and Prevention. Results from the national adolescent student health survey. *MMWR Morb Mortal Wkly Rep* 1989;38:147.

11. Blum RW, Resnick M, Geer L, et al. *The state of adolescent health in Minnesota.* Minneapolis: University of Minnesota Adolescent Health Program; 1989.

12. Centers for Disease Control and Prevention. Youth risk behavior surveillance: United States, 1995. *MMWR Morb Mortal Wkly Rep* 1996;45(SS-4):1.

13. McIntire MS, Angle CR, Struempler LJ. The concept of death in Midwestern children and youth. *American Journal of Diseases of Children* 1972;123:527.

14. Brent DA. Depression and suicide in children and adolescents. *Pediatr Rev* 1993;14:380.

15. Kachur SP, Potter LB, Powell KE, et al. Suicide: epidemiology, prevention, and treatment. *Adolescent Medicine: State of the Art Reviews* 1995;6:171.

16. Hodgman CH, McAnarney ER. Adolescent depression and suicide: rising problems. *Hosp Pract* 1992;27:73.

17. Holinger PC. The causes, impact, and preventability of childhood injuries in the United States: childhood suicide. *American Journal of Diseases of Children* 1990;144:670.

18. Sloan JH, Rivara FP, Reay DT, et al. Firearm regulations and rates of suicide: a comparison of two metropolitan areas. *N Engl J Med* 1990;322:369.

19. Brent DA, Perper JA, Allman CJ, et al. The presence and accessibility of firearms in the homes of adolescent suicides: a case-control study. *JAMA* 1991;266:2989.

20. Kellerman AL, Rivara FP, Somes G, et al. Suicide in the home in relation to gun ownership. *N Engl J Med* 1992;327:467.

21. Brent DA, Perper JA, Moritz G, et al. Firearms and adolescent suicide: a community case-control study. *American Journal of Diseases of Children* 1993;147:1066.

22. Sells CW, Blum RW. Morbidity and mortality among US adolescents: an overview of data and trends. *Am J Public Health* 1996;86:513.

23. Crumley FE. Substance abuse and adolescent suicidal behavior. *JAMA* 1990;263:3051.

24. Bukstein OG, Brent DA, Perper JA, et al. Risk factors for completed suicide among adolescents with a lifetime history of substance abuse: a case-control study. *Acta Psychiatr Scand* 1993;88:403.

25. Centers for Disease Control and Prevention. Fatal and nonfatal suicide attempts among adolescents: Oregon, 1988–1993. *MMWR Morb Mortal Wkly Rep* 1995;44:312.

26. Strasburger VC. *Adolescents and the media: medical and psychological impact.* Thousand Oaks, CA: Sage; 1995.

27. Reeve A, Strasburger VC. Is it "real" or is it psychosomatic? Principles of psychosomatic medicine in adolescence. In: Greydanus DE, Wolraich M, eds. *Behavioral pediatrics.* New York: Springer-Verlag; 1992:352.

28. deWilde EJ, Kienhorst ICWM, Diekstra RFW, et al. The relationship between adolescent suicidal behavior and life events in childhood and adolescence. *Am J Psychiatry* 1992;149:45.

29. McClure GMG. Suicide in children and adolescents in England and Wales 1960–1990. *Br J Psychiatry* 1994;165:510.

30. Hawton K, Catalan J. *Attempted suicide: a practical guide to its nature and management.* 2nd ed. Oxford, England: Oxford University Press; 1987.

31. Brent DA. Suicide and suicidal behavior in children and adolescents. *Pediatr Rev* 1989;10:269.

32. Tishler CL. Adolescent suicide: assessment of risk, prevention, and treatment. *Adolescent Medicine: State of the Art Reviews* 1992;3:51.

33. Berlin IN. Suicide among American Indian adolescents: an overview. *Suicide Life Threat Behav* 1987;17:218.

34. Davidson LE. Suicide clusters and youth. In: Pfeffer CR, ed. *Suicide among youth: perspectives on risk and prevention.* Washington, DC: American Psychiatric Press; 1989:83.

35. Grossman DC, Milligan BC, Deyo RA. Risk factors for suicide attempts among native American adolescents. *American Journal of Diseases of Children* 1990;144:439.

36. Thompson JW, Walker RD. Adolescent suicide among American Indians and Alaska natives. *Psychiatric Annals* 1990;20:128.

37. Shaffer D, Gould M, Hicks RC. Worsening suicide rate in black teenagers. *Am J Psychiatry* 1994;151:1810.

38. Brent DA, Perper JA, Allman CJ. Alcohol, firearms, and suicide among youth. *JAMA* 1987;257:3369.

39. Boyd JH, Moscicki EK. Firearms and youth suicides. *Am J Public Health* 1986;76:1240.

40. Sloan JH, Rivara FP, Reay DT, et al. Firearm regulations and rates of suicide: a comparison of two metropolitan areas. *N Engl J Med* 1990;322:369.

41. Wintemute GJ, Teret SP, Kraus JF, et al. The choice of weapons in firearm suicides. *Am J Public Health* 1988;78:824.
42. Sadowski LS, Cairns RB, Earp JA. Firearm ownership among nonurban adolescents. *American Journal of Diseases of Children* 1989;143:1410.
43. Christoffel KK, Christoffel T. Handguns as a pediatric problem. *Pediatr Emerg Care* 1986;2:343.
44. Berman AL, Schwartz RH. Suicide attempts among adolescent drug users. *American Journal of Diseases of Children* 1990;144:310.
45. Denny KM. Russian roulette: a case of questions not asked? *J Am Acad Child Adolesc Psychiatry* 1995;34: 1682.
46. Garfinkel BD, Froese A, Hood J. Suicide attempts in children and adolescents. *Am J Psychiatry* 1982;139: 1257.
47. Brent DA, Perper JA, Moritz G, et al. Suicide in adolescents with no apparent psychopathology. *J Am Acad Child Adolesc Psychiatry* 1993;32:494.
48. Shaffer D. The epidemiology of teen suicide: an examination of risk factors. *J Clin Psychiatry* 1988;49 (Suppl):36.
49. Riggs S, Alario AJ, McHorney C. Health risk behaviors and attempted suicide in adolescents who report prior maltreatment. *J Pediatr* 1990;116:815.
50. Brent DA, Perper JA, Goldstein CE, et al. Risk factors for adolescent suicide: a comparison of adolescent suicide victims with suicidal inpatients. *Arch Gen Psychiatry* 1988;45:581.
51. Shafii M, Carrigen S, Whittinghill JR, et al. Psychological autopsy of completed suicide in children and adolescents. *Am J Psychiatry* 142:1061, 1985;.
52. Brent DA, Perper JA, Moritz G, et al. Psychiatric risk factors for adolescent suicide: a case-control study. *J Am Acad Child Adolesc Psychiatry* 1993;32:521.
53. Marttunen MJ, Henriksson MM, Aro HM, et al. Suicide among female adolescents: characteristics and comparison with males in the age group 13 to 22 years. *J Am Acad Child Adolesc Psychiatry* 1995;34:1297.
54. King CA, Raskin A, Gdowski CL, et al. Psychosocial factors associated with urban adolescent female suicide attempts. *J Am Acad Child Adolesc Psychiatry* 1990;29:289.
55. Greene JW, Walker LS, Hickson G, et al. Stressful life events and somatic complaints in adolescents. *Pediatrics* 1985;75:19.
56. Schonberg SK. Can adolescent suicide attempters be distinguished from at-risk adolescents? *Pediatrics* 1991; 88:636.
57. Pastore DR, Fisher M, Friedman SB. Violence and mental health problems among urban high school students. *J Adolesc Health* 1996;18:320.
58. Hoberman HM, Garfinkel BD. Completed suicide in youth. *Can J Psychiatry* 1988;33:494.
59. Harkavay J, Asnis G. Suicide attempts in adolescence: prevalence and implications. *N Engl J Med* 1985;313: 1290.
60. Swedo SE, Rettew DC, Kuppenheimer M, et al. Can adolescent suicide attempters be distinguished from at-risk adolescents? *Pediatrics* 1991;88:620.
61. Greydanus DE, Pratt HD. Emotional and behavioral disorders of adolescence. Parts I and II. *Adolescent Health Update* 1995;7(3):1, 8(1):1.
62. Remafedi G, Farrow J, Deisher R. Risk factors for attempted suicide in gay and bisexual youth. *Pediatrics* 1991;87:869.
63. Slap GB, Vorters DF, Chaudhuri S, et al. Risk factors for attempted suicide during adolescence. *Pediatrics* 1989;84:762.
64. Pfeffer CR. Life stress and family risk factors for youth fatal and nonfatal suicidal behavior. In: Pfeffer CR, ed. *Suicide among youth: perspectives on risk and prevention*. Washington, DC: American Psychiatric Press; 1989:143.
65. Gould MS, Shaffer D. The impact of suicide in television movies. *N Engl J Med* 1986;315:690.
66. Phillips DP, Carstensen LL. Clustering of teenage suicides after television news stories about suicide. *N Engl J Med* 1986;315:685.
67. Gould MS, Davidson L. Suicide contagion among adolescents. *Advances in Adolescent Mental Health* 1988;3: 29.
68. Gould MS, Shaffer D, Kleinman M. The impact of suicide in television movies: replication and commentary. *Suicide Life Threat Behav* 1988;18:90.
69. Davidson LE, Rosenberg ML, Mercy JA, et al. An epidemiologic study of risk factors in two teenage suicide clusters. *JAMA* 1989;262:2687.
70. Wass H, Miller MD, Stevenson RG. Factors affecting adolescents' behavior and attitudes toward destructive rock lyrics. *Death Studies* 1989;13:287.
71. Ballenger J, Goodwin FK, Major LF. Alcohol and central serotonin metabolism in man. *Arch Gen Psychiatry* 1979;36:224.
72. Mann JJ, DeMeo MD, Keilp JG, et al. Biological correlates of suicidal behavior in youth. In: Pfeffer CR, ed. *Suicide among youth: perspectives on risk and prevention*. Washington, DC: American Psychiatric Press; 1989:185.

73. Cooper SJ, Kelley CB, King DJ. 5-Hydroxyindoleacetic acid in cerebrospinal fluid and prediction of suicidal behaviour in schizophrenia. *Lancet* 1992;340:940.

74. Nordstrom P., Samuelsson M, Asberg B, et al. CSF 5-HIAA predicts suicide risk after attempted suicide. *Suicide Life Threat Behav* 1994;24:1.

75. Asberg M, Nordstrom P, Traskman-Bendz L. Cerebrospinal fluid studies in suicide. *Ann NY Acad Sci* 1987; 487:243.

76. Pandey GN, Pandey SC, Janicak PG, et al. Platelet serotonin-2 receptor binding sites in depression and suicide. *Biol Psychiatry* 1990;28:215.

77. Centers for Disease Control and Prevention. Adolescent suicide and suicide attempts: Santa Fe County, New Mexico, January 1985–May 1990. *MMWR Morb Mortal Wkly Rep* 1991;40:329.

78. Brent DA, Perper JA, Moritz G, et al. Psychiatric sequelae to the loss of an adolescent peer to suicide. *J Am Acad Child Adolesc Psychiatry* 1993;32:509.

79. Brent DA, Perper JA, Moritz G, et al. Psychiatric impact of an adolescent sibling to suicide. *J Affect Disord* 1993;28:249.

80. Hodgman CH. Adolescent depression and suicide. *Adolescent Medicine: State of the Art Reviews* 1990;1:81.

81. Rotheram MJ. Evaluation of imminent danger for suicide. *Am J Orthopsychiatry* 1987;57:102.

82. Litt IF, Curskey WR, Rudd S. Emergency room evaluation of the adolescent who attempts suicide: compliance with follow-up. *J Adolesc Health* Care 1983;4:106.

83. Marks A. Management of the suicidal adolescent on a nonpsychiatric adolescent unit. *J Pediatr* 1979;95:305.

84. Centers for Disease Control and Prevention. *Youth prevention programs: a resource guide*. Atlanta, GA: U.S. Department of Health and Human Services, Public Health Service, Centers for Disease Control and Prevention; 1992.

85. Christoffel KK, Naureckas SM. Firearm injuries in children and adolescents: epidemiology and preventive approaches. *Curr Opin Pediatr* 1994;6:519.

86. Webster DW, Wilson MEH. Gun violence among youth and the pediatrician's role in primary prevention. *Pediatrics* 1994;94(Suppl):617.

87. Loftin C, McDowall D, Wiersma, et al. Effects of restrictive licensing of handguns on homicide and suicide in the District of Columbia. *N Engl J Med* 1991;325:1615.

88. Loftin C, McDowall D, Wiersma B. Evaluating effects of changes in gun laws. *Am J Prev Med* 1993;9 (Suppl):39.

89. Price RH, Cowen EL, Lorion RP, et al. The search for effective prevention programs: what we learned along the way. *Am J Orthopsychiatry* 1989;59:49.

90. Shaffer D, Garland A, Vieland V, et al. The impact of curriculum-based suicide prevention programs for teenagers. *J Am Acad Child Adolesc Psychiatry* 1991;30:588.

91. Shaffer D, Vieland V, Garland A, et al. Adolescent suicide attempters: response to suicide prevention programs. *JAMA* 1990;264:3151.

92. Shaffer D, Garland A, Fisher P, et al. Suicide crisis centers: a critical reappraisal with special reference to the prevention of youth suicide. In: Goldston FE, Heinicke CM, Pynoos RS, et al, eds. *Prevention of mental health disturbance in childhood*. Washington, DC: American Psychiatric Press; 1990:135.

93. Miller HL, Coombs DW, Leeper JD, et al. An analysis of the effects of suicide prevention facilities on suicide rates in the United States. *Am J Public Health* 1984;74:340.

94. King GD. An evaluation of the effectiveness of a telephone counseling center. *Am J Community Psychol* 1977;5:75.

95. Phillips DP, Carstensen LL, Paight DJ. Effects of mass media news stories on suicide, with new evidence on the role of story content. In: Pfeffer CR, ed. *Suicide among youth: perspectives on risk and prevention*. Washington, DC: American Psychiatric Press; 1989:101.

SUGGESTED READING

Adler RS, Jellinek MS. After teen suicide: Issues for pediatricians who are asked to consult to schools. *Pediatrics* 1990;86:982.

Berman AL, Jobes DA. Suicide prevention in adolescents (age 12–18). *Suicide Life Threat Behav* 1995;25:143.

Bostic JQ, Wilens TE. How should pediatricians approach the depressed adolescent? *Adolescent Medicine: State of the Art Reviews* 1997;8(3):517.

Brent DA. Depression and suicide in children and adolescents. *Pediatr Rev* 1993;14:380.

Garland AF, Zigler E. Adolescent suicide prevention: current research and social policy implications. *Am Psychol* 1993;48:169.

Gould M.S., Davidson L. Suicide contagion among adolescents. *Advances in Adolescent Mental Health* 1988;3:29.

Grossman DC. Risk and prevention of youth suicide. *Pediatr Ann* 1992;21:448.

Hodgman CH, McAnarney ER. Adolescent depression and suicide: rising problems. *Hosp Pract* 1992;27:73.

Holinger PC, Offer D, Barter JT, et al, eds. *Suicide and homicide among adolescents.* New York: Guilford Press; 1994.

Kachur SP, Potter LB, Powell KE, et al. Suicide: epidemiology, prevention, and treatment. *Adolescent Medicine: State of the Art Reviews* 1995;6:171.

Kellerman AL, Rivara FP, Somes G. Suicide in the home in relation to gun ownership. *N Engl J Med* 1992;327: 467.

Ladame F. Suicide prevention in adolescence: an overview of current trends. *J Adolesc Health* 1992;13:406.

Miller D. Adolescent suicide: etiology and treatment. *Adolesc Psychiatry* 1993;19:361.

Moscicki EK. Epidemiology of suicidal behavior. *Suicide Life Threat Behav* 1995;25:22.

Orr DP. Helping parents of suicidal or depressed adolescents. *Adolescent Medicine: State of the Art Reviews* 1991; 2:335.

Pfeffer CR, ed. *Suicide among youth: perspectives on risk and prevention.* Washington, DC: American Psychiatric Press; 1989.

Sells CW, Blum RW. Morbidity and mortality among US adolescents: an overview of data and trends. *Am J Public Health* 1996;86:513.

Slap GB, Vorters DF, Khalid N, et al. Adolescent suicide attempters: do physicians recognize them? *J Adolesc Health* 1992;13:286.

Tishler CL. Adolescent suicide: assessment of risk, prevention, and treatment. *Adolescent Medicine: State of the Art Reviews* 1992;3:51.

ADOLESCENT DEPRESSION AND RELATED DISORDERS

Depression is both a symptom and an illness. This explains some of the difficulty in understanding it or in researching its prevalence. Virtually all human beings experience depression at some point in their lives—so-called "situational" or "reactive" depression. As a part of the grieving process, it is even normal and beneficial. However, these depressions are transient and reality based. A variety of symptoms are common in adolescents and may accelerate in a downward spiral of loss of self-esteem and reality testing [1,2] (Table 12). A number of depressive syndromes have been described in adolescence [3]. Many experts believe that the incidence of depression and depressive symptoms is increasing significantly among children and adolescents [4,5].

Physicians need to become aware of the common signs and symptoms and the prospective treatment of adolescent depression and other psychiatric disorders. Under the new rules of managed care, primary care practitioners are being asked to treat more patients with milder psychiatric illness rather than immediately referring them [2].

Prevalence

Although depressive symptoms are extremely common during adolescence, clinical depression is somewhat rarer [2]. Distinguishing between normal adolescent mood swings and serious clinical depression can be surprisingly difficult at times, especially when large surveys of adolescents reveal significant depressive symptomatology [6]. For example, in the National Adolescent Health Survey, 45% of teenagers reported difficulty coping with either home or school situations, 24% reported feeling sad and hopeless, and 13% responded that they often had nothing to look forward to [7]. The true test is that downward mood swings in teenagers are usually short-lived, do not result in changes in school performance or relationships with peers, and are not associated with profound pessimism. Depressed mood occurs about eight times more frequently than serious depression [8].

Estimates of the prevalence of depression among adolescents vary widely [9–11], but when signs and symptoms are used to make the diagnosis, as in one study, perhaps as many as 13% to 28% of teens are mildly depressed, 7% moderately depressed, and 1.3% severely depressed [12]. The lifetime incidence of significant depression is said to be approximately 13% to 18% [8,9]. Many depressed adolescents are not suicidal, and many suicidal adolescents are not depressed [4]. Overall, suicidal tendencies develop in about 15% of depressed individuals [13].

Thorough and comprehensive reviews of adolescent depression, acting-out behavior, psychosomatic illness, and eating disorders are beyond the intended scope of this book. Nevertheless, physicians need to know the rudiments of dealing with such adolescents. For further, more detailed discussion, readers are referred to the Suggested Reading list at the end of each section.

TABLE 12. *Symptoms of adolescent depression*

Mood changes:	Feeling depressed or bored
	Diminished pleasure in most activities
	Self-destructive behavior
	Irritability
	Avoiding old friends
Changes in thinking:	Diminished ability to think clearly or to concentrate
	Deterioration in school work
	Increased self-criticism
	Preoccupation with thoughts about health, suicide, or death
	Feelings of hopelessness or pessimism
Changes in bodily function:	Increased *or* decreased appetite
	Significant weight loss *or* weight gain
	Increased *or* decreased sleeping
	Chronic fatigue or lack of energy

Adapted from *Diagnostic and statistical manual of mental disorders.* 3rd ed., revised (DSM-IIIR). Washington, DC: American Psychiatric Association; 1987.

Risk Factors

Family history is often positive for someone with either a psychiatric disorder or depression [5,14]. In one study of relatives of teenagers with bipolar depression, 35% of parents and 77% of relatives overall suffered from depression as well [15]. In a separate study, the risk of depression in a teenager was 27% if one parent had a major depression, 74% if both did [16]. Such data increase the basis for the genetic contribution to depression.

As in suicidal behavior, depression is often associated with an actual or perceived loss [5]. In addition, parental dysfunction and inconsistent discipline seem contributory as well [13]. Other associated risks include chronic illness, including cancer and orthopedic problems, eating disorders, conduct disorders, substance abuse, anxiety disorders, and borderline personality disorders [12,17]. In general, adolescents who have a depressive illness are more likely to use alcohol or other drugs, attempt suicide, have academic problems, and display other behavior disorders [8,18]. In one unusual study, smoking was found to be used as a self-medication for depression and anxiety by teenage girls [19].

Etiology

A number of biochemical theories of depression exist, including a key role for neurotransmitters such as dopamine, norepinephrine, and serotonin [20]. For example, depressed patients have increased levels of serotonin-2 receptors, and those who have suicidal ideation or have made suicide attempts have levels that are even higher [21]. Psychological theories include a psychoanalytical model of "anger turned inward" and poor self-esteem, produced by a negative childhood environment, and a cognitive model, in which self-destructive thinking causes depression [1]. Developmental and hormonal changes during puberty may also play a significant role [22].

Overall, a final common pathway hypothesis seems most likely. Environmental events, such as personal loss, chemicals, or illnesses could result in a biologic dysfunction of neurotransmitters [23]. Depressed young people are known to be exposed to greater family discord than nondepressed control subjects, and several biochemical abnormalities have been isolated (e.g., decreased growth hormone secretion, blunted prolactin response to 5-hydroxytryptophan, and insulin-induced hypoglycemia, all of which suggest abnormal noradrenergic or serotonergic pathways) [5]. In this way, anxiety and depression may be first cousins, with anxiety being mediated through the noradrenergic system and depression through the serotonergic system [13]. Other evidence raises the possibility of a dominant gene with incomplete penetrance, as well as specific chromosomal defects in depressed patients [1,4].

Diagnosis

Distinguishing between the normal vicissitudes of adolescence and pathologic sadness can be difficult, especially for the busy clinician more used to dealing with sore throats and otitis media. On the other hand, such an ability can be life saving at times and requires more of the art of medicine than the science. There is no single diagnostic test (Table 13). Vegetative signs—loss of appetite, weight loss, increased sleeping, decreased energy—can be present but are less common in adolescents than in adults [24]. More frequently, teenagers may complain of feeling empty, bored, or irritable [2]. In addition, some teenagers may exhibit so-called "masked depression," a term that is now outdated but is still useful to describe risk-taking and self-destructive behaviors that may mask an underlying depression [5]. Consequently, the adolescent appears full of aggression, energy, or bravado rather than withdrawn and silent.

Frequently, the history contains important clues. Parental discord or divorce, family dysfunction, physical or sexual abuse, loss of friends or an absence of close friends, death of acquaintances, and drug or alcohol abuse, all may be symptomatic of depression. School performance is often a sensitive indicator. Other normal developmental tasks may be affected as well. A major upheaval in parent–teen relations, running away, poor control of a chronic disease, unexplained new somatic complaints, or new onset of substance abuse or promiscuous sexual behavior may all be symptomatic of adolescent depression. A variety of medical disorders can also mimic depressive illness during adolescence (Table 14).

Because clinical interviews alone frequently may miss teenagers with significant problems, a number of sensitive self-questionnaires have been devised and tested [1,10,25,26] (Table 15). Biologic tests have been used as well, including the thyroid-stimulating hormone test, the growth hormone test, and the rapid eye movement test. All remain research tools [27].

Only the dexamethasone suppression test (DST) has achieved any widespread acceptance, and its interpretation is somewhat controversial, especially in adolescents [28,29]. If a dose of dexamethasone fails to suppress cortisol production, the test is said to be positive and indicative of a biologic or endogenous suppression (Table 16). However, alcoholism, anorexia nervosa, obesity, Cushing's syndrome, and protein malnutrition can also produce a false-positive DST. Moreover, many teenagers with depression do not have a positive test. Therefore, the DST is useful if it is positive (high specificity) but is not useful if it is negative (low sensitivity); in one study, DST specificity was 80% but sensitivity was only 47% [28].

Above all, consultation with a knowledgeable colleague in adolescent psychiatry, psychology, or social work is recommended if the clinician has any doubt about the diagnosis, treatment, or risk of suicide.

Treatment

The issue of how best to treat adolescent depression is still unsettled. Although widely used, antidepressants may not be any more effective than simple counseling, family therapy, or psychotherapy [5]. In addition, the placebo effect is powerful in treating such cases and may be equal to antidepres-

---

TABLE 13. *Diagnosis of major depression in adolescents*

Patients with major depression experience five (or more) of the following symptoms daily over a 2-week period in episodes sufficiently severe to represent a change from previous functioning:

- Depressed or irritable mood most of the day, nearly every day
- Diminished interest or pleasure in most activities
- Significant weight loss or gain, or decrease in appetite
- Insomnia or hypersomnia nearly every day
- Psychomotor agitation or retardation
- Fatigue or loss of energy
- Feelings of worthlessness or excessive guilt
- Diminished ability to think or concentrate, or indecisiveness
- Recurrent thoughts of death; suicidal ideation or suicide attempt

---

From Greydanus DE, Pratt HD. Emotional and behavioral disorders of adolescence: Part I. *Adolescent Health Update* 1995;7(3):1, with permission. Criteria are adapted from American Psychiatric Association, DSM-IV, 1994.

TABLE 14. *Medical illnesses that can mimic depression*

Infections
Influenza
Encephalitis
Pneumonia
Hepatitis
Syphilis
AIDS

Neurologic disorders
Epilepsy
Subarachnoid hemorrhage
Cerebrovascular accidents
Multiple sclerosis
Wilson's disease

Endocrine disorders
Hypothyroidism
Hyperthyroidism
Hyperparathyroidism
Hypopituitarism

Medications
Antihypertensives
Benzodiazepines
Corticosteroids
Oral contraceptives
Clonidine
Digitalis
Barbiturates

Other
Alcohol abuse
Anemia
Uremia
Drug abuse and withdrawal

Adapted from Yaylayan S, Viesselman JO, Weller EB, et al. Depressive mood disorders in adolescents. *Adolescent Medicine: State of the Art Reviews* 1992;3:41.

sants [29,30]. Both pharmacologic and psychological treatments seem to result in improvement in about two thirds of cases. Certainly, antidepressants should be used with considerable caution and selectivity.

Psychological Therapy

Counseling may be undertaken by the practitioner in milder cases and in conjunction with a psychiatrist in more severe cases. Discussing interpersonal issues and strategies has been shown to be superior to no treatment at all in two controlled trials [30]. Attempts at environmental manipulation may be more important than treating the affective symptoms. For example, intervention with abusive or punitive parents or new strategies of dealing with the patient's chronic illness may be needed [31]. Involving the teenager's parents can be crucial [32]. Because depression often includes the feelings of helplessness, hopelessness, and powerlessness, attempts must be made to alter these perceptions in whatever way possible [1].

One advance that may be effective with teenagers is cognitive therapy, in which they are encouraged to correct maladaptive views of themselves and their environment [33–35]. In one excellent study of 1,652 high school students, teenagers at high risk for the development of a future depressive disorder were randomized to receive either 15 sessions of cognitive group prevention therapy or no therapy. After 1 year, an affective disorder was twice as likely to have developed in the teens who had not received therapy (25.7% vs. 14.5%) [35].

TABLE 15. *Checklist tests for depression*

Test	Acronym	Age (y)	Items	Comments
Beck Depression Inventory	BDI	13–adult	27	Adult reading level but most widely used
Children's Depression Inventory	CDI	7–17	27	Based on BDI; can be read to younger patients
Children's Depression Scale	CDS	9–18	66	Wider range of questions than other tests
Children's Depression Rating Scale	CDRS	5–15	16	Good coverage of biologic symptoms
Reynolds' Adolescent Depression Scale	RADS	8–13	30	Good normative data

From Hodgman CH. Adolescent depression and suicide. *Adolescent Medicine: State of the Art Reviews* 1990;1:81. With permission.

Counseling and psychotherapy are usually appropriate for initial treatment and particularly for adjustment disorders, situational or reactive depressions, and mood disorders [1].

Pharmacotherapy

Pharmacologic treatment may be appropriate after counseling or psychotherapy for at least 1 month has yielded little or no improvement in the patient's status. In addition, antidepressants may be initially indicated if symptoms such as sleep disturbance, withdrawal, and self-criticism are prominent. Finally, some patients with depression may require medication before they can benefit from psychotherapy. For years, clinicians were limited primarily to the use of tricyclic antidepressants, which several studies have shown to have no superiority over placebo treatment in adolescent patients [5,36,37]. However, more recent reports show that serotonin-specific reuptake inhibitors (SSRIs) are substantially effective for treating adolescent depression [38–40].

Who should be administering the antidepressants is another controversial issue. Some adolescent medicine specialists insist that primary clinicians are capable of such therapy [13], but we maintain some skepticism, even given constraints imposed by managed care. It is a rare physician, even one with extensive training in adolescent medicine, who has the experience in adolescent psychiatry or the skill to be administering such drugs. Therefore, consultation with an adolescent psychiatry colleague may be appropriate [40]. Such consultation can be by telephone (after the initial visit), and the clinician and psychiatrist can certainly comanage the patient.

Because tricyclic antidepressants do not have proven efficacy and have significant anticholinergic side effects and cardiovascular toxicity (in overdose), the newer SSRIs have now become the initial drugs of choice for treatment of depression [40–42]. These include fluoxetine (Prozac), sertraline (Zoloft), and paroxetine (Paxil) [43–46]. All are believed to inhibit the presynaptic reuptake of serotonin, thereby leaving more neurotransmitter available to bind to postsynaptic receptors [47].

The SSRIs are more likely than tricyclic antidepressants to cause nausea, vomiting, headache, insomnia, and nervousness; however, they do not cause weight gain, anticholinergic effects, or orthostatic hypotension and are safer in overdosage. The most troublesome side effects of SSRIs are anor-

TABLE 16. *Dexamethasone suppression test*

1. **Day 1:**   0800: Serum cortisol level
                      2300: Dexamethasone 1 mg p.o.
2. **Day 2:**   0800, 1600, 2300: Serum cortisol level
3. **An abnormal test result is indicated by the failure of the serum cortisol levels from day 2 to be suppressed far below the level noted at 0800 of day 1.**

From Greydanus DE. Depression in adolescence: a perspective. *Journal of Adolescent Health Care* 1986;7(Suppl):109S. Copyright © 1986 by the Society for Adolescent Medicine. Reprinted by permission of Elsevier Science Publishing Company.

gasmia and other sexual dysfunction. One case has been reported of long-term sertraline treatment simulating hypothyroidism in an adolescent, with daytime somnolence, lack of energy, and insomnia [48].

If one SSRI is ineffective, switching to a different one may be useful. Adolescents are usually started at a lower dose and increased, to minimize side effects (Tables 17, 18). One alternative drug is bupropion (Wellbutrin), a unique antidepressant that is highly effective in the treatment of depression, eating disorders, and attention deficit/hyperactivity disorder. It is especially useful in patients with concurrent attention deficit/hyperactivity disorder and depression [40]. Bupropion has, however, been associated with seizures; therefore, no single dose should exceed 100 to 150 mg.

Tricyclic antidepressants are powerful drugs with many risks [18], and now represent second-line therapy [40,47,49]. Primary among the risks is overdosage and death. In families where younger children are at home, tricyclic drugs are commonly ingested accidentally. Toxicity is possible at any level; serum levels do not correlate well with symptoms of toxicity; and drug levels may vary as much as sevenfold from patient to patient on identical doses.

All tricyclic drugs are similar in their effectiveness, and their mechanism of action is to prevent reuptake of catecholamines at the synaptic level, thereby improving mood. Imipramine (Tofranil) and amitriptyline (Elavil) have been used most extensively. A single bedtime dose is preferable, and a therapeutic trial may require 4 to 6 weeks. Side effects commonly experienced are dry mouth, drowsiness, orthostatic hypotension, weight gain, and urinary retention.

The tricyclic drugs all have a quinidine-like effect on the heart—slowing intracardiac conduction, as manifested by increased PR intervals and QT intervals. Patients need baseline electrocardiograms and monitoring for first-degree heart block, tachycardia, and hypertension [50]. Unfortunately, both patients and their physicians often keep to lower doses of the drugs to avoid unpleasant side effects, but this may also lead to inadequate treatment.

TABLE 17. *Use of antidepressant medications in adolescents*[a]

Medication	Starting dose	Average daily dose	Consultation dose	Side effects
First-line drugs				
Fluoxetine (Prozac)	10–20 mg	20–40 mg	40 mg+	Anorexia, weight loss, agitation, insomnia, tremor, GI distress, sweating, syncope; *severe drug interactions* with lithium, tricyclic antidepressants, others
Sertraline (Zoloft)	25–50 mg	50–100 mg	100 mg+	
Paroxetine (Paxil)	20 mg	20–40 mg	40 mg+	
Second-line drugs				
Imipramine	25 mg bid or 50 mg qhs	100–125 (divided doses)	125 mg+	Sedation, anticholinergic effects (dry mouth, blurry vision, hypotension, urinary retention, constipation; conduction delays (increased PR interval, prolonged QT interval); *sudden withdrawal:* nausea, emesis, fatigue, increased depression; *overdose:* seizures, arrhythmias, coma, death
Amitriptyline	25 mg bid or 50 mg qhs	50 mg bid or 100 mg qhs	125 mg+	
Nortriptyline	10 mg bid or 25 mg	25 mg tid–qid	100 mg+	
Doxepin	25 mg qod	75–125 mg (divided doses)	125 mg+	

[a]All doses are oral and are suggestions; exact doses may vary. Psychiatric consultation is suggested at or above the "consultation dose."

Adapted from Greydanus DE, Pratt HD. Emotional and behavioral disorders of adolescence: Part I. *Adolescent Health Update* 1995;7(3):1, with permission.

TABLE 18. *Costs of some antidepressants*

Drug	Usual dosage	Wholesale cost (1 mo)
SSRIs		
Fluoxetine (Prozac)	20 mg qd	$64.75
Nefazodone (Serzone)	200 mg bid	$49.68
Paroxetine (Paxil)	20 mg qd	$54.60
Sertraline (Zoloft)	50 mg qd	$58.23
Tricyclics		
Imipramine	200 mg qd	Average generic price = $9.88
Aminoketones		
Bupropion (Wellbutrin)	100 mg tid	$67.60

SSRI, selective serotonin reuptake inhibitor.
Adapted from The Medical Letter. Nefazodone for depression.
The Medical Letter 1995;37(946):33.

REFERENCES

1. Hodgman CH. Adolescent depression and suicide. *Adolescent Medicine: State of the Art Reviews* 1990;1:81.
2. Sherry SL, Jellinek MS. The many guises of depression. *Contemporary Pediatrics* 1996;13:63.
3. American Psychiatric Association. *Diagnostic and statistical manual of mental disorders.* 4th ed. Washington, DC: American Psychiatric Association Press; 1994.
4. Hodgman CH, McAnarney ER. Adolescent depression and suicide: rising problems. *Hosp Pract* 1992;27:73.
5. Brent DA. Depression and suicide in children and adolescents. *Pediatr Rev* 1993;14:380.
6. Roberts RE, Lewinsohn PM, Seeley JR. Symptoms of DSM-III-R major depression in adolescence: evidence from an epidemiological survey. *J Am Acad Child Adolesc Psychiatry* 1995;34:1608.
7. Centers for Disease Control and Prevention. Results from the National Adolescent Student Health Survey. *MMWR Morb Mortal Wkly Rep* 1989;38:147.
8. Elster AB, Kuznets NJ. *AMA guidelines for adolescent preventative services (GAPS): recommendations and rationale.* Baltimore: Williams & Wilkins; 1994.
9. Fleming J, Offord D. Epidemiology of childhood depressive disorders: a critical review. *J Am Acad Child Adolesc Psychiatry* 1990;29:571.
10. Cappelli M, Clulow MK, Goodman JT, et al. Identifying depressed and suicidal adolescents in a teen health clinic. *J Adolesc Health* 1995;16:64.
11. Greydanus DE, Pratt HD. Emotional and behavioral disorders of adolescence. Parts I and II. *Adolescent Health Update* 1995;7(3):1, 8(1):1.
12. Kaplan SL, Hong GK, Weinhold C. Epidemiology of depressive symptoms in adolescents. *Journal of the American Academy of Child Psychiatry* 1984;27:91.
13. Greydanus DE. Depression in adolescence: a perspective. *Journal of Adolescent Health Care* 1986;7 (Suppl):109S.
14. Williamson DE, Ryan ND, Birmaher B, et al. A case-control family history study of depression in adolescents. *J Am Acad Child Adolesc Psychiatry* 1995;34:1596.
15. Strober M, Carlson G. Bipolar illness in adolescents with major depression. *Arch Gen Psychiatry* 1984;39: 549.
16. Gershon ES, Hamovit J, Gruoff JJ, et al. A family study of schizoaffective, bipolar I, bipolar II, unipolar, and normal control probands. *Arch Gen Psychiatry* 1982;39:1157.
17. Hodgman CH. Recent findings in adolescent depression and suicide. *Developmental and Behavioral Pediatrics* 1985;6:162.
18. Crumley FE. Substance abuse and adolescent suicidal behavior. *JAMA* 1990;263:3051.
19. Patton GC, Hibbert M, Rosier MJ, et al. Is smoking associated with depression and anxiety in teenagers? *Am J Public Health* 1996;86:225.
20. Rothschild AJ. Biology of depression. *Med Clin North Am* 1988;72:765.
21. Pandey GN, Pandey SC, Janicak PG, et al. Platelet serotonin-2 receptor binding sites in depression and suicide. *Biol Psychiatry* 1990;28:215.
22. Angold A, Worthman CW. Puberty onset of gender differences in rates of depression: a developmental, epidemiologic and neuroendocrine perspective. *J Affect Disord* 1993;29:145.
23. Freedman DX, Glass RM. Psychiatry. *JAMA* 1984;252:2223.
24. Kutcher SP, Marton P. Parameters of adolescent depression: a review. *Psychiatr Clin North Am* 1989;12:895.
25. Schubiner H, Robin A. Screening adolescents for depression and parent–teenager conflict in an ambulatory medical setting: a preliminary investigation. *Pediatrics* 1990;85:813.

26. Smith MS, Mitchell J, McCauley EA, et al. Screening for anxiety and depression in an adolescent clinic. *Pediatrics* 1990;85:262.
27. Potter WZ, Rudorfer MV, Manji H. The pharmacologic treatment of depression. *N Engl J Med* 1991;325:633.
28. Casat CD, Arana GW, Powell K. The DST in children and adolescents with a major depressive disorder. *Am J Psychiatry* 1989;146:503.
29. Yaylayan S, Viesselman JO, Weller EB, et al. Depressive mood disorders in adolescents. *Adolescent Medicine: State of the Art Reviews* 1992;3:41.
30. Gourash L, Puig-Antich J. Medical and biologic aspects of adolescent depression. *Seminars in Adolescent Medicine* 1986;2:299.
31. Sanford M, Szatmari P, Spinner M, et al. Predicting the one-year course of adolescent major depression. *J Am Acad Child Adolesc Psychiatry* 1995;34:1618.
32. Brown-Jones LC, Orr DP. Enlisting parents as allies against depression. *Contemporary Pediatrics* 1996;13:67.
33. Wilkes JCR, Rush AJ. Adaptation of cognitive therapy for depressed adolescents. *J Am Acad Child Adolesc Psychiatry* 1988;27:381.
34. Kaplan CA, Thompson AE, Searson SM. Cognitive behaviour therapy in children and adolescents. *Arch Dis Child* 1995;73:472.
35. Clarke GN, Hawkins W, Murphy M, et al. Targeted prevention of unipolar depressive disorder in an at-risk sample of high school adolescents: a randomized trial of a group cognitive intervention. *J Am Acad Child Adolesc Psychiatry* 1995;34:312.
36. Geller B, Cooper TB, Graham DL, et al. Double-blind, placebo-controlled study of nortriptyline in depressed adolescents using a "fixed plasma level" design. *Psychopharmacol Bull* 1990;26:85.
37. Strober M, Freeman R, Rigali J. The pharmacotherapy of depressive illness in adolescence: I. an open label trial of imipramine. *Psychopharmacol Bull* 1990;26:80.
38. Kye C, Ryan N. Pharmacologic treatment of child and adolescent depression. *Child and Adolescent Psychiatric Clinics of North America* 1995;4:261.
39. Emslie GJ, Rush AJ, Weinberg WA, et al. A double-blind, randomized placebo-controlled trial of fluoxetine in depressed children and adolescents. *Arch Gen Psychiatry* 1997 (in press).
40. Bailey R, Hendren RL. A primer of adolescent psychopharmacology. *Adolescent Medicine: State of the Art Reviews* 1997;8(1):33.
41. The Medical Letter. Drugs for psychiatric disorders. *The Medical Letter* 1994;36(933):89.
42. Bruhat A, Belmin J, Floquet F, et al. Initial choice of antidepressant therapy in primary care. *JAMA* 1996;276:1301.
43. The Medical Letter. Paroxetine for treatment of depression. *The Medical Letter* 1993;35(892):24.
44. The Medical Letter. Fluoxetine (Prozac) revisited. *The Medical Letter* 1990;32(826):83.
45. The Medical Letter. Sertraline for treatment of depression. *The Medical Letter* 1992;34(870):47.
46. Auster R. Sertraline: a new antidepressant. *Am Fam Physician* 1993;48:311.
47. Shrand JA, Jellinek MS. Psychopharmacology in mood and anxiety disorders. *Contemporary Pediatrics* 1995;12:21.
48. Harel Z, Biro FM, Tedford WL. Effects of long term treatment with sertraline (Zoloft) simulating hypothyroidism in an adolescent. *J Adolesc Health* 1995;16:232.
49. Lapierre YD, Raval KJ. Pharmacotherapy of affective disorders in children and adolescents. *Psychiatr Clin North Am* 1989;12:951.
50. Wilens T, Biederman J, Baldessarini J, et al. The cardiovascular effects of tricyclic antidepressants in children and adolescents. *J Am Acad Child Adolesc Psychiatry* 1996;35:1485.

SUGGESTED READINGS

Birmaher B, Ryan ND, Williamson DE, et al. Childhood and adolescent depression: a review of the past 10 years, parts I and II. *J Am Acad Child Adolesc Psychiatry* 1996;35:1427, 1575.
Brage DG. Adolescent depression: a review of the literature. *Arch Psychiatr Nurs* 1995;9:45.
Brent DA. Depression and suicide in children and adolescents. *Pediatr Rev* 1993;14:380.
Brown-Jones LC, Orr DP. Enlisting parents as allies against depression. *Contemporary Pediatrics* 1996;13:67.
Greydanus DE, Pratt HD. Emotional and behavioral disorders of adolescence. Parts I and II. *Adolescent Health Update* 1995;7(3):1, 8(1):1.
Bailey R, Hendren RL. A primer of adolescent psychopharmacology. *Adolescent Medicine: State of the Art Reviews* 1997;8(1):33.
Iglehart JK. Managed care and mental health. *N Engl J Med* 1996;334:131.
Orr DP. Helping parents of suicidal or depressed adolescents. *Adolescent Medicine: State of the Art Reviews* 1991;2:335.
Shrand JA, Jellinek MS. Psychopharmacology in office practice. *Contemporary Pediatrics* 1995;12:106.
Shrand JA, Jellinek MS. Psychopharmacology in mood and anxiety disorders. *Contemporary Pediatrics* 1995;12:21.
Sherry SL, Jellinek MS. The many guises of depression. *Contemporary Pediatrics* 1996;13:63.

The Medical Letter. Drugs for psychiatric disorders. *The Medical Letter* 1994;36(933):89.

Vanderhoff BT, Miller KE. Major depression: assessing the role of new antidepressants. *Am Fam Physician* 1997;55:249.

OUT-OF-CONTROL BEHAVIORS

What Constitutes Out-of-Control Behavior?

Adolescent behaviors constitute a spectrum, ranging from complete compliance to normal rebelliousness and questioning to out-of-control activities, including running away, prostitution, delinquency, and marked substance abuse. Frequently, the pediatrician is the initial person to make the important assessment of where the teenager fits in this spectrum. Parents often may underestimate the amount of control that they still have over their adolescents, or loss of control may exist in one particular area but not be complete.

Normal rebelliousness is reflected in clothing style, music tastes, and grooming fads that usually annoy and irritate parents but do not signify anything more than the teenager's desire to acknowledge his or her separate identity. The peer group's opinions become paramount, especially over those of the parents. The teenager even may vigorously defend one of his or her peer's use of drugs, for example, scaring the parents into thinking that he or she, too, is using drugs. The teen who argues, "Using drugs is each person's decision, and you don't have the right to impose your own opinion on someone else," is merely defending his or her right to independent thought, not necessarily condoning drug use [1].

Often, significant disagreement between the value systems of parents and teenagers does not exist, but dissent and challenges to authority are common and may lead parents to think that the apple is falling farther from the tree than they would like. The role modeling that occurs during adolescence is frequently silent. Teenagers' abuse of their parents' views represents more of a coping mechanism than a true rebellion. When firm limits are established by parents, they will inevitably be tested and perhaps even violated. Teenagers need to learn about their own abilities and their own powers. Such negativistic behavior must be seen by parents as being adaptive and healthy, even though it is annoying and sometimes worrisome.

Moderate rebelliousness is demonstrated by the adolescent who experiments with drugs, frequently breaks curfews, or provokes arguments at school or home. At this stage, such teenagers need firm limits set to keep their behavior from proceeding into more serious forms of self-destruction. For example, important research by Jessor [2] has shown that most teenagers mature out of drug use. In a follow-up study of a 1969 cohort of teenagers who were in their mid- to late 20s by 1981, he found a strong developmental shift in the direction of conventionality, accompanied by decreased use or discontinuation of drugs. More than half of teenage problem drinkers did not drink heavily as adults. Nearly one half of the women and one fourth of the men had stopped using marijuana [2]. In a sense, one crucial task for the physician of an adolescent is to see them through adolescence with as little permanent trauma as possible.

By contrast, out-of-control behavior usually represents an expression of anger, hostility, extreme frustration, or depression [1]. Substance abuse, unprovoked arguments with parents, or adoption of a life-style completely antithetical to the parents' own may signal impending trouble [3]. At the extremes, teenagers may run away, attempt homicide or engage in self-destructive behaviors, and risk being injured, arrested, or hospitalized. Sometimes such behavior represents a masked depression or underlying anxiety disorder. As one teenager remarked: "I guess I was really depressed. I really didn't like me very much. I treated my body just like a trashcan" [1].

Epidemiologic Features

Runaways

An estimated 1 to 2 million teenagers run away each year [4,5]. Although most return home within a week, 5% are gone for more than a year [6]. Add to this the number of homeless street youth and the total number of permanently displaced teenagers approaches 1 to 2 million [5,7]. Unlike the flower children of the 1960s, today's runaway is equally likely to be lower class or middle class, and no one race predominates. Although the median age for running away is 16 years [6], 10- to 12-year-olds run away as frequently as 17-year-olds [8]. Often, a history of parental neglect or abuse—either physical or sexual—precedes this behavior (50–70%) [6]. One national survey found that nearly half of all adolescents had been either pushed, shoved, slapped, beaten up, or hit with an object by their parents [9]. As might be expected, they are often suicidal [10]. In one study of homeless homosexual teenagers in Los Angeles, more than half reported a previous suicide attempt [11].

Teenage prostitutes are particularly likely to have lived in abusive homes. Over half report sexual abuse and incest as the reason for their leaving home [6]. Unfortunately, once they are on the street, half will be reabused by their pimps [6]. Adolescent male prostitutes are increasing in number as well, particularly since the mid-1980s. Over one third report conflicts over their homosexuality as their reason for running away from home. Their average age is 17 years, 1 year older than their female counterparts [6], although some researchers report an average age as low as 14 years [12].

Teenagers who run away are exposed to amplified adolescent health risks. Their nutrition is generally poor [5,13]. In two different studies, 70% to 97% of runaways used illegal drugs [4,10]. Runaway female adolescents experience sexual intercourse 2 to 4 years earlier than their counterparts at home, often as early as age 12 years [14–16]. In one study, 22% exchanged sex for drugs and 20% reported having more than 100 lifetime partners [15]. Less than half of boys and one third of girls used a condom the last time they had intercourse [16]. Runaway boys may have a higher incidence of homosexual encounters [17,18]. In one study in Los Angeles, the incidence of pelvic inflammatory disease, hepatitis, drug abuse, trauma, and rape among runaways was found to be three to nine times greater than average [18]. As a result of survival sex, multiple partners, and low rates of condom use, runaway youth have human immunodeficiency virus antibody prevalence rates that range from 4% to 12%, 10 times higher than the seropositivity rate found in age-matched adolescents entering the Job Corps [5,19].

Juvenile Offenders, Gangs, and Incarcerated Youth

In 1989, nearly two million arrests involved young people less than 18 years of age, with nearly half a million arrests in the under-15 age group. This represents a sixfold increase in teenage arrests from 1955 [8]. Expressed differently, juvenile court statistics indicate that 2.9% of teenagers appear in court each year for significant offenses, and an estimated one in nine young people will make a court appearance before their 18th birthday [20]. However, given the estimated prevalence of minor offenses such as shoplifting and vandalism, only a minority of adolescents committing illegal acts are detected [20].

From the perspective of the 1950s or 1960s, these figures are increasingly dramatically. Not only are the number of arrests increasing, but the number of violent crimes as well (29% since the mid-1980s) [8]. In 1990, 2,555 murders were committed by teenagers younger than 18 years of age, with 283 of these committed by teens younger than 15 years [8]. Although these account for only 14% and 1.5%, respectively, of the total murders reported in the United States, these statistics are alarming nonetheless. Between 1985 and 1994, the number of juveniles arrested for murder increased 150%, whereas the number of arrests for weapons charges and assault doubled [21]. Some experts believe that by 2010, between 150,000 and 200,000 juvenile offenders will be confined [21].

Most recently, however, these trends have slowed, if not reversed. The latest FBI data show that overall violent crime decreased 4% in 1995, with the greatest decline (7%) among 10- to 14-year-olds. Juvenile arrests for murder have also decreased 14% from 1994 to 1995 (*Associated Press*, December 13, 1996).

Most teenage offenders are raised in poverty and come from stressful or disorganized homes [8]. But middle-class youth have equal rates of status offenses (juvenile crimes) and minor delinquent acts. Although African-American teenagers account for 30% of arrests while comprising 15% of the population, actual rates of delinquent behavior as obtained through confidential self-reports are equal among African-American and white teens [8].

Many experts believe that multiple stresses contribute to delinquency, including physical abuse, poor parenting or communication, low self-esteem, learning disabilities, medical risk factors, and psychopathology [22–25]. Psychiatric illness is highly prevalent, particularly conduct disorders and major depression (20–60% of teens), and an estimated 70% of juvenile offenders have attention deficit/hyperactivity disorder or learning disabilities [8]. Early lead exposure has also been shown to increase the risk for antisocial and delinquent behavior [26].

Incarcerated youth show very high rates of sexual activity at a young age and sexually transmitted disease [6,27,28]. In a large study of 1,801 teens in 39 different correctional facilities, 62% reported onset of sexual intercourse by age 12 years [28]. Of 2,500 girls admitted annually to the Los Angeles County detention homes, 90% are ages 15 to 17 and most are sexually active. Routine screening has shown positivity rates of nearly 17% of girls for gonorrhea, 2.2% for pelvic inflammatory disease, 27% for trichomoniasis, and 19% for bacterial vaginosis [6]. On admission to detention facilities, 10% to 15% of girls are diagnosed as being pregnant [8]. Suicide attempts or suicidal ideation are also extremely common [28].

Many incarcerated youth are involved with gangs, 47% in the most recent study [28]. Drug and alcohol use, fighting, and gang membership seem to be interrelated. Youth gangs are common in American cities with populations over 10,000 people, especially where large minority groups live [29]. Estimates are difficult to find, but one author suggests that there are 1.5 million gang members in 2,100 such cities across the country [30]. Although gangs are commonly associated with blacks and Hispanics and with dysfunctional families, there are many examples of white, middle-class gangs [29,31]. Aside from gang-related violence and other criminal activities, gangs seem to be a major element in drug use and drug distribution, which again has important public health implications related to intravenous drug use and AIDS [29,32].

Clinical Approach

Practitioners are frequently the first professionals called on to assess an out-of-control adolescent. Often, this is in the context of an emergency or crisis, even though the behavior has been occurring for months or years [33]. Family members may now want to pass their responsibilities on to someone outside of the family who can take control of the situation. Thus, they may be annoyed if their unrealistic expectations are not fulfilled by the physician [33].

The differential diagnosis is usually not difficult, and an assessment can be made based on interviews with the adolescent and the parents (Table 19). Management of the patient and the family can be far more arduous. Mild rebellion can be dealt with through counseling. The goal here is to keep the parents from overreacting or interfering with normal developmental processes and to preserve the teenagers' sense of independence and self-esteem while keeping them free from self-injury. Moderate rebellion may require a consultation with a knowledgeable adolescent psychiatrist or psychologist to

TABLE 19. *Differential diagnosis: acting-out behavior*

	Acute psychosis	Suicidal behavior	Conduct disorder
Symptoms	Bizarre behavior Hallucinations	None or depression	School or legal problems
Predisposing factors	Family history Drug use Organic illness	Acute loss Drug use Impulsiveness Access to gun Isolation	Unstable home Drug use Sociopathic personality traits
History	Strange ideas and behavior Sleep problems Poor school performance	Sadness Low self-esteem Sleep problems Poor school performance Withdrawal	Chronic school and behavior problems
Evaluation	Strange ideas Disorganized thoughts Inappropriate responses	Feelings of sadness or hopelessness Suicidal intent and method Environmental stress	Blames others Little anxiety about behavior
Management	Hospitalize Psychiatry consult	Hospitalize Psychiatry consult	Outpatient or inpatient therapy Psychiatry consult

Adapted from Easson WM. Crisis intervention in children and adolescents. *Am Fam Physician* 1989;40:166.

investigate the possibility of an underlying depression or personality disorder. Therapy then can be conducted by the clinician or the mental health professional, or both.

Severe rebellion or out-of-control behavior ordinarily requires inpatient treatment, largely because of the risk that the teenager will run away or continue the self-destructive behaviors if kept in an outpatient treatment mode [3]. In addition, newer drugs can be tried, like clonidine for impulse control disorders and valproate or carbamazepine for aggressive disorders [34].

If the parents have, in fact, not lost control of their teenager, the prognosis is good, given timely and effective intervention. If their control is tenuous, immediate referral to an adolescent psychiatrist or psychologist is warranted. Alternatively, some parents have found solace in the "tough love" approach, which enables them to set clear and consistent limits but does not necessarily involve expelling the teenager from the household, as is commonly thought [35]. If the teenager is out of control, it is likely that the next degree of control will eventually have to be exercised by the juvenile authorities. Parents can sometimes petition the court to provide "surrogate" supervision, through a "Child in Need of Supervision" (CINS) declaration [1]. However, CINS petitions should not take the place of attempts at therapy. The risk of such petitions is that the teenager will feel rejected by the family, who is now willing to give up responsibility for his care and welfare.

The clinician confronted with a patient who has been arrested for a misdemeanor or felony may find herself in a dilemma. Families will want the physician to "defend" the youngster and will often offer up the promise of counseling, should the teenager be set free. However, once the charges are dismissed, the parents' view of the need for counseling shifts dramatically. A better alternative is for the physician to assist the teenager by providing counseling through the arrest and judicial proceedings, rather than serving as a primary advocate for him [1].

Although one third of juvenile detention centers fail to have regular medical clinics and half have no mental health services, primary care physicians may not always be able or willing to provide health care services directly. However, they can serve as advocates for appropriate policies in detention centers and as community leaders who advocate for the development of alternatives to detention centers, such as group homes, day treatment programs, and job training programs for disadvantaged youth [8]. Although it may be tempting to bow to public pressure to adjudicate juvenile offenders as adults, pediatricians and family physicians who care about adolescents should be on the front lines of advocating for more creative and less punitive solutions to treat these unfortunate teenagers.

REFERENCES

1. Friedman SB, Sarles RM. "Out of control" behavior in adolescents. *Pediatr Clin North Am* 1980;27:97.
2. Jessor R. A psychosocial perspective on adolescent substance use. In: Litt IF, ed. *Adolescent substance abuse: report of the Fourteenth Ross Roundtable on Critical Approaches to Common Pediatric Problems.* Columbus, OH: Ross Laboratories; 1983:21.
3. Jankowski JJ. Rebelliousness and out-of-control behavior. In: Dershewitz RA, ed. *Ambulatory pediatric care.* Philadelphia: JB Lippincott; 1988:206.
4. AMA Council on Scientific Affairs. Health care needs of homeless and runaway youths. *JAMA* 1989;262:1358.
5. Morey MA, Friedman LS. Health care needs of homeless adolescents. *Curr Opin Pediatr* 1993;5:395.
6. Manov A, Lowther L. A health care approach for hard-to-reach adolescent runaways. *Nurs Clin North Am* 1983;18:333.
7. Robertson JM. Homeless adolescents: a hidden crisis. *Hospital and Community Psychiatry* 1988;39:475.
8. Yancy WS. Juvenile delinquency: considerations for pediatricians. *Pediatr Rev* 1995;16:12.
9. Gelles RJ. Family violence and adolescents. *Adolescent Medicine: State of the Art Reviews* 1990;1:45.
10. Yates G, MacKenzie R, Pennbridge J, et al. A risk profile comparison of homeless youth involved in prostitution and homeless youth not involved. *Journal of Adolescent Health Care* 1991;12:545.
11. Kruks G. Gay and lesbian homeless/street youth: Special issues and concerns. Journal of Adolescent Health Care 1991;12:515.
12. Nightingale R. Adolescent prostitution. *Seminars in Adolescent Medicine* 1985;1:165.
13. Kufeldt K, Nimmo M. Youth on the street: abuse and neglect in the eighties. *Child Abuse Negl* 1987;11:531.
14. Hein K, Cohen M, Marks A, et al. Age at first intercourse among homeless adolescent females. *J Pediatr* 1978;93:147.
15. Rotheram-Borus MJ, Mayer-Bahlburg H, Koupman C, et al. Lifetime sexual behaviors among runaway males and females. *J Sex Res* 1992;29:15.
16. Anderson JE, Freese TE, Pennbridge JN. Sexual risk behavior and condom use among street youth in Hollywood. *Fam Plann Perspect* 1995;26:22.
17. Hein K. AIDS in adolescence. *NY State J Med* 1987;87:290.

18. Yates GL, MacKenzie R, Pennbridge J, et al. A risk profile comparison of runaway and non-runaway youth. *Am J Public Health* 1988;78:820.
19. St. Louis ME, Hayman CR, Miller C. HIV infection in disadvantaged adolescents in the U.S.: Findings from the Job Corps screening program. *JAMA* 1991;266:2387.
20. Weiner IB. Juvenile delinquency. *Pediatr Clin North Am* 1975;22:673.
21. Traub J. The criminals of tomorrow. *The New Yorker*, November 4, 1996:50.
22. Levine MD, Karniski WM, Palfrey JS, et al. A study of risk factor complexes in early adolescent delinquency. *American Journal of Diseases of Children* 1985;139:50.
23. Lewis DO, Pincus JH, Lovely R, et al. Biopsychosocial characteristics of matched samples of delinquents and nondelinquents. *J Am Acad Child Adolesc Psychiatry* 1987;26:744.
24. Henggeler SW. *Delinquency in adolescence.* Newbury Park, CA: Sage; 1989.
25. Famularo R, Kinscherff R, Fenton T, et al. Child maltreatment histories among runaway and delinquent children. *Clin Pediatr* 1990;29:713.
26. Needleman HL, Riess JA, Tobin MJ, et al. Bone lead levels and delinquent behavior. *JAMA* 1996;275:363.
27. Weber FT, Elfenbein DS, Richards NL, et al. Early sexual activity of delinquent adolescents. *Journal of Adolescent Health Care* 1989;10:398.
28. Morris RE, Harrison EA, Knox GW, et al. Health risk behavioral survey from 39 juvenile correctional facilities in the United States. *J Adolesc Health* 1995;17:334.
29. Greydanus DE, Farrell EG, Sladkin K, et al. The gang phenomenon and the American teenager. *Adolescent Medicine: State of the Art Reviews* 1990;1:55.
30. Miller W. Youth gangs: a look at the numbers. *Children Today* 1982;11:10.
31. Lowney J. The Wall Gang: a study of interpersonal process and deviance among twenty-three middle-class youths. *Adolescence* 1984;19:527.
32. Cos RP. An exploration of the demographic and social correlates of criminal behavior among adolescent males. *J Adolesc Health* 1996;19:17.
33. Easson WM. Crisis intervention in children and adolescents. *Am Fam Physician* 1989;40:166.
34. Bailey R, Hendren RL. A primer of adolescent psychopharmacology. *Adolescent Medicine: State of the Art Reviews* 1997;8(1):33.
35. Newton B. Tough love: help for parents with troubled teenagers—reorganizing the hierarchy in disorganized families. *Pediatrics* 1985;76(Suppl):691.

SUGGESTED READING

Arkin CF, Gilman JB. Rebellious adolescents: is toughlove the answer? *Adolescent Medicine: State of the Art Reviews* 1997;8(3):495.
Blau GM, Gullotta TP, eds. *Adolescent dysfunctional behavior: causes, interventions, and prevention.* Thousand Oaks, CA: Sage; 1996.
Brown RT. Health needs of incarcerated adolescents. *Bull NY Acad Med* 1993;70:208.
Farrow J, Deisher R, Brown R, et al, eds. Health and health needs of homeless and runaway youth: position paper of the Society for Adolescent Medicine. *Journal of Adolescent Health Care* 1993;13:717.
Greydanus DE, Farrell EG, Sladkin K, et al. The gang phenomenon and the American teenager. *Adolescent Medicine: State of the Art Reviews* 1990;1:55.
Kazdin AE. *Conduct disorders in childhood and adolescence.* Thousand Oaks, CA: Sage; 1995.
Morey MA, Friedman LS. Health care needs of homeless adolescents. *Curr Opin Pediatr* 1993;5:395.
Myers WC, Burket RC. Current perspectives on adolescent conduct disorder. *Adolescent Medicine: State of the Art Reviews* 1992;3:61.
Peters RD, McMahon RJ, eds. *Preventing childhood disorders, substance abuse, and delinquency.* Thousand Oaks, CA: Sage; 1996.
Rodriguez LJ. *Always running: la vida loca—gang days in L.A.* Willamantic, CT: Curbstone Press; 1993.
Traub J. The criminals of tomorrow. *The New Yorker,* November 4, 1996:50.
Yancy WS. Juvenile delinquency: considerations for pediatricians. *Pediatr Rev* 1995;16:12.

PSYCHOSOMATIC DISORDERS

It is more important to know what sort of person has a disease than to know what sort of disease a person has.
—Hippocrates

Evaluation and treatment of adolescents with psychosomatic disease represents one of the biggest challenges for clinicians interested in adolescent medicine [1,2]. No other set of disorders calls for the same diagnostic and management skills. Dealing successfully with psychosomatic illness represents the "art" of medicine at its finest. Although there is science present, it is in its infancy. An accurate diagnosis made here represents a real diagnostic coup and a major benefit to the patient and the family. An inaccurate diagnosis can result in repeated and expensive testing, "doctor-shopping," and occasionally even unnecessary surgery.

Basic Principles

Psychosomatic illness is an unfortunate term. All illnesses have both a physiologic and a psychological component to them. "Psychosomatic" seems to imply that there is a mind–body separation that, in fact, does not exist. Our popular culture seems to acknowledge that connections exist between emotions and bodily processes, even if modern medicine is more ambivalent. For example, such expressions as *all choked up, gut reaction, pissed off, you're going to give me a heart attack, you make me sick, I'm so angry I can't see straight* all have a certain psychophysiologic truth to them. And yet, the term *psychosomatic* is frequently used pejoratively, as if to say the pains were imaginary.

There are three basic principles of making the diagnosis of a psychosomatic disorder:

1. Organic disease must be ruled out.
2. There must be positive evidence for psychosocial dysfunction.
3. Ideally, when the psychosocial dysfunction improves, the symptoms of the illness should also improve.

Every medical student in America is taught the first principle. Unfortunately, the teaching about psychosomatic disease frequently begins and ends here. *Psychosomatic illness is not what the patient is left with when no organic illness can be discovered.* In other words, psychosomatic disease is as much a diagnosis of *inclusion* as of *exclusion.* All too frequently, adolescents are told that the pains are "all in your head."

The second principle can be even more difficult to abide by than the first, simply because the patient is usually not aware of any psychosocial dysfunctioning. In fact, the symptom or symptom complex may be keeping the patient from having to experience or deal with psychosocial stress. *If patients could identify the sources of their stress or anxiety, they would not, subconsciously, have to resort to somatization.* For example, acute chest pains develop in a 16-year-old during the period that his parents separate and decide to divorce. The appearance of these symptoms may allow the teenager to rechannel his distress about the divorce into (for him) a more acceptable pathway. Assuming the sick role means that he is not responsible for what is happening to him, nor must he behave in the same way as if he were well [3,4]. His symptoms may draw concerned attention from both parents and distract them from their own plans. Furthermore, it is far more acceptable to have a physical illness in our society than to suffer emotional distress. If he were able to verbalize and acknowledge his feelings— "My parents are getting a divorce, and I'm angry and frustrated and can't believe this is all happening"—it is unlikely that a psychosomatic picture would develop.

If the symptoms are indeed stress related, then they should ideally respond to measures that either reduce the stress or allow the patient to cope with it better. For example, the teenager with chest pains could either begin discussing his feelings about the divorce with a counselor or, when the divorce proceeds smoothly, he might realize that the family relationships have actually improved since his parents separated. A number of methods can be tried (see section on Diagnosis and Management).

Epidemiologic Features

Social, emotional, or behavioral problems may constitute up to one fourth of a pediatrician's practice [5–9] (Table 20). The stresses on today's adolescents are unparalleled in the history of American society [10–12] (see Tables 8, 9):

- As many as 40% of all American children will experience the divorce of their parents by age 18 years, and as many as half will spend part of their childhood with only one parent.
- More than two and a half million children have lost at least one of their parents through death.
- Each year, nearly 18% of children move with their families to a new home.
- An estimated 27% of women and 16% of men report having been sexually abused as children [13].
- Because of the high rates of early sexual intercourse and of drug use, today's teenagers have to develop coping strategies earlier than ever before.

TABLE 20. *Epidemiology of psychosocial problems*

Study	No. children surveyed	Prevalence of problems[a]
Goldberg (1979)	3,742	5%
Starfield (1980)	47,145	5–15%
Nader (1981)	671	24%
Goldberg (1984)	18,351	5%
Starfield (1984)	2,591	25%

[a]Behavioral, educational, or social problems.
From Boyce WT. Stress and child health: an overview. *Pediatr Ann* 1985;14:539, with permission.

- Teenagers' concerns about the threat of nuclear war or pollution of the environment may cause them to be skeptical about their future [12].
- An unprecedented number of American children and adolescents now live in poverty and have a bleak economic future as adults.
- The media, especially television and movies, offer teens conflicting and confusing information about the adult world [11].

In fact, the adolescent (and young adult) suicide rate may be serving as a very crude index of stress as experienced by young people in contemporary society.

In a seven-center study of psychosomatic illness in outpatient clinics, one researcher found an incidence of 8% to 10% [6]. The rate was highest among lower socioeconomic groups and female patients, and peaked during the early teen years. The latter is not surprising, given young adolescents' concerns with their bodies [14]. Over half of teenagers either think about their health often or worry about it all the time [15]. As many as 10% of teenagers report frequent chest pains, nausea, fatigue, weakness, or headaches. And 14% of 12- to 17-year-olds report frequent anxiety, with 20% of teens reporting often feeling depressed or miserable [14].

Two studies surveyed large numbers of teenagers and documented frequent somatic symptoms. A study of more than 1,500 middle school students found that 24% reported headaches and 13% reported abdominal pains either daily or several times a week [16]. In a Finnish study of 1,429 students in 10 different schools, 44% of girls and 28% of boys reported frequent or rather frequent occurrence of two or more somatic symptoms during the previous 6 months. Somatic symptoms were correlated with serious illness or injury in the family, parental discord, absence of a parent from the home, trouble with siblings, failing grades in school, and break-ups of relationships with the opposite sex [17].

Scientific Basis for Stress-Induced Disease: An Introduction

Establishing the precise mechanisms and routes of the mind–body connection has not been easy. Nevertheless, a considerable body of literature now attests to the physiologic basis of stress-induced disease [18–20].

A landmark study in 1962 demonstrated that stress can alter the susceptibility of individuals to disease, and that infections represent a good example [21]. The incidence of streptococcal illness increased consistently in children with medium and high levels of stress (as assessed independently) [21]. Other studies of children have found a correlation between amount of stress and injuries, duration of illness, and hospitalizations [22–24] (Fig. 6). Two studies of adults and one of children have demonstrated that the amount of social support may help to mediate stress [23,25,26] (Fig. 7). Greater ego strength has been correlated with a shorter recovery period from infectious mononucleosis [27].

At the organ level, psychiatric "stress interviews" have been shown to induce pressure and motility abnormalities in the sigmoid colon [28,29]. Similar findings were generated by an infamous experiment in which medical student volunteers underwent sigmoidoscopy, and a bowel carcinoma was "accidentally discovered" [30] (Fig. 8). When the hoax was explained, the readings returned to baseline [28].

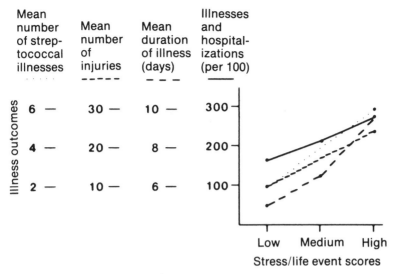

FIG. 6. Results of four studies in which health outcome correlated with extent of stress. (Boyce WT. Stress and child health: an overview. *Pediatr Ann* 1985;14:539, with permission.)

The exact biologic basis for these types of findings is an area of active and exciting research [20,31–34]. Immune responses are blunted under certain conditions, including stress and psychiatric illness [35]. For example, rats treated with cyclophosphamide and saccharine-flavored water demonstrate a decreased antibody response to an antigen. Once conditioned to this stress, the rats later demonstrate a decreased antibody response to antigen when challenged with saccharine-flavored water alone [35].

One important mediator may be salivary IgA, which is the first line of defense against respiratory infection. In one study of dental students, levels of secretion decreased during examinations but recovered afterward [36]. In a study of Harvard college students, researchers found that students with

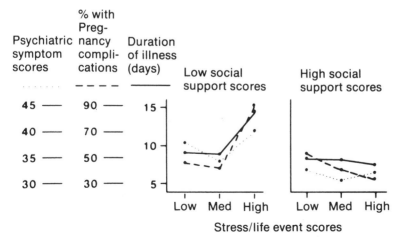

FIG. 7. How social support can mediate the effects of stress and improve health outcome. (Boyce WT. Stress and child health: an overview. *Pediatr Ann* 1985;14:539, with permission.)

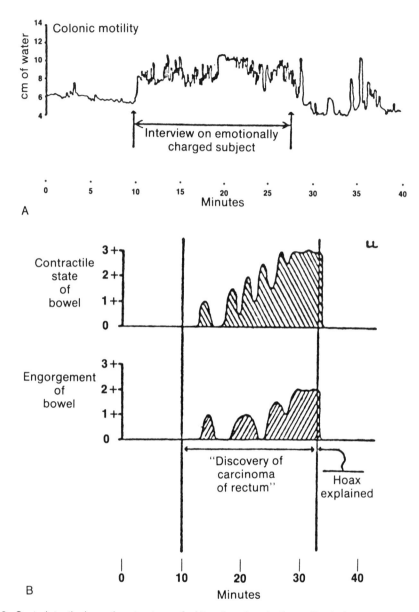

FIG. 8. Gastrointestinal reactions to stress. **A:** Alterations in colonic motility during a stress interview. **B:** Sigmoidoscopic observations before, during, and after a normal medical student volunteer was informed—as a hoax—that he had a carcinoma of the rectum. (Drossman DA, Powell DW, Sessions JT Jr. The irritable bowel syndrome. *Gastroenterology* 1977;73:811, with permission.)

greater need of power or control in their lives had a higher frequency of and more prolonged infections after final examinations. This correlated with higher urinary epinephrine levels and lower amounts of secretory IgA in their pharynx [37]. Interestingly, a Swedish study found that increased epinephrine secretion in response to stress is more frequently negatively associated with performance and self-esteem in women than in men—a finding that might explain why adolescent girls seem more vulnerable to psychosomatic disorders than boys [38].

On a cellular level, two main systems have been recognized that mediate stress responses: the hypothalamic–pituitary–adrenal axis (HPA) and the locus ceruleus–norepinephrine–autonomic nervous system [33]. Receptors on cell surfaces of lymphocytes and thymocytes exist for a broad range of hormones and neurotransmitters, including corticosteroids, beta-adrenergic agents, and endorphins [39]. Social stressors can trigger the HPA system; psychological stressors can also cause thymic involution and alter immunologic functions such as lymphocyte proliferation and natural killer (NK) cell activity [34]. Lymphocyte response to mitogen stimulation and absolute numbers of both B and T cells have been shown to be decreased in depressive illness [32]; in two separate studies, levels of NK cell activity were diminished in college students who reported high levels of stress and anxiety [40] and in medical students who were socially isolated or undergoing examinations [29]. One study also found that intense exercise causes increases in NK cell number and a transient leukocytosis [41]. Other studies have demonstrated that the individual's own temperament and his or her response to the stress are the key events, rather than the stress itself, which has important implications for treatment [32,39].

Diagnosis and Management

Although making a psychosomatic diagnosis can be satisfying to the practitioner (if not to the family and patient), it is fraught with anxiety as well [1,2]. "How can I be sure I'm not missing *X*, *Y*, or *Z*?" becomes a frequent thought, even after office hours. Often, such thoughts lead to "just one more test" or another consultation. Because there is no one test for psychosomatic illness, there is no safety in making the diagnosis; it hinges on adhering to the three basic principles mentioned at the beginning of the section.

Furthermore, the diagnosis is elusive because even though the symptoms are stress related, the patient and the family often have no concept of what stress the patient is experiencing, or how dysfunctional his response to the stress is. Therefore, questions like, "Are you aware of any stresses in your life?" or "What stressful thing happens each time your stomach hurts?" are a waste of time [14]. Identifying the relationship between the physical symptoms and the psychological stress requires great finesse, patience, and thoroughness. Often, the connection will not be apparent during the first visit, no matter how thorough a history is taken. And, of course, many patients and their families resent the implication that the pains are "all in my head."

Clinicians need to maintain a high index of suspicion that chronic pains are psychosomatic in origin. In particular, chronic headaches, chest pains, or abdominal pains frequently have either a psychogenic origin or at least a significant component. Other factors that may alert the physician to a psychosomatic diagnosis are [1,2]:

- The patient's reaction to the symptoms, which may be curiously disproportionate to his or her actual disability. For instance, a teenager with chronic abdominal pain may describe his symptoms in great detail and with great relish. This probably represents a variation on *la belle indifference* that Charcot originally described in conversion hysteria [42].
- A past history of multiple somatic complaints.
- Dysfunctional features in key areas of normal adolescent development: family, peers, and school.
- A history of multiple visits to different physicians.
- Presence, within the family, of a role model with chronic or recurrent symptoms.
- Presence of a "psychosomatic family" (e.g., rigid, "enmeshed," and overprotective). Such families tend to avoid conflict and encourage expression of feelings by the somatic route [43].

Ordinarily, there is no urgency in diagnosing rare medical disorders; they usually make their presence known eventually. The astute clinician follows and reassesses the patient frequently, rather than pursuing an immediate "shotgun" approach to testing. Many investigators have commented on the need to proceed with the organic and the psychological investigations simultaneously. This accomplishes several objectives. For reluctant patients and their families, the psychological evaluation is better tolerated because it, too, is seen as a diagnostic test. On the other hand, an appropriate diagnostic workup assures the patient, the family, and the physician that no medical disorder is being overlooked.

In the typical scenario, the medical workup is done first; then, when it is negative, the patient is shuttled off to see a psychiatrist. Understandably, most patients resent this, and *it is antitherapeutic*. When both aspects of the workup are pursued simultaneously, the physician can reassure the patient that the tests are all normal but that the psychological profile reveals significant stress and probably represents the source of the problem. Patients are able to accept this diagnostic style more readily.

Yet despite this approach, patients and their families are often reluctant to accept the diagnosis of a stress-related disorder. A number of options still exist. Even resistant families will accept the notion of tension headaches: the pains are real, but they are induced by stress. Likewise, diarrhea occurring around examination time is a common experience for many people. Families who still deny this association usually accept the fact that the teenager's symptoms are, themselves, stressful to the teenager and the parents, and this should merit some discussion and exploration. Sometimes the symptoms need to be placed in perspective: after all, it is far better to have tension headaches then a medulloblastoma, or psychosomatic abdominal pains rather than ulcerative colitis. Finally, there is the option that an organic illness could be found later on, should further testing be required.

Chronic Abdominal Pain

Case 1

A 15-year-old white boy is admitted by his physician for abdominal pain of 3 weeks' duration. The pain is sharp, intermittent, located in the right lower quadrant. There is no associated nausea, vomiting, fever, weight loss, or diarrhea. Past medical history reveals a similar episode at age 12, requiring a 10-day hospitalization. At that time, a barium enema, upper gastrointestinal series, stools for occult blood and ova and parasites, and erythrocyte sedimentation rate were all normal [44].

Since age 12, he has developed normally and is a well nourished, athletic-looking Tanner 5 male. His weight is 160 lb and he is 5 ft, 8 in tall. Physical examination is normal except for minimal tenderness in the right lower quadrant. Several observers note the patient's *belle indifference* to his pain.

This patient underwent a 2-week hospitalization (total cost: $9,000). All tests were normal and included a lactose tolerance test, upper gastrointestinal series, two barium enemas, pelvic and abdominal ultrasonography, sigmoidoscopy, gastroscopy, and colonoscopy. In addition, the patient underwent therapeutic trials of prednisone, cimetidine, and metronidazole, all of which proved ineffective. After 2 weeks, the patient was discharged from the hospital with no diagnosis established; and he was still complaining of abdominal pains! He was referred to an adolescent medicine specialist for counseling.

At first, the patient was extremely resistant to counseling. He was angry with his doctors for referring him and believed that they had simply not found the right test to perform; consequently, they now thought the pains were all in his head. Despite this and his difficulty expressing his feelings, he seemed to be a likable, intelligent 15-year-old. He could identify no obvious stresses in his life, nor could his family.

Only after six counseling sessions did the complete story emerge: the patient had been raised by his mother and maternal grandmother. When talking about the latter, he became very quiet and maintained poor eye contact. At age 12, he returned home from school to witness his grandmother having a fatal myocardial infarction right in front of him. He was the only one home at the time and was terrified. On reflection, his mother stated that he had refused to go to the funeral and had never really mourned the loss. His first hospitalization for abdominal pain occurred 3 weeks after her death, and he was readmitted to hospital 3 years later, near the anniversary of her death.

After this information was revealed, the patient went home and talked at length about his grandmother, weeping frequently. His abdominal pains gradually subsided during the next 6 weeks of counseling and did not recur during the subsequent 4 years of follow-up (during which time he entered college as a premed major). The total cost of counseling was approximately $350.

Case 2

A 17-year-old white girl is admitted to hospital with a 2-month history of intermittent abdominal pain and vomiting. The pain is mid-epigastric, comes in daily paroxysms, and is accompanied by nausea and vomiting. Her weight has decreased 20 lb in 2 months. There is no associated fever, diarrhea, urinary symptoms, or vaginal discharge, and no history of induced vomiting or distorted self-image. Her last menstrual period was 6 weeks before, and she had been having sexual intercourse with her boyfriend without benefit of contraception.

Her admitting physician believes the pains are psychosomatic in origin, despite not having done a pelvic examination or pregnancy test and despite her lack of psychosocial dysfunction. She is a high school senior, a straight-A student who has many friends and enjoys a close relationship with her family.

On examination, she looks somewhat emaciated. Her weight is 98 lb, and she is 5 ft 4 in tall. She is at Tanner 5 for breast and pubic hair development, her vital signs are normal, and there are no abnormalities found on general examination. However, a pelvic examination reveals a 10-cm mass in her right adnexa, confirmed by ultrasonography. Urine and serum pregnancy tests are negative. At laparotomy, she is found to have a torsion of the right ovary, requiring right salpingo-oophorectomy. A month later, she has returned to her previous weight of 120 lb.

Comment. The incidence of chronic abdominal pain in children and adolescents is high, accounting for as many as 5% of all pediatric office visits [45]. Estimates are that 10% to 15% of school-age children suffer from recurrent abdominal pain, although the exact prevalence among teenagers is unknown [46]. Some experts believe that recurrent abdominal pain is rare in children younger than 5 years or older than 15 years [47].

In Apley's landmark study of 1,000 unselected British schoolchildren, aged 4 to 15 years, 10% fit the criteria—at least three episodes of pain, severe enough to restrict normal activities, occurring over a period of at least 3 months [48]. One hundred of these youngsters were hospitalized for an intensive diagnostic workup. Only 8% were found to have organic lesions. Other studies have found similar figures [46,49,50]. Therefore, the clinician confronted with a teenager with chronic abdominal pain can say, with perhaps 95% accuracy, that the pains are likely to be psychosomatic.

As Case 2 illustrates, however, not only must the definition be fulfilled, but also common sense should dictate the extent of the workup: sexually active female teens should be considered pregnant until proven otherwise and need a thorough pelvic examination to rule out the possibility of pelvic inflammatory disease. Disturbing signs and symptoms, like a 20-pound weight loss, should inevitably lead to a more aggressive workup.

"Common children and adolescents have common diseases" is a useful axiom in practice. The incidence of inflammatory bowel disease is quite low, for example: only 15% of all cases of ulcerative colitis occur before the age of 20 years, with an overall incidence of 4 to 7 cases per 100,000, and Crohn's disease has an incidence of 1 to 3 cases per 100,000 [51–53]. More important, adolescence represents the second most rapid period of growth in a human's life. If the patient in Case 1 were to have had any chronic illness from age 12 to 15, it is unlikely that his growth and development would have proceeded normally. Such patients represent a good in vivo assay of any chronic disease and often suffer a delay in their sexual development as well as their height and weight. Adolescent patients with inflammatory bowel disease often have some abnormality in their basic laboratory tests as well (Table 21). In one of the largest follow-up studies, 161 pediatric patients were studied for 5 years; one third were teenagers. Half had a rapid cure, three fourths eventually improved, and only three patients ultimately had an organic diagnosis (all had Crohn's disease) [50].

A basic workup for chronic abdominal pain probably should include a complete blood count, erythrocyte sedimentation rate, urinalysis, and stools for occult blood and, in selected cases, ova and parasites. Sexually active young women require a pelvic examination, cultures, and a pregnancy test. Other tests may be required according to the findings on history and physical examination [46,47].

TABLE 21. *Laboratory abnormalities in inflammatory bowel disease*

Test	Ulcerative colitis (%) [N = 22]	Crohn's disease (%) [N = 52]
Erythrocyte sedimentation rate > 20 mm/h	90	87
Hematocrit < 33 mg%	38	50
Leukocytes > 10,000/mm	33	70
Iron < 50 μg/dl	68	58
Albumin < 3.3 g/dl	46	54
Folate < 3.6 ng/dl	34	40

From Motil KJ, Grand RJ. Ulcerative colitis and Crohn disease in children. *Pediatr Rev* 1987;9:109. Copyright © 1987. Reprinted with permission of *Pediatrics*.

Probably the most common cause of chronic abdominal pain is chronic constipation, which is usually easily diagnosable with a careful history and physical examination.

Another common cause is *lactase deficiency*. As children age, some lose activity of their lactase. At some point, intake of milk or milk products may exceed the capacity of the enzyme. Unabsorbed disaccharides enter the colon, where they are fermented by bacteria, with liberation of short-chain organic acids and hydrogen gas. Symptoms usually begin within 2 hours after ingestion of lactose, but the timing may vary considerably. In addition, a history of symptoms associated with milk ingestion may not distinguish lactose malabsorbers from other children with chronic abdominal pains [54]. Symptoms may include bloating, lower abdominal pains, increased flatus, and cramps, but not necessarily diarrhea [55]. The incidence is highest in Asian, Mexican-American, Native American, Jewish, Mediterranean, and black populations (60–85%) and lowest in Northern European whites (10–15%) [56]. Certainly, performing a breath hydrogen test is far less painful and costly than numerous invasive procedures [57]. Many experts believe that lactose intolerance is a significant cause of recurrent abdominal pain [46].

Irritable bowel syndrome (IBS) is another confusing aspect when classifying these patients: Is IBS the adult equivalent of chronic abdominal pain in children or adolescence? One prospective study of 227 children and adolescents aged 5 to 18 years with recurrent abdominal pain revealed that more than half fulfilled adult criteria for IBS [58]. An estimated 15% to 20% of adults have symptoms compatible with IBS [59]. A study of 507 adolescents found that 14% of high school and 6% of middle school students reported IBS-type symptoms recurrently, and those who did had higher anxiety and depression scores than asymptomatic students [60]. In general, although there are numerous theories about the pathophysiology of IBS, none is currently predominant [59]. However, newer research at the University of California, Los Angeles finds that patients with IBS have intestinal nerve cells that are unusually sensitive to pain and that brain filtering mechanisms may also play an important role [61]. What is clear is that the diagnosis of IBS requires not only recurrent abdominal pain but a dysfunctional pattern of elimination as well (i.e., diarrhea, constipation, or alternating diarrhea and constipation) [62].

Two trends bear watching in the future. First, researchers have tried to establish a link between recurrent abdominal pain in children and adolescents and infection with *Helicobacter pylori*. *H. pylori* is now the suggested cause of chronic gastritis and peptic ulcer disease in children and adults [63,64]. Is it possible that it causes chronic abdominal pain as well? One study has found a statistically significant increase in anti-*H. pylori* IgG antibodies in children with recurrent pain (17.4%) compared with control subjects (10.5%) [65]. However, a review of 45 studies in the medical literature found weak or no evidence of an association with recurrent abdominal pain [66]. A second study also detected no relationship between *H. pylori* seropositivity and recurrent abdominal pain [67].

Second, some researchers believe that a significant number of patients with recurrent abdominal pain have peptic esophagitis [62]. In one study, more than half of 27 consecutively diagnosed abdominal pain patients underwent pH probes and were found to have significant gastroesophageal reflux. Most responded to treatment with antireflux medications [68,69].

Finally, one other caveat: chronic abdominal pain caused by chronic appendicitis is probably a myth. As the authors of one gastroenterology textbook colorfully state:

> Pain in the right iliac fossa is a common manifestation of anxiety in young women and may have replaced the swooning of the Victorian era. A nagging pain, often *continuous* with occasional stabs, develops, often after worry such as an upset love affair. Fear of appendicitis may have been made worse by the suggestion of a `grumbling appendix'. . .. Many thousands of normal appendices are removed each year because of this. Sometimes the appendix is described as abnormally long or kinked—perhaps as a face-saving manoeuvre by the surgeon—or the pathologist reports minor inflammatory changes which are really variations of normal. . . [70].

Other authors agree [71,72]. Although appendicitis is the first disorder that parents will think of when their teenagers have abdominal symptoms, people carry only a 7% *lifetime* risk for development of it [73], and it should *not* be considered in the differential diagnosis of chronic abdominal pain.

Chronic Chest Pain

Case 3

A 16-year-old black girl is admitted to hospital with sudden onset of left precordial chest pain and difficulty breathing. She had experienced acute chest pains exactly 1 year previously and had been evaluated in the emergency room. At that time, a chest x-ray, electrocardiogram, and echocardiogram had been normal. The pains were attributed to an acute stress reaction: the patient's boyfriend had been driving to visit her and was killed in an automobile accident. Exactly 1 year later, the pains have returned, this time accompanied by severe dyspnea.

On examination, the patient is afebrile but has a pulse of 140 and a respiratory rate of 36. Her respirations are labored. On chest examination, air movement is diminished, although no rales, rhonchi, or wheezes are heard. The remainder of her examination is normal. Initially, her physicians think that she is suffering from psychosomatic chest pains secondary to an anniversary grief reaction. However, she is sufficiently dyspneic to warrant an arterial blood gas determination: pH 7.35, PO_2 68, PCO_2 38. The additional diagnosis of acute asthma is made, and the patient responds to oxygen therapy and standard doses of bronchodilators and steroids.

Comment. This case demonstrates the complexities of making a psychosomatic diagnosis. The patient had already had a thorough workup for her acute chest pains a year ago. When she came to the emergency room exactly 1 year later, it would have been easy to pass her symptoms off as being purely psychosomatic. Yet her physicians were willing to add one more test to the workup: an arterial blood gas. Certainly the new onset of her asthma could be said to be triggered by psychological stress, but most physicians would agree that asthma is a real organic disease, requiring acute medical intervention. Undiagnosed reactive airway disease is now well recognized as a cause of recurrent chest pain in adolescents [74]. Actually, this patient had two physiologic processes at work—acute chest pains, psychosomatic in origin, which responded well to only three sessions of counseling, and acute dyspnea, resulting from her asthma, which responded well to standard medical therapy.

Epidemiologically, chest pains are not as common as abdominal pains, but they have been reported in 3 per 1,000 children visiting an emergency room or outpatient clinic at a children's hospital [75]. Chest pain accounts for 650,000 visits annually for teenagers seen in primary care settings [76]. One survey of black adolescents found chest pain to be the seventh most common health problem [77], and a 1-year study of all children and adolescents seen for chest pain in the emergency room of Children's Hospital of Philadelphia found 407 patients [75]. The mean age of children with chest pain is 12 to 14 years. In 15% to 36% of children with chest pain, the symptom is present for longer than 6 months [75]. A number of prospective studies [75,78–82] and retrospective studies [83,84] have found the following approximate distribution of diagnoses:

Musculoskeletal disorder (including trauma and costochondritis)	35%
Idiopathic disorder	30%
Psychosomatic disorder (including hyperventilation and precordial catch syndrome)	25%
Miscellaneous (respiratory, cardiac, or breast abnormalities, esophagitis)	10%

Hyperventilation can be a particularly difficult disorder to diagnose because many patients are completely unaware of their behavior. However, more than half report anxiety, paresthesias, or lightheadedness [85]. Although having the patient hyperventilate to try to reproduce the symptoms is a common maneuver, in fact it may require 20 to 30 minutes of hyperventilation to produce pain [86]. Panic attacks may be closely related to hyperventilation and are characterized by massive autonomic nervous system discharge, associated with a feeling of overwhelming anxiety. A predisposition to panic attacks may be inherited [87,88].

Given the benign nature of the differential diagnoses [76], it may be surprising to learn that adolescents take their chest pains very seriously; more than 50% fear heart disease, and 12% fear cancer [81]. How the clinician inquires about the symptoms may be extremely important (Table 22).

Chronic Headaches

Case 4

A 13-year-old white boy is referred for evaluation of his headaches. They are frontal, have occurred nearly daily for the past 6 months, and are not associated with nausea, vomiting, auras, or neurologic symptoms. The headaches do not awaken the patient from sleep but are often present on arising. During the past 6 months, they have not increased or decreased in severity. The patient's parents feel that he has undergone a "complete personality change" in the past year. Previously a happy-go-lucky child who was very affectionate with them, he is now more sullen and moody and tends to avoid them. He dislikes their displays of affection. Frequently, he is critical of their views, whereas as a child he was

TABLE 22. *Importance of phrasing questions properly in evaluating psychosomatic chest pain*

	"What do you think caused your pain?"	"What were you *afraid* caused your pain?"
Heart attack	4% ⎫	44% ⎫
Heart disease	6% ⎬ 12%	12% ⎬ 68%
Cancer	2% ⎭	12% ⎭
Gas	7%	0%
Don't know	61%	23%
Miscellaneous	20%	9%

From Pantell RH, Goodman BW Jr. Adolescent chest pain: a prospective study. *Pediatrics* 1983;71:881. Copyright © 1983. Reprinted with permission of *Pediatrics.*

very respectful. They want him to have a computed tomography (CT) scan because they fear he may have a brain tumor.

Physical examination reveals a pleasant, Tanner stage 2 young man who relates well to the examiner. Early bilateral gynecomastia is present, but the remainder of the physical examination is normal. A complete neurologic examination is also normal. Psychologically, the teenager is bright but somewhat isolated from his peers. He has just moved to a new school, is self-conscious about his gynecomastia, and dislikes one of his teachers. He feels that his parents are overly critical of him and still "treat me like a baby." He displays considerable animation when he talks and denies suicidal ideation. He is very interested in electronics but has no friends to share his interest with. He believes that his parents will be disappointed if he does not go to law school.

After the initial visit, he is asked to keep a headache diary for a month (Fig. 9). When he returns, the frequency of headaches is noted to be approximately three to four times weekly, occurring most often

Date _____   Name _____

CIRCLE ANSWER

1. How long did headache last?
      1   2   3   4   5   >6 hours
2. Vomiting?   How many times?
      Yes   No   _____
3. Did child practice relaxation exercise?
      Yes   No
4. Child slept to relieve headache?
      Yes   No
5. Drug given during headache?
      Aspirin   Tylenol   Midrin   Fiorinal
      Cafergot   Other   _____
6. How severe was the headache?
      0   1   2   3   4   5   6   7   8   9   10
7. If school day, did you stay home?
      Yes   No

FIG. 9. Sample headache diary. (Olness KN, MacDonald JT. Recurrent headaches in children. *Pediatr Rev* 1987;8:307. (Copyright 1987. Reproduced by permission of the American Academy of Pediatrics.)

during the week, especially on mornings when he either has gym or history (with the disliked teacher). His physical and neurologic examinations remain normal. Four additional sessions of counseling are set up, incorporating the parents into the process as well. After a month, the parents have a better understanding of normal adolescence, the teenager's academic schedule has been reorganized, he has been appropriately counseled about his gynecomastia, a new best friend has appeared, and the headaches have disappeared.

Comment. Headaches are extremely common during childhood and adolescence [89,90]. Epidemiologic studies report incidences as high as 21% to 55% of all children [91]. Migraine headaches occur in 4% to 10% [92,93]. Data from the 1988 National Health Interview Survey indicate that 4.6% of teenagers suffer from frequent or severe headaches [94].

Unlike with abdominal or chest pains, there is no basic workup here, and walking the tightrope between doing too few diagnostic tests and too many is more difficult. Physicians may believe that by ordering CT scans and electroencephalograms (EEGs) they will be thorough and reassure the family, whereas in fact they may be alarming the teenager who has simple tension headaches.

The fear of missing an early brain tumor is nearly universal among physicians, yet brain tumors occur only rarely during adolescence, with an estimated incidence of 2 to 3 cases per 100,000 [95]. Despite the advent of high-tech scans, a careful neurologic examination is still the best method of screening and identifies all but 5% to 6% of patients with brain tumors [96] (Tables 23, 24). In one unique study of children with headaches secondary to brain tumors, 85% of patients manifested neurologic or ocular abnormalities within 2 months of the onset of their headaches [97]. Two thirds of patients were awakened from sleep with headaches, and over three fourths of patients had associated vomiting [97]. Brain tumor headaches are usually intermittent, deeply aching, exacerbated by exertion and change in position, and commonly occur nocturnally [98].

Patients with chronic headaches do not require an immediate referral to a neurologist, particularly one who is going to automatically order a CT scan and EEG. Time should be spent eliciting a careful medical and social history. For example, headaches that remit on weekends or in a different environment should lead to an investigation of situational stressors. Depressed teenagers should demonstrate other supporting features, such as a decline in school performance, sleep difficulties, or an abnormal score on a depression inventory [99]. On the other hand, disorders such as chronic sinusitis and refractive errors should also be considered. One series of chronic headache patients found a 10% incidence of abnormal sinus films, and the patients' headaches responded to medical therapy for sinusitis [100]. Neuroimaging (e.g., magnetic resonance imaging, CT scans) should be reserved for those patients with specific neurologic findings and who have life-threatening or acutely reversible conditions [101].

Treatment

A variety of treatment options are available and must be tailored to fit each teenager's and family's unique psychological profile [1,2,12,89]. Frequently, several methods can be combined. Repeated diagnostic testing only impedes the healing process if the symptoms are, in fact, psychologically based. A carefully crafted initial workup, which includes some means of assessing the teenager and his family's psychological functioning, serves as a prelude to successful treatment [1,2,102].

TABLE 23. *Features of brain tumor headaches in children*

Recent onset of headaches (within past 4 mo)
Presence or onset of neurologic abnormality, especially ocular findings (papilledema, decreased acuity, or loss of vision)
Persistent vomiting
Increasing severity of headache
Headache awakening child from sleep

Adapted from Honig PJ, Charney EB. Children with brain tumor headaches. *American Journal of Diseases of Children* 1982; 136:121.

TABLE 24. *Checklist: differential diagnosis of headaches*

History	Headache type		
	Migraine	Tension	Organic
Acute onset	+	−	±
Daily frequency	−	+	±
Nausea or vomiting	+	−	±
Fever	−	−	±
Neurologic signs	±	−	+
Family history of headache	±	±	±
Signs of depression	−	+	−
Stress at school or home	±	+	−
Appears ill during headache	+	−	+

Modified from Olness KN, MacDonald JT. Recurrent headaches in children: diagnosis and treatment. *Pediatr Rev* 1987;8:307. Copyright © 1987. Reprinted with permission of *Pediatrics.*

Counseling and Psychotherapy

As previously discussed, pediatricians are well placed to perform office counseling if they wish to do so. In particular, older, more insightful adolescents who have a strong bond with their physician are ideal candidates for counseling. Younger, more immature boys may require an alternative method. Counseling can focus on the source of the stress and discuss alternative ways of coping with it. Simple reassurance and good advice are not useful. To relinquish the symptom, the patient requires another strategy that is less costly psychologically. Patients with more severe types of personality disturbance or marked anxiety states may require assessment or treatment by a skilled adolescent psychiatrist.

Relaxation Training

In suggestive or highly motivated teenagers, teaching them to learn to identify certain bodily cues that signal tension and then relax the muscles involved can be useful. Guided imagery or self-hypnosis accomplishes the same goal. This is particularly useful in teenagers who have chronic tension headaches or migraines or who are undergoing chemotherapy [103–106].

Biofeedback

For patients who are particularly somatically oriented and not insightful or verbal, biofeedback can be ideal. It is also tolerated by families who continue to deny the psychosomatic nature of the teenager's disorder but nevertheless want to see the symptoms brought under control. The teenager is connected to a machine that measures galvanic skin response or temperature, and the conditions of stress and relaxation are systematically rehearsed. Teenagers with chronic headaches, chest pains, or abdominal pains may find this technique useful.

Environmental and Behavioral Interventions

Anticipatory guidance is important during times of major biologic or psychological change; when stressors can be anticipated and planned for, they are less likely to cause distress [12]. Physicians can also help teenagers with two different coping strategies, "emotion-focused" coping (dealing with one's feelings without changing the stressor) and "problem-focused" coping (changing the stress) [12].

Changing a teenager's environment may be difficult, but sometimes minor alterations can be useful. Speaking with a particularly difficult teacher, asking for an alternative class, or arranging for tutoring can sometimes be effective. In more extreme situations, such as physical or sexual abuse, the teenager may require temporary shelter, and the physician may need to report the situation to the local health authorities. Behavioral interventions include such techniques as "time out" when the symptom occurs, or providing a positive reinforcement system when the symptom is absent. Such techniques are designed to alter the "cost-effectiveness" of the symptom.

Family Therapy

In situations in which the teenager or his or her symptom is scapegoated by the family, therapy is indicated for the entire group. More severe symptoms, conversion reactions [107], and noncompliance with medical treatment protocols may all necessitate family-oriented intervention. Families that are "enmeshed," overprotective, rigid, or lack appropriate ways of resolving conflicts may either ignore the teenager's symptom or require it to keep the family intact [108]. Such therapy should probably be undertaken by someone with more expertise than the pediatrician or family practitioner (e.g., social worker, psychologist, psychiatrist).

REFERENCES

1. Strasburger VC, Reeve A: Chronic pains during adolescence: Principles of diagnosis and management. *Adolescent Medicine: State of the Art Reviews* 1991;2:677.
2. Reeve A, Strasburger VC. Is it "real" or is it psychosomatic? Principles of psychosomatic medicine in adolescence. In: Greydanus DE, Wolraich M, eds. *Behavioral pediatrics.* New York: Springer-Verlag; 1992: 352.
3. Parsons T. Definitions of health and illness in light of American values and social structure. In: Jaco E, ed. *Physicians and illness: a sourcebook in behavioral science and health.* 2nd ed. New York: Free Press; 1972.
4. Stark T, Blum R. Psychosomatic illness in childhood and adolescence. *Clin Pediatr* 1986;25:549.
5. Goldberg ID, Regier DA, McInerny TK, et al. The role of the pediatrician in the delivery of mental health services to children. *Pediatrics* 1979;63:898.
6. Starfield B, Gross E, Wood M, et al. Psychosocial and psychosomatic diagnoses in primary care of children. *Pediatrics* 1980;66:159.
7. Nader PR, Ray L, Brink SG. The new morbidity: use of school and community health care resources for behavioral, educational, and social–family problems. *Pediatrics* 1981;67:53.
8. Goldberg ID, Roghmann KJ, McInerny TK, et al. Mental health problems among children seen in pediatric practice: prevalence and management. *Pediatrics* 1984;73:278.
9. Starfield B, Katz H, Gabriel A, et al. Morbidity in childhood: a longitudinal view. *N Engl J Med* 1984;310: 824.
10. Boyce WT. Stress and child health: an overview. *Pediatr Ann* 1985;14:539.
11. Strasburger VC. *Getting your kids to say no in the '90s when you said yes in the '60s.* New York: Fireside/Simon & Schuster; 1993.
12. Greene JW, Werner MJ, Walker LS. Stress and the modern adolescent. *Adolescent Medicine: State of the Art Reviews* 1992;3:13.
13. National Resource Center on Child Sexual Abuse. *The incidence and prevalence of child sexual abuse.* Huntsville, AL: NRCCSA, 1994.
16. Beiter M, Ingersoll G, Ganser J, et al. Relationships of somatic symptoms to behavioral and emotional risk in young adolescents. *J Pediatr* 1991;118:473.
17. Poikolainen K, Kanerva R, Lonnqvist J. Life events and other risk factors for somatic symptoms in adolescence. *Pediatrics* 1995;96:59.
18. Ader R, Felten DL, Cohen N, eds. *Psychoneuroimmunology.* 2nd ed. San Diego, CA: Academic Press; 1991.
19. Boyce WT, Barr RG, Zeltzer LK, eds. Collection of papers from the William T. Grant Foundation Research Consortium on the Developmental Psychobiology of Stress. *Pediatrics* 1992;90(Suppl):483.
20. Liang SW, Boyce WT. The psychobiology of childhood stress. *Curr Opin Pediatr* 1993;5:545.
21. Meyer RJ, Haggerty RJ. Streptococcal infection in families: factors affecting individual susceptibility. *Pediatrics* 1962;29:539.
22. Padilla ER, Rohsenow DJ, Bergman AB. Predicting accident frequency in children. *Pediatrics* 1976;58:223.
23. Boyce WT, Jensen EW, Cassel JC, et al. Influence of life events and family routines on childhood respiratory tract illness. *Pediatrics* 1977;60:609.
24. Beautrais AL, Fergusson DM, Shannon FT. Life events and child morbidity: a prospective study. *Pediatrics* 1982;70:935.
25. Lin N, Simeone RS, Ensel WM. Social support, stressful life events, and illness: a model and an empirical test. *J Health Soc Behav* 1979;20:108.
26. Nuckolls KB, Cassel J, Kaplan BH. Psychosocial assets, life crisis, and the prognosis of pregnancy. *Am J Epidemiol* 1972;95:431.

27. Greenfield NS, Roessler R, Crosley AP. Ego strength and length of recovery from infectious mononucleosis. *J Nerv Ment Dis* 1959;128:125.

28. Almy TP, Kern F, Tulin M. Alteration in colonic function in man under stress: II. experimental production of sigmoid spasm in health persons. *Gastroenterology* 1949;12:425.

29. Tucker H, Schuster MM. Irritable bowel syndrome: newer pathophysiologic concepts. *Adv Intern Med* 1982; 27:183.

30. Drossman DA, Powell DW, Sessions JT Jr. The irritable bowel syndrome. *Gastroenterology* 1977;73:811.

31. Plaut SM, Friedman SB. Biological mechanisms in the relationship of stress to illness. *Pediatr Ann* 1985;14: 563.

32. Editorial. Depression, stress, and immunity. *Lancet* 1987;1:1467.

33. Chrousos GP, Gold PW. The concepts of stress and stress system disorders. *JAMA* 1992;267:1244.

34. Zakowski SG, McAllister CG, Deal M, et al. Stress, reactivity, and immune function in healthy men. *Health Psychol* 1992;11:223.

35. Ader R. *Psychoneuroimmunology.* New York: Academic Press; 1981.

36. Jemmott JB, Borysenko JZ, Borysenko M, et al. Academic stress, power motivation, and decrease in secretion rate of salivary secretory immunoglobulin A. *Lancet* 1983;1:1400.

37. McClelland DC, Floor E, Davidson RJ, et al. Stressed power motivation, sympathetic activation, immune function, and illness. *Journal of Human Stress* 1980;6:11.

38. Lambert WW. Catecholamines excretion in young children and their parents as related to behavior. *Scand J Psychol* 1969;10:306.

39. Boyce WT, Barr RG, Zeltzer LK. Temperament and the psychobiology of childhood stress. *Pediatrics* 1992; 90(Suppl):483.

40. Locke SE, Kraus L, Leserman J, et al. Life change stress, psychiatric symptoms, and natural killer cell activity. *Psychosom Med* 1984;46:441.

41. Boas SR, Joswiak ML, Nixon PA, et al. Effects of anaerobic exercise on the immune system in eight- to seventeen-year-old trained and untrained boys. *J Pediatr* 1996;129:846.

42. Sherry DD, McGuire T, Mellins E, et al. Psychosomatic musculoskeletal pain in childhood: clinical and psychological analyses of 100 children. *Pediatrics* 1991;88:1093.

43. Menuchin S, Baker L, Rosman BL, et al. A conceptual model of psychosomatic illness in children. *Arch Gen Psychiatry* 1975;32:1031.

44. Strasburger VC. Why adolescent medicine? Four illustrative cases. *Clin Pediatr* 1984;23:12.

45. Arnhold RG, Callos ER. Composition of a suburban pediatric office practice: an analysis of patient visits during one year. *Clin Pediatr* 1966;5:722.

46. Hyams JS. Chronic abdominal pain. *Adolescent Medicine: State of the Art Reviews* 1995;6:305.

47. Oberlander TF, Rappaport LA. Recurrent abdominal pain during childhood. *Pediatr Rev* 1993;14:313.

48. Apley J. *The child with abdominal pains.* London: Blackwell Scientific Publications, 1975.

49. Liebman WM. Recurrent abdominal pain in children. *Clin Pediatr* 1978;17:149.

50. Stickler GB, Murphy DB. Recurrent abdominal pain. *American Journal of Diseases of Children* 1979;133: 486.

51. Motil KJ, Grand RJ. Ulcerative colitis and Crohn disease in children. *Pediatr Rev* 1987;9:109.

52. Kirschner BS. Inflammatory bowel disease in children. *Pediatr Clin North Am* 1988;35:189.

53. Markowitz JF. Inflammatory bowel disease: the pediatrician's role. *Contemporary Pediatrics* 1996;13:25.

54. Barr RG, Levine MD, Watkins JB. Recurrent abdominal pain of childhood due to lactose intolerance. *N Engl J Med* 1979;300:1449.

55. Barr RG. Abdominal pain in the adolescent female. *Pediatr Rev* 1983;4:281.

56. Lebenthal E, Rossi TM, Nord KS, et al. Recurrent abdominal pain and lactose absorption in children. *Pediatrics* 1981;67:828.

57. Coleman WL, Levine MD. Recurrent abdominal pain: the cost of the aches and the aches of the cost. *Pediatr Rev* 1986;8:143.

58. Hyams JS, Treem WR, Justinich CJ, et al. Characterization of symptoms in children with recurrent abdominal pain: resemblance to irritable bowel syndrome. *J Pediatr Gastroenterol Nutr* 1995;20:209.

59. Bonis PAL, Norton RA. The challenge of irritable bowel syndrome. *Am Fam Physician* 1996;53:1229.

60. Hyams JS, Burke G, Davis PM, et al. Abdominal pain and irritable bowel syndrome in adolescents: a community-based study. *J Pediatr* 1996;129:220.

61. Maugh TH II. Studies find major clues to disorder. Los Angeles Times News Service, *Albuquerque Journal*, September 23, 1996:C1.

62. McGregor RS. Chronic complaints in adolescence: chest pain, chronic fatigue, headaches, abdominal pain. *Adolescent Medicine: State of the Art Reviews* 1997;8(1):15.

63. Bourke BG, Sherman PM. Peptic ulcer disease in adolescents. *Adolescent Medicine: State of the Art Reviews* 1995;6:341.

64. Wyllie R. *Helicobacter pylori* disease in childhood. *Clin Pediatr* 1995;34:463.

65. Chong SKF, Lou Q, Asnicar MA, et al. *Helicobacter pylori* infection in recurrent abdominal pain in childhood: comparison of diagnostic tests and therapy. *Pediatrics* 1995;96:211.

66. Macarthur C, Saunders N, Feldman W. *Helicobacter pylori*, gastroduodenal disease, and recurrent abdominal pain in children. *JAMA* 1995;273:729.
67. O'Donohoe JM, Sullivan PB, Scott R, et al. Recurrent abdominal pain and *Helicobacter pylori* in a community-based sample of London children. *Acta Paediatr* 1996;85:961.
68. Van der Meer. Gastroesophageal reflux in children with recurrent abdominal pain. *Acta Paediatr* 1992;81:137.
69. Camilleri M. Nonulcer dyspepsia: a look into the future. *Mayo Clin Proc* 1996;71:614.
70. Bouchier IAD, Allan RN, Hodgson HJF, et al. *Textbook of gastroenterology.* London: Bailliere Tindall; 1984.
71. Sleisinger MH. *Gastrointestinal disease: pathology, diagnosis, and management.* 2nd ed. Philadelphia: WB Saunders; 1978.
72. Bain HW. Chronic vague abdominal pain in children. *Pediatr Clin North Am* 1974;21:991.
73. Wagner JM, McKinney WP, Carpenter JL. Does this patient have appendicitis? *JAMA* 1996;276:1589.
74. Wiens L, Sabath R, Ewing L, et al. Chest pain in otherwise healthy children and adolescents is frequently caused by exercise-induced asthma. *Pediatrics* 1992;90:350.
75. Selbst SM, Ruddy RM, Clark BJ, et al. Pediatric chest pain: a prospective study. *Pediatrics* 1988;82:319.
76. Anzai AK, Merkin TE. Adolescent chest pain. *Am Fam Physician* 1996;53:1682.
77. Brunswick A, Boyle J, Tarica C. Who sees the doctor? A study of urban black adolescents. *Soc Sci Med* 1979; 13A:45.
78. Asnes R, Santulli R, Bemporad J. Psychogenic chest pain in children. *Clin Pediatr* 1981;20:788.
79. Brown R. Costochondritis in adolescents. *Journal of Adolescent Health Care* 1981;1:198.
80. Driscoll D., Glicklich L, Gallen W. Chest pain in children: a prospective study. *Pediatrics* 1976;57:648.
81. Pantell R, Goodman B. Adolescent chest pain: a prospective study. *Pediatrics* 1983;71:881.
82. Reynolds JL. Precordial catch syndrome in children. *South Med J* 1989;82:1228.
83. Brenner J, Berman M. Chest pain in childhood and adolescence. *Journal of Adolescent Health Care* 1983;3:271.
84. Selbst SM. Chest pain in children. *Pediatrics* 1985;75:1068.
85. Herman P, Stickler GB, Lucas AR. Hyperventilation syndrome in children and adolescents: long-term follow-up. *Pediatrics* 1981;67:183.
86. Lum LC. Hyperventilation: the tip and the iceberg. *J Psychosom Res* 1975;19:375.
87. Pary R, Lewis S. Identifying and treating patients with panic attacks. *Am Fam Physician* 1992;46:841.
88. Weinstein RS. Panic disorder. *Am Fam Physician* 1995;52:2055.
89. Brown RT. Psychosomatic problems in adolescents. *Adolescent Medicine: State of the Art Reviews* 1992;3: 87.
90. Smith MS. Comprehensive evaluation and treatment of recurrent pediatric headache. *Pediatr Ann* 1995;24:450.
91. Olness KN, MacDonald JT. Recurrent headaches in children: diagnosis and treatment. *Pediatr Rev* 1987;8:307.
92. Deubner DC. An epidemiologic study of migraine and headache in 10-20 year olds. *Headache* 1977;17:172.
93. Linet MS, Stewart WF, Celentano DD, et al. An epidemiologic study of headache among adolescents and young adults. *JAMA* 1989;261:2211.
94. Newacheck PW, Taylor WR. Childhood chronic illness: prevalence, severity, and impact. *Am J Public Health* 1992;82:364.
95. Altman AJ, Schwartz AD. *Malignant diseases of infancy, childhood, and adolescence.* Philadelphia: WB Saunders; 1978.
96. Barlow CF. Headaches and brain tumors. *American Journal of Diseases of Children* 1982;136:99.
97. Honig PJ, Charney EB. Children with brain tumor headaches. *American Journal of Diseases of Children* 1982;136:121.
98. Suwanwela N, Phanthumchinda K, Kaoropthum S. Headache in brain tumor: a cross-sectional study. *Headache* 1994;34:435.
99. Martin SE, Smith MS. Psychosocial factors in recurrent pediatric headache. *Pediatr Ann* 1995;24:469.
100. Faleck H, Rothner AD, Erenberg G, et al. Headache and subacute sinusitis in children and adolescents. *Headache* 1988;28:96.
101. Coutin IB, Glass SF. Recognizing uncommon headache syndromes. *Am Fam Physician* 1996;54:2247.
102. Wells LA. Functional disorders in children and adolescents: diagnostic considerations. *Mayo Clin Proc* 1996;71:259.
103. Benson H. *The relaxation response.* New York: William Morrow; 1975.
104. Werder DS, Sargent JD. A study of childhood headache using biofeedback as a treatment alternative. *Headache* 1984;24:122.
105. Olness K, MacDonald J. Self-hypnosis and biofeedback in the management of juvenile migraine. *Journal of Developmental and Behavioral Pediatrics* 1981;2:168.
106. McGrath PJ, Reid GJ. Behavioral treatment of pediatric headache. *Pediatr Ann* 1995;24:486.
107. Gold MA, Friedman SB. Conversion reactions in adolescents. *Pediatr Ann* 1995;24:296.
108. Minuchin S, Roman B, Baker L. *Psychosomatic families.* Cambridge, MA: Harvard University Press; 1978.

SUGGESTED READING

Amaya-Jackson L, March JS. Post-traumatic stress disorder in adolescents: risk factors, diagnosis, and intervention. *Adolescent Medicine: State of the Art Reviews* 1995;6:251.

Anzai AK, Merkin TE. Adolescent chest pain. *Am Fam Physician* 1996;53:1682.

Apley J. *The child with abdominal pains.* London: Blackwell Scientific Publications; 1975.

Bonis PAL, Norton RA. The challenge of irritable bowel syndrome. *Am Fam Physician* 1996;53:1229.

Brown RT. Psychosomatic problems in adolescents. *Adolescent Medicine: State of the Art Reviews* 1992;3:87.

Dalton CB, Drossman DA. Diagnosis and treatment of irritable bowel syndrome. *Am Fam Physician* 1997;55: 875.

Emery RE, Coiro MJ. Divorce: consequences for children. *Pediatr Rev* 1995;16:306.

Gold MA, Friedman SB. Conversion reactions in adolescents. *Pediatr Ann* 1995;24:296.

Greene JW, Werner MJ, Walker LS. Stress and the modern adolescent. *Adolescent Medicine: State of the Art Reviews* 1992;3:13.

Hodgman CH. Conversion and somatization in pediatrics. *Pediatr Rev* 1995;16:29.

Hyams JS. Chronic abdominal pain. *Adolescent Medicine: State of the Art Reviews* 1995;6:305.

Kaufman KL, Brown RT, Graves K, et al. What, me worry? A survey of adolescents' concerns. *Clin Pediatr* 1993;32:8.

Liang SW, Boyce WT. The psychobiology of childhood stress. *Curr Opin Pediatr* 1993;5:545.

Li BUK. Cyclic vomiting: new understanding of an old disorder. *Contemporary Pediatrics* 1996;13:48.

Lynn RB, Friedman LS. Irritable bowel syndrome. *N Engl J Med* 1993;329:1940.

Markowitz JF. Inflammatory bowel disease: the pediatrician's role. *Contemporary Pediatrics* 1996;13:25.

Martin SE, Smith MS. Psychosocial factors in recurrent headaches in children and adolescents. *Pediatr Ann* 1995; 24:469.

McGregor RS. Chronic complaints in adolescence: chest pain, chronic fatigue, headaches, abdominal pain. *Adolescent Medicine: State of the Art Reviews* 1997;8(1):15.

Oberlander TF, Rappaport LA. Recurrent abdominal pain during childhood. *Pediatr Rev* 1993;14:313.

Phillips S, Anthony BJ, Tepper V. Use of psychometrics with adolescent patients. *Adolescent Medicine: State of the Art Reviews* 1992;3:111.

Reeve A, Strasburger VC. Is it "real" or is it psychosomatic? Principles of psychosomatic medicine in adolescence. In: Greydanus DE, Wolraich M, eds. *Behavioral pediatrics.* New York: Springer-Verlag; 1992:352.

Ryan CW. Evaluation of patients with chronic headache. *Am Fam Physician* 1996;54:1051.

Smith MS, ed. Headaches. *Pediatr Ann* 1995;24:444.

Smith MS. Comprehensive evaluation and treatment of recurrent pediatric headache. *Pediatr Ann* 1995;24: 450.

Stylianos S, Stein JE, Flanigan LM, et al. Laparoscopy for diagnosis and treatment of recurrent abdominal pain. *J Pediatr Surg* 1996;31:1158.

Weinstein RS. Panic disorder. *Am Fam Physician* 1995;52:2055.

Wells LA. Functional disorders in children and adolescents: diagnostic considerations. *Mayo Clin Proc* 1996;71: 259.

EATING DISORDERS AND OBESITY

Anorexia Nervosa

Anorexia nervosa is the perfect model to convince skeptical clinicians of the existence of real organic consequences of psychosomatic disorders. Anorexia nervosa represents a complicated web of events that begins on a societal level, extends through the family to the individual, and eventually becomes expressed through the hypothalamic–pituitary–adrenal axis in life-threatening consequences. Key features of the disorder include:

- A marked disturbance in body image
- Fear of fatness and an obsessional desire to lose weight
- Obsession with food, occasionally accompanied by binging and purging behaviors
- Significant weight loss, usually 15% or more below ideal body weight
- Amenorrhea, either primary or secondary
- Increased physical activity
- A stubborn denial of illness

Many patients lack all of the classic criteria, but still merit treatment for an eating disorder [1].

The term *anorexia nervosa* is somewhat misleading because patients experience real hunger and obsession with food but deny their initial urges. Mortality rates range from 2% to 8% [2,3].

Epidemiologic Features

The incidence of eating disorders has increased two- to fivefold since the mid-1960s [3,4]. Currently, there is one new case per year for every 100 to 150 middle-class and upper-class white adolescent women [5]. The most typical patient is white, female, of middle or upper class, and between the ages of either 12 to 14 or 17 to 18 years [6]. However, increasing numbers of cases are being diagnosed in all social and economic classes [1,7,8]. Eating disorders are highly prevalent among female athletes; reportedly, many suffer from the "female athletic triad" of menstrual dysfunction, osteoporosis, and disordered eating [9–11]. Only 5% to 10% of cases involve young men, and the diagnosis is more difficult as a result [12–14].

Etiology

Anorexia nervosa is a complex syndrome with a multicentric etiology [1,6,15–17]. Social mores, family dynamics, and biologic and psychological vulnerability all interact to produce a downward spiral of pathologic drive to lose weight, malnutrition, and physiologic disturbances.

American culture and the ideal media image of women are key contributors [18,19]. As the incidence of eating disorders has increased, society's ideal body type has become progressively slimmer. A 1980 study of *Playboy* centerfolds and Miss America winners over the past 25 years revealed a progressive decrease in bust and hip measurements, for example [20]. In a male-dominated society, women frequently define themselves in terms of how attractive they appear to men [21]. (Similarly, a survey of 895 adolescent boys found that 42% were dissatisfied with their weight—they wanted to *increase* their weight and musculature [22].) Women's magazines are filled with shapely, computer-enhanced images of models whose average weight is 23% less than the average woman's [23,24]. Contemporary American television also contributes to the problem by glorifying thinness in its portrayal of young women. Yet, paradoxically, the poor nutritional habits and junk food depicted in most programming and commercials are guaranteed to induce obesity [25,26].

Family studies indicate that the patient may be the identified problem in already troubled families [27,28]. The "psychosomatic family" is often at work here, with its mechanisms of enmeshment, overprotection, rigidity, and inability to resolve conflicts or display feelings [28]. Alternatively, one parent may also be suffering from an eating disorder [4]. As with suicidal behavior, there is also an association between this syndrome and major affective disorders within families, particularly in first-degree relatives [1,29]. As one expert eloquently states:

> Children should be made to feel wanted, loved, and valued but not possessed, overprized, or indulged. They should be expected to perform well, not for their parents' fulfillment and satisfaction and that of others, but rather for their own gratification, inner satisfaction, pride, and sense of accomplishment. Parents must be there, accessible, accepting, and available (the *three A's* of good parenting and doctoring) but cannot become subservient to or totally enmeshed in the lives of their children. That winding and difficult path between over-involvement on one side and apathy or disinterest on the other is a difficult one for parents to follow [5, p. 46].

Hypotheses about individual psychological mechanisms have varied through the decades [30]. In the 1940s, the psychoanalytic theory was in vogue, and anorexia nervosa was viewed as a patient's aversion to normal sexuality, with unconscious fantasies about food as representing oral impregnation [31]. More recently, the disorder has been seen as a complex psychoneurotic syndrome with many distinctive neuroendocrine changes. Some researchers have speculated about the resemblance between anorectic women and long-distance runners [32], although further studies have shown that the former do have significantly greater psychopathology as measured by personality inventories [33]. Ballet dancers, models, and elite athletes are known to be at increased risk [10,11,34]. Up to half of all anorectic patients may fulfill the criteria for a major depressive or anxiety disorder [1,35].

The biochemistry of eating disorders is still in its infancy, but cerebrospinal fluid (CSF) concentrations of neuropeptide Y have been shown to be significantly elevated in anorectic patients, even after restoration of normal weight [36,37].

Diagnosis

The physician in practice needs to be most knowledgeable about how to diagnose, rather than manage or treat, anorexia nervosa. Although primary care clinicians can be valuable members of the multidisciplinary team approach used in treatment, most would probably prefer to refer such patients to an adolescent medicine specialist and psychiatrist.

The syndrome often begins when a young teenage girl sees herself as being overweight and begins dieting. Typically, this is a middle-class overachiever and perfectionist who has always been a model child. Of course, dieting is endemic among female adolescents and, itself, represents a substantial risk factor [38–41]: one 1989 study of 326 girls aged 13 to 18 years found that half were "extremely fearful" of being overweight and one third were "preoccupied with body fat," despite the fact that only 17% were overweight for their height [42]. Two earlier studies found that only 14% of adolescent girls were satisfied with their weight, and 67% to 78% wanted to weigh less [43,44]. Even children as young as 8 years want to be thinner (45% in one study) and have already tried dieting (37%) [45,46].

In fact, dieting may account for much of the gender difference in prevalence of eating disorders; women are far more likely to diet than men [41]. What separates the casual or even the recurrent dieter from the anorectic is a profound distortion in self-image, a preoccupation with thinness, and an extreme change in eating habits. Patients with anorexia nervosa continue to diet well past the normal end point, and they actually perceive themselves to be fat even when they are severely underweight. Even at weights of 80 or 90 lb, such patients often pinch their scrawny hips and say that they just need to lose a few more pounds "right here." Although they deny hunger, they are in fact obsessed with food and often spend considerable time in the kitchen, preparing food for others. In addition, obsessive athletic activity allows them to keep their weight under control. Patients with restrictive anorexia nervosa severely curtail their caloric intake, whereas those with the binge-eating/purging form regularly engage in self-induced vomiting or misuse of laxatives, diuretics, or enemas [47]. The latter begin to resemble bulimics in being older and less isolated socially but having greater family and behavioral instability [5].

Such behavior would appear clearly abnormal to most normal people, but anorectics cleverly disguise their weight loss by wearing bulky clothes, even in summertime, and often exercise surreptitiously, such as by repetitive muscle contractions. Even when followed closely in an outpatient setting or when confined on an inpatient unit, these patients frequently binge to meet the weight requirements set and avoid discovery or further loss of privileges [48]. In addition, their behavior allows them to achieve a sense of control and power that they previously lacked. The ability to control one's weight precisely can be extremely seductive.

Thus, the diagnosis is made based on a constellation of historical findings, in combination with a careful physical examination and a few laboratory tests (Table 25). In most cases, an extensive workup is not needed. Because patients with anorexia nervosa exhibit a spectrum of disease and progress at different rates, the clinician should not necessarily wait for all the "official" criteria listed in the *Diagnostic and Statistical Manual of Mental Disorders*, 4th edition (DSM-IV) to appear before suspecting the diagnosis and deciding to intervene [1,6] (Table 26). The differential diagnosis is not usually difficult in typical patients (Table 27), because teenagers who suffer from anorexia secondary to depression or a chronic disease have a normal self-image and are quite concerned about their weight loss.

Amenorrhea is a constant feature of the syndrome, although it may antedate the weight loss in up to 25% of patients [49,50]. Interestingly, patients resume their normal prepubertal pattern of follicle-stimulating hormone and luteinizing hormone release [51]. With the accompanying estrogen deficiency, osteoporosis can be a significant, long-term problem (reversibility and adequate treatment remain unknown) [52–54]. The inability to maintain normal body temperature may result from either a hypothalamic defect, a loss of body fat, or both [55]. Decreased conversion of thyroxine to triiodothyronine results in bradycardia, cold intolerance, and dry skin and hair, and may be adaptive, lowering the metabolic rate in the face of a diminished energy supply [5,56]. Multiple electrolyte disturbances can exist, including azotemia from increased protein catabolism, total body sodium and potassium depletion, and hypokalemia if diuretics, cathartics, or self-induced vomiting are used. The gastrointestinal findings of delayed gastric emptying and decreased intestinal motility may produce constipation and a sense of fullness, and interfere with refeeding attempts [5].

Complications from anorexia nervosa are related to those of starvation. Even diminished CSF and gray and white matter volumes have been found [57]. Mortality is usually related to cardiac arrhythmias, precipitated by decreased myocardial mass and electrolyte imbalance [58].

Treatment

Patients with anorexia nervosa are among the most difficult of all adolescents to treat. They require a multidisciplinary approach, with input from a primary care physician, psychiatrist, nutritionist, and

TABLE 25. *Anorexia nervosa: common physical examination and laboratory findings*

General:	Loss of subcutaneous fat
	Loss of scalp or pubic hair
	Presence of lanugo hair
	Cold, mottled hands and feet
Vital signs:	Low body temperature
	Bradycardia
	Hypotension (esp. postural)
Gastrointestinal:	Decreased bowel sounds
Hematologic:	Normal or low erythrocyte sedimentation rate
	Decreased white blood cell count
	Anemia
	Thrombocytopenia
Endocrine:	Low follicle-stimulating hormone/luteinizing hormone
	Low normal triiodothyronine, thyroxine, thyroid-stimulating hormone
	Decreased estradiol
	Normal or high cortisol
Hepatic:	Early: elevated cholesterol
	Late: decreased cholesterol
Renal:	Normal or elevated blood urea nitrogen
	Hematuria, pyuria, proteinuria
Electrolytes:	Metabolic alkalosis, decreased Na, Cl, K if patient has been vomiting or using laxatives or diuretics
Electrocardiogram:	Low voltage
	Sinus bradycardia
	Low or inverted T waves
	Prolonged QTc
Chest x-ray:	Thin cardiac sillouette

Adapted from Joffe A. Too little, too much: eating disorders in adolescents. *Contemporary Pediatrics* 1990;7:114.

skilled nursing [6,59–61]. "Divide and conquer" is the subconscious watchword of many such patients, and many clinicians have found themselves in the uncomfortable role of being "the bad guy," forced to set the treatment limits and reinforcement schedules [29]. Consequently, practitioners who are interested in treating anorexia nervosa require specialized training and experience and availability of other skilled personnel. Otherwise, referral to a nearby adolescent medical or psychiatric facility with expertise in this area is strongly recommended.

Treatment methods range from individual to group and family psychotherapy, and from behavior modification techniques to pharmacotherapy. To date, treatment of anorexia nervosa and bulimia ranks as one of the most unsatisfactory in clinical medicine [5]. However, many disappointing data come from adult psychiatry programs, where patients may be referred only after many years of illness and treatment. Reports from adolescent medicine programs tend to be far more optimistic. The recently published Rochester experience followed 49 adolescents with anorexia nervosa for an average of 6 to 7 years after treatment on an inpatient unit. Average body weight had increased from 72% to 96% of ideal, menstruation began or resumed in 80% of patients, and no young women had difficulty with pregnancies. Overall, 86% of their patients were thought to have a satisfactory outcome [48,62]. (However, almost half of their patients acquired binge eating patterns during or after hospitalization,

TABLE 26. *Diagnostic criteria: anorexia nervosa*

1. Refusal to maintain body weight above normal height for weight (e.g., weight less than 85% expected).
2. Intense fear of gaining weight or becoming fat, despite being underweight.
3. Disturbance in body perception—feels fat despite being underweight.
4. Absence of at last three consecutive menstrual periods (primary or secondary amenorrhea).

Adapted from American Psychiatric Association. *Diagnostic and statistical manual of mental disorders.* 4th ed., revised. Washington, DC: American Psychiatric Association; 1994.

TABLE 27. *Differential diagnosis: anorexia nervosa*

Organic disease

Endocrine:	Hyperthyroidism
	Hypothyroidism
	Diabetes
	Addison's disease
Central nervous system:	Tumor
Gastrointestinal:	Inflammatory bowel disease
	Gastroesophageal reflux
Genitourinary:	Pregnancy
Neoplastic:	Any malignancy

Psychiatric disease
Depression
Anxiety disorder
Schizophrenia
Thought disorder
Substance abuse
Posttraumatic stress disorder

Adapted from Levine RL. Eating disorders in adolescents: a comprehensive update. *International Pediatrics* 1995;10:327.

presumably because of the emphasis on "making weight" to retain privileges.) An earlier, more short-term study of 63 adolescents treated on a general adolescent medical service found a 71% satisfactory outcome rate [63].

One of the most crucial questions is when to hospitalize a teenager with anorexia nervosa. Although various weight ranges are reported in the literature (e.g., weight loss greater than 30% over 3 months; continued or rapid weight loss despite treatment), the clinician would be wise not to wait for an exact number but to consider the entire clinical picture. Patients with families in crisis, suicidal ideation, unusual presentations, or out-of-control behaviors may require hospitalization, regardless of their weight. Additional indications are listed in Table 28.

Details of inpatient management are available in the literature [1,29,62,64]. Nutritional rehabilitation is the first and primary concern [1,65]. Unfortunately, health insurers and managed care companies are intensifying their attempts to shorten inpatient stays or refusing altogether to fund inpatient treatment [66]. With such a disorder as anorexia nervosa, this may turn out to be "penny-wise and pound-foolish," both literally and figuratively.

TABLE 28. *Indications for hospitalizing an adolescent with anorexia nervosa*

1. Severe malnutrition (weight < 75% ideal body weight)
2. Dehydration
3. Electrolyte disturbances
4. Physiologic instability
   - Severe bradycardia
   - Hypotension
   - Hypothermia
   - Orthostatic changes
5. Acute food refusal
6. Acute medical complication of malnutrition (e.g., pancreatitis, syncope, cardiac failure)
7. Acute psychiatric emergencies (e.g., suicidal ideation, acute psychosis)
8. Failure of outpatient treatment

Adapted from Fisher M, Golden NH, Katzman DK, et al. Eating disorders in adolescents: a background paper. *J Adolesc Health* 1995;16:420.

If the adolescent's weight loss is mild or moderate (e.g., 10–20% below ideal body weight), outpatient management can be tried first, assuming that the social situation is stable. Individual and family therapy is usually the first choice for treatment. A variety of drugs have been tried, but their exact role remains unclear [67]. Antidepressants have been most popular, but in most studies they have no proven superiority over placebo therapy [5]. Cyproheptadine (Periactin) is one attractive alternative. It is an antihistamine and serotonin antagonist that can stimulate appetite and has few side effects. In restrictive anorectics, it has proven more effective than placebo in producing weight gain and improving depression [68].

Prognosis

Traditionally, anorexia nervosa is believed to carry a guarded prognosis. In the psychiatric literature, an estimated one third to one half of patients have some degree of psychological dysfunction after 2 years, and one fourth do not regain their menses or attain 75% of their ideal body weight [69–71]. As mentioned previously, the pediatric literature is somewhat more optimistic [1,48,58,63]. All agree that the best prognosis exists for teenagers diagnosed and treated early, before abnormal eating and behavior patterns become established, marked weight loss occurs, and the patients become accustomed to a persistently low body weight [72].

Bulimia

Bulimia is episodic binge eating, often accompanied by purging, and is very prevalent among adolescent and young adult women. Although only 1% to 5% of adolescent girls meet the DSM-IV criteria for bulimia, as many as 10% to 50% reportedly engage in occasional self-induced vomiting or binge eating [1,40,73]. Bulimia nervosa is a syndrome seen mostly in older adolescents and young adults and includes the following features [47]:

- Repeated attempts to lose weight by self-induced vomiting, severe food restriction, or abuse of laxatives or ipecac
- Wide fluctuations in weight
- Fear of a loss of control surrounding eating behaviors
- Depressive symptoms, especially after binging

Although the pediatrician is unlikely to encounter many patients with bulimia nervosa, the family practitioner may [74]. In addition, both pediatricians and family practitioners may witness the spectrum of abnormal eating behaviors leading up to the disorder. It is extremely common among younger teenagers.

Epidemiologic Features

Using fixed DSM-IV criteria (Table 29), an estimated 1% to 5% of adolescent and college women and up to 0.4% of young men suffer from bulimia nervosa [6,75–77]. However, many more college men (41–60%) and women (26–79%) demonstrate occasional bulimic behaviors (e.g., binging and

TABLE 29. *Diagnostic criteria: bulimia*

1. Recurrent episodes of binge eating
2. A feeling of lack of control over eating behavior.
3. Regularly engaging in either self-induced vomiting, use of laxatives or diuretics, strict dieting or fasting, or vigorous exercise to prevent weight gain.
4. At least two binging episodes a week for at least 3 months.
5. Persistent overconcern with body shape and weight.

Adapted from American Psychiatric Association. *Diagnostic and statistical manual of mental disorders.* 4th ed., revised. Washington, DC: American Psychiatric Association; 1994.

purging to achieve desired weight for wrestlers, group binging among college women) [40,78,79]. In addition, 13% of adolescents report engaging in some sort of purging behavior at some time [40,80]. Obviously, the prevalence is heavily dependent on how the syndrome is defined and whether symptoms or the full-blown disorder are being assessed. A clearer picture comes from a survey of female adolescents in two private schools, one a boarding school and the other a day school: 18% had at least *one symptom* of an eating disorder [81]. Most bulimic patients are white and of middle or upper class, with the incidence of bulimia nervosa decreasing to 1.9% in a community population of young women [82].

Etiology

Bulimia is a relatively newly described disorder, and so its definition is still being revised and refined. As such, far less is understood about its etiology than about anorexia nervosa. As in that disease, adolescents with bulimia have a high prevalence of depression (35%) and of affective disorders in first-degree relatives (50% or more) [83]. Again, society is thought to play a key role: weight control is synonymous with self-control and attractiveness. Children as young as 6 years rate pictures of endomorphs negatively, and pudgy children are frequently subjected to ridicule and exclusion [84].

Adolescent girls in particular are unhappy with their weight [42–44]. Female appearance is so important, in fact, that when pictures of women are manipulated to increase their bust size, they are viewed as being less intelligent and competent than with smaller busts [85]. Bulimic patients tend to be impulsive and suggestible, and the media may certainly be suggesting inappropriate body images [41]. It is not surprising, then, that some researchers believe that most women are at risk for development of some degree of eating disorder [69,86].

Psychologically, the bulimic patient differs from the anorectic patient. In the former, there is an increased history of childhood maladjustment and family psychiatric disorders [87]. Bulimics describe their mothers as being more emotionally distant than enmeshed and seem to experience greater rejection and blame as youngsters [88]. Bulimic women are also more prone to have been obese, are more extroverted, and are more likely to abuse alcohol, steal, be sexually active, or attempt suicide than patients with anorexia nervosa [89]. The association between bulimia and a history of childhood sexual abuse remains controversial [90]. Bulimia therefore appears to be more of a disorder in regulation of affect and impulse control [30].

From a biologic perspective, because serotonin seems to play a key role in mediating satiety (and decreasing one's desire for carbohydrates), a number of researchers have studied its metabolism in bulimic patients [29,30,91]. Such patients demonstrate lower levels of CSF serotonin levels than restrictive anorectics; one hypothesis is that binging on carbohydrates represents an attempt to self-medicate to increase brain serotonin levels [92,93]. CSF concentrations of neuropeptide YY are also elevated in bulimic patients and may contribute to the drive to overfeed [36].

Diagnosis

The typical patient with bulimia is female, in her late teens or early twenties, slightly overweight, and has a history of unsuccessful dieting. At some point, she becomes aware of being able to control her weight through self-induced vomiting or the use of cathartics [21]. Unlike the anorectic patient, who almost by definition is asexual and isolated, this young woman is usually extroverted and has heterosexual relationships. However, she rapidly becomes preoccupied with planning for her binges, which are usually solitary and involve junk food. She may have other impulsive behaviors as well, such as drug use or shoplifting [94]. She may binge recurrently or binge and purge using syrup of ipecac, laxatives, or diuretics. After binging, she feels out of control and ashamed, yet she is unable to tell significant others or her physician about her behavior [95]. Overall, her personality is more labile than an anorectic's, and she is more likely to attempt suicide.

Unless a patient confesses to such behavior or a specific question is asked and answered truthfully, bulimia is unlikely to be discovered until it has become a chronic problem [74]. A number of clinical clues exist as a result of the recurrent vomiting and use of cathartics [56,96,97] (Table 30):

• Hypertrophy of the parotid gland
• Dental enamel erosion

TABLE 30. *Clinical clues to the diagnosis of bulimia*

History:	Abdominal bloating or pain
	Muscle aches or stiffness
	Weakness
Skin:	Calluses on knuckles from self-induced vomiting
	Edema of feet or hands
Oral:	Dental caries
	Erosion of enamel
	Parotid hypertrophy
Renal:	Hematuria, pyuria, or proteinuria
Electrolytes:	Metabolic alkalosis
	Decreased Na, Cl, K
Electrocardiogram:	Wandering atrial pacemaker
	Prolonged QTc
Chest x-ray:	Mediastinal emphysema

Adapted from Joffe A. Too little, too much: eating disorders in adolescents. *Contemporary Pediatrics* 1990;7:114.

- Sudden, severe chest or abdominal pain, secondary to a ruptured esophagus or Mallory-Weiss tear
- Peripheral edema
- Hypokalemia

Treatment

Counseling or therapy with bulimic patients is unlikely to fall within the purview of the average practicing physician. Referral to an expert in psychotherapy with young women with eating disorders probably is indicated [98]. Such patients may be difficult to keep in therapy because of their low frustration tolerance [21]. Nevertheless, the clinician can play an important role in the medical follow-up of the patient, especially in monitoring the patient's weight and electrolyte status, and in providing family support. Because of the known association between bulimia and depression, psychiatrists have been more aggressive with using antidepressants [99]. Many controlled studies find improvements (reduction in binging, improvement in mood, less preoccupation with weight) with use of tricyclic antidepressants [100]. Fluoxetine (Prozac) has also been demonstrated to be effective [100,101]. However, studies also show that psychotherapy is most important and that drugs alone are not effective [100,102].

Prognosis

Several studies examining short- and long-term outcomes for bulimic patients have been published [103–108]. In general, approximately 50% of patients report no binging or purging behavior 2 to 10 years after cognitive behavioral therapy, 20% remain persistently symptomatic, and 30% seem to have remissions and relapses [104]. Surprisingly, in one 20-month follow-up of 628 bulimic women, 25% showed improvement in their symptoms, regardless of whether they were in therapy, although all continued to show psychological distress surrounding their eating behavior [108]. At present, the picture remains unclear. Of the bulimic patients who present for treatment, a significant proportion probably do not recover quickly [109]. Certainly bulimic patients who have an affective disorder or features of anorexia nervosa fare more poorly. Finally, there is a significantly increased risk of early death from either suicide or electrolyte imbalance [110].

EVALUATION AND MANAGEMENT OF ADOLESCENT OBESITY

Obesity remains one of the most significant and prevalent disorders during adolescence, yet it is notoriously refractory to successful intervention [111–113]. In 1986, health care costs for obesity were estimated at $39 billion, and another $30 billion is spent annually by people attempting to lose or control their weight [114].

Now, in the 1990s, remarkable progress is being made in understanding the pathogenesis of obesity, spawning new efforts at treatment. However, much still depends on the motivation of the adolescent and family. Patients identified as obese or overweight solely by the practitioner and in need of treatment may be particularly frustrating and noncompliant, much the same as teenagers identified as needing contraception but unwilling to seek medical attention themselves. Nonetheless, the health consequences of obesity are so significant that attempts at intervention are still worthwhile and occasionally even may be successful. Certainly, *prevention* of obesity should rank as a primary concern for all practitioners dealing with children and adolescents.

Definition

Surprisingly, the indices for identifying overweight or obese adolescents have not been standardized [115]. Typically, overweight patients are identified as exceeding some index of body mass or relative weight compared with reference norms. Weight-for-age growth charts are not very useful because they ignore body habitus and lean tissue mass. Currently, body mass index (BMI) is the preferred method of assessing obesity [115].

It is calculated as:

Weight (kg)/height (m^2)

A BMI exceeding the 85th percentile is arbitrarily chosen to define obesity [111]. Guidelines suggest that people should try to maintain a BMI below 25.

The triceps skinfold thickness is also a useful means of assessing adolescents, and it measures body fat directly, but the measure does not track into adulthood as well as the BMI. The waist-to-hip circumference ratio commonly used in adults may also prove useful in adolescents, but more so for girls than boys [111].

Prevalence

According to Cycle 3 of the National Health and Nutrition Examination Survey (NHANES III), which examined nearly 1,500 adolescents between 1988 and 1991, the prevalence of obesity (defined as BMI greater than 85th percentile) in 12- to 19-year-olds is now 21%, an increase of 6% since the early 1980s [116,117] (Table 31). Even more alarming, the prevalence appears to be steadily increasing [114]. An estimated 30% of adults in the United States are overweight and 12% are obese [118]. Compared with other Western nations, the United States has the highest percentage of overweight and obese adults [119]. In 1996, for the first time ever in the United States, overweight people outnumber normal-size ones. Cycle 4 of the NHANES, conducted on 30,000 people from 1991 to 1994, found that 59% of American men and 49% of women have BMIs greater than 25, an increase of nearly 20% from 10 years earlier [120].

Although racial differences exist, socioeconomic factors are far more significant, especially in women. Excess weight is 7 to 12 times more common in women from lower socioeconomic classes [121]. In black children, two studies show reduced resting energy expenditure compared with their white peers [122,123].

Medical Morbidity

Hypertension, hyperlipidemia, and hyperinsulism are well known risk factors associated with obesity, whether it occurs in children, adolescents, or adults. Moreover, tracking studies indicate that obese children or adolescents with any of these complications tend to carry them into adulthood. In addition, excellent longitudinal data now exist that demonstrate that adolescent obesity increases mortality and morbidity in adulthood [124–126]. In a 55-year follow-up study of subjects in the Third Harvard Growth Study [1922–1935], men who were overweight (BMI>75th percentile) during their high school years had higher mortality rates than men who were lean. Both men and women had increased morbidity from several diseases if they were obese as adolescents. However, only 10% of obese adult men had the onset of their obesity during adolescence, compared with 30% of obese adult women [125]. Specifically, medical risks include the following [127–129]:

TABLE 31. *Prevalence of being overweight[a]*
among adolescents

Sex/survey	Sample size	Incidence (%)
Male		
NHANES II	1,351	15
NHANES III	717	20
Female		
NHANES II	1,241	15
NHANES III	739	22
Total		
NHANES II	2,592	15
NHANES III	1,456	21

NHANES, National Health and Nutrition Examination Survey (NHANES II: 1976–1980, NHANES III: 1988–1991).
[a]Defined as body mass index $\geq$23.0 for men aged 12–14 years; $\geq$24.3 for men aged 15–17 years; $\geq$25.8 for men aged 18–19 years; $\geq$24.8 for women aged 15–17 years; and $\geq$25.7 for women aged 18–19 years.
Adapted from Centers for Disease Control and Prevention. Prevalence of overweight among adolescents: United States, 1988–91. *MMWR Morb Mortal Wkly Rep* 1994;43:818.

- Compared with normal subjects, obese adults carry a five- to sixfold increased risk of hypertension, a nearly threefold greater risk of diabetes, and a 1.5-fold increased risk of hypercholesterolemia.
- Obesity ranks as the most common identifiable cause of hypertension in children and adolescents. At the same time, obese adolescents whose blood pressure is initially elevated show a return to normal values after weight loss has been achieved [130,131].
- The well known cardiovascular risk factors of elevated low-density lipoproteins and decreased high-density lipoproteins are associated with obesity [132,133].
- Obese adolescents are particularly prone to such orthopedic disorders as slipped capital femoral epiphyses and Legg-Calvé-Perthes disease.
- Morbidly obese children and adolescents are at risk for central respiratory dysfunction, Pickwickian syndrome, and major neurocognitive defects [134].

In adults, some newer data have revolutionized thinking about obesity [132,135]. Apparently, the distribution of body fat is far more significant than its relative amount. The android/male/abdominal distribution, with a higher waist-to-hip ratio ("beer belly"), carries a far greater risk of diabetes and cardiovascular disease than the gynoid/female/pelvic distribution [136–139] (Table 32).

TABLE 32. *Classification of body fat distribution*

Android	Gynoid
Upper body	Lower body
Apple-shape	Pear-shape
Abdominal	Gluteal
Central	Peripheral
Subscapular skinfold thickness > 25	Subscapular skinfold thickness > 25
Waist-to-hip girth ratio > 0.85	Waist-to-hip girth ratio < 0.85

From Kaplan NM. The deadly quartet: upper-body obesity, glucose intolerance, hypertriglyceridemia, and hypertension. *Arch Intern Med* 1989;149:1514. Copyright © 1989, American Medical Association. Reprinted with permission.

Psychological Morbidity

American society dislikes fat people [140]. In the media, obese children and adults typically have been comic characters, clumsy and gluttonous. Few TV stars are obese, Roseanne and Queen Latifah being the notable exceptions, and 90% of obese characters on television are black, despite the greater prevalence of obesity among whites [141,142]. Food is frequently used to bribe people or to facilitate social introductions on TV, rather than to satisfy hunger, and 88% of all characters are thin or average in body build [141]. There are few obese people to be found in TV commercials [142]. As one researcher summarizes the problem: "Television presents viewers with two sets of conflicting messages. One suggests that we eat in ways almost guaranteed to make us fat; the other suggests that we strive to remain slim" [141].

By age 7, children have already learned norms of cultural attractiveness [143]. Young children will choose a playmate with a major physical handicap over one who is obese [144]. An adolescent's self-concept is sufficiently tenuous that any physical characteristic that causes him to be different and noticed by his peers can potentially become a major problem, particularly in lowering self-esteem [145–147].

One study seems to confirm that being obese not only can have social and psychological consequences, but educational and economic ones as well. A group of researchers studied more than 10,000 16- to 24-year-olds in 1981 for 7 years and found that overweight women [140]:

- Had completed fewer years of school (0.3 years less)
- Were less likely to be married (20% less likely)
- Had lower household incomes ($6,710 per year less)
- Had greater rates of household poverty (10% higher)

Risk Factors for Development of Obesity

The nature-versus-nurture controversy exists throughout the scientific literature on obesity. According to some researchers, twin studies and studies of adopted children and their biologic and adoptive parents demonstrate that up to 70% to 80% of the variance in skinfold thickness can be attributed to heredity rather than environment [148–151].

By contrast, other researchers claim that the family environment is paramount and that, for example, genetics cannot explain the significant association of fatness in spouses, nor the resemblance between overweight owners and their pets [152]. In addition, such factors as family size, socioeconomic class, and education have been correlated with obesity [111,152]. Interestingly, obesity is more common among single children than in larger families [153]. Therefore, 25% is probably a more accurate estimate of genotypic influence, versus 75% from environmental factors [111,119,154].

Of course, the distinction between environmental and genetic influence becomes blurred when looking at the biologic family. Parental obesity is well known as a risk factor for childhood obesity, with a correlation coefficient of approximately 0.25.; the risk increases according to whether both parents are lean, one is obese, or both are [155]. Expressed differently, a child with two obese parents has an 80% chance of being obese, a 40% chance if only one parent is obese, and only a 14% chance if both parents are of normal weight [156].

Because obesity represents an imbalance in the equation between energy expenditure and energy intake, diet and physical activity are extremely important factors [114,157,158]. A sedentary life-style has become the norm in the United States, and increasing amounts of data demonstrate that teenagers are not as physically active as they once were [114,158]. In the 1990 Youth Risk Behavior Survey, barely one third of students in grades 9 through 12 reported being vigorously active three or more times per week [159,160]. Most adults fail to achieve even a moderate level of physical activity as well (defined as expending 150 calories of energy per day or 1,000 calories per week) [161]. Added to this is the fact that the fat intake of children and adolescents in the United States continues to exceed 35% of daily caloric intake [111].

One environmental factor that appears to have an important role in obesity is television viewing. Using data from the National Health Examination Survey, researchers found that watching television was directly related to the risk of obesity [162]. In addition, after prior obesity, television was the most important predictor of obesity in adolescents, and a dose–response effect could be demonstrated: the more TV viewed, the greater the risk of obesity [142]. Only two studies have failed to find this association [163,164]. Most studies have documented a profound influence of television on the prevalence of obesity; up to 60% of obesity was attributable to excess television viewing time in the most recent study [165]. There could be many reasons for this effect [165–167]:

- Television frequently advertises high-caloric snack foods [168].
- TV characters exhibit poor nutritional behaviors [141].
- Children are more likely to snack while watching TV [152].
- Watching television displaces other, more active outdoor activities such as sports [164,165].
- Children's metabolic rate during TV viewing is actually lower than at rest [169].

One of the most significant risk factors for children and adolescents is that once they become obese, they are likely to remain obese for the rest of their lives. The likelihood of persistent obesity increases steadily with age and, to a far lesser extent, the duration of obesity [111]. For example, an obese adolescent, overweight for 2 years, is more likely to become an obese adult than an obese 10-year-old, overweight since age 2 [127]. Of superobese adults (greater than 160% of ideal body weight), 50% to 75% were obese as children [152]. Or, expressed differently, the odds against achieving an ideal body weight are 4 to 1 at age 12 and 28 to 1 at age 20 years [170]. Boys can lose fat during their growth spurt, and girls can rearrange it, but significant obesity during childhood or adolescence is a major concern.

Causes of Secondary Obesity

Most adolescent obesity—probably 99% or more—is *primary* in origin and *is not associated with any identifiable endocrine abnormality* [111,127,152,171,172]. In particular, knowledge of a few normal growth dynamics during adolescence allows the practitioner to avoid unnecessary overtesting (Table 33): obese preadolescents tend to enter puberty earlier than their leaner peers, whereas most endocrine causes of obesity are associated with poor growth, particularly in height. For example, patients with hypothyroidism, Cushing's disease, and growth hormone deficiency would all present with short stature as well as obesity. Other clues depend on the clinical disease—for example, cold intolerance, constipation, and lethargy in hypothyroidism; and striae, central obesity, hypertension, and "moon facies" in Cushing's disease.

Use of Tanner staging, growth charts, and calculation of the BMI enables the clinician to make a rapid assessment concerning the need for further diagnostic testing. In general, any female adolescent who is having absolutely normal, regular menstrual periods is unlikely to be hypothyroid. An obese female adolescent who is Tanner stage 4 or 5, in the 75th percentile for height, and has normal menses does not ordinarily require thyroid function tests, despite the entreaties of her mother that "it must be something glandular."

TABLE 33. *Organic causes of obesity*

Dysmorphic syndromes
   Prader-Willi
   Laurence-Moon-Biedl
   Turner's syndrome

Central nervous system
   Trauma
   Tumor
   Postinfectious

Endocrine
   Hypothyroidism
   Insulinoma
   Cushing's syndrome
   Exogenous steroids
   Polycystic ovary syndrome
   Growth hormone deficiency
   Pseudohypoparathyroidism (type I)

Adapted from Dietz WH, Robinson TN. Assessment and treatment of childhood obesity. *Pediatr Rev* 1993;14:337.

Etiology

An extraordinary amount of research is now taking place on obesity, with a variety of new findings and insights, including the discovery of a possible "obesity gene" and its product, a possible "satiety factor" [173–175].

Obesity represents an unbalanced physiologic equation: energy intake outstrips energy expenditure, and the excess is stored as fat. In fact, the imbalance may be surprisingly small—perhaps only 50 calories per day, resulting in a net weight gain above expected of only 5 pounds per year [152,176]. This represents the use of 2% milk rather than 1% milk, or the addition of 1 teaspoon of butter to a dinner roll [177]. Therefore, overeating is a relatively infrequent cause of obesity [178]. In addition, there appears to be a homeostasis mechanism that opposes changes from usual weight [176,179], but is biased in favor of keeping people overweight rather than underweight [178].

Most energy expenditure (70%) comes from supplying the basal metabolic rate, and food intake and physical activity account for only 15% each of the total energy equation [154] (Fig. 10). This may help to explain why losing weight is so difficult and why simply increasing exercise may not represent an automatic guarantee of weight loss. Basal metabolic rates vary from individual to individual, even among people with the same lean body mass or surface area, but rates do tend to be similar among family members [180]. Interestingly, basal metabolic rate *increases* as body weight increases [180]. Therefore, although obese people may expend less energy (e.g., choosing an escalator instead of stairs), they also use more energy per given physical activity [181,182]. One theory is that obese people have an altered metabolic response to food, mediated through either the sympathetic nervous system or brown adipose tissue [183].

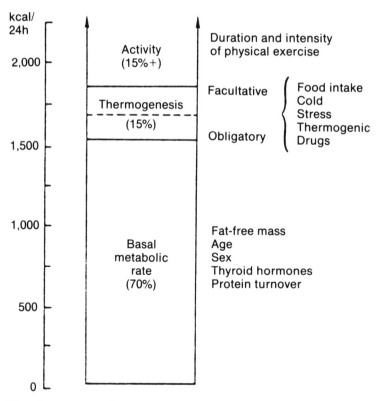

FIG. 10. Partition of energy expenditures for the average person, based on 2,500 kcal per day. Activity is variable and can be increased, but usually represents no more than 15% to 30% of calories expended per day. (Bray GA, Gray DS. Obesity: I. pathogenesis. *West J Med* 1988;149:429. With permission.)

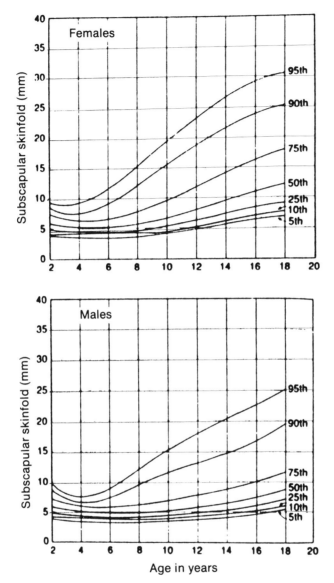

FIG. 11. Percentiles of subscapular skinfold thicknesses for children aged 2 to 18 years. Patients with measures greater than 75th percentile should be considered "at risk" for obesity-related morbidity. (Rosenbaum M, Leibel RL. Obesity in childhood. *Pediatr Rev* 1989;11:43. Copyright 1989. Reproduced with permission of the American Academy of Pediatrics.)

Fat cells have always been a source of controversy in the research literature [158]. In the mid-1960s, researchers started to define obesity at a cellular level and showed that fat may be packaged in two different ways: either in small droplets in many fat cells (hyperplasia), or in large droplets in a few fat cells (hypertrophy) [184]. Do obese people have larger fat cells, more of them, or both? The answer seems to be that mildly obese patients have hypertrophy of fat cells, whereas superobese patients have both cell hypertrophy and hyperplasia.

Because a fat cell cannot be lost once it is formed, this theory has important implications: identification and prevention of obesity in early childhood becomes critical [127]. Childhood obesity is hy-

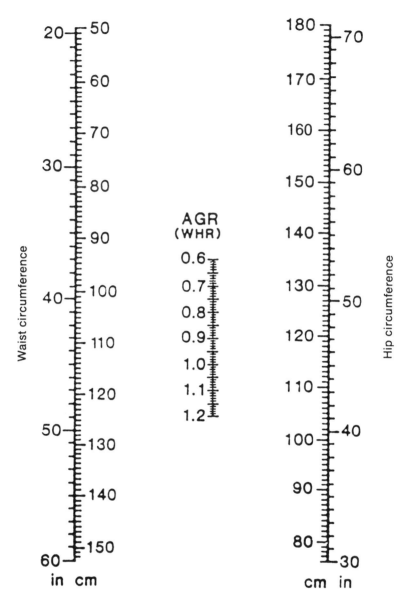

FIG. 12. Nomogram for determining waist-to-hips ratio. (Bray GA. Classification and evaluation of the obesities. *Med Clin North Am* 1989;73:161. With permission.)

perplastic and progresses to hyperplastic adult obesity. On the other hand, adult obesity can be either hypertrophic or hyperplastic or both [158]. As it happens, weight reduction is most difficult in hyperplastic obesity because fat cells cannot be eliminated.

The first year of life, the period of adiposity rebound between ages 5 and 7 years, and the years around puberty may represent extremely susceptible periods [115]. These are times when physiologic alterations may increase the later prevalence of obesity. By the end of the first year, the size of the fat cell has nearly doubled, whereas the number of cells has not changed. Fat cells then decrease in size in lean children and increase in size in obese children. Fat cell hyperplasia occurs throughout childhood as well—more in obese children than in lean children—but usually ends during adolescence. After puberty, obesity mainly occurs through hypertrophy of cells, not hyperplasia [136].

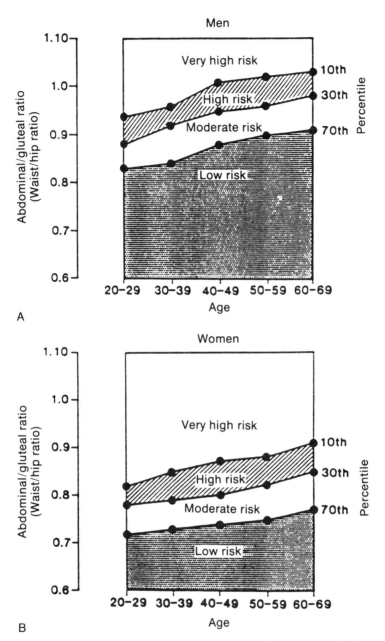

FIG. 13. Relative risk associated with waist-to-hips ratio for men **(A)** and women **(B)**. (Bray GA. Classification and evaluation of the obesities. *Med Clin North Am* 1989;73:161. With permission.)

Toward a Coherent Theory of Obesity

How does all of this information get combined into a coherent explanation of the pathophysiology of obesity? Since 1990, much progress has been made in elucidating how the body gains, loses, and stores fat. The body seems to have a "set point" for body fat, sometimes called the "adipostat," located somewhere in the brain [178]. The set point influences two types of largely voluntary behavior: eating and physical activity. Exactly how the body "measures" its own fat stores has been a mystery for many years, but in 1994 an "obesity gene" was discovered [185] that probably produces a "satiety factor" known as the "ob protein" or "leptin," which can then signal the central nervous system [175,186].

Leptin is produced in adipose tissue and acts in a feedback loop that may affect the appetite and satiety centers of the brain, thus regulating body fat mass. In humans, researchers were surprised to find a strong *positive* correlation between serum leptin concentrations and the percentage of body fat, the BMI, and basal serum insulin concentrations, thus indicating a possible *decreased* sensitivity of either adipose tissue or the hypothalamus in obese people to the protein [158,174].

Like a thermostat, the adipostat can be reset by a variety of factors, primarily drugs, diet, and physical activity. As people grow more sedentary with age, the adipostat veers upward. In addition, the set point is under heavy genetic influence. Obese people often have lower resting metabolic rates *before* they become obese [158,177].

Diagnosis

The easiest and most readily available method of gauging obesity in adolescents is either direct measurement of skinfold thickness at various sites using calipers, or calculation of the BMI [187]. Skinfold measurements are made by grasping the subcutaneous skin between the thumb and forefinger, placed 6 to 8 cm apart, and stretching it just enough to permit the calipers to compress the

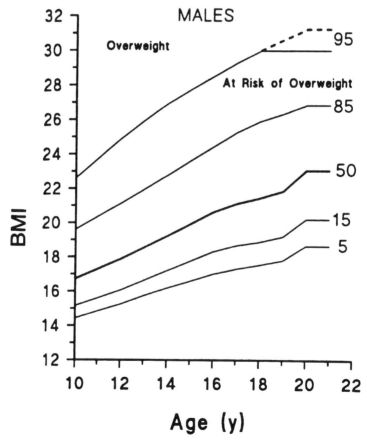

FIG. 14. Nomograms for body mass index for male **(A)** and female **(B)** adolescents. (Himes JH, Dietz WH. Am J Clin Nutr. American Society for Clinical Nutrition, 1994;59:312.)

tissue [127]. Several measurements should be taken, and the mean used. Subscapular skinfold thickness is most reliable, but triceps skinfold measurements are also commonly used (Fig. 11). Given what is now known about fat distribution and subsequent medical risk, it is also possible that measurement of the abdominal (waist) to gluteal (hips) ratio should be included in any assessment (Figs. 12, 13). Percentile grids for BMI in adolescents are now available as well [115] (Fig. 14).

Few laboratory tests are indicated in the routine evaluation of adolescents with obesity, with the exception of a serum lipid profile.

Treatment

A comprehensive look at different treatment methods is beyond the scope of this book (and probably beyond the interests of most practitioners), but several reviews are available [187–200]. Furthermore, a few basic principles of nutritional counseling and behavioral treatment are all that a practitioner needs to know. Without access to a large, multidisciplinary team of nutritionists, psychologists, nurse specialists, and physicians, the average practitioner would be wise to limit attempts at intervention to the general principles described here and to refer morbidly obese adolescents to specialized programs. Some consolation may exist in the fact that even large and expensive programs produce many patients who rapidly regain their lost weight [111,190,191] (Fig. 15, Table 34). Rates of recidi-

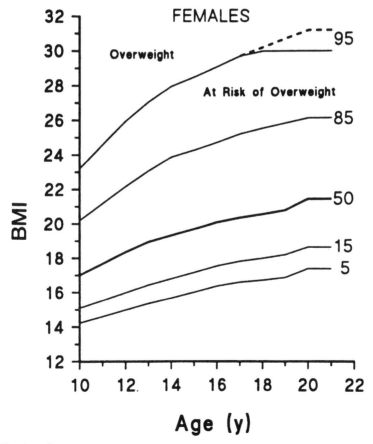

FIG. 14. *(Continued)*

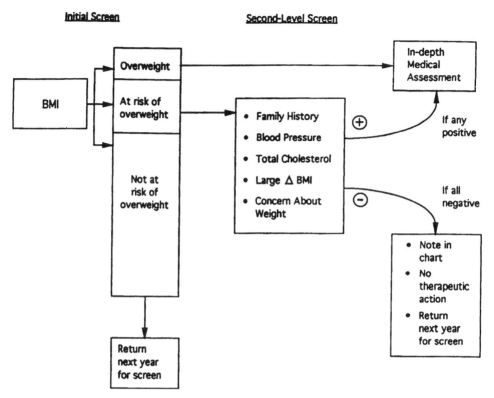

Initial Screen   **Second-Level Screen**

FIG. 15. Recommended screening for overweight adolescents. (Himes JH, Dietz WH. *Am J Clin Nutr* 1994;59:312. American Society for Clinical Nutrition.)

vism in long-term studies of children and adolescents approach 80% to 90%, [113,127]. Involving parents in the treatment may produce better results than focusing on the adolescent alone.

Prevention

As discussed previously, *prevention* of childhood obesity is the key element in avoiding adolescent obesity [201]. For clinicians, this means avoidance of the Gerber baby syndrome (i.e., "a fat baby is a healthy baby") and careful scrutiny of growth curves. One crude index of leanness is to aim for weight percentiles that are equal to or less than height percentiles as a child grows. Although low-fat diets may be harmful [202] especially during infancy, early introduction of cereal should be avoided; and babies should not be fed more than 16 to 24 fluid ounces of milk after solids are well tolerated. Given the observation that obesity may be produced by the ingestion of only an additional 50 calories per day over a long period of time, attention to seemingly trivial sources of energy imbalance such as snack foods or time spent watching television probably is justified [152,165].

Motivation for Change

Motivation is a key ingredient in being able to intervene in adolescent obesity. Patients who seek treatment probably have a better prognosis than those who are identified on routine examinations. Motivation factors are also reflected in initial 1-week weight loss, frequency of attendance at a weight loss program, and one's own belief that weight can be controlled—all predictors of success [190]. In addition, as previously discussed, prevention of childhood obesity is paramount and far preferable to attempts at intervention once obesity has occurred.

TABLE 34. *Assessment of obesity treatments*

Treatment	Rate of weight loss	Risk	Cost	Long-term efficacy
Conventional diet	+	Low	$–$$	Low
Very–low-calorie diet	+ +	Moderate	$$–$$$	Low/moderate
Starvation	+ +	High	$–$$$$	Low
Behavior modification	+	Low	$–$$	Moderate
Self-help groups	+	Low	$	Low/moderate
Exercise	±	Low/moderate	$–$$	Low/moderate
Appetite suppressants	+	Low/moderate	$–$$	Low

Adapted from Bray GA, Gray DS. Obesity: II. treatment. *West J Med* 1988;149:555.

Counseling

Counseling should highlight the following areas of concern and potential remedy:

- Psychological and family impact
- Diet
- Dieting
- Exercise
- Drugs
- Behavior modification
- A diet journal
- Support groups

Psychological and Family Impact. A detailed history should be elicited, including the teenager's reaction to his or her weight problem, age at onset of obesity, cultural context, activity level, amount of television viewed per day, and dietary intake. Often, a prospective record of intake over several days affords some insight into eating habits. In addition, the teenager and family should be asked to what they attribute the obesity, because intervention then can be appropriately oriented [111].

In fact, the family—not the patient—may be the logical focus of treatment efforts [111]. Studies show that weight reduction occurs more reliably when the mother and child are jointly involved [103]. In addition, children whose parents are divorced or separated do not lose weight as readily as those from intact families [104].

Diet. Many practical measures allow a healthier diet without making the teenager feel like a culinary outcast:

- Reducing the fat content of the diet to 35% of total calories accomplishes several goals: fat (9 kcal/g) is more calorically dense than carbohydrate (4 kcal/g), whereas carbohydrates produce greater satiety and consume more energy when being converted to adipose tissue [152].
- Such simple measures as trimming fat from meats, removing skin from poultry, switching from butter to margarine, avoiding gravy, and using low-fat mayonnaise are relatively easy to do.
- Concentrated sweets, such as candy, cookies, ice cream, and potato chips, should be avoided. But tasty, low-fat cookies that contain nontropical oils are becoming widely available (from Keebler, Pepperidge Farm, Healthy Choice, Nabisco), and reduced-fat ice cream and ice milk both can be acceptable substitutes for popular brands that contain up to 30% butterfat.
- Use of skim or low-fat milk in place of whole milk and diet soda instead of regular soda should also be strongly encouraged [135].
- Foods from all five food groups (e.g., milk, meat, bread, fruits, and vegetables) should be consumed as part of a balanced diet. Increasing fiber in the diet may also be useful [205].
- Consumption of "junk food" need not be entirely eliminated, but certainly should be severely curtailed [132] (Table 35).

All of these measures are more likely to succeed if they are made a part of the entire family's nutritional pattern, rather than isolating the teenager as having a "problem" that requires special meals.

TABLE 35. *Caloric and fat content of selected fast food*

Food	Calories	Fat (g)
McDonald's		
Big Mac	530	28
Quarter Pounder	430	21
Hamburger	270	9
Small french fries	210	10
Large french fries	450	22
Chicken McNuggets	430	26
Fajita chicken salad	250	10
with lite vinaigrette dressing		
Hard Rock Cafe		
Hamburger	660	36
Onion Rings	890	65
Pizza Hut		
Cheese pizza, 2 slices	446	20
Pepperoni pizza, 2 slices	640	38
Arby's		
Roast beef sandwich	552	28
Jr. roast beef sandwich	233	11
Taco Bell		
Tacos (2)	360	22
Taco Bell salad w/o salsa	838	55
Kentucky Fried Chicken		
KFC Original Recipe, half breast	360	20
KFC Rotisserie Gold, 1/4	199	6

Adapted from *USA Today,* October 20, 1994, p. 7D, and Hurley J, Schmidt S. Hard artery cafe? *Nutrition Action Health Letter* 1996; 23:1.

Dieting. Recurrent dieting may produce short-term success but long-term failure (Fig. 16). This is especially true in diets that restrict carbohydrates. Such diets lead to a sodium diuresis and weight loss through extracellular and intracellular fluid loss, not loss of body fat [190]. Because obese patients have greater metabolic rates than lean patients, the former can be expected to lose weight *faster* if calories are restricted [111].

In general, any caloric deprivation during early adolescence (and rapid pubertal growth) should be avoided. Theoretically, early adolescence represents an ideal time for intervention: using the growth spurt as an ally, and keeping caloric intake constant result in production of a relatively leaner body mass as height increases, at least in boys. If a diet is undertaken during adolescence, it should be carefully controlled and supervised. A 30% restriction in caloric intake, or approximately 500 kcal/day, ordinarily results in a weight loss of about 1 pound per week and does not compromise growth [135,172].

A number of fad diets are ill-advised: low-carbohydrate diets can cause ketosis and dehydration; liquid protein diets can lead to electrolyte and cardiac dysfunction; liquid formula diets tend to be monotonous and constipating; and special combination diets (e.g., the grapefruit diet) tend to be monotonous and unbalanced [170,195,206]. Newer liquid diets have become available that appear to be safer (e.g., Optifast and Medifast); however, patients quickly regain most of their lost weight and such diets appear to offer no advantages over a more conservative long-term program of modification of eating and exercise habits [107].

Exercise. Although exercise accounts for only approximately 15% of basal metabolic expenditure, increasing physical activity can have many beneficial side effects: a gradual increase in metabolic rate, an increase in lean muscle mass at the expense of adipose tissue, and a decrease in food intake [112,190,193,208] (Table 36). It can also improve a teenager's sense of well-being, the so-called "fitness factor" [209]. In general, however, restriction of caloric intake is more effective than exercise alone [198]. In superobese adolescents, physical activities that do not involve significant weight bearing (e.g., swimming or bicycling) are preferable to high-impact activities like aerobics or jogging.

TABLE 36. *Approximate energy expenditure for activities*

Activity category	Relative value
Resting	
Sleeping, reclining	1.0
Very light	
Seated or standing activities, typing, driving, cooking, sewing, playing cards	1.5
Light	
Walking on a level surface 2.5–3.0 mph, house-cleaning, golf, child care	2.5
Moderate	
Walking 3.5–4 mph, carrying a load, skiing, cycling, tennis	5.0
Heavy	
Walking with load uphill, basketball, climbing, football, soccer	7.0

Adapted from Hergenroeder AC, Phillips S. Advising teenagers and young adults about weight gain and loss through exercise and diet: practical advise for the physician. In: Shenker IR, ed. *Adolescent medicine.* Chur, Switzerland: Harwood Academic Publishers; 1994:113.

Drugs. Appetite suppressants are about to become a burgeoning industry in the United States, but they remain controversial [199]. For decades, anorexic drugs have been used, legally and illegally, to treat obesity. Amphetamines were the prototypical drugs but were quickly found to be potent, addictive, and associated with unacceptable side effects (e.g., hypertension and tachycardia) [190]. High school seniors in the class of 1995 reported a lifetime use rate of over 15% for stimulants, much of which are probably used as appetite suppressants [210]. In the National Adolescent Student Health Survey, 16% of adolescent girls reported using diet pills (usually pseudoephedrine) in the previous year [211].

In 1994, a National Institutes of Health workshop concluded that drugs should play a role in weight control [113]. Short-term drug therapy has been found to be effective; however, long-term drug therapy remains problematic because its efficacy has not yet been demonstrated and side effects are unknown [187,198].

In April, 1996, the U.S. Food and Drug Administration approved dexfenfluramine (Redux) for treatment of obesity.* Dexfenfluramine stimulates serotonin release and inhibits reuptake; in animals, increased serotonin suppresses appetite [198]. It is often combined with phentermine, which inhibits the reuptake of norepinephrine and has a stimulating effect (the so-called Fen–phen regimen) [200,212]. Multiple studies demonstrate its dramatic effectiveness in producing short-term weight loss, but patients often regain the lost weight [198,200]. In one study of 404 obese patients treated for 1 year, nearly two thirds lost at least 5% of their body weight, with one fifth losing 15% [213]. In another 6-month trial, patients averaged a 9.7-kg weight loss, compared with an average 4.9-kg weight loss in the control group [214]. Patients likely to benefit from the use of anorexic drugs have BMIs greater than 30 [199].

Side effects of dexfenfluramine therapy can include nausea, dry mouth, fatigue, drowsiness, and dizziness [200]. Unfortunately, use of anorexic drugs such as dexfenfluramine is associated with a rare but often fatal side effect, the development of primary pulmonary hypertension, as well as valvular heart disease in women [215]. When anorexic drugs are used for more than 3 months, the odds ratio for development of primary pulmonary hypertension was 23.1 [216]. Although the overall risk is extremely small (28 cases per million person-years) and the risks of obesity are substantial, we believe that a conservative approach is advisable until more is known about long-term effects. At this time, dexfenfluramine should probably be reserved for morbidly obese adolescent patients who have

---

*Fenfluramine was withdrawn from the market in September 1997. Phentermine may still be used in combination with Prozac (Phen-Pro).

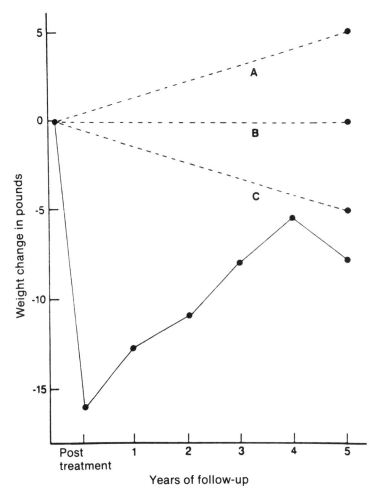

FIG. 16. Results of behaviorally based weight loss programs (solid line). Lines A, B, and C represent hypothetical groups receiving no treatment. A shows the natural history of untreated obese patients; B shows stable weight; and C shows gradual weight loss. (Brownell KD, Kramer FM. Behavioral management of obesity. *Med Clin North Am* 1989;73:185. With permission.)

failed other treatment modalities, and used only with appropriate informed consent and a research-type protocol [217]. Other critics disagree and believe that the benefits of weight loss using drugs like dexfenfluramine outweigh the risks [199].

Another, more common selective serotonin reuptake inhibitor that has been used frequently for depression is fluoxetine (Prozac). Its effectiveness in treating obese patients seems to be limited to 6 months or less, and weight is often regained. Successful use also requires behavioral and nutritional counseling. Furthermore, the number of potential side effects at the usual 60-mg dose required (nausea, diarrhea, sweating, nervousness, tremor, insomnia, somnolence, delayed or absent orgasm) make this an unlikely candidate for most obese teenagers [192].

In the past, thyroid hormone has also been used to increase metabolic rate and induce weight loss. However, it is associated with increased protein catabolism, calcium loss from bone, and cardiovascular risks and is not indicated for such use.

Several experimental drugs are under study, including lipase inhibitors, which interfere with food absorption, and selective beta-adrenergic agents, which could accelerate metabolic rates [218].

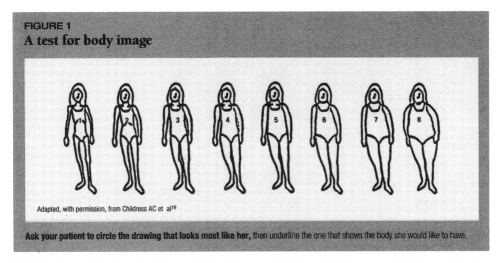

FIGURE 1
A test for body image

Adapted, with permission, from Childress AC et al[19]

Ask your patient to circle the drawing that looks most like her, then underline the one that shows the body she would like to have.

FIG. 17. One test for female adolescents' body image. (Childress AC, Brewerton TD, Hodges EL, et al. The Kids' Eating Disorder Survey [KEDS]: a study of middle school students. *J Am Acad Child Adolesc Psychiatry* 1993;32:843. Reproduced from Stashwick C. When you suspect an eating disorder. *Contemporary Pediatrics* 1996;13:124.)

Behavior Modification. Several studies have documented the effectiveness of behavior modification over an extended period of time [191,194,219]. The goal is to change the nature of eating behavior and the circumstances surrounding it. Current behavior modification programs use the principles of self-monitoring, stimulus control, positive reinforcement, good nutrition, exercise, social support, and cognitive change [191]:

- *Self-monitoring* involves keeping a food diary of what is eaten, when, and under what circumstances.
- *Stimulus control* tries to reduce behaviors that are linked with eating—watching television, for example. In addition, exposure to food is reduced by keeping it out of sight as much as possible and reducing time spent at meals. Patients are instructed to eat slowly, to eat three to five regular meals a day, to eat only in one place, and to avoid eating when depressed or just because food is available. Attempts are made to discontinue automatic behaviors, such as eating two slices of toast in the morning. Instead, the patient begins with eating one slice of toast and then decides if a second slice is desired.
- *Positive reinforcement* includes rewards from family or friends as well as from one's self. This could include purchasing a desired item or going to a movie if certain goals are met.
- *Good nutrition* is stressed, and patients are instructed to set a daily goal of 1,500 calories for boys and 1,200 calories for girls.
- *Exercise* is increased by simple measures (e.g., walking up stairs instead of taking an elevator) and through daily walking.
- *Social support* from family is crucial in the patient's efforts to lose weight and maintain the loss. For example, one study of obese adolescents found that successful weight-losers felt they had more personal control over their weight, more family problems associated with their obesity, and greater willingness of family members to share the same diet [220].
- *Cognitive methods* represent the newest addition to behavior modification schemes. Efforts are made to change patients' self-image and beliefs about their excess weight (Fig. 17).

A Diet Journal. Keeping a journal in which both food intake and feelings are recorded can assist the patient and the counselor in their ongoing discussions.

Support Groups. With their unique need for peer approval and support, adolescents are excellent candidates for inclusion in support groups [196]. Groups such as Teenage Obesity Programs (TOPS),

Weight Watchers, or Shapedown may allow teenagers to gain valuable self-esteem and encouragement from their peers [147]. An evaluation of the Shapedown program showed that teens lost an average of over 5 kg compared with control subjects, had increases in self-esteem, and maintained their weight loss for at least 1 year [221] A similar program, entitled Weight Winners, documented an 11% weight loss within a 9-month follow-up period [222].

REFERENCES

1. Fisher M, Golden NH, Katzman DK, et al. Eating disorders in adolescents: A background paper. *J Adolesc Health* 1995;16:420.
2. Herzog DB, Keller MB, Lavori PW. Outcome in anorexia nervosa and bulimia nervosa. *J Nerv Ment Dis* 1988;176:131.
3. Levine RL. Eating disorders in adolescents: a comprehensive update. *Int Pediatr* 1995;10:327.
4. Zerbe KJ. Eating disorders: the apple doesn't fall far from the tree. *Contemporary Pediatrics* 1996;13:65.
5. Comerci GD. Eating disorders in adolescents. *Pediatr Rev* 1988;10:37.
6. Kreipe RE. Eating disorders among children and adolescents. *Pediatr Rev* 1995;16:370.
7. Pate JE, Pumariega AJ, Hester C, et al. Cross-cultural patterns in eating disorders: a review. *J Am Acad Child Adolesc Psychiatry* 1992;5:802.
8. Robinson TN, Killen JD, Litt IF, et al. Ethnicity and body dissatisfaction: are Hispanic and Asian girls at increased risk for eating disorders? *J Adolesc Health* 1996;19:384.
9. Merritt D. Recognizing and treating weight disorders in adolescents: the thick and thin of it. *NASPAG News* 1996;10(3):1.
10. Rome ES, Imrie RK, Rybicki LA, et al. Prevalence of abnormal eating attitudes and behaviors in hospital-based primary and tertiary care clinics: a window of opportunity? *Journal of Pediatric and Adolescent Gynecology* 1996;9:133.
11. Tofler IR, Stryer BK, Micheli LJ, et al. Physical and emotional problems of elite female gymnasts. *N Engl J Med* 1996;335:281.
12. Kulig JW, Siqueira LM. Diagnosis of anorexia nervosa in the adolescent male. *Journal of Adolescent Health Care* 1983;4:31.
13. Farrow JA. The adolescent male with an eating disorder. *Pediatr Ann* 21:760, 1992;.
14. Hobbs WL, Johnson CA. Anorexia nervosa: an overview. *Am Fam Physician* 1996;54:1273.
15. Comerci GD, ed. Eating disorders in adolescents. *Pediatr Ann* 1992;21:707.
16. Woodside DB. Anorexia nervosa and bulimia nervosa in children and adolescents. *Curr Opin Pediatr* 1993;5:415.
17. Harper G. Eating disorders in adolescence. *Pediatr Rev* 1994;15:72.
18. Levine MP, Smolak L, Hayden H. The relation of sociocultural factors to eating attitudes and behaviors among middle school girls. *Journal of Early Adolescence* 1994;14:471.
19. Strasburger VC. *Adolescents and the media: medical and psychological impact.* Thousand Oaks, CA: Sage; 1995.
20. Garner DM, Garfinkel PE, Schwartz D, et al. Cultural expectations of thinness in women. *Psychol Rep* 1980; 47:483.
21. Herzog DB, Copeland PM. Eating disorders. *N Engl J Med* 1985;313:295.
22. Moore DC. Body image and eating behavior in adolescent boys. *American Journal of Diseases of Children* 1990;144:475.
23. Kilbourne J. Killing us softly: gender roles in advertising. *Adolescent Medicine: State of the Art Reviews* 1993;4:635.
24. Goldner EM, Leung SP. *Shaping the future: freedom from eating disorders.* Vancouver, BC: St. Paul's Hospital; 1995.
25. Dietz WH. You are what you eat: what you eat is what you are. *Journal of Adolescent Health Care* 1990; 11:76.
26. Kaufman L. Prime-time nutrition. *Journal of Communication* 1980;30:37.
27. Yager J. Family issues in the pathogenesis of anorexia nervosa. *Psychosom Med* 1982;44:43.
28. Minuchin S, Rosman BL, Baker L. *Psychosomatic families: anorexia nervosa in context.* Cambridge, MA: Harvard University Press; 1978.
29. Joffe A. Too little, too much: eating disorders in adolescents. *Contemporary Pediatrics* 1990;7:114.
30. Yates A. Current perspectives on the eating disorders: I. history, psychological and biological aspects. *J Am Acad Child Adolesc Psychiatry* 1989;28:813.
31. Waller JV, Kaufman MR, Deutsch F. Anorexia nervosa: a psychosomatic entity. *Psychosom Med* 1940;2:3.
32. Yates A, Leehey K, Shisslak CM. Running: an analogue of anorexia? *N Engl J Med* 1983;308:251.
33. Blumenthal JA, O'Toole LC, Chang JL. Is running an analogue of anorexia nervosa? An empirical study of obligatory running and anorexia nervosa. *JAMA* 1984;252:520.
34. Frisch RE, Wyshak G, Vincent L. Delayed menarche and amenorrhea in ballet dancers. *N Engl J Med* 1980;303:17.

35. Herzog DB. Are anorexic and bulimic patients depressed? *Am J Psychiatry* 1984;141:1594.
36. Kaye WH, Berrettini W, Gwirtsman H, et al. Altered cerebrospinal fluid neuropeptide Y and peptide YY immunoreactivity in anorexia and bulimia nervosa. *Arch Gen Psychiatry* 1990;47:548.
37. Kaye WH. Neurotransmitters and anorexia nervosa. In: Brownell KD, Fairburn CG, eds. *Eating disorders and obesity: a comprehensive handbook*. New York: Guilford Press; 1995:255.
38. Patton GC, Johnson-Sabine E, Wood K, et al. Abnormal eating attitudes in London schoolgirls: a prospective epidemiological study: outcome at twelve month follow-up. *Psychol Med* 1990;20:383.
39. Story M, Rosenwinkel K, Himes JH, et al. Demographic and risk factors associated with chronic dieting in adolescents. *American Journal of Diseases of Children* 1991;145:994.
40. Whitaker AH. An epidemiologic study of anorectic and bulimic symptoms in adolescent girls: implications for pediatricians. *Pediatr Ann* 1992;21:752.
41. Halmi KA. Changing rates of eating disorders: what does it mean? *Am J Psychiatry* 1995;152:1256.
42. Moses N, Banilivy MM, Lifshitz F. Fear of obesity among adolescent girls. *Pediatrics* 1989;83:393.
43. Eisele J, Hertsgaard D, Light HK. Factors related to eating disorders in young adolescent girls. *Adolescence* 1986;21:283.
44. Moore DC. Body image and eating behavior in adolescent girls. *American Journal of Diseases of Children* 1988;142:1114.
45. Maloney MJ, McGuire J, Daniels SR, et al. Dieting behavior and eating attitudes in children. *Pediatrics* 1989;84:482.
46. Mellin LM, Irwin CE Jr, Scully S. Prevalence of disordered eating in girls: a survey of middle-class children. *J Am Diet Assoc* 1992;92:851.
47. American Psychiatric Association. *Diagnostic and statistical manual of mental disorders*. 4th ed. Washington, DC: American Psychiatric Association; 1994.
48. Kreipe RE, Churchill BH, Strauss J. Long-term outcome of adolescents with anorexia nervosa. *American Journal of Diseases of Children* 1989;143:1322.
49. Drossman DA, Ontjes DA, Heizer W.D. Anorexia nervosa. *Gastroenterology* 1979;77:1115.
50. Golden NH, Shenker IR. Amenorrhea in anorexia nervosa: etiology and implications. *Adolescent Medicine: State of the Art Reviews* 1992;2:503.
51. Boyar RM, Katz J, Finkelstein JW, et al. Anorexia nervosa: immaturity of the 24-hour luteinizing hormone secretory pattern. *N Engl J Med* 1974;291:861.
52. Rigotti NA, Nussbaum SR, Herzog DB, et al. Osteoporosis in women with anorexia nervosa. *N Engl J Med* 1984;311:1601.
53. Bachrach LK, Guido D, Katzman DK, et al. Decreased bone density in adolescent girls with anorexia nervosa. *Pediatrics* 1990;86:440.
54. Mehler PS. Bone density in amenorrheic athletes and in anorexia nervosa. *JAMA* 1996;276:1384.
55. Vigersky RA, Andersen AE, Thompson RH, et al. Hypothalamic dysfunction in secondary amenorrhea associated with simple weight loss. *N Engl J Med* 1977;297:1141.
56. Gupta MA, Gupta AK, Haberman HF. Dermatologic signs in anorexia nervosa and bulimia nervosa. *Arch Dermatol* 1987;123:1386.
57. Katzman DK, Lambe EK, Mikulis DJ, et al. Cerebral gray matter and white matter volume deficits in adolescent girls with anorexia nervosa. *J Pediatr* 1996;129:794.
58. Kreipe RE, Harris JP. Myocardial impairment resulting from eating disorders. *Pediatr Ann* 1992;21:760.
60. Kreipe RE, Golden NH, Katzman DK, et al. Eating disorders in adolescents: a position paper of the Society for Adolescent Medicine. *J Adolesc Health* 1995;16:476.
61. American Psychiatric Association. Practice guidelines for eating disorders. *Am J Psychiatry* 1993;150:207.
62. Kreipe RE, Uphoff M. Treatment and outcome of adolescents with anorexia nervosa. *Adolescent Medicine: State of the Art Reviews* 1992;3:519.
63. Nussbaum M, Shenker R, Baird D, et al. Follow-up investigation in patients with anorexia nervosa. *J Pediatr* 1985;106:835.
64. Fichter MM. Inpatient treatment of anorexia nervosa. In: Brownell KD, Fairburn CG, eds. *Eating disorders and obesity: a comprehensive handbook*. New York: Guilford Press; 1995:336.
65. Schebendach J, Nussbaum MP. Nutrition management in adolescents with eating disorders. *Adolescent Medicine: State of the Art Reviews* 1992;3:541.
66. Silber TJ. Eating disorders and health insurance. *Arch Pediatr Adolesc Med* 1994;148:785.
67. Hsu LKG. The treatment of anorexia nervosa. *Am J Psychiatry* 1986;143:573.
68. Halmi KA, Eckert ED, LaDu TJ, et al. Anorexia nervosa: treatment efficacy of cyproheptadine and amitriptyline. *Arch Gen Psychiatry* 1986;43:177.
69. Schwartz DM, Thompson M. Do anorectics get well? Current research and future needs. *Am J Psychiatry* 1981;138:319.
70. Hsu LKG, Crisp AH, Harding B. Outcome of anorexia nervosa. *Lancet* 1979;1:61.
71. Lacey H. Bulimia nervosa, binge eating, and psychogenic vomiting: a controlled treatment study and long-term outcome. *Br Med J* 1983;286:1609.
72. Bryant-Waugh RJ, Bryan DL, Rosamund L, et al. Do doctors recognise eating disorders in children? *Arch Dis Child* 1992;67:103.

73. Stein DM. The prevalence of bulimia: a review of the empirical research. *J Nutr Educ* 1991;23:205.
74. Bursten MS, Gabel LL, Brose JA et al . Detecting and treating bulimia nervosa: how involved are family physicians? *J Am Board Fam Pract* 1996;9:241.
75. Schotte DE, Stunkard AJ. Bulimia vs. bulimic behaviors on a college campus. *JAMA* 1987;258:1213.
76. Drewnowski A, Yee DK, Krahn DD. Bulimia in college women. *Am J Psychiatry* 1988;145:753.
77. Timmerman MG, Wells LA, Chen S. Bulimia nervosa and associated alcohol abuse among secondary school students. *J Am Acad Child Adolesc Psychiatry* 1990;29:118.
78. Halmi KA, Falk JR, Schwartz E. Binge eating and vomiting: a survey of a college population. *Psychol Med* 1981;11:697.
79. Marchi M, Cohen P. Early childhood eating behaviors and adolescent eating disorders. *J Am Acad Child Adolesc Psychiatry* 1990;29:112.
80. Killen JD, Taylor CB, Telch MJ, et al. Self-induced vomiting and laxative and diuretic use among teenagers. *JAMA* 1986;225:1447.
81. Hendren RL, Barber JK, Sigafoos A. Eating-disordered symptoms in a nonclinical population: a study of female adolescents in two private schools. *J Am Acad Child Adolesc Psychiatry* 1986;25:836.
82. Fairburn CG, Cooper PJ. The clinical features of bulimia nervosa. *Br J Psychiatry* 1984;144:238.
83. Swift WJ, Andrews D, Barklage NE. The relationship between affective disorder and eating disorders: a review of the literature. *Am J Psychiatry* 1986;143:290.
84. Dietz WH. Childhood obesity: prevalence and effects. In: Brownell KD, Fairburn CG, eds. *Eating disorders and obesity: a comprehensive handbook*. New York: Guilford Press; 1995:438.
85. Kleinke CL, Staneski RA. First impressions of female bust size. *J Soc Psychol* 1980;110:123.
86. Thompson DA, Berg KM, Shatford LA. The heterogenicity of bulimic symptomatology: cognitive and behavioral dimensions. *Int J Eat Disord* 1987;6:215.
87. Strober M. Family-genetic perspectives on anorexia nervosa and bulimia nervosa. In: Brownell KD, Fairburn CG, eds. *Eating disorders and obesity: a comprehensive handbook*. New York: Guilford Press; 1995:212.
88. Humphrey LL. Relationships within subtypes of anorexics, bulimics, and normal families. *J Am Acad Child Adolesc Psychiatry* 1988;27:544.
89. Garfinkel PE, Garner DM, Goldbloom DS. Eating disorders: implications for the 1990's. *Can J Psychiatry* 1987;32:624..
90. Pope HG, Hudson JI. Is childhood sexual abuse a risk factor for bulimia nervosa? *Am J Psychiatry* 1992;149:455.
91. Yates A. Biologic considerations in the etiology of eating disorders. *Pediatr Ann* 1992;21:739.
92. Kaye WH, Ebert MH, Raleigh M, et al. Abnormalities in CSF monoamine metabolism in anorexia nervosa. *Arch Gen Psychiatry* 1984;41:350.
93. Kaye WH, Ebert MH, Gwirtsman H.E. Differences in brain serotoninergic metabolism between bulimic and non-bulimic patients with anorexia nervosa. *Am J Psychiatry* 1984;141:1598.
94. Herzog DB. Bulimia in the adolescent. *American Journal of Diseases of Children* 1982;136:985.
95. Abraham SF, Beumont PJV. How patients describe bulimia or binge eating. *Psychol Med* 1982;12:625.
96. Fisher M. Medical complications of anorexia and bulimia nervosa. *Adolescent Medicine: State of the Art Reviews* 1992;3:487.
97. Mitchell JE. Medical complications of bulimia nervosa. In: Brownell KD, Fairburn CG, eds. *Eating disorders and obesity: a comprehensive handbook*. New York: Guilford Press; 1995:271.
98. Fairburn CG. Short-term psychological treatments for bulimia nervosa. In: Brownell KD, Fairburn CG, eds. *Eating disorders and obesity: a comprehensive handbook*. New York: Guilford Press; 1995:344.
99. Mitchell PB. The pharmacologic management of bulimia nervosa: a critical review. *Int J Eat Disord* 1988; 7:29.
100. Walsh BT. Pharmacotherapy of eating disorders. In: Brownell KD, Fairburn CG, eds. *Eating disorders and obesity: a comprehensive handbook*. New York: Guilford Press; 1995:313.
101. Fluoxetine Bulimia Nervosa Study Group. Fluoxetine in the treatment of bulimia nervosa. *Arch Gen Psychiatry* 1992;29:139.
102. Agras WS, Rossiter EM, Arnow B, et al. Pharmacologic and cognitive-behavioral treatment for bulimia nervosa: a controlled comparison. *Am J Psychiatry* 1992;49:82.
103. Collings S, King M. Ten-year follow-up of 50 patients with bulimia nervosa. *Br J Psychiatry* 1994;164:80.
104. Hsu LKG. Outcome of bulimia nervosa. In: Brownell KD, Fairburn CG, eds. *Eating disorders and obesity: a comprehensive handbook*. New York: Guilford Press; 1995:238.
105. Mitchell JE, Pyle RL, Hatsukami D, et al. A two-to-five year follow-up study of patients treated for bulimia. *Int J Eat Disord* 1988;8:157.
106. Cox GL, Merkel WT. A qualitative review of psychosocial treatments for bulimia. *J Nerv Ment Dis* 1989; 177:77.
107. Yager J. The treating of eating disorders. *J Clin Psychiatry* 1988;49:18.
108. Yager J, Landsverk J, Edelstein C.K. A 20-month follow-up of 628 women with eating disorders. *Am J Psychiatry* 1987;144:1172.
109. Lustick MJ. Bulimia in adolescents: a review. *Pediatrics* 1985;76(Suppl):685.
110. Comerci GD. Eating disorders in adolescents. *Pediatr Rev* 1988;10:37.

111. Dietz WH, Robinson TN. Assessment and treatment of childhood obesity. *Pediatr Rev* 1993;14:337.
112. Hergenroeder AC, Phillips S. Advising teenagers and young adults about weight gain and loss through exercise and diet: practical advice for the physician. In: Shenker, IR, ed. *Adolescent medicine*. Switzerland: Harwood Academic Publishers; 1994:113.
113. Adkinson RL, Hubbard VS. Report on the NIH workshop on pharmacologic treatment of obesity. *Am J Clin Nutr* 1994;60:153.
114. Pi-Sunyer FX. The fattening of America. *JAMA* 1994;272:238.
115. Himes JH, Dietz WH. Guidelines for overweight in adolescent preventive services: recommendations from an expert committee. *Am J Clin Nutr* 1994;59:307.
116. Centers for Disease Control and Prevention. Prevalence of overweight among adolescents: United States, 1988–91. *MMWR Morb Mortal Wkly Rep* 1994;43:818.
117. Troiano RP, Flegal KM, Kuczmarski RJ, et al. Overweight prevalence and trends for children and adolescents. *Arch Pediatr Adolesc Med* 1995;149:1085.
118. Kuczmarski RJ, Fleagal KM, Campbell SM, et al. Increasing prevalence of overweight among US adults: the National Health and Nutrition Examination Surveys, 1960 to 1991. *JAMA* 1994;272:205.
119. Bray GA, Gray DS. Obesity: I. pathogenesis. *West J Med* 1988;149:429.
120. Associated Press. Most Americans are overweight. *The New York Times,* October 16, 1996:B6.
121. Goldblatt PB, Moore ME, Stunkard AJ. Social factors in obesity. *JAMA* 1965;192:1039.
122. Morrison JA, Alfaro MP, Khoury P, et al. Determinants of resting energy expenditure in young black girls and young white girls. *J Pediatr* 1996;129:637.
123. Kaplan AS, Zemel BS, Stallings VA. Differences in resting energy expenditure in prepubertal black children and white children. *J Pediatr* 1996;129:643.
124. Mossberg HO. 40-year follow-up of overweight children. *Lancet* 1989;2:491.
125. Must A, Jacques PF, Dallal GE, et al. Long-term morbidity and mortality of overweight adolescents: a follow-up of the Harvard Growth Study of 1922 to 19@REF: 35.   *N Engl J Med* 1992;327:1350.
126. Nieto FJ, Szklo M, Comstock GW. Childhood weight and growth rate as predictors of adult mortality. *Am J Epidemiol* 1992;136:201.
127. Rosenbaum M, Leibel RL. Obesity in childhood. *Pediatr Rev* 1989;11:43.
128. Gortmaker SL, Dietz WH Jr, Cheung LW. Inactivity, diet and the fattening of America. *J Am Diet Assoc* 1990;90:1247.
129. Pi-Sunyer FX. Medical hazards of obesity. *Ann Intern Med* 1993;119:655.
130. Hemsley SE Jr, Berkowitz RI, Stallings VA, et al. Weight reduction and blood pressure change in morbidly obese adolescent females [abstract]. *J Adolesc Health* 1995;16:147.
131. Rocchini AP, Katch V, Anderson J, et al. Blood pressure in obese adolescents: effect of weight loss. *Pediatrics* 1988;82:16.
132. Heald FP. Fast food and snack food: beneficial or deleterious? *J Adolesc Health* 1992;13:380.
133. Steinberger J, Moorehead C, Katch V, et al. Relationship between insulin resistance and abnormal lipid profile in obese adolescents. *J Pediatr* 1995;126:690.
134. Rhodes SK, Shimoda KC, Waid LR, et al. Neurocognitive deficits in morbidly obese children with obstructive sleep apnea. *J Pediatr* 1995;127:741.
135. Bandini LG. Obesity in the adolescent. *Adolescent Medicine: State of the Art Reviews* 1992;3:459.
136. Bray GA. Classification and evaluation of the obesities. *Med Clin North Am* 1989;73:161.
137. Donahue RP, Abbott RD, Bloom E, et al. Central obesity and coronary heart disease in men. *Lancet* 1987;1:821.
138. Kaplan NM. The deadly quartet: upper-body obesity, glucose intolerance, hypertriglyceridemia, and hypertension. *Arch Intern Med* 1989;149:1514.
139. Ostlund RE Jr, Staten M, Hohrt WM, et al. The ratio of waist-to-hip circumference, plasma insulin level, and glucose intolerance as independent predictors of the HDL_2 cholesterol level in older adults. *N Engl J Med* 1990;322:229.
140. Gortmaker SL, Must A, Perrin JM, et al. Social and economic consequences of overweight in adolescence and young adulthood. *N Engl J Med* 1993;329:1008.
141. Kaufman L. Prime-time nutrition. *Journal of Communication* 1980;30:37.
142. Dietz WH. You are what you eat: what you eat is what you are. *Journal of Adolescent Health Care* 1990;11:76.
143. Feldman W, Feldman E, Goodman JT. Culture versus biology: children's attitudes towards thinness and fitness. *Pediatrics* 1988;81:190.
144. Staffieri JR. A study of social stereotype of body image in children. *J Pers Soc Psychol* 1967;7:101.
145. Stunkard A, Mendelson M. Obesity and the body image: I. characteristics of disturbances in the body image of some obese persons. *Am J Psychiatry* 1967;123:1296.
146. Baum CG, Forehand R. Social factors associated with adolescent obesity. *J Pediatr Psychol* 1984;9:293.
147. Willis ED, McCoy B, Berman M. The effect of a weight management program on self esteem and body image in obese youth. *American Journal of Diseases of Children* 1990;144:417.
148. Stunkard AJ, Sorensen TIA, Harris C, et al. Adoption study of human obesity. *N Engl J Med* 1986;314:193.
149. Stunkard AJ, Foch TT, Hrubec Z. A twin study of human obesity. *JAMA* 1986;256:51.

150. Stunkard AJ, Harris JR, Pedersen NL, et al. The body-mass index of twins who have been reared apart. *N Engl J Med* 1990;322:1483.
151. Kleinman RE, ed. *Pediatric nutrition handbook.* 4th ed. Elk Grove Village, IL: American Academy of Pediatrics; 1997.
152. Dietz WH Jr. Prevention of childhood obesity. *Pediatr Clin North Am* 1986;33:823.
153. Ravelli GP, Belmont L. Obesity in nineteen-year-old men: family size and birth order associations. *Am J Epidemiol* 1979;109:66.
154. Bray GA. Adolescent overweight may be tempting fate. *N Engl J Med* 1992;327:1379.
155. Garn SM, Clark DC. Trends in fatness and the origins of obesity. *Pediatrics* 1976;57:443.
156. Boodman SG. Childhood obesity not all matter of genetics. *The Washington Post,* June 26, 1995.
157. Leibel RL. Obesity: a game of inches. *Pediatrics* 1995;95:131.
158. Winick M. Editorial: understanding and treating obesity. *Am J Public Health* 1996;86:925.
159. Centers for Disease Control and Prevention. Vigorous physical activity among high school students: United States, 1990. *MMWR Morb Mortal Wkly Rep* 1992;41:33.
160. Heath GW, Pratt M, Warren CW, et al. Physical activity patterns in American high school students: results from the 1990 Youth Risk Behavior Survey. *Arch Pediatr Adolesc Med* 1994;148:1131.
161. U.S. Department of Health and Human Services. *Physical activity and health: a report of the Surgeon General.* Atlanta, GA: U.S. Department of Health and Human Services, Public Health Service, CDC, National Center for Chronic Disease Prevention and Health Promotion, 1996.
162. Dietz WH, Gortmaker SL. Do we fatten our children at the TV set? Television viewing and obesity in children and adolescents. *Pediatrics* 1985;75:807.
163. Robinson TN, Hammer LD, Killen JD, et al. Does television viewing increase obesity and reduce physical activity? Cross-sectional and longitudinal analyses among adolescent girls. *Pediatrics* 1993;91:273.
164. DuRant RH, Baranowski T, Johnson M, et al. The relationship among television watching, physical activity, and body composition of young children. *Pediatrics* 1994;94:449.
165. Gortmaker SL, Must A, Sobol AM, et al. Television viewing as a cause of increasing obesity among children in the United States, 1986–1990. *Arch Pediatr Adolesc Med* 1996;150:356.
166. Dietz WH, Gortmaker SL. TV or not TV: fat is the question. *Pediatrics* 1993;91:499.
167. Strasburger VC. *Adolescents and the media: medical and psychological impact.* Thousand Oaks, CA: Sage; 1995.
168. Cotugna N. T.V. ads on Saturday morning children's programming *Journal of Nutrition Education* 1988;20:125.
169. Klesges RC, Shelton ML, Klesges LM. Effects of television on metabolic rate: potential implications for childhood obesity. *Pediatrics* 1993;91:281.
170. Neinstein LS. *Adolescent health care: a practical guide.* 3rd ed. Baltimore: Williams & Wilkins; 1996.
171. Avery ME, First LR. *Pediatric medicine.* Baltimore: Williams & Wilkins; 1989.
172. Comerci GD, Kilbourne KA, Harrison GG. Eating disorders: obesity, anorexia nervosa, and bulimia. In: Hofmann AD, Greydanus DE, eds. *Adolescent medicine.* 2nd ed. Norwalk, CT: Appleton & Lange; 1989:441.
173. Lindpaintner K. Finding an obesity gene: a tale of mice and man. *N Engl J Med* 1995;332:679.
174. Considine RV, Sinha MK, Heiman ML, et al. Serum immunoreactive-leptin concentrations in normal-weight and obese humans. *N Engl J Med* 1996;334:292.
175. Rohner-Jeanrenaud F, Jeanrenaud B. Obesity, leptin, and the brain. *N Engl J Med* 1996;334:324.
176. Leibel RL, Rosenbaum M, Hirsch J. Changes in energy expenditure from altered body weight. *N Engl J Med* 1995;332:621.
177. Dietz WH. Is reduced metabolic rate associated with obesity? *J Pediatr* 1996;129:621.
178. Bennett WI. Beyond overeating. *N Engl J Med* 1995;332:673.
179. Leibel RL. Obesity: a game of inches. *Pediatrics* 1995;95:131.
180. Bogardus C, Lillioja S, Ravussin E, et al. Familial dependence of resting metabolic rate. *N Engl J Med* 1986;315:96.
181. Brownell KD, Stunkard AJ, Albaum JM. Evaluation and modification of exercise patterns in the natural environment. *Am J Psychiatry* 1980;137:1540.
182. Maffels C, Schutz Y, Schena F, et al. Energy expenditure during walking and running in obese and nonobese prepubertal children. *J Pediatr* 1993;123:193.
183. Segal KR, Gutin B, Albu J, et al. Thermic effects of food and exercise in lean and obese men of similar lean body mass. *Am J Physiol* 1985;15:E110.
184. Hirsch J. Cell number and size as a determinant of subsequent obesity. In: Winick M, ed. *Childhood obesity.* New York: John Wiley & Sons; 1975:000.
185. Zhang Y, Proenca R, Maffei M, et al. Positional cloning of the mouse *obese* gene and its human homologue. *Nature* 1994;372:425.
186. Rink TJ. In search of a satiety factor. *Nature* 1994;372:406.
187. Berkowitz RI. Treating adolescent obesity. *Adolescent Medicine: State of the Art Reviews* 1997;8(1), (in press).
188. Brownell KD, Foreyt JP, eds. *Handbook of eating disorders: physiology, psychology, and treatment of obesity, anorexia, and bulimia.* New York: Basic Books; 1986.
189. Atkinson RL. Low and very low calorie diets. *Med Clin North Am* 1989;73:203.
190. Bray GA, Gray DS. Obesity: II. treatment. *West J Med* 1988;149:555.
191. Brownell KD, Kramer FM. Behavioral management of obesity. *Med Clin North Am* 1989;73:185.

192. The Medical Letter. Fluoxetine (Prozac) and other drugs for treatment of obesity. *The Medical Letter* 1994;36(936):107.
193. Brownell KD. Exercise in the treatment of obesity. In: Brownell KD, Fairburn CG, eds. *Eating Disorders and obesity: a comprehensive handbook.* New York: Guilford Press; 1995:473.
194. Wilson GT. Behavioral approaches to the treatment of obesity. In: Brownell KD, Fairburn CG, eds. *Eating disorders and obesity: a comprehensive handbook.* New York: Guilford Press; 1995:479.
195. Dwyer J. Popular diets. In: Brownell KD, Fairburn CG, eds. *Eating disorders and obesity: a comprehensive handbook.* New York: Guilford Press; 1995:491.
196. Cormillot A. Commercial and self-help approaches to weight management. In: Brownell KD, Fairburn CG, eds. *Eating disorders and obesity: a comprehensive handbook.* New York: Guilford Press; 1995:498.
197. Heshka S, Heymsfield SB. Pharmacological treatment of obesity. In: Brownell KD, Fairburn CG, eds. *Eating disorders and obesity: a comprehensive handbook.* New York: Guilford Press; 1995:504.
198. Boisaubin EV. Treatment for obesity. *JAMA* 1996;276:445.
199. Manson JE, Faich GA. Pharmacotherapy for obesity: do the benefits outweigh the risks? *N Engl J Med* 1996;335:659.
200. The Medical Letter. Dexfenfluramine for obesity. *The Medical Letter* 1996;38(979):64.
201. Stunkard AJ. Prevention of obesity. In: Brownell KD, Fairburn CG, eds. *Eating disorders and obesity: a comprehensive handbook.* New York: Guilford Press; 1995:572.
202. Pugliese MT, Weyman-Daum M, Moses N, et al. Parental health beliefs as a cause of nonorganic failure to thrive. *Pediatrics* 1987;80:175.
203. Brownell KD, Kelman JH, Stunkard AM. Treatment of obese children with and without their mothers: changes in weight and blood pressure. *Pediatrics* 1983;71:515.
204. Dietz WH Jr. Family characteristics affect rates of weight loss in obese children. *Nutr Res* 1983;3:43.
205. Kimm SYS. The role of dietary fiber in the development and treatment of childhood obesity. *Pediatrics* 1995;96:1010.
206. Wadden TA. Very-low-calorie diets: appraisal and recommendations. In: Brownell KD, Fairburn CG, eds. *Eating disorders and obesity: a comprehensive handbook.* New York: Guilford Press; 1995:484.
207. The Medical Letter. Formula diets for obesity. *The Medical Letter* 1989;31:22.
208. Eliakim A, Barstow TJ, Brasel JA, et al. Effect of exercise training on energy expenditure, muscle volume, and maximal oxygen uptake in female adolescents. *J Pediatr* 1996;129:537.
209. Blair SN. Evidence for success of exercise in weight loss and control. *Ann Intern Med* 1993;119(Suppl):702.
210. Johnston LD, O'Malley PM, Bachman JG. *Monitoring the future study.* Ann Arbor, MI: News and Information Services of the University of Michigan; December, 1995.
211. Centers for Disease Control and Prevention Results from the National Adolescent Student Health Survey. *MMWR Morb Mortal Wkly Rep* 1989;38:147.
212. The Medical Letter. Fluoxetine (Prozac) and other drugs for treatment of obesity. *The Medical Letter* 1994;36(936):107.
213. Guy-Grand B, Apfelbaum M, Crepaldi G, et al. International trial of long-term dexfenfluramine in obesity. *Lancet* 1989;2:1142.
214. O'Connor HT, Richman RM, Steinbeck KS, et al. Dexfenfluramine treatment of obesity: a double blind trial with post trial follow-up. *International Journal of Obesity.* 1995;19:181.
215. Nightingale SL. Health advisory on concomitant fenfluramine and phentermine use. *JAMA* 1997;278:379.
216. Abenhaim L, Moride Y, Brenot F, et al. Appetite suppressant drugs and the risk of primary pulmonary hypertension. *N Engl J Med* 1996;335:609.
217. National Task Force on the Prevention and Treatment of Obesity. Long-term pharmocotherapy in the management of obesity. *JAMA* 1996;276:1907.
218. Drent MD, van der Veen EA. Lipase inhibition: a novel concept in the treatment of obesity. *International Journal of Obesity* 1993;17:241.
219. Stunkard AJ. Conservative treatments for obesity. *Am J Clin Nutr* 1987;45:1142.
220. Uzark KC, Becker MH, Dielman TE, et al. Perceptions held by obese children and their parents: implications for weight control intervention. *Health Educ Q* 1988;15:185.
221. Mellin LM, Slinkard LA, Irwin CE Jr. Adolescent obesity intervention: validation of the SHAPEDOWN program. *J Am Diet Assoc* 1987;87:333.
222. Hoerr SL, Nelson RA, Essex-Sorlie D. Treatment and follow-up of obesity in adolescent girls. *Journal of Adolescent Health Care* 1988;9:28.

SUGGESTED READING

Eating Disorders

Andersen AE. Eating disorders in males. In: Brownell KD, Fairburn CG, eds. *Eating disorders and obesity: a comprehensive handbook.* New York: Guilford Press; 1995:177.
Beumont PJV. The clinical presentation of anorexia and bulimia nervosa. In: Brownell KD, Fairburn CG, eds. *Eating disorders and obesity: a comprehensive handbook.* New York: Guilford Press; 1995:151.

Brownell KD, Fairburn CG, eds. *Eating disorders and obesity: a comprehensive handbook*. New York: Guilford Press; 1995.

Bruch H. *The golden cage: the enigma of anorexia nervosa*. Cambridge, MA: Harvard University Press; 1978.

Comerci GD. Medical complications of anorexia nervosa and bulimia nervosa. *Med Clin North Am* 1990;74:1293.

Comerci GD, ed. Eating disorders in adolescents. *Pediatr Ann* 1992;21:707.

Comerci GD. Eating disorders: evolving, controvertible, and irresolute issues. *Pediatr Ann* 1992;21:711.

Crisp AH. *Anorexia nervosa: let me be*. London: Academic Press; 1980.

Farrow JA. The adolescent male with an eating disorder. *Pediatr Ann* 1992;21:769.

Fisher M. Medical complications of anorexia and bulimia nervosa. *Adolescent Medicine: State of the Art Reviews* 1992;3:487.

Fisher M, Golden NH, Katzman DK, et al. Eating disorders in adolescents: a background paper. *J Adolesc Health* 1995;16:420.

Garfinkle PE. Classification and diagnosis of eating disorders. In: Brownell KD, Fairburn CG, eds. *Eating disorders and obesity: a comprehensive handbook*. New York: Guilford Press; 1995:125.

Goldbloom DS, Kennedy SH. Medical complications of anorexia nervosa. In: Brownell KD, Fairburn CG, eds. *Eating disorders and obesity: a comprehensive handbook*. New York: Guilford Press; 1995:266.

Golden NH, Shenker IR. Amenorrhea in anorexia nervosa: Etiology and implications. *Adolescent Medicine: State of the Art Reviews* 1992;3:503.

Harper G. Eating disorders in adolescence. *Pediatr Rev* 1994;15:72.

Hobbs WL, Johnson CA. Anorexia nervosa: an overview. *Am Fam Physician* 1996;54:1273.

Hsu LKG. *Eating disorders*. New York: Guilford Press; 1990.

Hsu LKG. Outcome of bulimia nervosa. In: Brownell KD, Fairburn CG, eds. *Eating disorders and obesity: a comprehensive handbook*. New York: Guilford Press; 1995:238.

Joffe A. Too little, too much: eating disorders in adolescents. *Contemporary Pediatrics* 1990;7:114.

Kilbourne J. Killing us softly: gender roles in advertising. *Adolescent Medicine: State of the Art Reviews* 1993;4:635.

Kreipe RE. Eating disorders among children and adolescents. *Pediatr Rev* 1995;16:370.

Kreipe RE, Golden NH, Katzman DK, et al. Eating disorders in adolescents: a position paper of the Society for Adolescent Medicine. *J Adolesc Health* 1995;16:476.

Kreipe RE, Harris JP. Myocardial impairment resulting from eating disorders. *Pediatr Ann* 1992;21:760.

Kreipe RE, Uphoff M. Treatment and outcome of adolescents with anorexia nervosa. *Adolescent Medicine: State of the Art Reviews* 1992;3:519.

Levine RL. Eating disorders in adolescents: a comprehensive update. *Int Pediatr* 1995;10:327.

Lucas AR. The eating disorder "epidemic": more apparent than real? *Pediatr Ann* 1992;21:746.

Mitchell JE. Medical complications of anorexia nervosa. In: Brownell KD, Fairburn CG, eds. *Eating disorders and obesity: a comprehensive handbook*. New York: Guilford Press; 1995:271.

Nussbaum MP, Dwyer JT, eds. Adolescent nutrition and eating disorders. *Adolescent Medicine: State of the Art Reviews* 1992;3:377.

Sargent J. Teaching housestaff about eating disorders. *Pediatr Ann* 1992;21:720.

Schebendach J, Nussbaum MP. Nutrition management in adolescents with eating disorders. *Adolescent Medicine: State of the Art Reviews* 1992;3:541.

Silber TJ. Eating disorders and health insurance. *Arch Pediatr Adolesc Med* 1994;148:785.

Stashwick C. When you suspect an eating disorder. *Contemporary Pediatrics* 1996;13:124.

Steinhausen HC. The course and outcome of anorexia nervosa. In: Brownell KD, Fairburn CG, eds. *Eating disorders and obesity: a comprehensive handbook*. New York: Guilford Press; 1995:234.

Whitaker AH. An epidemiologic study of anorectic and bulimic symptoms in adolescent girls: implications for pediatricians. *Pediatr Ann* 1992;21:752.

Woodside DB. Anorexia nervosa and bulimia nervosa in children and adolescents. *Curr Opin Pediatr* 1993;5:415.

Yates A. Biologic considerations in the etiology of eating disorders. *Pediatr Ann* 1992;21:739.

Zerbe KJ. Eating disorders: The apple doesn't fall far from the tree. *Contemporary Pediatrics* 1996;13:65.

Obesity

Bandini LG. Obesity in the adolescent. *Adolescent Medicine: State of the Art Reviews* 1992;3:459.

Bennett WI. Beyond overeating. *N Engl J Med* 1995;332:673.

Berkowitz RI. Treating adolescent obesity. *Adolescent Medicine: State of the Art Reviews* 1997;8(1):181.

Brownell KD, Fairburn CG, eds. *Eating disorders and obesity: a comprehensive handbook*. New York: Guilford Press; 1995.

Carek PJ, Sherer J, Carson DS. Management of obesity: medical treatment options. *Am Fam Physician* 1997;55:551.

Dietz WH Jr. You are what you eat: what you eat is what you are. *Journal of Adolescent Health Care* 1990;11:76.

Dietz WH. Childhood obesity: prevalence and effects. In: Brownell KD, Fairburn CG, eds. *Eating disorders and obesity: a comprehensive handbook*. New York: Guilford Press; 1995:438.

Dietz WH, Robinson TN. Assessment and treatment of childhood obesity. *Pediatr Rev* 1993;14:337.

Dwyer JT. Great expectations: overview of adolescent nutrition for the year 200 and beyond. *Adolescent Medicine: State of the Art Reviews* 1992;3:377.

Gortmaker SL, Must A, Sobol AM, et al. Television viewing as a cause of increasing obesity among children in the United States, 1986–1990. *Arch Pediatr Adolesc Med* 1996;150:356.

Leibel RL. Obesity: a game of inches. *Pediatrics* 1995;95:131.

Manson JE, Faich GA. Pharmacotherapy for obesity: do the benefits outweigh the risks? *N Engl J Med* 1996;335:659.

Nussbaum MP, Dwyer JT, eds. Adolescent nutrition and eating disorders. *Adolescent Medicine: State of the Art Reviews* 1992;3(3):377.

Pi-Sunyer FX. Medical hazards of obesity. *Ann Intern Med* 1993;119:655.

Rickert VL, ed. *Adolescent nutrition: assessment and management.* New York: Chapman & Hall; 1996.

Rosenbaum M, Leibel RL, Hirsch J. Medical progress obesity. *N Engl J Med* 1997;337:396.

Skiba A, Loghmani E, Orr DP. Nutritional screening and guidance for adolescents. *Adolescent Health Update* 1997;9(2):1.

Winick M. Editorial: understanding and treating obesity. *Am J Public Health* 1996;86:925.

8

Substance Use and Abuse

In the United States of America in the 1990s, a person who watches television cannot help but see at least one public service announcement a day decrying the use of alcohol or drugs by teenagers. The public perception seems to be that no other problem facing our nation is quite so pervasive and dangerous as adolescent substance abuse. The accuracy of this perception is one of the things this chapter explores. In addition, we attempt to give the clinician a brief summary of the major drugs of abuse, some guidelines on assessing teenagers' risk of abuse, some tips on counseling and referring adolescents who seem to have a problem, and methods of helping teens avoid getting involved with alcohol, tobacco, and illicit drugs.

Epidemiologic Features

Many American teenagers use alcohol, tobacco, and illicit drugs regularly. Table 1 shows the latest figures for use of all classes of drugs by high school students in the 30 days before the survey. This statistic is more reflective of true substance misuse/abuse problems than lifetime use rates or use in the past year. Use in the month before the survey and daily use are the real indicators of a problem. Table 2 shows daily use rates since 1975. These data come from the annual survey of substance use by Lloyd Johnston [1] of the University of Michigan. The 1997 survey assessed over 15,000 high school seniors nationwide. The key points from Johnston's annual survey are as follows [1]:

1. After peaking in the late 1970s and the early 1980s, the monthly use of marijuana, stimulants, hallucinogens, sedatives and other tranquilizers, and alcohol has declined regularly until 1993, when an upward trend began.
2. Monthly use of cocaine peaked in 1985 and declined until 1993, when a slightly increased use rate was noted. Monthly use of the "crack" form of cocaine by high school seniors declined from 1988 to 1992. The rate has risen slightly to 1.8% by 1995. Heavy crack users are not going to be represented in a survey of high school seniors, however, because use of this substance is not conducive to finishing one's education.
3. The use of cigarettes in the past month has declined slightly, but the percentage of high school seniors who are current users (3 4%) was the higher in 1996 than at any time since 1979.
4. The percentage of high school seniors who used alcohol in the prior 30 days has declined from a peak of 72% in 1980 to 50.8% in 1996, a 1% increase since 1993. Over 30% of high school seniors reported recent bouts of heavy drinking (five or more drinks in a row during the previous 2 weeks) in 1996, compared with 41% in 1983.

There are other facts of interest. For example, current use of amphetamines is 4.1%, down from a high of 12% in 1980; "ice," or crystal methamphetamine, has appeared on the scene, mainly on the West Coast, with a 30-day use rate among high school seniors of 1.1% nationally. Thirty-day use rates of inhalants (e.g., aerosols, glue, nitrous oxides, amyl and butyl nitrate) is higher among 8th graders than among 10th and 12th graders. The 30-day use rate has risen in this young group from 4.4% in 1991 to over 6% in 1995.

The worrisome trend of increasing substance use rates since 1992 has attracted national political attention, and is cause for concern. Still, regular use of illicit substances by adolescents is considerably lower today than it was 15 to 20 years ago. However, a significant proportion of teenagers continues to use substances excessively, to their own detriment and to the detriment of society as a whole. Also, these data do not reflect those adolescents who drop out of high school before their senior year. Because most dropouts are at higher risk for problem behaviors than are the teenagers who finish high school, the survey data may be underestimating significantly the extent of adolescent use of drugs and alcohol.

Morbidity caused by these substances is due not only to their direct effects but, more important, to the consequences of their use. These include violence (e.g., accidents, suicides, and homicides) as well as negative effects of these substances on cognitive and psychosocial development of adolescents.

The three leading causes of death among adolescents in the United States are accidents, suicide, and homicide. More than one in five 16- to 20-year-old drivers involved in fatal motor vehicle accidents from 1982 to 1990 were drunk [2]. There is a significant relationship between substance abuse, particularly alcohol, and suicide [3,4]. Many homicides are committed when one or both parties are intoxicated [5]. In addition, in large urban centers, the increased rate of homicide is related to the drug trade [6]. Overall, it has been noted that the use of alcohol and other drugs is correlated with an increase in the risk of violent behavior [7,8]. Tables 3 through 6 reflect this relationship.

Another morbid consequence of substance use and abuse is its effect on personality development in adolescents. When an adolescent becomes dependent on chemicals for avoiding problems and for coping with stresses, his or her psychosocial development ceases. A person may be considered to develop psychosocially in a series of steps based on overcoming problems, which forces further personality development. Drugs and alcohol interfere with that process. When these youths become detoxified and drug free, they are left with the personality development of, for example, a 13-year-old in the body of an 18-year-old. Catch-up growth is possible, but it is a lengthy and painful process.

Patterns of Use and Abuse

Before the late 1960s and 1970s, problem drug use was confined primarily to adults. It was not until the "baby boomer" generation reached adolescence and young people became disillusioned by the Vietnam war that drug use and abuse became a true phenomenon of adolescence. That period was one of rejection of then-current societal norms and of adult values as exemplified by the antiwar, civil rights, and feminist movements. Many youths got caught up in countercultural activities. The "drop out and turn on," "make love, not war," and other movements were spearheaded by young adults, especially those in and just graduated from college. The use of drugs, particularly marijuana and hallucinogens such as lysergic acid diethylamide (LSD), was popularized by people of this age group, and only as time went on did use trickle down to younger adolescents. Drug use by young adults was not usually for escaping problems but, as promoted by such gurus as the late Dr. Timothy Leary, was for reaching a higher level of consciousness and a greater comprehension of humankind's role in both the world and the universe. As the use of drugs trickled down to younger cohorts of users, these lofty aspirations were forgotten or discarded. Mind-altering substances were used solely for the sake of getting "stoned." By getting stoned, or intoxicated, youths could escape from everyday cares and avoid problems. Even worse, youths who had low self-esteem and who were depressed could make the pain go away for at least a little while.

An added factor that seems predictive of increased use is a decrease in the perceived harmfulness of drugs. The proportion of students seeing drugs as harmful has declined since the early 1990s. The percentage of 12th graders who perceived regular marijuana use as a great risk declined from 71% in 1991 to 61% in 1995. This correlates with the increase noted in marijuana use over the same time period. It has been suggested that this decrease in perceived danger of marijuana use may reflect the ambiguity of parents who used marijuana in the 1960s and 1970s and who are unsure about saying "no" to their own children.

Adding to the difficulty of comprehending the substance use and abuse problems in this country is the national hypocrisy about alcohol. On the issue of illicit drugs, most people are in agreement that they are uniformly harmful, but on the issue of alcohol, no national consensus has ever been reached. While some of our government leaders tell our kids to "just don't do it," those same preteens and teenagers watch advertisements on television telling them that beer will lead to sexual success and that "the night belongs to Michelob." The United States is the country that tells teenagers never to take even one drink, while at least 30% of 18-year-olds, and significant proportions of younger ones, get drunk almost every Friday and Saturday night. For every "just say no" ad that teens see, they will see 25 to 50 beer and wine ads [9]. Beer and wine manufacturers spend almost $2 billion per year on

TABLE 1. *Long-term trends in 30-day prevalence of use of various types of drugs for 12th graders*

	Percentage of the year's class who used in last 30 days (approximate *N*)									
	1975 (9,400)	1976 (15,400)	1977 (17,100)	1978 (17,800)	1979 (15,500)	1980 (15,900)	1981 (17,500)	1982 (17,700)	1983 (16,300)	1984 (15,900)
Any illicit drug[a,b]	30.7	34.2	37.6	38.9	38.9	37.2	36.9	32.5	30.5	29.2
Any illicit drug other than marijuana[a,b]	15.4	13.9	15.2	15.1	16.8	18.4	21.7	17.0	15.4	15.1
Marijuana and hashish	27.1	32.2	35.4	37.1	36.5	33.7	31.6	28.5	27.0	25.2
Inhalants[c]	NA	0.9	1.3	1.5	1.7	1.4	1.5	1.5	1.7	1.9
Inhalants, adjusted[c,d]	NA	NA	NA	NA	3.2	2.7	2.5	2.5	2.5	2.6
Amyl and butyl nitrites[e,f]	NA	NA	NA	NA	2.4	1.8	1.4	1.1	1.4	1.4
Hallucinogens	4.7	3.4	4.1	3.9	4.0	3.7	3.7	3.4	2.8	2.6
Hallucinogens, adjusted[g]	NA	NA	NA	NA	5.3	4.4	4.5	4.1	3.5	3.2
LSD	2.3	1.9	2.1	2.1	2.4	2.3	2.5	2.4	1.9	1.5
PCP[e,f]	NA	NA	NA	NA	2.4	1.4	1.4	1.0	1.3	1.0
Cocaine	1.9	2.0	2.9	3.9	5.7	5.2	5.8	5.0	4.9	5.8
Crack[h]	NA	NA	NA	NA	NA	NA	NA	NA	NA	NA
Other Cocaine[i]	NA	NA	NA	NA	NA	NA	NA	NA	NA	NA
Heroin[j]	0.4	0.2	0.3	0.3	0.2	0.2	0.2	0.2	0.2	0.3
Other opiates[k]	2.1	2.0	2.8	2.1	2.4	2.4	2.1	1.8	1.8	1.8
Stimulants[b,k]	8.5	7.7	8.8	8.7	9.9	12.1	15.8	10.7	8.9	8.3
Crystal meth. (ice)[l]	NA	NA	NA	NA	NA	NA	NA	NA	NA	NA
Sedatives[k,m]	5.4	4.5	5.1	4.2	4.4	4.8	4.6	3.4	3.0	2.3
Barbiturates[k]	4.7	3.9	4.3	3.2	3.2	2.9	2.6	2.0	2.1	1.7
Methaqualone[k,m]	2.1	1.6	2.3	1.9	2.3	3.3	3.1	2.4	1.8	1.1
Tranquilizers[k]	4.1	4.0	4.6	3.4	3.7	3.1	2.7	2.4	2.5	2.1
Alcohol[n]	68.2	68.3	71.2	72.1	71.8	72.0	70.7	69.7	69.4	67.2
Been drunk[l]	NA	NA	NA	NA	NA	NA	NA	NA	NA	NA
Cigarettes	36.7	38.8	38.4	36.7	34.4	30.5	29.4	30.0	30.3	29.3
Smokeless tobacco[e,o]	NA	NA	NA	NA	NA	NA	NA	NA	NA.4	NA
Steroids[l]	NA	NA	NA	NA	NA	NA	NA	NA	NA	NA

NA, not available.

[a]Use of "any illicit drug" includes any use of marijuana, lysergic acid diethylamide (LSD), other hallucinogens, crack, other cocaine, or heroin, *or* any use of other opiates, stimulants, barbiturates, methaqualone (excluded since 1990), or tranquilizers not under a doctor's orders.

[b]Beginning in 1982, the question about stimulant use (i.e., amphetamines) was revised to get respondents to exclude the inappropriate reporting of nonprescription stimulants. The prevalence rate dropped slightly as a result of this methodologic change.

[c]Data based on four of five forms in 1976–1988; *N* is four fifths of *N* indicated. Data based on five of six forms in 1989–1996; *N* is five sixths of *N* indicated.

[d]Adjusted for underreporting of amyl and butyl nitrites.

[e]Data based on one form; *N* is one fifth of *N* indicated in 1979–1988 and one sixth of *N* indicated in 1989–1996.

[f]Question text changed slightly in 1987.

[g]Adjusted for underreporting of phencyclidine (PCP).

[h]Data based on one of five forms in 1986; *N* is one fifth of *N* indicated. Data based on two forms in 1987–1989; *N* is two fifths of *N* indicated in 1987–1988 and two sixths of *N* indicated in 1989. Data based on six forms in 1990–1996.

[i]Data based on one form in 1987–1989; *N* is one fifth of *N* indicated in 1987–1988 and one sixth of *N* indicated in 1989. Data based on four of six forms in 1990–1996; *N* is four sixths of *N* indicated.

[j]In 1995 the heroin question was changed in half of the questionnaire forms. Separate questions were asked for use with injection and without injection. Data presented here represent the combined data from all forms.

advertising. Even worse, cigarette manufacturers spent $3.27 billion on advertising and promotions in 1988 alone! Eighty-four million dollars were spent by tobacco companies to sponsor and promote sporting events [10]. Sales of cigarettes and smokeless tobacco products to children and adolescents resulted in annual revenues of $1.26 billion for tobacco companies [11]. Far more money is received by the U.S. government from cigarette and tobacco tax revenues on sales to children than is spent on prevention activities. Faced with conflicting messages and with these economic realities, it is little wonder that many adolescents disregard adult admonitions altogether and do whatever they please [9]. In 1996, some hope in the fight against tobacco use appeared with the enactment of U.S. Food and

TABLE 1. (Cont.) *Long-term trends in 30-day prevalence of use of various types of drugs for 12th graders*

												Percentage of the year's class who used in last 30 days (approximate N)
1985 (16,000)	1986 (15,200)	1987 (16,300)	1988 (16,300)	1989 (16,700)	1990 (15,200)	1991 (15,000)	1992 (15,800)	1993 (16,300)	1994 (15,400)	1995 (15,400)	1996 (14,300)	1995–1996 change[p]
29.7	27.1	24.7	21.3	19.7	17.2	16.4	14.4	18.3	21.9	23.8	24.6	+0.8
14.9	13.2	11.6	10.0	9.1	8.0	7.1	6.3	7.9	8.8	10.0	9.5	−0.5
25.7	23.4	21.0	18.0	16.7	14.0	13.8	11.9	15.5	19.0	21.2	21.9	+0.7
2.2	2.5	2.8	2.6	2.3	2.7	2.4	2.3	2.5	2.7	3.2	2.5	−0.7s
3.0	3.2	3.5	3.0	2.7	2.9	2.6	2.5	2.8	2.9	3.5		
1.6	1.3	1.3	0.6	0.6	0.6	0.4	0.3	0.6	0.4	0.4	0.7	+0.3
2.5	2.5	2.5	2.2	2.2	2.2	2.2	2.1	2.7	3.1	4.4	3.5	−0.9s
3.8	3.5	2.8	2.3	2.9	2.3	2.4	2.3	3.3	3.2	4.6		
1.6	1.7	1.8	1.8	1.8	1.9	1.9	2.0	2.4	2.6	4.0	2.5	−1.5sss
1.6	1.3	0.6	0.3	1.4	0.4	0.5	0.6	1.0	0.7	0.6	1.3	+0.7s
6.7	6.2	4.3	3.4	2.8	1.9	1.4	1.3	1.3	1.5	1.8	2.0	+0.2
NA	NA	1.3	1.6	1.4	0.7	0.7	0.6	0.7	0.8	1.0	1.0	0.0
NA	NA	4.1	3.2	1.9	1.7	1.2	1.0	1.2	1.3	1.3	1.6	+0.3
0.3	0.2	0.2	0.2	0.3	0.2	0.2	0.3	0.2	0.3	0.6	0.5	−0.1
2.3	2.0	1.8	1.6	1.6	1.5	1.1	1.2	1.3	1.5	1.8	2.0	+0.2
6.8	5.5	5.2	4.6	4.2	3.7	3.2	2.8	3.7	4.0	4.0	4.1	+0.1
NA	NA	NA	NA	NA	0.6	0.6	0.5	0.6	0.7	1.1	1.1	0.0
2.4	2.2	1.7	1.4	1.6	1.4	1.5	1.2	1.3	1.8	2.3		
2.0	1.8	1.4	1.2	1.4	1.3	1.4	1.1	1.3	1.7	2.2	2.1	−0.1
1.0	0.8	0.6	0.5	0.6	0.2	0.2	0.4	0.1	0.4	0.4	0.6	+0.2
2.1	2.1	2.0	1.5	1.3	1.2	1.4	1.0	1.2	1.4	1.8	2.0	+0.2
65.9	65.3	66.4	63.9	60.0	57.1	54.0	51.3	51.0	NA	NA	NA	NA
								48.6	50.1	51.3	50.8	−0.5
NA	NA	NA	NA	NA	NA	31.6	29.9	28.9	30.8	33.2	31.3	−1.9
30.1	29.6	29.4	28.7	28.6	29.4	28.3	27.8	29.9	31.2	33.5	34.0	+0.5
NA	11.5	11.3	10.3	8.4	NA	NA	11.4	10.7	11.1	12.2	9.8	−2.4
NA	NA	NA	NA	0.8	1.0	0.8	0.6	0.7	0.9	0.7	0.7	0.0

(Continued)

[k] Only drug use that was not under a doctor's orders is included here.

[l] Data based on two of six forms; N is two sixths of N indicated. Steroid data based on one of six forms in 1989–1990; N is one sixth of N indicated in 1989–1990. Steroid data based on two of six forms since 1991; N is two sixths of N indicated since 1991.

[m] Sedatives: data based on five forms in 1975–1988, six forms in 1989, one form in 1990 (N is one sixth of N indicated in 1990), and six forms of data adjusted by one-form data beginning in 1991. Methaqualone: data based on five forms in 1975–1988; six forms in 1989, and one of six forms beginning in 1990 (N is one sixth of N indicated beginning in 1990).

[n] Data based on five forms in 1975–1988 and on six forms in 1989–1992. In 1993, the question text was changed slightly in three of six forms to indicate that a "drink" meant "more than a few sips." The data in the upper line for alcohol came from the three forms using the original wording (N is three sixths of N indicated), whereas the data in the lower line came from the three forms containing the revised wording (N is three sixths of N indicated). Data for 1994–1996 were based on all six forms.

[o] Prevalence of smokeless tobacco was not asked of 12th graders in 1990 and 1991. Before 1990, the prevalence question on smokeless tobacco was located near the end of one 12th-grade questionnaire form, whereas after 1991 the question was placed earlier and in a different form. This shift could explain the discontinuities between the corresponding data.

[p] Level of significance of difference between the two most recent classes: s = 0.05, ss = 0.01, sss = 0.001.

From Johnston LS, O'Malley PM, Bachman JG. *National survey results on drug use from the Monitoring the Future Study, 1975–1996.* Rockville, MD: National Institute of Drug Abuse; 1996, with permission.

Drug Administration rules that limit the ability of tobacco companies to advertise to children. The effectiveness of such actions remains to be seen.

Today, adolescents encounter drugs and inappropriate alcohol use at ever earlier ages. Longitudinal surveys suggest that those who misuse and abuse drugs begin in fifth or sixth grades and progress in a somewhat predictable sequence from cigarettes, alcohol, and marijuana, to drugs such as cocaine, narcotics, and stimulants [12]. Of course, use of cigarettes, alcohol, or marijuana can occur without progression to other drugs of abuse. Adolescents can use just alcohol or marijuana sporadically without getting hooked on either, but with use comes the danger of abuse and, with regular use, abuse of other, more harmful drugs becomes increasingly more likely. For these reasons, cigarettes, alcohol, and marijuana have been called *gateway* drugs. Two signs that may be helpful to the practitioner are the use of

TABLE 2. *Long-term trends in 30-day prevalence of daily use of various types of drugs for 12th graders*

	Percentage of the year's class who used daily in last 30 days (approximate *N*)									
	1975 (9,400)	1976 (15,400)	1977 (17,100)	1978 (17,800)	1979 (15,500)	1980 (15,900)	1981 (17,500)	1982 (17,700)	1983 (16,300)	1984 (15,900)
Marijuana and hashish	6.0	8.2	9.1	10.7	10.3	9.1	7.0	6.3	5.5	5.0
Inhalants[a]	NA	*	*	0.1	*	0.1	0.1	0.1	0.1	0.1
Inhalants, adjusted[a,b]	NA	NA	NA	NA	0.1	0.2	0.2	0.2	0.2	0.2
Amyl and butyl nitrites[c,d]	NA	NA	NA	NA	*	0.1	0.1	0.0	0.2	0.1
Hallucinogens	0.1	0.1	0.1	0.1	0.1	0.1	0.1	0.1	0.1	0.1
Hallucinogens, adjusted[e]	NA	NA	NA	NA	0.2	0.2	0.1	0.2	0.2	0.2
LSD	*	*	*	*	*	*	0.1	*	0.1	0.1
PCP[c,d]	NA	NA	NA	NA	0.1	0.1	0.1	0.1	0.1	0.1
Cocaine	0.1	0.1	0.1	0.1	0.2	0.2	0.3	0.2	0.2	0.2
Crack[f]	NA	NA	NA	NA	NA	NA	NA	NA	NA	NA
Other cocaine[g]	NA	NA	NA	NA	NA	NA	NA	NA	NA	NA
Heroin[h]	0.1	*	*	*	*	*	*	*	0.1	*
Other opiates[i]	0.1	0.1	0.2	0.1	*	0.1	0.1	0.1	0.1	0.1
Stimulants[i,j]	0.5	0.4	0.5	0.5	0.6	0.7	1.2	0.7	0.8	0.6
Crystal meth. (ice)[k]	NA	NA	NA	NA	NA	NA	NA	NA	NA	NA
Sedatives[i,l]	0.3	0.2	0.2	0.2	0.1	0.2	0.2	0.2	0.2	0.1
Barbiturates[i]	0.1	0.1	0.2	0.1	*	0.1	0.1	0.1	0.1	*
Methaqualone[i,l]	*	*	*	*	*	0.1	0.1	0.1	*	*
Tranquilizers[i]	0.1	0.2	0.3	0.1	0.1	0.1	0.1	0.1	0.1	0.1
Alcohol										
Daily[m]	5.7	5.6	6.1	5.7	6.9	6.0	6.0	5.7	5.5	4.8
Been drunk daily[k]	NA	NA	NA	NA	NA	NA	NA	NA	NA	NA
5+drinks in a row in last 2 weeks	36.8	37.1	39.4	40.3	41.2	41.2	41.4	40.5	40.8	38.7
Cigarettes										
Daily	26.9	28.8	28.8	27.5	25.4	21.3	20.3	21.1	21.2	18.7
Half-pack or more per day	17.9	19.2	19.4	18.8	16.5	14.3	13.5	14.2	13.8	12.3
Smokeless tobacco[c,n]	NA	NA	NA	NA	NA	NA	NA	NA	NA	NA
Steroids[k]	NA	NA	NA	NA	NA	NA	NA	NA	NA	NA

NA, not available.

[a]Data based on four of five forms in 1976–1988; *N* is four fifths of *N* indicated. Data based on five of six forms in 1989–1996; *N* is five sixths of *N* indicated.

[b]Adjusted for underreporting of amyl and butyl nitrites.

[c]Data based on one form; *N* is one fifth of *N* indicated in 1979–1988 and one sixth of *N* indicated in 1989–1996.

[d]Question text changed slightly in 1987.

[e]Adjusted for underreporting of phencyclidine (PCP).

[f]Data based on one of five forms in 1986; *N* is one fifth of *N* indicated. Data based on two forms in 1987–1989; *N* is two fifths of *N* indicated in 1987–1988 and two sixths of *N* indicated in 1989. Data based on six forms in 1990–1996.

[g]Data based on one form in 1987–1989; *N* is one fifth of *N* indicated in 1987–1988 and one sixth of *N* indicated in 1989. Data based on four of six forms in 1990–1996; *N* is four sixths of *N* indicated.

[h]In 1995 the heroin question was changed in half of the questionnaire forms. Separate questions were asked for use with injection and without injection. Data presented here represent the combined data from all forms.

[i]Only drug use that was not under a doctor's orders is included here.

[j]Beginning in 1982, the question about stimulant use (i.e., amphetamines) was revised to get respondents to exclude the inappropriate reporting of nonprescription stimulants. The prevalence rate dropped slightly as a result of this methodologic change.

[k]Data based on two of six forms; *N* is two sixths of *N* indicated. Steroid data based on one of six forms in 1989–1990; *N* is one sixth of *N* indicated in 1989–1990. Steroid data based on two of six forms since 1991; *N* is two sixths of *N* indicated since 1991.

cigarettes by girls and the use of marijuana by boys. These practices seem to augur poorly for future avoidance of other drugs [5]. It also should be noted that adolescents who report having consumed alcohol in the past month are 10 times more likely than nondrinkers to use marijuana and 11 times more likely to use cocaine [13]. A group that should be of special concern is the old-for-grade adolescent. This group has an increased risk for substance use [14].

TABLE 2. (Cont.) *Long-term trends in 30-day prevalence of daily use of various types of drugs for 12th graders*

							Percentage of the year's class who used daily in last 30 days (approximate N)					
1985 (16,000)	1986 (15,200)	1987 (16,300)	1988 (16,300)	1989 (16,700)	1990 (15,200)	1991 (15,000)	1992 (15,800)	1993 (16,300)	1994 (15,400)	1995 (15,400)	1996 (14,300)	1995–1996 change[o]
4.9	4.0	3.3	2.7	2.9	2.2	2.0	1.9	2.4	3.6	4.6	4.9	+0.3
0.2	0.2	0.1	0.2	0.2	0.3	0.2	0.1	0.1	0.1	0.1	0.2	+0.1
0.4	0.4	0.4	0.3	0.3	0.3	0.5	0.2	0.2	NA	NA		
0.3	0.5	0.3	0.1	0.3	0.1	0.2	0.1	0.1	0.2	0.2	0.4	+0.2
0.1	0.1	0.1	*	0.1	0.1	0.1	0.1	0.1	0.1	0.1	0.1	0.0
0.3	0.3	0.2	*	0.3	0.3	0.1	0.1	0.1	NA	NA		
0.1	*	0.1	*	*	0.1	0.1	0.1	0.1	0.1	0.1	*	0.0
0.3	0.2	0.3	0.1	0.2	0.1	0.1	0.1	0.1	0.3	0.3	0.3	+0.1
0.4	0.4	0.3	0.2	0.3	0.1	0.1	0.1	0.1	0.1	0.2	0.2	+0.1
NA	NA	0.1	0.1	0.2	0.1	0.1	0.1	0.1	0.1	0.1	0.2	0.0
NA	NA	0.2	0.2	0.1	0.1	0.1	*	0.1	0.1	0.1	0.1	0.0
*	*	*	*	0.1	*	*	*	*	*	0.1	0.1	+0.1
0.1	0.1	0.1	0.1	0.2	0.1	0.1	*	*	0.1	0.1	0.2	+0.1
0.4	0.3	0.3	0.3	0.3	0.2	0.2	0.2	0.2	0.2	0.3	0.3	+0.1
NA	NA	NA	NA	NA	0.1	0.1	0.1	0.1	*	0.1	0.1	0.0
0.1	0.1	0.1	0.1	0.1	0.1	0.1	0.1	0.1	*	0.1		
0.1	0.1	0.1	*	0.1	0.1	0.1	*	0.1	*	0.1	0.1	0.0
*	*	*	0.1	*	*	*	0.1	0.0	0.1	0.1	0.0	−0.1
*	*	0.1	*	0.1	0.1	0.1	*	*	0.1	*	0.2	+0.2sss
5.0	4.8	4.8	4.2	4.2	3.7	3.6	3.4	2.5	NA	NA	NA	NA
								3.4	2.9	3.5	3.7	+0.2
NA	NA	NA	NA	NA	NA	0.9	0.8	0.9	1.2	1.3	1.6	+0.3
36.7	36.8	37.5	34.7	33.0	32.2	29.8	27.9	27.5	28.2	29.8	30.2	+0.4
19.5	18.7	18.7	18.1	18.9	19.1	18.5	17.2	19.0	19.4	21.6	22.2	+0.6
12.5	11.4	11.4	10.6	11.2	11.3	10.7	10.0	10.9	11.2	12.4	13.0	+0.6
NA	4.7	5.1	4.3	3.3	NA	NA	4.3	3.3	3.9	3.6	3.3	−0.2
NA	NA	NA	NA	0.1	0.2	0.1	0.1	0.1	0.4	0.2	0.3	+0.1

(Continued)

[l]Sedatives: data based on five forms in 1975–1988, six forms in 1989, one form in 1990 (N is one sixth of N indicated in 1990), and six forms of data adjusted by one-form data beginning in 1991. Methaqualone: data based on five forms in 1975–1988; six forms in 1989, and one of six forms beginning in 1990 (N is one sixth of N indicated beginning in 1990).

[m]Data based on five forms in 1975–1988 and on six forms in 1989–1992. In 1993, the question text was changed slightly in three of six forms to indicate that a "drink" meant "more than a few sips." The data in the upper line for alcohol came from the three forms using the original wording (N is three sixths of N indicated), whereas the data in the lower line came from the three forms containing the revised wording (N is three sixths of N indicated). Data for 1994–1996 were based on all six forms.

[n]Prevalence of smokeless tobacco was not asked of 12th graders in 1990 and 1991. Before 1990, the prevalence question on smokeless tobacco was located near the end of one 12th-grade questionnaire form, whereas after 1991 the question was placed earlier and in a different form. This shift could explain the discontinuities between the corresponding data.

[o]Level of significance of difference between the two most recent classes: s = 0.05, ss = 0.01, sss = 0.001. Asterisk (*) indicates less than 0.05%. Any apparent inconsistency between the change estimate and the prevalence estimates for the two most recent classes is due to rounding error.

From Johnston LS, O'Malley PM, Bachman JG. *National survey results on drug use from the Monitoring the Future Study, 1975–1996*. Rockville, MD: National Institute of Drug Abuse; 1996, with permission.

The stages of progression (Table 7) from casual use to addiction follow a somewhat predictable pattern in those who become regular users or who become addicted [15–19]. In stage 1, adolescents learn that drugs can make them feel good or at least can relieve some psychic pain. Stage 2 is characterized by regular use, and the variety of drugs used increases. Here adolescents learn that the euphoria produced by drugs is followed by feelings of depression and anxiety, and so they actively seek the drug-induced euphoria. In stages 3 and 4, adolescents regularly seek the "high"; they become preoccupied with staying high and actively seek drugs. Tolerance develops, so larger quantities are consumed and

TABLE 3. *Use of alcohol among 6th to 8th graders according to engagement in violent behavior*

Behavior	Engaged in behavior (%)	Never engaged in behavior (%)
Carrying a gun to school	66.6	19.0
Taking part in gang activities	52.0	15.7
Thinking of suicide often/a lot	51.6	18.8
Threatening to harm another person	40.5	12.4
Getting in trouble with police	47.2	14.0

Adapted from Office of National Drug Control Strategy. *National drug control strategy: executive summary.* Washington, DC: Executive Office of the President; 1995.

TABLE 4. *Use of marijuana among 6th to 8th graders according to engagement in violent behavior, 1993–1994*

Behavior	Engaged in behavior (%)	Never engaged in behavior (%)
Carrying a gun to school	56.2	6.2
Taking part in gang activities	31.9	4.3
Thinking of suicide often/a lot	29.9	6.8
Threatening to harm another person	19.8	3.3
Getting in trouble with police	28.2	3.1

Adapted from Office of National Drug Control Strategy. *National drug control strategy: executive summary.* Washington, DC: Executive Office of the President; 1995.

TABLE 5. *Use of alcohol among 9th to 12th grades according to engagement in violent behavior, 1993–1994*

Behavior	Engaged in behavior (%)	Never engaged in behavior (%)
Carrying a gun to school	80.2	48.6
Taking part in gang activities	77.2	46.7
Thinking of suicide often/a lot	73.0	49.1
Threatening to harm another person	69.5	41.0
Getting in trouble with police	75.3	41.9

Adapted from Office of National Drug Control Strategy. *National drug control strategy: executive summary.* Washington, DC: Executive Office of the President; 1995.

TABLE 6. *Use of marijuana among 9th to 12th graders according to engagement in violent behavior, 1993–1994*

Behavior	Engaged in behavior (%)	Never engaged in behavior (%)
Carrying a gun to school	66.2	21.5
Taking part in gang activities	57.2	19.6
Thinking of suicide often/a lot	49.8	22.8
Threatening to harm another person	41.9	15.6
Getting in trouble with police	51.8	14.8

Adapted from Office of National Drug Control Strategy. *National drug control strategy: executive summary.* Washington, DC: Executive Office of the President; 1995.

TABLE 7. *The stages of substance abuse*

Stage 1: sampling; potential for abuse
Stage 2: experimentation; learning the euphoria is followed by depression and anxiety
Stage 3: regular use; seeking the euphoria
Stage 4: regular use; preoccupation with the high
Stage 5: burnout

Adapted from Comerci GD. Recognizing the five stages of substance abuse. *Contemporary Pediatrics* 1985;5:57.

stronger drugs may be tried. Drugs are now used when teens are alone as well as when they are with others, and illegal activities such as stealing and prostitution are initiated to obtain the money to support the habit. In stage 5, adolescents enter burnout: in this stage, adolescents need drugs not to get high but just to feel normal. They engage in further risk-taking behaviors to maintain the habit, and mental and physical deterioration sets in. Drugs are used all the time, and paranoia, flashbacks, aggressive behavior, and amnesia can occur.

Most adolescents who use drugs do not go through all these phases. For example, 21% of all high school seniors used marijuana in the 30 days before the survey in 1995, but only 4.6% used this drug daily [1]. However, the risk for progression to stage 2 or 3 is always present, and it is frequently up to the health care provider to detect use and abuse initially.

One pattern of use worth mentioning is that of adolescents who use alcohol and other substances only on the weekends and who do so regularly with the primary purpose of getting drunk or stoned. They are not regular users, at least on a daily basis, and are not addicted. Their weekday performance is not hampered, but they have to get high on weekends to have a good time. These teens are at extreme risk for morbid consequences of their substance misuse, such as automobile accidents, property damage, and sexual activity that they would normally avoid if sober. These are the adolescents who exemplify the phrase, "Party 'til you puke." Much of their behavior is based on their need to flaunt adult values, but some of it can be seen to be a reflection of adult behavior. This group of teenagers is at very high risk for negative consequences of their behavior, but they are not frequently detected by either the health care system or other adult authorities. We discuss them further in the section on alcohol. Each of the following sections on specific substances of abuse mentions acute intoxication and management.

Specific Substances of Abuse

Tobacco

Tobacco accounts for more morbidity and death than any other substance. Approximately 3,000 young people become regular tobacco users each day [20]. More than 90% of preschoolers recognize cigarettes, and as many as 55% think they will smoke when they grow up [20]. As stated previously, the percentage of teens who continue to use tobacco regularly has not declined appreciably in the last 15 years, and actually the 30-day use rate for cigarettes has risen from 1992 to 1995 [1]. Teenagers spend over a billion dollars per year on tobacco products, whereas the tobacco companies spend more than $6 billion on cigarette and smokeless tobacco advertising and promotion [21,22]. If tobacco use is to be prevented, prevention must start with children and adolescents, because almost all smokers begin use before the age of 18 years [23,24].

Women are a particular target group for smoking prevention efforts. Smoking rates have declined even less for women than they have for men [25], and girls are smoking at the same increasing rate as boys [1]. Smoking during pregnancy has negative consequences to the developing fetus, and smoking while taking oral contraceptive pills increases the risks of cardiovascular disease, at least among women older than 35 years. One group that seems to be at particularly increased risk for initiating smoking is high school girls who do not have plans for further education. Minorities and blue-collar workers have higher smoking rates than do whites and white-collar workers. However, the trends in all groups are similar [25].

Public health education efforts to increase knowledge of the negative health consequences of smoking appear to have been successful. However, many smokers are not aware or deny that smoking has other negative health consequences. In addition to their feelings of invulnerability, many adolescent smokers believe that they will be able to stop smoking whenever they want. This belief illustrates the fact that many adolescents are unaware of the addictive nature of tobacco [26]. Furthermore, it is the addictive nature of tobacco that may enable tobacco to be a "gateway" into the use of other drugs; tobacco users have a 15-fold increase in their likelihood of progression to the use of marijuana and other illegal drugs [20,27,28].

Particular mention should be made of smokeless tobacco use among adolescents. In earlier days of our republic, the use of smokeless forms of tobacco was prevalent. Spittoons were everywhere. However, as smoking became more popular, use of smokeless forms of tobacco declined. It is only recently that use of smokeless tobacco (i.e., chewing tobacco and snuff) has increased significantly [1]. Among high school seniors, about 4% use smokeless tobacco products daily, and over 12% had used these substances in the month before the survey [1]. The use of smokeless tobacco has been shown to be primarily a phenomenon of white male adolescents [29,30]. First use of smokeless tobacco seems to occur at an earlier age than does cigarette smoking [31–33]. Users report first use being influenced by family use patterns and by advertisements [33]. Cigarette smoking correlates well with the use of smokeless tobacco [33].

Most users are aware that chewing tobacco and snuff are harmful, but many believe that they are less dangerous than cigarettes. Actually, smokeless tobacco does have several negative consequences: 1) a significant increase in the rates of oral cancer [34,35], 2) leukoplakia and gum recession, and 3) addiction to nicotine. Tobacco poses a continuing threat to American youth, despite massive public health education campaigns that have been launched against it since the early 1960s. Although a slightly lower percentage of adolescents are using tobacco products today than in 1975, many adolescents are still affected. Several changes are needed to eliminate this threat to our youth. These include better detection of at-risk children, better formulated antitobacco education efforts in schools and in the media, and countering of the strong national tobacco lobby. The recent changes in rules governing tobacco advertising should help [36].

Alcohol

Of all substances that adolescents ingest illicitly, alcohol is by far the most significant. Many reasons exist for the use, misuse, and abuse of alcohol, and alcohol remains a significant threat to our adolescents. The use rates for alcohol steadily declined from the late 1970s until 1993, when a slow rise began, one that is continuing as this text goes to press [1]. A most alarming statistic is that almost 30% of high school seniors get drunk every week or two. Even more alarming is the fact that 24% of 10th graders and 14.5% of 8th graders participate in the same behavior. Older adolescents are not immune to the problems of alcohol misuse and abuse by any means. A significant proportion of college students misuse and abuse alcohol and suffer for it [37,38]. It is safe to say that alcohol poses a large public health problem for American's youth.

Why do American adolescents misuse and abuse alcohol? Table 8 shows many reasons given by adolescents. One important factor is parental use and attitudes [39]. Children model behavior they see at home. In addition, children inherit genetic propensities for alcohol addiction [40,41]. Peer use is another important influence. Parental factors play a more important role in children and younger adolescents, whereas peers have more of an influence with older teens [35,39,42–44]. The initiation of alcohol use appears to be less influenced by peers than is the maintenance of alcohol use [43,45,46]. This is because adolescents tend to seek peer groups whose members have similar needs.

Another social factor that significantly influences adolescents' attitudes toward alcohol is the media [9,47,48]. Although the United States has been successful in deleting tobacco advertising from broadcast media, alcohol advertising abounds [9]. This is particularly true with advertising for sporting events. Football and baseball cannot be viewed without also viewing beer commercials. The image that these commercials almost uniformly convey is that of the young, attractive male adult who either is successful beyond his wildest dreams with attractive young women, or deserves a reward for effort well spent. Although some beer makers advertise warnings against drinking and driving, the fact remains that they do it in a context that glamorizes beer drinking [49].

The final social factor that should be mentioned is our inconsistent cultural attitude toward alcohol. On the one hand, European societies have a generally permissive attitude, whereas in the United States we glorify alcohol use in the media but, on the other hand, we tell our youth to "just say no." We have age limitations when youth can legally drink in public. Nevertheless, we do nothing to prepare them to assume this adult privilege in a responsible fashion. It is no wonder that so

---

TABLE 8. *Why do teenagers drink?*

AS:
    Socialization
    Recreation
    Rite of passage
FOR:
    Acceptance
    Pleasure
    Experimentation and risk taking
IN:
    Self-exploration
    Response to impulse
    Rebellion
    Acting out against parents (perceived as restrictive)
TO:
    Prove sexual prowess
    Reduce stress
    Relieve anxiety, depression, fear, boredom, and pain of stressful
      home situation
    Conform and fit in
    Solve personal problems

Adapted from Morrison SF, Rogers PD, Thomas MH. Alcohol and adolescents. *Pediatr Clin North Am* 1995;42:371.

many of our adolescents use alcohol irresponsibly. For many youths, saying "no" is not considered an option.

The physical effects of alcohol on adolescents are no different from those on adults. The substance is absorbed from the stomach and small intestine in 2 to 6 hours. Food can delay the absorption of alcohol. Almost all alcohol is metabolized in the liver by alcohol dehydrogenase to acetaldehyde, and then by aldehyde dehydrogenase and acetyl coenzyme A to carbon dioxide and water. The rate-limiting step in this metabolism is the conversion of alcohol to acetaldehyde. Regular drinkers of large amounts of alcohol develop tolerance to increasing amounts. This is due in part to increased enzyme activity in the liver, but predominantly to central nervous system adaptation [50]. Ethanol diffuses rapidly into all body compartments, so the blood level reflects the tissue level.

Ethanol is a central nervous system (CNS) depressant, with different parts of the brain responding varyingly. In low doses, it is a stimulant and a relaxant. At these levels, it causes decreases in higher cortical functions and impaired judgment. Many of the pleasurable perceptions induced by alcohol are mediated by dopamine receptors [51]. With increasing levels, slurred speech and ataxia occur, and at still higher levels (more than 350 mg/dl), lethargy, stupor, and coma occur. The lethal dose is the same for alcoholic and nonalcoholic subjects [52]. Blackouts do occur in adolescent alcoholics, but acute alcoholic withdrawal symptoms and severe CNS effects, such as encephalopathy, are rare.

Heavy drinkers also suffer significant gastrointestinal effects such as gastritis. Alcohol's effects on the liver include elevation of serum lipids [53], impairment of mitochondrial function, and, eventually, hepatitis and fatty infiltration. Pancreatitis is another sequela of alcohol abuse.

The psychological effects of alcohol are a primary source of trouble in adolescents. As stated previously, adolescents with significant substance abuse problems suffer what can be termed a *developmental arrest*. Drinking becomes a problem behavior for adolescents when it interferes with the normal developmental tasks of adolescence [54,55]. Depression is a significant problem in adolescent substance abusers. The question is which comes first. The available evidence suggests that depression more commonly precedes the substance problem, with the substance being the self-administered medication [56]. The most significant and visible damage done by alcohol is through the morbid behaviors it facilitates. Adolescents are more prone to have high-risk sex when under the influence of alcohol [57,58]. The connection between alcohol and the morbid consequences of accidents, homicides, and suicides is well known [59–61].

Prevention is discussed more fully later, but it is important to note that without a major overhaul of societal attitudes toward alcohol use in general and by adolescents in particular, the problem will not change appreciably. The fact is that adolescents in many other countries do not have the problem that American youth have. When alcohol is consumed with meals as a beverage, when its use as an intoxicant is not acceptable, and when children are taught to use it responsibly, there are few adolescent alcohol problems.

Marijuana

There is no more popular illicit drug used in the United States than marijuana. Marijuana use was a phenomenon of young adults who were trying to "mellow out" in the 1960s, and it did not become a significant drug of abuse for adolescents until the 1970s. Marijuana was introduced into Western medicine in 1839, but has been a significant drug of recreation, of religion, and of medicine in the East for centuries [62]. Monthly and daily use rates of marijuana decreased from highs of 37% and 10.7%, respectively, to 11.9% and 1.9% in 1992. However, the rates have increased steadily and dramatically since then. In 1995, they were 21.2% for use within the past month and 4.6% for daily use. These rates are four or more times greater than those for any other illicit drug. An interesting parallel can be drawn between the increasing use rates for marijuana and the decreasing disapproval rates for its use. In 1990, the disapproval rate by high school seniors for marijuana use was over 80%, and the rate in 1995 was 66.7% [1]. Figure 1 shows this phenomenon graphically.

Marijuana as used today is composed of the crumbled, cured leaves, flowers, and small stems of the resin-producing varieties of the hemp plant, *Cannabis sativa*. The resin produced by these plants contains approximately 60 substances, called *cannabinoids*, of which the most prevalent and psychoactive is delta-9-tetrahydrocannabinol (THC). The concentration of THC in a plant depends on the variety and on conditions of growth and storage. The potency of street "pot" has increased threefold since the early 1960s because of improved growth methods, and the United States produces most of the marijuana it uses [56].

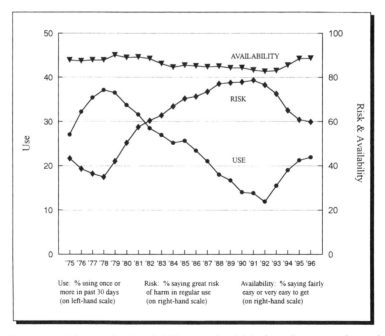

FIG. 1. Marijuana: trends in perceived availability, perceived risk of regular use, and prevalence of use in past 30 days for 12th-graders. (From Johnston LS, O'Malley PM. *Drug use, drinking, and smoking: national survey results from high school, college, and young adult populations 1975–1996.* Rockville, MD: National Institute of Drug Abuse; 1996, with permission.)

The preferred method of use is marijuana cigarettes, which are either purchased whole or made by the user with loose marijuana and cigarette papers. Other methods include smoking with a pipe or water pipe, or with water-cooled smoking chambers called *bongs*. It is often purchased in 4- to 5-g bags ("nickel" bags) or in ready-made cigarettes. Marijuana can also be eaten. As with all street drugs, the purchaser can never be sure of the product being purchased. Marijuana frequently contains phencyclidine (PCP) and can be diluted with (usually) oregano or any type of dried and crumbled leaves.

When marijuana is smoked, a large amount of smoke is sucked into the mouth, inhaled deeply, and held as long as possible in the lungs. Using this technique, approximately 50% of the THC in the marijuana is delivered into the bloodstream [63]. Other forms of this drug that are used include hashish, the dried resin of the plant, and hash oil, a viscous, black liquid derived from mashing marijuana with organic solvents. The latter substance contains 20% to 30% THC, compared with approximately 4% to 7% in one marijuana cigarette. It is applied to the cigarette paper before the cigarette is smoked. Teens who occasionally smoke marijuana usually share a cigarette ("joint").

The intoxicating dose of THC is 0.035 mg/kg for a 70-kg adult [63]. As few as two high-potency marijuana cigarettes per day can deliver a dose of more than 40 mg THC, a very high dose indeed. With regular use, tolerance to THC can develop. Most of the drug is metabolized in the liver. THC is intensely lipophilic; much of it is stored in fatty tissue such as adipose, brain, and gonadal tissue. Stored THC is released sporadically and slowly; the half-life is approximately 3 days. The high occurs several minutes after smoking, and effects can last 2 to 3 hours. Oral ingestion gives approximately one-third the effect of smoked marijuana. Urine testing for metabolites of THC can be positive for up to 3 days after one casual use and up to 4 weeks after cessation in daily users.

The high of marijuana can be masked much more easily than that of alcohol, so a user can appear normal. The user experiences euphoria, but feelings of depersonalization can occur. There is an intensification of visual, auditory, and tactile sensations, and one's sense of the passage of time is distorted. After several hours, lethargy increases, and an intense hunger can occur (the "munchies"). There is usually no hangover effect.

Marijuana can produce adverse psychological effects, especially in the novice, casual user. These can include feelings of panic, delusions, hallucinations, illusions, and full-blown psychotic episodes. Flashbacks are uncommon. Coordination and reaction time are impaired. Consequently, the operation of machines, such as cars, is dangerous. This impairment may persist from 12 to 24 hours after use [64–66]. There is also an impairment of short-term memory. In addition, heavy marijuana use is related to neuropsychological impairment for at least a day after last use [67]. Marijuana smoke, when not cooled in a water pipe or bong, is harsh and causes irritation to the respiratory membranes. Marijuana smoke contains more carcinogens and more tar than tobacco smoke. The inhalation of the smoke is deeper and it is retained in the lungs longer. In addition, the marijuana cigarettes are smoked down to the very end (the last little bit is known as a "roach"), so every bit of harmful substance is inhaled. Therefore, histologic changes can occur in the lungs, and respiratory mucosa is frequently found to be inflamed and irritated. Chronic marijuana smokers are prone to bouts of bronchitis and may have exacerbations of asthma. Functional and pathologic investigations of the pulmonary system in marijuana smokers have found abnormalities [68–70]. Other harmful physical effects have been claimed for marijuana, but these have never been proven conclusively. There are suggestions that use of marijuana by pregnant women can have harmful effects on the fetus [71].

The chronic, frequent use of marijuana can result in negative consequences such as the amotivational syndrome [63], characterized by symptoms similar to stage 5 of any substance abuse: loss of interest in life, loss of desire to work or to perform in school, fatigue, impaired concentration, development of slovenly personal habits, and a life-style centering on procurement of the drug of choice. One of the major dangers of marijuana use is its role as a gateway to multiple drug abuse. This is not to say that marijuana, by some intrinsic property of its own, automatically leads to the abuse of other more toxic drugs. Rather, the use of marijuana is one of the behaviors of the adolescent who seeks ever-increasing levels of emotional anesthesia to deal with the pain of no perceived love and low self-esteem. As such, frequent use of marijuana can be a marker of a teen heading for further significant problems.

Cocaine

For thousands of years, peoples of the Andean highlands in South America have chewed the leaves of a common shrub, the coca plant, as a tonic. The tonic derived from the shrub is cocaine, which has become the most dangerous illicit drug available in the United States today. It has engendered an industry in which the profits are astronomical and the dangers are deadly to the drug's users, manufacturers, and those who try to stop its manufacture and distribution. The abuse of cocaine has reached epidemic proportions in some inner cities and has generated a whole syndrome of neonatal addiction and maternal deprivation.

The earliest evidence of the use of the coca plant is a 3-inch ceramic head of a man with the characteristic chewer's bulge in his cheek, circa 1500 BC, which is displayed in a museum in Ecuador [72]. By 1862, German chemists had isolated from leaves from Peru an alkaloid that they labeled *cocain* [72]. The first epidemic of stimulant abuse in the 1890s centered on cocaine, and the drug was glamorized, to some extent, by its use by the fictional master detective, Sherlock Holmes. Initially, cocaine was perceived as harmless and was an original ingredient in the formula for Coca-Cola. It was finally removed from the soft drink in the early 1900s and replaced by the current stimulant, caffeine. America recently has had its fifth epidemic of stimulant abuse since the 1890s [73]. The 1890 epidemic was followed by one of cocaine abuse in the 1920s, by amphetamine in the 1950s, and by methamphetamine in the 1960s. This latest epidemic began in the late 1970s. The senior high school class of 1976 had a 2% monthly use rate of cocaine, which increased to 3.9% in the class of 1978, 5.8% in 1981, and 6.7% in 1985. By 1992 and 1993, however, this rate had dropped to 1.3%. There has been a subsequent increase, and the monthly use rate for 1995 was 1.8% of high school seniors [1].

The financial and political consequences of this current cocaine epidemic are significant. Cocaine costs approximately $5,000 per kilogram to produce. In the United States, a kilo may wholesale for $30,000. An ounce of adulterated cocaine bought on the street can cost approximately $1,000. With 60 cents for baking soda, it can be converted into crack worth nearly $7,000 [72]. The worth of the cocaine industry to the South American cartels that control its growth, manufacture, and shipment is in the billions of dollars, and the political havoc created is significant. It was only during the 1980s that cocaine began to be perceived as especially harmful [73]. This is a pattern similar to those of the previous epidemics of stimulant abuse.

Cocaine and amphetamines are very similar in structure and effect. The major difference is in the duration of action; cocaine has an effective half-life of approximately 45 minutes, whereas that of amphetamine is from 4 to 8 hours. High-dose effects of both drugs are virtually indistinguishable [73]. Stimulants produce a sense of well-being and heightened awareness. There is an increase in energy level, a decrease in social inhibition, a heightened perception of sexual pleasure, and a decrease in anxiety [74–76]. The high is intensified by increased frequency and amount of use. Without external or internal constraints, the user seeks more frequent and higher highs to the exclusion of other life activities. Most cocaine users do not become addicted. Many adults "snort" cocaine recreationally (nasal inhalation). The people who are dependent show tolerance for cocaine, compulsive drug acquisition and use, and withdrawal symptoms [77]. Large and frequent doses, usually administered by intravenous injection, produce a euphoria so intense that it has been compared to orgasm. Once this feeling is experienced, it is sought again and again. The craving between binges is so intense that it supersedes any other need and becomes the sole driving factor in the addict's life. A hallmark of the cocaine addict is use of the drug in binges rather than on a daily basis. This is different from the alcohol addict [73], and has been called *compulsive abuse*. It requires large amounts of the drug, and is therefore expensive. The need for the money to buy the drug fuels a substantial proportion of the crime in many inner cities today. Cocaine may be the most addictive of all drugs of abuse currently available. One researcher notes, "Cocaine reinforces cocaine-seeking behavior to an extent not seen with any other psychoactive agent" [78].

Cocaine is available in two forms: *cocaine hydrochloride*, a powder that is water soluble and that is usually snorted or dissolved in water and injected, and the alkaloid base known as *cocaine freebase* or *crack*. This is usually smoked. When cocaine is injected with heroin it is called a *speedball*, and deaths associated with the use of this combination are increasing [79]. The increased availability of crack has intensified the problem of cocaine addiction. Crack has a low per-dose price compared with the powder, which makes it accessible to and desired by adolescents and by the poor. It is smoked, thereby giving an incredibly intense but very short-lived high. The intensity of the craving produced by crack is such that it may shorten the time lag from first use to addiction to a matter of weeks.

The complications of cocaine use, other than addiction, can be classified as behavioral or organic. Behavioral complications are the direct result of both the intense high while on the drug and the intense low when off it. The high can give a feeling of invulnerability that can lead to risk-taking behaviors that, in turn, can produce significant morbidities. The lows can simulate severe depression and can lead to further risk-taking behaviors engendered by the need to obtain more drug, including robbery and prostitution. The need to have the drug can also draw adolescents into the cocaine-selling business, thereby exposing them to situations where violent death is a real possibility.

Acute intoxication can produce delirium, confusion, and paranoia (Fig. 2). As with any stimulant intoxication, hypertension and tachycardia occur. Mydriasis is present, as is hyperpyrexia. Apnea can follow tachypnea; seizures, which are treatable with intravenous diazepam, can happen. Cardiac arrhythmias, myocardial ischemia, and infarction are all possible [80]. Chest pain, therefore, can be a sign of cocaine intoxication or, when recurrent, of cocaine abuse. The emergency management of acute cocaine intoxication is outlined in Table 9.

Medical complications of cocaine abuse can be local or systemic. Local complications include upper respiratory symptoms due to nasal administration, which may consist of congestion, epistaxis, or apparent colds or allergies that last for weeks or months. Smoking crack can cause chronic cough, hemoptysis, expectoration of a black, nonbloody material, and chest pain [81]. Intravenous injection, of course, can produce tracks, skin abscesses, hepatitis, human immunodeficiency virus (HIV) infection with its consequences, and subacute bacterial endocarditis. Chronic systemic symptoms include weight loss, lethargy, and impotence.

Four typical situations may be encountered by the clinician who sees adolescents [82]:

1. The patient with early and intermittent cocaine use may present with short-lived mood swings and personality changes. Upper respiratory symptoms may be prominent.
2. Regular use two to three times weekly by snorting produces an intensified picture of the aforementioned situation with the addition of dropping school grades, change in peer group, and other symptoms of the drug-abusing adolescent.
3. Chronic, almost daily smoking of crack produces a teenager who is withdrawn, has wild mood swings, is depressed frequently, is paranoid, and has multiple physical complaints. Lethargy and hypersomnolence occur when cocaine is not available.
4. The full-blown picture of acute cocaine intoxication is the final possibility.

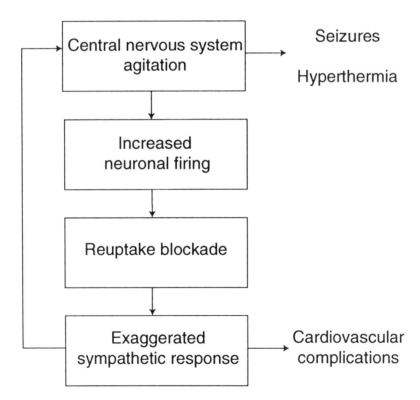

FIG. 2. A model of cocaine toxicity. (From Hollander JE. The management of cocaine-associated myocardial ischemia. *N Engl J Med* 1995;333:1267, with permission.)

TABLE 9. *Emergency medical management of cocaine intoxication*

Respiratory management
Support ventilation as needed
Naloxone if opiates are suspected
Metabolic management
Aggressive treatment of acidosis
Management of arrhythmias
Phenytoin or cardioversion
Lidocaine may not be used
Seizure management
Diazepam or lorazepam
Hypertension management
Nitroprusside or labetalol
Hyperthermia
Cooling blanket
Antipyretics or phenothiazines may not be used

From Farrar HC, Kearns GL. Cocaine: clinical pharmacology and toxicology. *J Pediatr* 1989;5:665.

The treatment of cocaine abuse should begin with a full assessment, which can be begun in the clinician's office but usually needs to be completed by a trained substance abuse professional. With an understanding of the neurochemical basis for cocaine's effects, primarily dealing with the dopamine reuptake transporter, there is reason to hope for drugs that will be able to treat cocaine dependence and toxicity effectively [77,83]. For the primary clinician, the key to detecting adolescents who use cocaine is a high index of suspicion.

Other Stimulants

The prototypical stimulants are the amphetamines, which include several related compounds differing only in relative potency and half-life. These include amphetamine (Benzedrine), methamphetamine (Desoxyn), dextroamphetamine (Dexedrine), and benzphetamine (Didrex) [84]. As with other illicit drugs, their monthly use rate has risen from 2.8% in the class of 1992 to 4% in the class of 1995. A new stimulant has appeared in the last few years and is causing increased concern because of its increased potency and addictive potential: crystal methamphetamine, *crystal meth* or *ice*. It has spread from Hawaii to the West Coast, with usage rates of 1.1% monthly among high school seniors, up from 0.5% in 1992 [1]. The high of ice is supposedly as intense as that of crack, but it lasts much longer.

Other stimulants are primarily the look-alike drugs. These are capsules that are created to look like prescription amphetamine capsules but are over-the-counter substances that do not contain amphetamines. They do contain phenylpropanolamine, ephedrine, caffeine, or lidocaine. Over-the-counter diet medications containing phenylpropanolamine are also abused for their stimulant effects. Another drug that can be abused is methylphenidate (Ritalin). Stimulants all have similar effects. They heighten awareness, cause restlessness and agitation, increase feelings of invulnerability, increase ability to concentrate (at lower doses), and, at higher doses, can cause hypertension, seizures, and strokes. There have been reports of idiosyncratic reactions to look-alike drugs in which teens have had hypertensive crises, strokes, and have even died [85–91]. Cerebral vasculitis after the use of phenylpropanolamine also has been reported [92,93].

The easy availability of the amphetamine analogs means that a potentially large number of teens could abuse these drugs. It is prudent for the clinician to make his or her adolescent patients aware of the potential dangers of stimulants, because most teens are not.

Before leaving this topic, mention should be made of "designer drugs." Designer amphetamines are chemical modifications of commonly abused drugs that are manufactured in illicit laboratories and sold for recreational use. These compounds, which are not illegal until they can be found, characterized, and placed on controlled substances lists by the Drug Enforcement Agency, can be more potent and less expensive than the original substance, thereby becoming extremely profitable. These drugs have been used all over the country [94,95]. These drugs include MDMA, or ecstasy, and MDEA, or eve. Both are Schedule 1 drugs, and both are used for their euphoric and inhibition-decreasing properties. MDMA has been called the "love drug." MDMA more recently has been used at "raves" (all-night dance marathons that are facilitated by the drug's "upper" qualities) [96]. The sympathomimetic qualities of these drugs make them arrhythmogenic, and, combined with vigorous dancing, they have been associated with severe toxicity and even death. A designer version of the decongestant and "diet" medication, pheylpropanolamine, has been formulated and is called "U4ia." This drug is hallucinogenic and stimulatory, with all the attendant dangers [95].

Hallucinogens

The monthly use rate of the class of drugs commonly known as *hallucinogens* had decreased among adolescents from a high of more than 5% in the senior class of 1979 to less than 3% a decade later, but it has risen in the early 1990s, so that now 4.6% of high school seniors report use in the month preceding the survey [1]. The primary drug in this category is LSD. Hallucinogens, especially LSD, were introduced into American youth culture in the 1960s and early 1970s by young adults who were seeking more than just another drug for intoxication. These were older adolescents and young adults who, in the wake of President Kennedy's assassination and of the Vietnam war, were seeking a more peaceful, humane, and loving world. They believed that by using substances such as LSD, a higher plane of consciousness could be reached through which their goals could be achieved.

The LSD "trip" was glorified by such cult gurus as the late Dr. Timothy Leary, and the wonders of acid trips were recounted in popular songs such as "White Rabbit" by Jefferson Airplane.

Later, in the 1970s, the use of hallucinogens spread to younger and younger adolescents until, by the 1980s, the typical users were secondary school students who were merely seeking to get high without any of the more philosophic goals of the young adults of the 1960s. As such, hallucinogens have become simply other drugs of abuse. In addition, a new kind of hallucinogen—PCP—was developed in the late 1970s. This drug is not nearly as benign as the prototype hallucinogens, and its use can have very severe consequences.

To be properly understood, the class of drugs known as hallucinogens must be divided into subcategories, LSD and related drugs in one class and PCP in the other. LSD is more precisely categorized as an "illusogen" [97]. It produces alterations of reality-based perceptions rather than perceptions of things that are not there (true hallucinations). Other drugs in the LSD group include psilocybin or psilocin, mescaline, nutmeg, morning glory, and jimsonweed. LSD is 100 to 1,000 times more powerful than these naturally occurring substances.

Although extremely potent, LSD is one of the safest drugs in terms of lethality. It can have effects in doses as low as 10 μg, yet is not fatal in doses hundreds of times greater [98]. Tolerance to repeated doses is both gained and lost rapidly. The drug is rapidly absorbed from the gastrointestinal tract, and sympathomimetic effects occur within a few minutes of ingestion. The psychological and behavioral effects are felt approximately 20 to 30 minutes later and peak at 2 to 4 hours. They are usually gone by 6 to 12 hours after the dose. LSD solution is sprayed or basted onto sheets of blotting paper that are dried, perforated, and often printed with special symbols or designs. The user chews and swallows the small section of the sheet of paper. Alternatively, the user soaks the paper, squeezes out the substance, and then ingests the liquid with a dropper [99].

The psychological effects of LSD center around distortions of reality. Synesthesias (e.g., "hearing" smells, "feeling" colors) occur occasionally. Visual perception is markedly altered. Colors and shapes are heightened and tend to meld into each other. Sense of touch is magnified, and the feeling of the passage of time is markedly distorted. Actual perceptual motor performance is impaired, but feelings of competence and true insight are generated. Thinking does not proceed in logical sequences. In bad trips (i.e., negative experiences), feelings of paranoia can be generated, and the user can feel panic that his or her personality is falling apart. In addition to these acute negative reactions, chronic problems such as flashbacks (having an illusionary experience without taking the drug), psychoses, depression, and chronic personality changes have occurred. Whether these chronic changes were due directly to the drug or to preexisting morbid states that were unmasked by the LSD is unknown. A bad trip could be due to a substance other than LSD that was present in the product ingested. Recovery from LSD toxicity takes 10 to 12 hours. No physical dependence syndrome is generated. It is worth screening the urine for other substances of abuse such as PCP when a patient with such a reaction is encountered. Otherwise, urine testing is not very reliable [98].

Other relatively benign hallucinogens include psilocybin and psilocin, the active ingredients in psychedelic mushrooms, mescaline from the peyote cactus, nutmeg, morning glory seeds, and jimsonweed. Other than the last substance, these are rarely encountered in most practices. Jimsonweed (*Datura stramonium*) grows wild throughout the United States and is well known to many adolescents. As few as 10 well chewed seeds can produce vivid hallucinations as well as the remainder of the anticholinergic syndrome ("mad as a hatter, hot as a hen, red as a beet, dry as a bone") [100–103].

Phencyclidine, originally a veterinary anesthetic, is used by humans purposely for its true hallucinogenic properties or inadvertently when it is surreptitiously substituted for LSD, marijuana, or other drugs [104]. Therefore, the actual use rate is higher than reported, and it may account for many bad trips and even deaths.

Also known as *angel dust* and *hog*, PCP was first introduced as a human anesthetic in 1963. Two years later, it was withdrawn because of postoperative reactions such as agitation, hallucinations, muscle rigidity, and seizures. PCP is a versatile substance in that it may be ingested, snorted, smoked, or taken intravenously. It can act as a stimulant, as a depressant, or as a hallucinogen, depending on dose and route of administration. PCP is sold in pure form as a powder, liquid, granules, capsules, or tablets. It is also dusted into tobacco and marijuana cigarettes. More recently, a new form of PCP use has come to the fore. PCP is dissolved in an organic solvent such as formaldehyde, brake fluid, or gasoline, and then cigarettes are dipped into the liquid and smoked. Because cigarettes made by the Nat Sherman Tobacconists firm are more tightly wrapped and have coarser paper, the amount of dissolved PCP that is absorbed is greater, so these "Sherms" are more desirable than regular cigarettes. This form of PCP has been called "wet" or "water" (H. Faigel, personal communication).

Similar to its close relative, ketamine, PCP is a dissociative anesthetic that causes the recipient to feel separated from the environment. With varying doses and routes, PCP can produce euphoria, dysphoria, paranoia, perceptual distortion, psychoses, aggressive and violent behavior, depression, seizures, coma, and death [105]. Deaths from PCP can result from delusional feelings of omnipotence, from self-directed or other-directed aggression, and from overdose with resultant convulsions and cerebral hemorrhage.

The most frequent neurologic signs seen with PCP are horizontal and vertical nystagmus, gait ataxia, dysarthria, muscle rigidity, major seizures, and, with large amounts, open-eyed coma. Anesthesia, hypertension, tachycardia, flushing, sweating, and ileus can also occur. Behavior is often bizarre, and flashbacks are more common than with LSD. A comatose patient with open eyes and horizontal and vertical nystagmus should be considered to have PCP overdose until proved otherwise [106]. Urine screen for PCP can remain positive for anywhere from 1 day to 2 weeks [107].

Phencyclidine intoxication can be treated with gastric emptying, activated charcoal, and cathartics. Violent behavior must be treated with restraints, and it is best to have the patient isolated in a quiet, dark room. "Talking down," as is done with LSD, does not work with PCP. Intramuscular haloperidol can be used for the severely agitated patient; chlorpromazine should not be used because of its anticholinergic and alpha-adrenergic blocking effects. Unfortunately, PCP is cheap and widely available. Its low price, ease of manufacture, and role as an adulterant of other drugs makes its use relatively common. Clinicians should always consider it as a possible cause of unusual symptoms in adolescents.

Inhalants

The use of inhaled substances to alter consciousness has been practiced since ancient times [108]. Table 10 gives the classification of these substances. The typical reasons for use of these substances include rapid onset of effects, quality and pattern of the high, low cost, easy availability, convenient packaging, and legality of possession [109].

Monthly use by high school seniors rose from approximately 2.5% in 1992 to 3.5% in 1995. What makes these compounds different from other substances of abuse is that the highest use rates are in eighth graders, with rates declining as teens get older [1]. Most commonly, the substance is placed in a plastic or paper bag and the fumes are inhaled. Alternatively, a rag or handkerchief is soaked in the substance and then inhaled through the cloth ("huffing") [110]. Liquids are frequently inhaled directly from the container.

The changes in consciousness are analogous to those induced by anesthesia. Subjectively, there is first excitation followed by euphoria and exhilaration. This is frequently accompanied by nausea and vomiting. With continued inhalation, CNS depression deepens and the user becomes more confused

TABLE 10. *Chemical classification of commonly abused inhalants*

Substance	Source	Structural group
Acetone, methylethyl ketone, methyl isobutyl ketone	Glues, adhesives, dyes, solvents	Ketones
Amyl nitrite, butyl, isobutyl nitrite	Room odorizers	Alkyl nitrites
Benzene, xylene, toluene shoe polish	Glues, solvents, paints, varnishes,	Aromatic hydrocarbons
Diethyl ether	Solvents	Ethers
Methylene chloride, carbone tetrachloride, trichloroethane, trichloroethylene, perchloroethylene, freons	Paint stripper, solvent (dry) cleaner, spot removers, typewriter correction fluid	Alkyl halides
Nitrous oxide	Aerosol propellant	Nitrous oxide
Propane, butane, gasoline, kerosene, mineral spirits, hexane	(Liquid) fuels, lighter fluid, paint thinner, solvent	Aliphatic hydrocarbons

Adapted from Henretig F. Inhalant abuse in children and adolescents. *Pediatr Ann* 1996;25:48.

and disoriented. Impulsive behavior can occur, with possible trauma as a result. As toxicity increases, ataxia develops and reflexes become depressed. Finally, stupor ensues, which may be accompanied by seizures or cardiorespiratory arrest [111,112]. Chronic neurologic effects can occur from sniffing of gasoline, toluene, glue, and naphtha fumes [113]. Other chronic problems can affect all major body systems, particularly cardiovascular, pulmonary, hepatic, and renal. Management is based on the individual substance inhaled and on general principles of managing the acutely intoxicated patient. Table 11 gives a summary of some of the clinical effects of various inhaled substances.

Narcotics

When most people think of the prototypical drugs of abuse, they think of opium-based narcotics. Physicians' fears of addicting patients to narcotic analgesics have led many to underdose patients who are suffering from severe pain. Although these drugs are still highly addictive when abused, they are used infrequently by teenagers, except possibly for adolescents who live in certain major urban centers, such as New York City. The 1995 monthly use rate for heroin use by high school seniors was 0.6%, double the rate from 1994 and all previous years since 1976. The monthly use rate for other opiates was 1.8%, a significant rise from the 1.1% of 1991 [1]. Even more disturbing, heroin and its image of the wasted waif have become "in" in both music and fashion circles. Recently, famous music stars have either died of heroin overdoses (Kurt Cobain of Nirvana and Jonathan Melvoin of Smashing Pumpkins) or have fought its effects publicly (Steven Tyler of Aerosmith) [114]. Heroin's increased popularity is

TABLE 11. *Summary of effects of commonly abused volatile substances*

Effects	Substance
Aplastic anemia, hepatorenal toxicity, leukemia	Benzene
Carbon monoxide production	Methylene chloride
Cardiac arrhythmias, hepatorenal toxicity, high risk for sudden death	Carbon tetrachloride (other halogenate hydrocarbons)
Cardiac arrhythmias, high risk for sudden death	Butane, propane
Encephalopathy, hepatorenal toxicity	Xylene
Encephalopathy, gastrointestinal syndrome, muscle weakness with electrolyte imbalance, renal tubular acidosis, other renal effects	Toluene
Methemoglobinemia, hypotension	Nitrites
Neuropathy and spinal cord syndrome (subacute combined degeneration)	Nitrous oxide
Peripheral neuropathy	Hexane

Adapted from Henretig F. Inhalant abuse in children and adolescents. *Pediatr Ann* 1996;25:48.

somewhat predictable given that increased heroin use follows periods of increased narcotics use. Also facilitating heroin's use is its increased availability and higher potency. In 1980, a typical $10 bag was 2% to 8% pure. In 1994, the average purity in New York City was 63%. Meanwhile, the price has dropped from $1.81/mg in 1988 to $0.37/mg in 1994. One of the causes is a significant increase in heroin production from countries such as Burma, Afghanistan, Laos, Pakistan, Colombia, and Mexico. An optimistic note may be the fact that the media picks up on increased use rates when they have already peaked, and the increased notoriety may presage a downturn in use [114].

Narcotics, strictly speaking, are agents that cause sleep, but their legitimate use is primarily for relief of severe pain. The opiate narcotics (to which the term *narcotic* will herein refer unless otherwise specified) exert their effects on the CNS and the intestines at specific opiate receptor sites. All of the drugs in this group are capable of causing respiratory depression, mood changes, mental clouding, and nausea and vomiting (Table 12). Anesthesia can occur at higher doses. Narcotics also produce miosis, reversible by atropine, and constipation [84]. The cardiovascular system is affected minimally. All narcotics cross the placenta and, therefore, have addicting potential for the fetus.

Addiction is not automatic with narcotics, but, with recurrent use, tolerance and craving for more occur in almost anyone. Table 13 lists various narcotics and their addictive potential. Narcotics can be administered in several ways, certain routes being preferred or necessary for certain compounds. For centuries, Asians have smoked opium from water pipes. Opium can be used in oral preparations, as can meperidine and others. Heroin is usually injected either under the skin or intravenously, which puts the user at risk for HIV infection, hepatitis, and subacute bacterial endocarditis, among others. Injectable drug users currently have the highest rates of new HIV infection, nearly twice that of gay men.

Addiction to narcotics is compounded by the fact that the preferred route of delivery for heroin is intravenous and the composition of these drugs, when purchased on the street, can vary considerably. The variability of both the dose of the desired drug in the current purchase and the adulterants that may be used puts the user at high risk for harmful reactions from overdose. The variations in purity contribute to the 3,000 to 4,000 annual deaths from heroin overdose, in many of which heroin was used with other drugs such as alcohol or cocaine ("speedballs").

Narcotic overdose can cause respiratory depression (leading to respiratory collapse), bradycardia, cardiopulmonary arrest, and death. Miosis is typical with narcotic overdose, but hypoxia can produce mydriasis, as can overdose with meperidine. Meperidine, in toxic amounts, can also produce excitation and seizure activity [84]. The narcotic antagonist naloxone can reverse the symptoms of narcotic

TABLE 12. *Opiates and nonopiate narcotics and other analgesics*

Generic name	Trade name
Opiate agonists	
Morphine[a]	Morphine
Codeine[a]	Codeine, Tylenol with Codeine, Fiorinal with Codeine
Dihydrocodeine	
Dihydrocodeinone hydrocodone	Vicodin
Dihydromorphinone hydrochloride	Dilaudid
Methadone[a]	Dolophine
Meperidine	Demerol
Opium[a]	Opium with belladonna
Oxymorphone	Numorphan
Propoxyphene[a]	Darvon
Oxycodone	Tylox, Percodan, Percocet
Heroin[b]	
Opiate partial agonists	
Pentazocine	Talwin
Nalbuphine	Nubain
Butorphanol tartrate	Sladol

[a]Available under the generic name.
[b]Not legal.
From King P, Coleman JH. Stimulants and narcotic drugs. *Pediatr Clin North Am* 1987;34:349.

TABLE 13. *Abuse potential of common opioids*

Drug	Route	Risk of abuse level
Codeine	Oral	Low
Heroin	Intravenous/intranasal	High
Hydromorphone	Oral	High
Methadone	Oral	High
Opium	Smoked	Moderate
Oxycodone	Oral	Moderate
Pentazocine	Intravenous/oral	Low
Propoxyphene	Oral	Moderate

Adapted from Ling W, Wesson DR. Drugs of abuse: opiates. *West J Med* 1990;152:565.

overdose [114], but it also produces withdrawal symptoms in chronic users. Naloxone has been added to tablets of pentazocine to prevent its use intravenously (naloxone is inactivated when taken orally, so the pentazocine can have its intended analgesic effect).

As with other drugs of abuse, breaking the law is common. These drugs are illegal to sell, buy, or possess, and, more important, to get the money to pay for a significant habit, users have to resort to stealing, dealing, or prostitution. The associated morbidity is high.

Sedatives and Tranquilizers

Monthly use of sedatives and tranquilizers has increased, just as it has with most other drugs of abuse. In 1995, sedatives were used in the past month by 2.3% of high school seniors, whereas tranquilizers had a use rate of 1.8% [1]. These drugs have a long history of abuse and retain a significant potential for such.

The classic drugs of abuse in this category are the barbiturates, methaqualone, and the benzodiazepines, a group that falls more properly into the category of the tranquilizers. Over-the-counter drugs that can mimic the effects of these substances include antihistamines. Sedatives and tranquilizers are CNS depressants. They cause somnolence, a feeling of placidity, and, in high doses, respiratory depression. Tolerance develops with continued use of the drugs. Long-term use is both physically and psychologically addictive. In addition, the dangerous effects of these drugs is additive with alcohol and other CNS-depressant drugs, a common combination [115–118].

Sedatives are frequently used by stimulant abusers to bring them down from their stimulant high. Users then find themselves needing both drugs to maintain even the semblance of normal life.

Acute intoxication with barbiturates presents primarily with respiratory and CNS depression. Hypotension, hypothermia, shock, and coma can occur with ingestion of large amounts [119]. Management centers around respiratory support and getting the substance out of the gastrointestinal tract by emesis if the patient is awake, by catharsis, and by use of activated charcoal. The primary danger of overdose with benzodiazepines is respiratory depression, although when taken alone they have a high median lethal dose (LD_{50}). Still, artificial ventilation may be needed in an emergency. As mentioned previously, one should always consider the possibility that another substance is present when confronted with an adolescent who is known to be suffering from a sedative or tranquilizer overdose, the most likely culprit being alcohol. A new benzodiazepine, flunitrazepam (Rohypnol; known on the street as "roofies") has caused a stir in Congress because of its alleged use as a sedative and amnesic on unsuspecting young women by college men who then proceed to have sex with their suddenly sedated and "willing" dates. This has led to the nickname "the date rape drug" for Rohypnol [120].

What the Primary Clinician Can Do

Detection

The clinician's primary roles in the care of the adolescent are those of detection and prevention of alcohol and drug misuse and abuse. Treatment should be left to professional counselors who specialize in this area.

The primary method of detecting adolescents who have a drug problem is through the standard history and physical examination. By taking the time necessary to delve into the "five boxes" sufficiently, clues that an adolescent is having a substance abuse problem should be readily apparent. The key warning signs are [15]:

- A decrease in school performance or attendance
- Mood swings more pronounced than usual in a particular teenager
- Recent change in the peer group to one totally out of character for that adolescent
- Increased interest in the drug culture as evidenced by possession of drug literature, paraphernalia, and clothing (heavy metal T-shirts, for example, although this alone is not diagnostic)
- A change to sloppy dress and poor grooming and hygiene
- A rebellious and paranoid flavor to interpersonal relationships with family and adult authority figures (Table 14)

Detection of substance misuse (e.g., inappropriate use on weekends at parties) may be more difficult than detecting the daily user. Questions relating to weekend activities, such as going to parties every Friday and Saturday night, presence of parents at parties, and whether friends get drunk a lot, are helpful in this regard.

Substance misuse and abuse are not isolated entities. They are usually part of a larger dysfunctional syndrome that involves many aspects of a teenager's life. Risk factors include history of parental substance abuse, living in a single-parent family, school problems such as learning disabilities, trouble with the law, early participation in sexual activity (particularly among white teenagers), sexual promiscuity, a history of being sexually abused, and a history of running away (Table 15).

As with any adolescent health problem, the parents should be questioned thoroughly. This is usually not difficult to manage, because, most often, it is the parents who have brought the adolescent to the clinician for concerns about substance use or abuse. The parents may have already detected one or more of the previously listed risk factors, and, when their memories are jogged, other clues may become apparent. Parents also usually know the family history better than the teenager. They are aware of family members who had or have substance abuse problems, and they may reveal previous problems the adolescent failed to mention. When school or legal authorities force an adolescent to come in for an assessment, however, his or her parents may deny, both verbally and psychologically, that the teenager has any problems. In this situation, it is prudent to review with the parents the hallmarks of this condition and urge them to examine the situation objectively.

Certain responses to the clinician's questions may indicate a problem, including deliberate vagueness about leisure-time habits, belligerence about being accused of using drugs, or, alternatively, an inappropriate lack of concern about such accusations, defense of the use of drugs by others, and an excessive amount of knowledge about drug paraphernalia and drug culture. In addition, adolescents may respond more honestly about friends' use of substances than about their own problem.

Physical examination usually is normal. That is because most teens are not truly addicted and, therefore, do not have the typical physical stigmata of addiction. If the adolescent is addicted, how-

---

TABLE 14. *Possible signs of drug use*

- Reddened eyes, use of eyedrops
- Distorted sense of time
- Use of breath fresheners, incense, room deodorizers
- Chronic cough, chest pain, hoarseness
- Fatigue, lack of energy
- Impaired memory or judgment
- Change in sleeping pattern
- Change in eating habits, increased or decreased appetite
- Change in appearance, less attention to cleanliness
- Change of friends
- Secretiveness, lying
- Missing money or items of value
- Loss of interest in school, hobbies, family activities
- Missing school, skipping classes, drop in grades
- Mood changes, irritability, hostility

TABLE 15. *Risk factors for substance abuse*

- Family management problems
- Childhood and early adolescent antisocial behavior
- Academic underachievement
- Little commitment to education
- Aberration, rebelliousness, lack of social bonding to society
- Friends who abuse drugs
- Favorable attitudes toward drug use
- Early first use of drugs
- Affective disorders

Adapted from Macdonald DI. *Drugs, drinking, and adolescence.* Chicago: Year Book; 1984; and American Academy of Pediatrics. Screening for drugs of abuse in children and adolescents. *Pediatrics* 1989;84:396.

ever, the examiner might detect scars or scabs between the fingers or toes (indicative of "skin popping," subcutaneous injection) or "tracks" in the antecubital fossae. Signs of intravenous drug use may also include jaundice or liver enlargement from hepatitis. Other physical stigmata of nonintravenous drug use may include nasal congestion, chronic cough, irritated palpebral membranes, and weight loss.

Frequently, the clinician finishes the visit without clear-cut conclusions about whether the adolescent does or does not have a substance use or abuse problem. The next step suggested by the parents is usually a urine test for drugs. Whether the clinician should order such a test is controversial. On the one hand, if drugs are present, a positive test gives at least one concrete indication that the adolescent has used a substance at least once, and the clinician can then proceed with educational, if not therapeutic, interventions. Certainly, the presence of drugs in the teenager's urine does not automatically mean that the patient is addicted or even moderately abusing the substance. On the other hand, the absence of substances in the test does not indicate lack of a problem. In the situation where the clinician is confronted with an obviously intoxicated patient, it is incumbent to obtain a urine sample for drug testing.

An additional factor that must be taken into account is the purpose for which the drug screening test is to be used. If the test is to be used for punitive purposes alone, such as scholastic expulsion, then there is grave concern about ordering such a test. The physician's role is to detect pathologic processes and to treat them, not to be an instrument of a punitive authority. In addition, the clinician must be the guardian of the adolescent's confidentiality and right to grant consent, breaching them only when it is clear that the teenager is not competent to make informed judgments. The Committee on Substance Abuse of the American Academy of Pediatrics (AAP) has stated that [121]:

- The Academy is opposed to the nontherapeutic use of psychoactive drugs by children and adolescents.
- The appropriate response to suspicion of drug abuse is referral of the child or adolescent to a qualified health care professional for evaluation, counseling, and treatment as needed.
- The role of pediatricians is one of prevention, diagnosis, counseling, and treatment, or appropriate referral for care.
- Voluntary screening may be a deceptive term, in that there often are negative consequences for those who decline to volunteer. Parental permission is not sufficient for involuntary screening of the older, competent adolescent, and the AAP opposes such involuntary screening. Consent from the older adolescent may be waived when there is reason to doubt competency or in those circumstances in which information gained by history or physical examination strongly suggests that the young person is at high risk of substance abuse.
- Diagnostic testing for the purpose of drug abuse treatment is within the ethical tradition of health care, and in the competent patient, it should be conducted noncovertly, confidentially, and with informed consent in the same context as for other medical conditions.
- Involuntary testing in a minor who lacks the capacity to make informed judgments may be done with parental permission. Parental permission is not sufficient for involuntary testing of the adolescent with decisional capacity, and the AAP opposes such involuntary testing. Suspicion that an ado-

lescent may be using a psychoactive drug does not justify involuntary testing, and it is not sufficient justification to rely solely on parental agreement to test the patient. Testing adolescents requires their consent unless: 1) a patient lacks decision-making capacity, or 2) there are strong medical indications or legal requirements to do so.

• Notwithstanding the Supreme Court ruling [122], students and student athletes should not be singled out for involuntary screening for drugs of abuse. Such testing should not be a condition for participation in sports or any school functions except for health-related purposes. Suspicion of drug use warrants a comprehensive evaluation by a qualified health care professional.

Drug screening should be done only for specific indications when there is sufficient suspicion of a problem and when the adolescent's rights are adequately safeguarded (Table 16). Every positive test should be followed by a second test to confirm the finding. Again, it must be stressed: *the adolescent's rights of consent and confidentiality and of knowing that the test results will be used only for his or her own benefit must be preserved.*

The most widely used tests include enzyme-multiplied immunoassay technique (EMIT), color-spot tests, thin-layer chromatography (TLC), gas–liquid chromatography (GLC), high-performance liquid chromatography (HPLC), and gas chromatography—mass spectrometry (GC/MS). Table 17 lists the commonly used analytic techniques, and Table 18 lists duration of detectability of suspected drugs in urine. Each technique has its advantages and limitations, and the clinician should be somewhat familiar with the ones most commonly used in his or her area. For example, some tests are so sensitive that the detection of a drug is somewhat meaningless and may do more harm than good. A test may be very specific for some drugs but not for others. To be of any use, the test must provide useful information for diagnosis and treatment. For more detailed information about the individual tests and their best use, the reader is referred to the work of MacKenzie and colleagues [123] and of Hoffman [124]. Hair analysis also can be used to detect drugs of abuse [125]. Finally, a home test kit for detection is now available. Parents can wipe down surfaces with which their children regularly come into contact to pick up microscopic traces of drugs and then mail the swab to the company, where it is assayed for six drugs, including marijuana and heroin. The results are mailed or phoned back to the parents in 10 days [126].

Prevention

Prevention can appear difficult, but armed with knowledge of the risk factors that may predispose adolescents to substance abuse, clinicians can learn to detect the early signs of potential problems in their patients [127]. Intervention can then commence with education about the negative effects of drugs and alcohol and the teaching of skills that the adolescent can use to avoid getting more involved with substance use. When family or individual problems exist that are beyond the capability of the individual practitioner to handle, having a network of colleagues in the psychosocial professions can provide an effective method of intervening. Developing a close liaison with schools that their patients attend can help the clinician intervene when educational problems surface. Most important, incorporating a program of child and family education about substance misuse and abuse, proper parenting

TABLE 16. *Absolute indications for drug screening on body fluids in adolescents*

• All adolescents with psychiatric symptoms
• High-risk adolescents (e.g., runaways, delinquents)
• Evaluation of all adolescents with mental state or performance changes
• Acute-onset behavioral states
• Monitoring abstinence
• Adolescents with recurrent respiratory ailments
• Adolescents with recurrent accidents or unexplained somatic symptoms

From MacKenzie RG, Cheng M, Haftel AJ. The clinical utility and evaluation of drug screening techniques. *Pediatr Clin North Am* 1987;34:423.

TABLE 17. *Comparison of commonly used analytic techniques*

Technique	Preanalysis treatment of sample	Major instrumentation	Drug identification	Can specimen be adulterated?	Limits of sensitivity	Instrumentation costs ($)	Confirmation required	Multiple drug analysis at once	Level of personal experience
TLC	Yes	No	Position on plate	No	1 μg/mL	—	Yes	Yes	High
Modified TOXI-LAB	Yes	No	Response to color reagents fluorescent pattern	No	0.2–5 μg/ml	500	Yes	Yes	Moderate
HPLC with scanning ultraviolet detector	Yes	Yes	Relative retention times; comparison of ultraviolet spectra with standards	No	0.02–10 μg/ml	20,000–50,000	No[a]	Yes	High
Dual-column capillary GC with nitrogen detectors	Yes	Yes	Relative retention times matched in both columns; comparison of peaks with standards	No	0.01–10 μg/ml	20,000–50,000	No[a]	Yes	High
Capillary GC/MS	Yes	Yes	Relative retention times; comparison of mass spectra with standards	No	0.001–5 μg/ml	20,000–200,000	No	Yes	High
EMIT	No	Yes	Variation in enzyme activity	Yes	0.025–5 μg/ml	7,000–100,000	Yes	No	Moderate
RIA	No	Yes	Variation of bound radiolabeled tracer	Yes	0.001–10 μg/ml	5,000–100,000	Yes	No	Moderate

TLC, thin-layer chromatography; modified TOXI-LAB, modified thin-layer chromatography; HPLC, high-performance liquid chromatography; GC, gas chromatography; GC/MS, gas chromatography/mass spectrometry; EMIT, enzyme-multiplied immunoassay technique; RIA, radioimmunoassay.

[a]Confirmation necessary only if results must meet a forensic challenge.

From Council on Scientific Affairs. Scientific issues in drug testing. *JAMA* 1987:257:3110, "Copyright 1987, American Medical Association," with permission.

TABLE 18. *Approximate duration of detectability of selected drugs in urine*

Drug	Approximate duration of detectability[a] (in days)
Amphetamine	2
Barbiturates: (short acting) pentobarbital/secobarbital	1[b]
Cannabinoids: 11-nor-Δ⁹-tetrahydrocannabinol-9-carboxylic acid	3[c], 5[d], 10[e], 21–27[f]
Cocaine metabolites: benzoylecgonine	2–3
Codeine	2
Methamphetamine	2
Morphine	2
Phencyclidine	8; 3 for casual use

[a]Interpretation of the duration of detectability must take into account many variables, such as drug metabolism and half-life, subject's physical condition, fluid balance and state of hydration, and route and frequency of ingestion. These are general guidelines only.

[b]Using therapeutic dosages.

[c]Single use.

[d]Moderate smoker (4 times/wk).

[e]Heavy smoker (smoking daily).

[f]Chronic heavy smoker.

Adapted from American Academy of Pediatrics and Center for Advanced Health Studies. Use of the laboratory. In: Schoenberg SK, ed. *Substance abuse: a guide for health professionals.* Elk Grove Village, IL: American Academy of Pediatrics; 1988:48.

techniques, effective decision making, and effective problem solving in patients' health maintenance visits can help avoid problems before they arise. Examples of questions to ask teens and their parents are shown in Tables 19 through 22. Physicians should remember the four "A"s. *Anticipate* that adolescents could be involved with alcohol, tobacco, and drugs. Risk behaviors such as the use of illicit substances and alcohol carry certain meanings for adolescents, and clinicians need to understand the perceived benefits that may apply to an adolescent at any particular stage of development. Then the following "A"s become more useful [128]: *Ask* about such use in ways mentioned previously; *Advise* and educate your adolescent patients and their parents; and *Assist* them to stop using when necessary, by referral or direct counseling [129].

Clinicians can have considerable impact on groups of adolescents as well. Despite the criticism and erosion of image that the health professions have encountered in recent years, physicians and nurses are still more respected by the public than almost any other profession. This respect can be translated

TABLE 19. *Questionnaire items relevant to substance abuse*

1. Do you smoke cigarettes?	Y_____	N_____
2. Do you smoke marijuana?	Y_____	N_____
3. Do you often feel "bummed out," down, or depressed?	Y_____	N_____
4. Do you ever use drugs or alcohol to feel better?	Y_____	N_____
5. Do you ever use drugs or alcohol when you are alone?	Y_____	N_____
6. Do your friends get drunk or get high at parties?	Y_____	N_____
7. Do you get drunk or get high at parties?	Y_____	N_____
8. Do your friends ever get drunk or get high at rock concerts?	Y_____	N_____
9. Do you ever get drunk or get high at rock concerts?	Y_____	N_____
10. Have your school grades gone down recently?	Y_____	N_____
11. Have you flunked any subjects recently?	Y_____	N_____
12. Have you had recent problems with your coaches or advisers at school?	Y_____	N_____
13. Do you feel that friends or parents just do not seem to understand you?	Y_____	N_____

From Schonberg SK, ed. *Substance abuse: a guide for health professionals.* Elk Grove Village, IL: American Academy of Pediatrics; 1988.

TABLE 20. *Open-ended questions intended to provide a basis for further exploration of advanced substance abuse*

1. What do your friends do at parties? Do you go to the parties? Do you drink? Get drunk? Get high?
2. Do you drive drunk? Stoned? Have you ridden with a driver who was drunk or stoned? Could you call home and ask for help? What would your parents say or do?
3. Do you go to rock concerts? Do you drink there? Do you get high? Who drives after the concert?
4. After drinking, have you ever forgotten where you had been or what you had done?
5. Have you recently dropped some of your old friends and started going with a new group?
6. Do you feel that lately you are irritable, "bitchy," or moody?
7. Do you find yourself getting into more frequent arguments with your friends? Brothers and sisters? Parents?
8. Do you have a girlfriend (boyfriend)? How is that going? Are you having more fights (arguments) with her (him) lately? Have you recently broken up?
9. Do you find yourself being physically abusive to others? To your brothers/sisters? To your mother or father?
10. Do you think your drinking (drug use) is a problem? Why?

From Schonberg SK, ed. *Substance abuse: a guide for health professionals.* Elk Grove Village, IL: American Academy of Pediatrics; 1988.

into a positive impact on school and community educational programs for youth and parents. Clinicians can make themselves available as consultants to the local schools, churches, and public health departments. They can seek positions on boards of education or community action committees to lend expertise, common sense, and direction to resolving these volatile issues. Through involvement in these types of activities, the individual practitioner can have a significant effect on children and adolescents far beyond the boundaries of his or her own practice. For example, the local clinician can bring scientific objectivity to programs that are popular but that have not been shown to be effective, such as DARE [130]. Last, practitioners can become involved in the political process, both in their own profession as well as in the public arena. It is important for the clinician to become known to local and state legislators as an expert from whom they can obtain insight and knowledge about these societal issues. Practitioners can testify at legislative committee hearings on laws that will have an impact on children and adolescents. Here is an opportunity to influence the lives of many more chil-

TABLE 21. *Questionnaire for adolescent patients suspected of or known to be abusing drugs or alcohol or both*

1. Have you ever been stopped for driving while intoxicated (drunk, stoned, high)?
2. Have you ever been arrested for possession of drugs, burglary, vandalism, shoplifting, or breaking and entering?
3. Have you ever had to go to an emergency room or doctor's office for a drug-related accident or illness (overdose)?
4. Have you ever overdosed or intentionally tried to kill yourself?
5. Have your grades recently gone down?
6. Did you receive any F's on your last report card?
7. Have you been expelled from school?
8. Have you ever been intoxicated or high (stoned) at school?
9. Have you ever been caught at school for drug or alcohol possession?
10. Have any of your friends been admitted to a drug treatment center?
11. What drugs, if any, have you used in the past? How much?
12. What drugs, if any, are you currently using? How much?
13. Have you ever experienced "blackouts" while drinking heavily? (For example, have you awoken unable to remember what happened the night before?)
14. Has your alcohol or drug use caused problems with your friends and/or family?
15. Have you ever gotten into trouble at work or at school because of alcohol or drug use?
16. Do you often wake up with a "hangover"?

From Schonberg SK, ed. *Substance abuse: a guide for health professionals.* Elk Grove Village, IL: American Academy of Pediatrics; 1988.

TABLE 22. *Questionnaire for the parent(s) of the adolescent suspected of or known to be abusing drugs or alcohol or both*

1. Does your son/daughter spend many hours alone in his/her bedroom apparently doing nothing?
2. Does your son/daughter resist talking to you or persistently isolate himself/herself from the family?
3. Has your daughter's/son's taste in music had a dramatic change to hard rock music?
4. Has there been a definite change in your son's/daughter's attitude at school? With his/her friends? At home?
5. Has your daughter/son shown recent pronounced mood swings with increased irritability and angry outbursts?
6. Does your son/daughter always seem to be unhappy and less able to cope with frustration than he/she used to be?
7. Has your daughter's/son's personality changed from being a considerate and caring person to being selfish, unfriendly, and unsympathetic?
8. Does your son/daughter always seem to be confused or "spacey"?
9. Have money or valuable articles recently disappeared from your home?
10. Has your daughter/son begun to neglect household chores and homework?
11. Has there been a change in your son's/daughter's friends from age-appropriate friends to older, "unacceptable" associates?
12. Has there been a change in your daughter's/son's appearance (e.g., sloppy dress and poor grooming and hygiene)?
13. Have there been excuses and alibis made, and has there been lying to avoid confrontation or getting caught?
14. Do you feel you have lost control of your son/daughter?
15. Has your daughter/son begun lying to cover up sources of money and possessions?

From Schonberg SK, ed. *Substance abuse: a guide for health professionals.* Elk Grove Village, IL: American Academy of Pediatrics; 1988.

dren and adolescents than anyone could hope to care for in an individual practice. These guidelines for clinicians follow, in large part, the recent recommendations by the AAP Committee on Substance Abuse [131].

Treatment is the province of the drug and alcohol treatment professional. Primary care clinicians rarely have either the time or the expertise to get involved directly. However, they *can* play a role when their patients are being followed on an aftercare or outpatient treatment basis. In those situations, they can take the role of case manager and coordinate all aspects of the adolescent's care. In addition, clinicians should familiarize themselves with the drug and alcohol treatment programs in their areas so that they can decide which ones are truly qualified to care for adolescents and which are the most effective. The clinician should consider referring adolescents only to programs that recognize the developmental needs of adolescents, above and beyond just getting them detoxified. In addition, the clinician should ensure that the program to which he or she refers patients has qualified psychological or psychiatric consultants who can treat the psychological problems of the substance-abusing adolescent. The AAP has issued a series of guidelines for pediatricians for selection of substance abuse treatment programs [132].

The use, misuse, and abuse of illicit psychoactive chemicals by adolescents is a major problem in the United States today. It is the authors' hope that, with sufficient knowledge and skills, the practicing clinician will begin to appreciate the positive impact that he or she can have in this area.

REFERENCES

1. Johnston LD, O'Malley PM, Bachman JG. Drug use, drinking, and smoking: national survey results from high school, college, and young adult populations, 1975–1996. Rockville, MD: National Institute of Drug Abuse; 1996.
2. National Highway Traffic Safety Administration. *Fatal accident reporting system 1990: a review of information on fatal traffic crashes in the United States.* DOT HS 807 794. Washington, DC: U.S. Department of Transportation; December, 1991.
3. Brent DA, Perper JA, Allman CJ. Alcohol, firearms, and suicide among youth: temporal trends in Allegheny County, Pennsylvania, 1960 to 1983. *JAMA* 1987;257:3369.
4. Crumley FE. Substance abuse and adolescent suicidal behavior. *JAMA* 1990;263:3051.
5. Christoffel KK. Violent death and injury in U.S. children and adolescents. *American Journal of Diseases of Children* 1990;144:697.

6. National Institute of Justice Research Preview. *Youth violence, guns, and illicit drug markets.* Washington, DC: U.S. Department of Justice, Office of Justice Programs; December, 1995.

7. Dukarm CP, Byrd RS, Auinger P, et al. Illicit substance use, gender, and the risk of violent behavior among adolescents. *Arch Pediatr Adolesc Med* 1996;150:797.

8. Office of National Drug Control Policy. *National drug control strategy: executive summary.* Washington, DC: Executive Office of the President; April, 1995.

9. Strasburger VC. Prevention of adolescent drug abuse: why "Just Say No" just won't work. *J Pediatr* 1989;114:676.

10. Centers for Disease Control and Prevention. Cigarette advertising: United States, 1988.*MMWR Morb Mortal Wkly Rep* 1990;39:261.

11. Difranza JR, Tye JB. Who profits from tobacco sales to children? *JAMA* 1990;263:2784.

12. MacDonald DI. *Drugs, drinking, and adolescence.* Chicago: Year Book; 1984.

13. Gans JE, Blyth DA, Elster AE, et al. *America's adolescents: how healthy are they?* Vol. 1, AMA Profiles of Adolescent Health Series. Chicago, IL: American Medical Association; 1991.

14. Byrd RS, Weitzman M, Doniger AS. Increased drug use among old-for-grade adolescents. *Arch Pediatr Adolesc Med* 1996;150:470.

15. Kandel DB, Logan, JA. Patterns of drug use from adolescence to young adulthood: I. periods of risk for initiation, continued use, and discontinuation. *Am J Public Health* 1984;74:660.

16. MacDonald DI. Patterns of alcohol and drug use among adolescents. *Pediatr Clin North Am* 1987;34:275.

17. Comerci GD. Recognizing the five stages of substance abuse. *Contemporary Pediatrics* 1985;5:57.

18. Schwartz RH, Cohen PR, Bair GO. Identifying and coping with a drug-using adolescent: some guidelines for pediatricians and parents. *Pediatr Rev* 1985;7:133.

19. MacDonald DI. Substance abuse. *Pediatr Rev* 1988;10:89.

20. A Report of the Surgeon General. *Preventing tobacco use among young people.* Washington, DC: U.S Department of Health and Human Services; 1994.

21. Federal Trade Commission. *Report to Congress for 1993 pursuant to the Federal Cigaret Labeling and Advertising Act.* Washington, DC: Federal Trade Commission; 1995.

22. Federal Trade Commission. *Report to Congress pursuant to the Comprehensive Smokeless Tobacco Health Education Act of 1986.* Washington, DC: Federal Trade Commission; 1995.

23. Escabedo LG, Marcus SD, Holtzman D, et al. Sports participation, age at smoking initiation, and the risk of smoking among US high school students. *JAMA* 1993;269:1391.

24. Centers for Disease Control and Prevention. *Reducing the health consequences of smoking: 25 years of progress. A report of the Surgeon General.* DHHS Publication No. (CDC) 89-84 11. Washington, DC: U.S Department of Health and Human Services, Public Health Service; 1989.

25. Centers for Disease Control and Prevention. The Surgeon General's 1989 report on reducing the health consequences of smoking: 25 years of progress (executive summary). *MMWR Morb Mortal Wkly Rep* 1989;38(Suppl S-2).

26. Kessler DA. Nicotine addiction in young people [Sounding Board]. *N Engl J Med* 1995;333:186.

27. Fischer P, Schwartz M, Richards J, et al. Brand logo recognition by children aged 3 to 6 years. *JAMA* 1991;226:3145.

28. Pierce J, Gilpin E, Burns D, et al. Does tobacco advertising target young people to start smoking? *JAMA* 1991;226:3154.

29. Boyd G. Use of smokeless tobacco among children and adolescents in the United States. *Prev Med* 1987;16:402.

30. Marty PJ, McDermott RJ, Williams T. Patterns of smokeless tobacco use in a population of high school students. *Am J Public Health* 1986;76:190.

31. Ary DV, Lichtenstein E, Severson HH. Smokeless tobacco use among male adolescents: patterns, correlates, predictors and the use of other drugs. *Prev Med* 1987;16:385.

32. Schaefer SD, Henderson AH, Glover ED, et al. Patterns of use and incidence of smokeless tobacco consumption in school-age children. *Arch Otolaryngol* 1985;111:639.

33. Riley WT, Barenie JT, Myers DR. Typology and correlates of smokeless tobacco use. *Journal of Adolescent Health Care* 1989;10:357.

34. McGuirt WF. Snuff dipper's carcinoma. *Arch Otolaryngol* 1983;109:757.

35. Millman RB, Botvain GJ. Substance use, abuse and dependence. In: Levine MD, Carey WB, Crocker AC, et al, eds. *Developmental–behavioral pediatrics.* Philadelphia: WB Saunders; 1983:683.

36. Centers for Disease Control and Prevention. State laws on tobacco control: United States, 1995. *MMWR Morb Mortal Wkly Rep* 1995;44(Suppl SS-6).

37. Wechsler H, Davenport A, Dowdall G, et al. Health and behavioral consequences of binge drinking in college. *JAMA* 1994;272:1672.

38. Werner MJ, Walker LS, Greene JW. Concurrent and prospective screening for problem drinking among college students. *J Adolesc Health* 1996;18:276.

39. Wilkes J, Callan VJ. Similarity of university students' and their parents attitudes toward alcohol. *J Stud Alcohol* 1984;45:326.

40. Knop J, Goodwin DW, Jensen P, et al. A 30-year follow-up study of the sons of alcoholic men. *Acta Psychiatr Scand* 1993;370:48.

41. Harford TC, Parker DA, Grant BF. Family history: alcohol use and dependence symptoms among young adults in the United States. *Alcohol Clin Exp Res* 1992;16:1042.
42. Bloom MD, Greenwald MA. Alcohol and cigarette use among early adolescents. *Drug Education* 1984;14:195.
43. Kandel DB. On processes of peer influences in adolescent drug use: a developmental perspective. *Advances in Alcohol and Substance Abuse* 1985;4:139.
44. Zucker R, Developmental aspects of drinking through the young adult years. In: Blane HT, Chapetz M, eds. *Youth, alcohol, and social policy*. New York: Plenum Press; 1979:91.
45. Chassin L, Tetzloff C, Hershey M. Self-image and social-image factors in adolescent alcohol use. *J Stud Alcohol* 1985;46:39.
46. Smart RG, Gray G, Bennett C. Predictors of drinking and signs of heavy drinking among high school students. *Int J Addict* 1978;13:1079.
47. Futch EJ, Lisman SA, Geller MI. An analysis of alcohol portrayal on prime-time television. *Int J Addict* 1984;19:403.
48. Singer DG. Alcohol, television and teenagers. *Pediatrics* 1985;76:668.
49. Postman N, Nystrom C, Strate L, et al. *Myths, men, and beer: an analysis of beer commercials on broadcast television, 1987*. Washington, DC: AAA Foundation for Traffic Safety; 1988.
50. Kissin B. Alcohol abuse and alcohol-related illnesses. In: Wyngaarden J, Smith L, eds. *Cecil textbook of medicine*. Philadelphia: WB Saunders; 1988:48
51. Morrison SF, Rogers PD, Thomas MH. Alcohol and adolescents. *Pediatr Clin North Am* 1995;42:371.
52. Rogers PD, Harris J, Jarmuskewicz J. Alcohol and adolescence. *Pediatr Clin North Am* 1987;34:289.
53. Glueck CJ, Heiss G, Morrison JA, et al. Alcohol intake, cigarette smoking and plasma lipids and lipoproteins in 12-19 year old children. *Circulation* 1981;69(Suppl):48.
54. Muramoto ML, Leshan L. Adolescent substance abuse. Recognition and early intervention. *Prim Care* 1993;20(1):141–154.
55. Morrison MA, Smith QT. Psychiatric issues of adolescent chemical dependence. In: *ASAM review course syllabus*. 1990:542.
56. Deykin EY, Levy JC, Wells V. Adolescent depression, alcohol and drug abuse. *Am J Public Health* 1987;77:178.
57. Piombo M, Piles M. The relationship between college females drinking and their sexual behaviors. *Women's Health Issues* 1996;6:221.
58. Fergusson DM, Lynskey MT. Alcohol misuse and adolescent sexual behaviors and risk taking. *Pediatrics* 1996;98:91.
59. Centers for Disease Control and Prevention. Update: alcohol-related traffic fatalities: United States, 1982–1993. *JAMA* 1994;272:1892.
60. Centers for Disease Control and Prevention. Update: Alcohol-related traffic crashes and fatalities among youth: United States, 1982–1994. *JAMA* 1995;274:1904.
61. Public Health Service. *Healthy people 2000: national health promotion and disease prevention objectives*. Washington, DC: U.S. Department of Health and Human Services, Public Health Service, Centers for Disease Control and Prevention; 1990.
62. Mikuriya TH. Historical aspects of Cannabis sativa in western medicine. *New Physician* 1969;18:902.
63. Schwartz RH. Marijuana: an overview. *Pediatr Clin North Am* 1987;34:305.
64. Moskowitz H. Marijuana and driving. *Accid Anal Prevent* 1976;8:21.
65. Moskowitz H, Peterson R. *Marijuana and driving: a review*. Rockville, MD: American Council on Marijuana and Other Psychoactive Drugs; 1982.
66. Moskowitz H, Sharma S, Zieman K. Duration of skills performance impairment. In: *Proceedings of the twenty-fifth conference of the American Association for Automotive Medicine, San Francisco, California*. 1981:87.
67. Pope HG, Yurgelun-Todd D. The residual cognitive effects of heavy marijuana use in college students. *JAMA* 1996;275:52.
68. Tashkin DP, Calvarese BM, Simmons MS, et al. Respiratory status of seventy-four habitual marijuana smokers. *Chest* 1980;78:699.
69. Morris RRL. Human pulmonary histopathology changes from marijuana smoking. *J Forensic Sci* 1985;30:345.
70. Wu T-C, Tashkin DP, Djahed B, et al. Pulmonary hazards of smoking marijuana as compared with tobacco. *N Engl J Med* 1988;318:347.
71. Dahl RE, Scher MS, Willimason DE, et al. A longitudinal study of prenatal marijuana use. *Arch Pediatr Adolesc Med* 1995;149:145.
72. White PT. Coca. *National Geographic* 1989;175(1):6.
73. Gawin FH, Ellinwood EH Jr. Cocaine and other stimulants. *N Engl J Med* 1988;318:1173.
74. Nathanson MH. The central action of beta-aminopropylbenzene (Benzedrine). *JAMA* 1937;108:528.
75. Lasagna L, von Felsinger JM, Beecher HK. Drug-induced mood changes in man: I. observations on healthy subjects, chronically ill patients, and postaddicts. *JAMA* 1955;157:1006.
76. VanDyke C, Ungerer J, Jatlow P, et al. Intranasal cocaine: dose relationships of psychological effects and plasma levels. *Int J Psychiatry Med* 1982;12:1.

77. Mendelson JH, Mellon K. Management of cocaine abuse and dependence. *N Engl J Med* 1996;334:965.

78. Cohen S. The cocaine problems. *Drug Abuse and Alcoholism Newsletter* 1983;12(10).

79. National Institute on Drug Abuse. *Epidemiologic trends in drug abuse. Vol. 1. Highlights and executive summary.* NIH Publication No. 95-3988. Washington, DC: Government Printing Office; 1995.

80. Hollander JE. The management of cocaine-associated myocardial ischemia. *N Engl J Med* 1995;333:1267.

81. Farrar HC, Kearns GL. Cocaine: clinical pharmacology and toxicology. *J Pediatr* 1989;113:665.

82. Tarr JE, Macklin M. Cocaine. *Pediatr Clin North Am* 1987;34:319.

83. Leshner AI. Molecular mechanisms of cocaine addiction. *N Engl J Med* 1996;335:128.

84. King P, Coleman JH. Stimulants and narcotic drugs. *Pediatr Clin North Am* 1987;34:349.

85. King J. Hypertension and cerebral hemorrhage after Timolets ingestion. *Med J Aust* 1979;2:258.

86. Bernstein E, Diskant B. Phenylpropanolamine, a potentially hazardous drug. *Ann Emerg Med* 1982;11:311.

87. Johnson DA, Etter HS, Reeves PM. Stroke and phenylpropanolamine use. *Lancet* 1983;2:970.

88. Kizer K. Intracranial hemorrhage associated with overdose of decongestant containing phenylpropanolamine. *Am J Emerg Med* 1984;2:180.

89. Mesnard JR, Ginn DR. Excessive phenylpropanolamine ingestion followed by subarachnoid hemorrhage. *South Med J* 1984;77:939.

90. Kikta DG, Devereaux MW, Krishan C. Intracranial hemorrhages due to phenylpropanolamine. *Stroke* 1985;16:510.

91. McDowell JR, LeBlanc HJ. Phenylpropanolamine and cerebral hemorrhage. *West J Med* 1985;142:688.

92. Forman HP, Levin S, Stewart B, et al. Cerebral vasculitis and hemorrhage in an adolescent taking diet pills containing phenylpropanolamine: case report and review of literature. *Pediatrics* 1989;83:737.

93. Fallis RJ, Fisher M. Cerebral vasculitis and hemorrhage associated with phenylpropanolamine. *Neurology* 1985;35:405.

94. Jerrard DA. Designer drugs: a current perspective. *J Emerg Med* 1990;8:733.

95. Ruttenber AJ. Stalking the elusive designer drugs: techniques for monitoring new problems in drug use. *J Addict Dis* 1991;11:71.

96. Randall T. Ecstasy-fueled rave parties become dances of death for English youths. *JAMA* 1992;268:1505.

97. Strassman RJ. Adverse reactions to psychedelic drugs: a review of the literature. *J Nerv Ment Dis* 1984;172:577.

98. Cohen S. The hallucinogens and the inhalants. *Psychiatr Clin North Am* 1984;7:681.

99. Schwartz RH. LSD makes a comeback. *Contemporary Pediatrics* 1996;13:71.

100. Levy R. Jimson weed poisoning: a new hallucinogen on the horizon. *Journal of the American College of Emergency Physicians* 1977;6:58.

101. Mahler D. The jimsonweed high. *JAMA* 1975;231:138.

102. Savott D, Roberts J, Siegel E. Anisocoria from jimsonweed. *JAMA* 1986;255:11.

103. Shervette R, Schydlower M, Lampe R, et al. Jimson "loco" weed abuse in adolescents. *Pediatrics* 1979;63:520.

104. Silber TJ, Iosefsohn M, Hicks JM, et al. Prevalence of PCP use among adolescent marijuana users. *J Pediatr* 1988;112:827.

105. Brown RT, Braden NJ. Hallucinogens. *Pediatr Clin North Am* 1987;34:341—347.

106. Hall AH, Kulig KW, Rumack BH. Acute management of common illicit drug intoxications. *Seminars in Adolescent Medicine* 1985;1:264.

107. Ungerleider J, DeAngelis GG. Hallucinogens. In: Lowinson J, Ruiz P, eds. *Substance abuse: clinical problems and perspectives.* Baltimore: Williams & Wilkins; 1981:154.

108. McHugh MJ. The abuse of volatile substances. *Pediatr Clin North Am* 1987;34:333.

109. Cohen S. Inhalant abuse: an overview of the problem. In: Sharp CW, Brehm ML, eds. *Review of inhalants: euphoria to dysfunction.* NIDA Monograph 15. Washington, DC: U.S. Government Printing Office; 1977:2.

110. Barnes GEL. Solvent abuse: a review. *Int J Addict* 1979;14:1.

111. Kulberg A. Substance abuse: clinical identification and management. *Pediatr Clin North Am* 1986;33:325.

112. Wyse DG. Deliberate inhalation of volatile hydrocarbons: a review. *Can Med Assoc J* 1973;108(1):71–74.

113. Henretig F. Inhalant abuse in children and adolescents. *Pediatr Ann* 1996;25:47.

114. Ford M, Hoffman RS, Goldfrank LR. Opioids and designer drugs. *Emerg Med Clin North Am* 1990;8:495.

115. McCurdy HH, Solomons ET, Holbrook J. Incidence of methaqualone in driving-under-the-influence (DUI) cases in the State of Georgia. *J Anal Toxicol* 1981;5:270.

116. Bailey DN. Methaqualone ingestion: present status. *J Anal Toxicol* 1981;5:279.

117. Gitelson S. Methaqualone–meprobamate poisoning. *JAMA* 1967;201:977.

118. Coleman JB, Barone JA. Abuse potential of methaqualone–diphenhydramine combination. *Am J Hosp Pharm* 1981;38:160.

119. Felter R, Izsak E, Lawrence HS. Emergency department management of the intoxicated adolescent. *Pediatr Clin North Am* 1987;34:399.

120. The Associated Press. House Oks penalty for using date-rape drugs. *The Columbus Dispatch*, October 5, 1996.

121. American Academy of Pediatrics, Committee on Substance Abuse. Testing for drugs of abuse in children and adolescents. *Pediatrics* 1996;98:305.
122. *Vernonia School District. 47J v Acton*, 94-590 Sct (9th Cir 1995).
123. MacKenzie RG, Cheng M, Haftel AJ. The clinical utility and evaluation of drug screening techniques. *Pediatr Clin North Am* 1987;34:423.
124. Hoffmann NG, Mee-Lee D, Arrowod AA. Treatment issues in adolescent substance use and addictions: options, outcome, effectiveness, reimbursement, and admission criteria. *Adolescent Medicine: State of the Art Reviews* 1993;4:371.
125. Mieczkowski T. *Hair analysis as a drug detector.* Washington, DC: U.S. Department of Justice, Office of Justice Programs, National Institute of Justice; October, 1995.
126. Hamilton K, Springen K, Kalb C. Dusting for kids' dope. *Newsweek* 1995;April 24:69.
127. Zarek D, Hawkins JD, Rogers PD. Risk factors for adolescent substance abuse: implications for pediatric practice. *Pediatr Clin North Am* 1987;34:481.
128. Levitt MZ, Selman RL, Richmond JB. The psychosocial foundations of early adolescents high-risk behavior: implications for research and practice. *Journal of Research on Adolescence* 1991;1:349.
129. Klein JD. Incorporating effective smoking prevention and cessation counseling into practice. *Pediatr Ann* 1995;24:646.
130. Ennet ST, Rosenbaum DP, Flewelling RL, et al. Long-term evaluation of drug abuse resistance education. *Addict Behav* 1994;19:113.
131. American Academy of Pediatrics, Committee on Substance Abuse. Role of the pediatrician in prevention and management of substance abuse. *Pediatrics* 1993;91:1010 .
132. Provisional Committee on Substance Abuse. Selection of substance abuse treatment programs. *Pediatrics* 1990;86:139.

SUGGESTED READING

Bergmann PE, Smith MD, Hoffmann NG. Adolescent treatment: implications for assessment, practice guidelines, and outcome management. *Pediatr Clin North Am* 1995;42:453.

Brown RT, Coupey SM. Illicit drugs of abuse. *Adolescent Medicine: State of the Art Reviews* 1993;4:321.

Committee on Substance Abuse, American Academy of Pediatrics. Role of the pediatrician in prevention and management of substance abuse. *Pediatrics* 1993;91:1010,.

Fergusson DM, Lynskey MT. Alcohol misuse and adolescent sexual behaviors and risk taking. *Pediatrics* 1996;98:91.

Gans JE, Shook KL, eds. *Policy compendium on tobacco, alcohol, and other harmful substances affecting adolescents: alcohol and other harmful substances.* Chicago: American Medical Association; 1994.

Henningfield JE. Nicotine medications for smoking cessation. *N Engl J Med* 1995;333:1196.

Henretig F. Inhalant abuse in children and adolescents. *Pediatr Ann* 1996;25:47.

Keller DA. Nicotine addiction in young people. *N Engl J Med* 1995;333:186.

Klein JD. Incorporating effective smoking prevention and cessation counseling into practice. *Pediatr Ann* 1995;24:646.

Knight JR. Adolescent substance use: screening, assessment, and intervention. *Contemporary Pediatrics* 1997;14:45.

Mendelson JH, Mellon K. Management of cocaine abuse and dependence. *N Engl J Med* 1996;334:965.

Morrison SF, Rogers PD, Thomas NJ. Alcohol and adolescents. *Pediatr Clin North Am* 1995;42:371.

Office of National Drug Control Policy. *National drug control strategy: executive summary.* Washington, DC: Executive Office of the President; April, 1995.

O'Malley PM, Johnston LD, Boehman JG. Adolescent substance abuse: epidemiology and implications for public policy. *Pediatr Clin North Am* 1995;42:241.

Schoemer K. Rockers, models, and the new allure of heroin. *Newsweek* 1996;August 26:50.

Schwartz RH. LSD makes a comeback. *Contemporary Pediatrics* 1996;13:71.

Strasburger VC. Prevention of adolescent drug abuse: why "Just Say No" just won't work. *J Pediatr* 1989;114:676.

Strasburger VC. Adolescents, drugs, and the media. *Adolescent Medicine: State of the Art Reviews* 1993;4:391.

The Medical Letter. Acute reactions to drugs of abuse. *The Medical Letter* 1996;38:43.

Werner MJ, Adger H Jr. Early identification, screening, and brief intervention for adolescent alcohol use. *Arch Pediatr Adolesc Med* 1995;149:1241.

White PT. Coca. *National Geographic* 1989;175(1):6.

Woolf AD, Shannon MW. Clinical toxicology for the pediatrician. *Pediatr Clin North Am* 1995;42:317.

9

Legal Issues

As if mastering the clinical aspects of adolescent medicine were not difficult enough, physicians must also contend with the complexities of the American legal system. Many physicians are concerned about the apparent epidemic of malpractice suits that currently exists (although pediatricians are far less likely to be sued than most other physicians). In a 1982 study of Connecticut pediatricians in practice, nearly two thirds expressed some or great concern about the legal aspects of treating adolescent patients [1]. Others may be too busy to investigate their own state's laws and regulations. For instance, the same survey revealed that only 1 of 79 physicians could correctly answer 17 true-or-false questions about common medicolegal concerns [1]. Fortunately, there is good news in the field of adolescent medicine and the law. By observing the following important general principles, physicians can successfully treat adolescents without incurring major legal risks:

1. Know the law, especially state agency regulations and state statutes.
2. Consult with local attorneys, state legal societies, hospital attorneys, and others if specific questions arise.
3. Document information carefully and thoroughly in the patient's chart. In malpractice cases, if something is not documented in the chart, it did not happen.
4. Never hesitate to obtain a second opinion, if needed.
5. When in doubt, do what is best for the patient. Such a strategy is unlikely to place a practitioner in legal jeopardy, because that is how the courts typically view the physician's role in providing good health care.

These principles notwithstanding, the reader is cautioned that this chapter is not intended to give specific legal advice. If legal advice is required, the services of a knowledgeable attorney should be sought.

Confidentiality

No single issue affects the clinician's ability to attract teenagers into his or her practice more than *confidentiality*. It is paramount in the minds of adolescent patients, even if they are being seen for a trivial illness, and must be dealt with in a forthright fashion [2–5].

In a 1993 survey of nearly 1,300 9th through 12th graders, 58% reported having health concerns that they wished to keep private from their parents, and 25% reported that they would forego health care in some situations if it meant their parents might find out. Although 86% said that they would go to their regular physician for a physical illness, only 57% would go for pregnancy, acquired immunodeficiency syndrome, or substance abuse concerns (Tables 1, 2). Finally, two thirds had concerns about the privacy of a school-based clinic [3]. Physician assurances of confidentiality do increase adolescents' willingness to disclose sensitive information regarding sex, substance abuse, and mental health issues [4]. However, only 56% of 1,210 primary care physicians in California reported discussing confidentiality with their patients. Female physicians and gynecologists were more likely to discuss it than other primary care physicians [5].

Increasingly, the courts, legislatures, and state agencies have recognized the adolescent's right to confidential health care [6]. Rather than representing an altruistic philosophy or extreme concern about adolescents' welfare, this policy is extremely practical and public health oriented: if a teenager believes that the physician will phone his or her parents after the teen leaves the office, he or she will

TABLE 1. *Perceptions of adolescents regarding health care*

Survey item	Yes	No
"There are some health concerns that I would not want my parents to know."	58%	39%
"There are some health concerns that I would not want my friends and classmates to know."	69%	28%
"Would you ever not go for health care because your parents might find out?"	25%	73%
"Since becoming a teenager, when you have gone to get health care has anyone talked to you about privacy?"	44%	54%

Adapted from Cheng TL, Savageau JA, Sattler AL, et al. Confidentiality in health care: a survey of knowledge, perceptions, and attitudes among high school students. *JAMA* 1993;269:1404.

not seek medical attention. From the public health perspective—with alarming numbers of teenage pregnancies, infections with sexually transmitted diseases (STDs), and widespread drug abuse—this is simply bad practice.

In 1989, the American Academy of Pediatrics, the American Academy of Family Physicians, and the American College of Obstetricians and Gynecologists joined together in a policy statement that says that all adolescents should "have an opportunity for examination and counseling apart from parents and the same confidentiality [should] be preserved between the adolescent patient and the provider as between the parent/adult and the provider" [7]. The American Medical Association joined the others in 1993 [8] (Table 3). This does *not* mean that physicians cannot or should not encourage adolescent patients to discuss medical problems, including sexual activity, pregnancy, abortion, or drug use, with their parents. It is also not an absolute privilege: confidentiality should be breached if the teenager is deemed at significant risk for harming himself or herself or others. Interestingly, in the case of depressed teenagers who may be contemplating suicide, breaching confidentiality may not alienate them as patients. However, in other situations (e.g., telling a 15-year-old's parents that she came in and asked for oral contraceptives) breaching confidentiality will result not only in loss of that particular patient, but in many more potential adolescent patients as well once the news is spread by word-of-mouth.

TABLE 2. *Attitudes of adolescents regarding confidentiality*

Health issue	Yes, should keep private	No, should not keep private
Having sex	78%	19%
Homosexuality	57%	38%
Pregnancy	56%	40%
Sexually transmitted disease	46%	50%
AIDS/human immunodeficiency virus infection	35%	60%
Alcohol/drug problem	35%	62%
Plan to run away	32%	66%
Sexual abuse	20%	77%
Physical abuse	18%	78%
Plan to commit suicide	15%	82%

Adapted from Cheng TL, Savageau JA, Sattler, AL, et al. Confidentiality in health care: a survey of knowledge, perceptions, and attitudes among high school students. *JAMA* 1993;269:1404.

TABLE 3. *Confidential health care: office practice and policies*

1. Routinely see teenagers alone for at least part of each office visit.
2. Periodically assess high-risk health behaviors.
3. Incorporate counseling on high-risk health behaviors into routine visits.
4. Decide whether gynecologic care will be done by the practitioner or by referral. If by referral, ensure that confidentiality will be maintained by the referral resource as well.
5. Routinely discuss confidential health care with the adolescent and whether parental involvement is possible.
6. Establish office procedures for adolescents to make their own appointments.
7. Establish alternative billing and payment options.
8. Train office personnel to be sensitive to adolescents.
9. Establish procedures to protect confidential information in the patient's chart, including the possibility of dual records.
10. Develop a list of low-cost referral resources, including Planned Parenthood clinics, community clinics for adolescents, and the like.

From Hofmann AD. Consent and confidentiality: critical issues in providing contraceptive care. In: Strasburger VC, ed. *Basic adolescent gynecology: an office guide.* Baltimore: Urban & Schwarzenberg, 1990:59. With permission.

Confidentiality also is routinely breached in reporting cases of STDs to the public health department, for example, and patients should be informed about this. However, reporting information to third-party payers should be done with sensitivity and caution, because parents will almost certainly see such information.

The easiest and most painless way to establish these principles in a clinical practice is to do it expectantly, when a child reaches age 10 or 12 years, rather than waiting for the issue to arise in a crisis situation. A form letter can be sent to parents informing them that their child, beginning with the 12th birthday, will begin qualifying for confidential adolescent health care [9] (see Chapter 5, this volume). This does not mean that "anything goes," but rather that the physician will be acting *in loco parentis*, in the best interests of both parent *and* child. Most parents will find this extremely reassuring—especially when they cannot yet conceive of *their* child having major problems—because they would undoubtedly rather have their teenager treated for an STD, for example, than have him or her suffer irreparable harm.

In actual practice, the issue of confidentiality usually does not arise except around sensitive issues such as sexual activity and drug use [10]. Nonetheless, the issue should be discussed early with both parents and adolescents, and adolescents should be informed in a way that they will understand (e.g., "Whatever you tell me will stay in this room, between us, unless you tell me that you are going to harm yourself or someone else"). Physicians can also use a variety of office practice techniques to ensure that confidential care will be provided and respected (Table 4). When it is established in advance, confidentiality is usually respected. Parents may call the physician to learn about a teenager's visit, but they will be more curious than angry. A simple reminder will then suffice, or a suggestion can be made to ask their son or daughter. On the other hand, if the parents first hear about confidential health

TABLE 4. *Recommendations for confidential health care for adolescents*

- Confidential health care for adolescents is essential.
- Physicians should allow emancipated and mature minors to consent for their own treatment.
- Physicians should involve parents in the medical care of their adolescents when it is in the best interests of the adolescent. When it is not, parental consent or notification should not be a barrier to care.
- Physicians should discuss their policies about confidentiality with parents and the adolescent patient.
- State and county medical societies should play a more active role in supporting confidential health services for teenagers. They also need to work to eliminate laws that restrict such care.
- Medical schools and training programs need to educate students and residents about issues surrounding consent and confidential health care.
- Health care financers need to develop systems that preserve confidentiality for adolescents.

Adapted from Council on Scientific Affairs, American Medical Association. Confidential health services for adolescents. *JAMA* 1993;269:1420.

care when they accidentally discover their daughter's packet of oral contraceptives, angry and threatening phone calls may ensue. In this situation, the physician should empathize with the parents' anger and immediately set up an appointment with the parents and teenager the next day to discuss the situation. After an overnight cooling-off period, the session can be directed more toward the problem—intergenerational conflict—and away from angry accusations against the physician [11].

Issues of Consent

Until the 1960s, in Western civilization, children and adolescents were viewed as the "property" of their parents [10]. As such, they could never consent to their own medical treatment. Since the 1960s, an increasing amount of legal attention has been directed to teenagers' legal rights within the health care system. As a general rule, parental consent for a minor (below the age of majority [i.e., 18 years old]) is always preferable, especially because it makes insurance reimbursement or billing more feasible. Nevertheless, many special circumstances have evolved in which consent may be obtained from a minor without parental consent or notification [10,12–14]. These circumstances may be delineated by state statute [15], executive order, regulations issued by state agencies, case law, or federal law. In instances where state and federal law conflict, the latter takes precedence [16].

Emergency Care

State laws are uniform in permitting emergency care to minors without parental consent [17]. How *emergency* is defined may vary from state to state, but, in general, the courts give wide latitude to the health professional, especially if documented efforts have been made to contact the parents. In particular, the emergency does not necessarily have to involve a threat to life or limb. It may involve pain or well-being. For example, if a teenager is involved in a motor vehicle accident and has a broken leg that requires reduction or a bleeding laceration that requires suturing, the physician should opt for doing what is best for the patient because that usually represents the wisest legal course as well [18].

Emancipated Minors

In certain instances, minors are considered to be emancipated from their parents and therefore capable of consenting to health care themselves. These circumstances may vary from state to state, but generally include a teenager who is:

- A member of the armed forces
- The parent of a child
- Married, widowed, or divorced
- Living separately from and financially independent of his or her parents
- Formally emancipated by virtue of a court order

In addition, a condition of *relative* emancipation exists when the minor's health is endangered and the state wishes to encourage intervention [6]. Virtually all states in the United States have statutes or regulations that permit a minor to consent for treatment related to [10]:

- Pregnancy
- Sexually transmitted disease (some states specify that this includes testing for human immunodeficiency virus; others have specific regulations or statutes permitting confidential testing [14])
- Alcohol or drug dependency

In such situations, consent for treatment covers only the specific condition involved. Clinicians must be careful not to bill the teenager's parents for such visits.

Mature Minors

Even in the absence of a minor consent statute, there have not been any judgments since 1955 in which a parent has recovered damages for treatment of a mature child, 15 years of age or older, who has given an informed consent [10]. This is because of the judicial doctrine of the "mature minor" that has evolved since the early 1970s [12]. Simply stated, a mature minor is one who is near the age of consent (i.e., 14–15 years or older) and who is capable of understanding the risks and benefits of any medical treatment and therefore can give an informed consent. The reasoning behind the doctrine is that a person who is 17 years and 364 days of age (a minor) possesses the same judgment capabilities as one who is 18 years and 1 day of age (an adult). In addition, numerous studies have shown that decision making by older adolescents is likely to be as competent as that of adults [13].

Determining the maturity of a minor has usually been left to the discretion of the physician. Clearly, a 14-year-old who is developmentally delayed and in the fourth grade at school would not qualify, but a 15-year-old who is a straight-A student in ninth grade, makes her own appointment, and wants to discuss the fact that she and her boyfriend may begin having sexual intercourse and need appropriate contraception, would certainly qualify. If there is any question in the physician's mind, a second opinion should be sought. Care should be exercised to document all of the circumstances in the case, including the medical situation and efforts made to contact the family, or reasons for not contacting them. In addition, the treatment should be necessary according to conservative medical opinion and be undertaken for the patient's benefit—not, for example, an organ donation or participation in a medical experiment that involves some element of risk. The minor should also be as fully informed as an adult would be and, when appropriate, sign a consent form as well.

Contraception

Practically speaking, the issue of adolescents' legal rights and their ability to consent for treatment arises only surrounding the areas of sexual activity and drug abuse [10]. Otherwise, although a 15-year-old mature minor certainly could agree to a hospitalization for a tonsillectomy, for example, no hospital admitting office would accept his consent alone for fear that the insurance company would not pay for the admission.

Numerous studies in the 1980s have shown that confidential health care is crucial if teenagers are to use family planning services [19–24]. Between one third and one half of teenagers state that they would not come to the clinic if their parents were informed. Of these, most would continue having intercourse but would use a less effective method of birth control; only 2% would stop having sex [19,20]. Another study revealed that although most teens were actually using contraceptives with at least one of their parents' knowledge, only 43% felt that they could communicate with their parents about sexual issues [20].

Interestingly, *adults* have only had the legal right to use contraception since 1965. In that year, the Supreme Court struck down a Connecticut law that made the prescription or use of contraceptives a criminal offense and asserted that adults have a constitutional "right to privacy," which includes the use of birth control [25]. In *Carey v. Population Services*, the Supreme Court held that the "right of privacy in connection with decisions affecting procreating extends to minors as well as to adults" [26]. The case overturned a New York statute that made it a criminal offense for drugstores to sell contraceptives to minors, regardless of age. In that opinion, Mr. Justice Stevens discussed the state's attempt to legislate public morality:

> Although the state may properly perform a teaching function, it seems to me that an attempt to persuade by inflicting harm on the listener is an unacceptable means of conveying a message that is otherwise legitimate . . . . It is as though a State decided to dramatize its disapproval of motorcycles by forbidding the use of safety helmets [26, p. 715].

More recently, a federal court of appeals in Michigan held in the case of *Doe v. Irwin* that a state-supported family planning clinic for adolescents was under no obligation to notify parents or obtain their consent before prescribing contraceptives to teenagers [27]. Further support for this principle can be found in federal regulations governing programs that receive funding under Title XIX and XX of the Social Security Act and Title X of the Family Planning Services Act [11]. In addition, about half of all states in the United States have specific statutes specifying that minors can consent for their own contraceptive care [15].

Most recently, the U.S. Supreme Court refused to overturn *Curtis v. School Committee of Falmouth*, a lower court decision that upheld the Falmouth, Massachusetts school district's decision to make condoms available in high schools [28]. (Most school-based clinics use a blanket parental permission form, however [13].) Opponents had argued that the program violated parents' rights and hindered families' religious freedom.

Therefore, it is currently safe to say that adolescents can be provided confidential birth control services on their own in any jurisdiction in the United States [11,17]. *No physician has ever been successfully sued for providing contraception to a minor; nor is there a record of such suits even being brought* [18]. (This may be because a lawsuit is a matter of public record, and no parent wants to advertise that his or her teenage daughter has been taking oral contraceptives.) An adolescent seeking contraception at a federally funded clinic has a constitutional right to obtain it. In an office setting, a private practitioner has the right to refuse to provide such treatment but incurs the obligation to refer the patient to an appropriate Planned Parenthood or public clinic [10]. Parental involvement is always desirable in such situations; however, parental notification is *not permissible* without the adolescent's knowledge and consent.

The issue of "immature minors" is somewhat moot: When 12- and 13-year-olds are sexually active, it is most often in the context of severe family dysfunction and adolescent acting-out behavior, and often the mother is aware or at least suspicious. In cases of suspected child abuse, however, all practitioners have a legal obligation to report their suspicions to the local health authorities [10]. (In return, they are immune from lawsuits brought by the parents.) A few states have tried to restrain adolescents from early sexual activity by requiring health personnel to report them. However, such attempts are invariably enjoined by the courts and have been unsuccessful to date [11]. Statutory rape laws do continue to apply to male partners. Most often, the girl's parents bring criminal charges against the partner. In such instances, physicians are not *required* to report cases to local authorities [11].

Finally, the Reagan Administration's attempt at a "squeal rule"—mandating that federally funded clinics must inform parents if teenagers seek birth control services—was enjoined in two federal courts of appeal in 1983 and later dropped [29,30].

Abortion

Abortion law is currently a battleground in the United States. Caught in the crossfire are America's teenagers—who account for 1.1 million pregnancies a year and 21% of all abortions [31]. If all the time, energy, and money fueling the debate were spent instead on preventing adolescent pregnancy, far more could be accomplished. At present, it is entirely possible that the controversy will have a significant chilling effect on adolescents, not only those seeking abortions, but those wanting to prevent pregnancy as well. According to a large 1992 study, most (61%) young women seeking abortions do so with their parents' knowledge (see Chapter 5, this volume). Of those who do not inform their parents, 30% have experienced violence at home, feared that violence would occur, or were afraid of being forced to leave home [32]. If abortions were banned altogether, one study estimates an additional 75,000 teen births in the United States per year [33].

A number of Supreme Court decisions in the 1970s and 1980s have delineated adolescents' rights in this area. Beginning with *Planned Parenthood of Central Missouri v. Danforth* in 1976, 3 years after *Roe v. Wade*, the Court stated that minors who were mature enough to become pregnant were also mature enough to be able to consent to an abortion [34]. However, the Court also pointed out that it was not giving teenagers blanket permission for abortion, "regardless of age or maturity." *In Bellotti v. Baird* in 1976 and 1979, the Court spelled out its current criteria for laws that *are* permissible regarding adolescents' right to consent for abortions:

> Every minor must have the opportunity—if she so desires—to go directly to a court without first consulting or notifying her parents. If she satisfies that court that she is mature and well enough informed to make intelligently the abortion decision on her own, the court must authorize her to act without parental consultation or consent. If she fails to satisfy the court that she is competent to make this decision independently, she must be permitted to show that an abortion nonetheless would be in her best interests. If the court is persuaded that it is, the court must authorize the abortion [35,36].

The Supreme Court reaffirmed this stance in 1983 in two further cases [37,38]. Basically, a state may require parental consent for abortion but *only* if it provides for this judicial bypass procedure as well. In states that have no specific statutes, the adolescent may consent to an abortion under the same guidelines as mature minors seeking medical treatment [10].

Parental *notification* about an adolescent's abortion is a related issue and is also extremely controversial. In *H.L. v. Matheson* in 1981, the Court upheld a Utah law that required notification of parents of an unemancipated, unmarried minor before an abortion is performed [39]. However, the ruling was actually quite limited in scope. The adolescent involved in the case made no claim to "mature minor" status; nor did the statute go any further than requiring a physician to give notice to parents "if possible" before performing an abortion [40]. Therefore, it appears that parental notification statutes will have to adhere to the same judicial bypass guidelines as parental consent statutes. Finally, emancipated minors unquestionably can give consent for their own abortion.

Although the Supreme Court's 1989 *Webster* decision was viewed as chipping away at abortion rights, it did not affect adolescents. Two more recent cases before the Court—*Hodgeson v. Minnesota* and *Ohio v. Akron Center for Reproductive Health*—have delineated the Court's thinking more clearly: states *can* require that a teenager notify both her parents before having an abortion as long as a judicial alternative exists (the decision in *Hodgeson*). Similarly, state laws that require notification of only one parent are also acceptable, as long as there is a judicial bypass system in place (*Ohio*) [41–43]. What remains unclear is whether a state can require notification of one parent without providing for a judicial bypass system [43]. To date, 33 states have some sort of parental notification laws, although in the past they have been variably enforced. In the absence of such a law in a physician's own state, no notification is necessary.

Do parental notification or consent laws work? Mississippi data for 1993 indicate that the state's parental consent requirement had little effect on abortion rates among teenagers except to increase the number of second trimester abortions [44]. Likewise, a Minnesota parental notification law increased late abortions; however, it did seem to decrease the rate of first trimester abortions [45]. Many physicians and organizations, including the American Academy of Pediatrics, believe that legislation that mandates parental involvement is counterproductive: not only does it fail to achieve better family communication, it is potentially harmful to high-risk teens and delays access to appropriate medical care [46].

REFERENCES

1. Strasburger VC, Eisner JM. Teenagers, physicians, and the law in Connecticut, 1982.*Conn Med* 1982;46:80.
2. Alan Guttmacher Institute. *Teenage pregnancy: the problem that hasn't gone away.* New York: Alan Guttmacher Institute; 1981.
3. Cheng TL, Savageau JA, Sattler AL, et al. Confidentiality in health care: a survey of knowledge, perceptions, and attitudes among high school students. *JAMA* 1993;269:1404.
4. Ford CA, Millstein SG, Halpern-Feisher B, et al. Confidentiality and adolescents' disclosure of sensitive information [Abstract]. *J Adolesc Health* 1996;18:111.
5. Ford CA, Millstein SG. Delivery of confidentiality assurances to adolescents by primary care physicians [Abstract]. *J Adolesc Health* 1996;18:112.
6. Gans JE, ed. *Confidential health services for adolescents.* Chicago: American Medical Association; 1993.
7. American Academy of Pediatrics. Policy statement: confidentiality in adolescent health care. *AAP News* 1989;April:9.
8. Council on Scientific Affairs, American Medical Association. Confidential health services for adolescents. *JAMA* 1993;269:1420.
9. Tolmas HC. Solutions: the role of the private practitioner. I. Continuity and communication. *Adolescent Medicine: State of the Art Reviews* 1990;1:145.
10. Holder AR. Legal issues in adolescent sexual health. *Adolescent Medicine: State of the Art Reviews* 1992;3:257.
11. Hofmann AD. Consent and confidentiality: critical issues in providing contraceptive care. In: Strasburger VC, ed. *Basic adolescent gynecology: an office guide.* Baltimore: Urban & Schwarzenberg; 1990:59.
12. Sigman GS, O'Connor C. Exploration for physicians of the mature minor doctrine. *J Pediatr* 1991;119:520.
13. Weisz VP, Melton GB. Legal issues in adolescent health care. In: Wallander JL, Siegel LJ, eds. *Adolescent health problems: behavioral perspectives.* New York: Guilford Press; 1995:72.
14. English A. Consent and confidentiality: adolescents' access to HIV services. *Family Life Educator* 1996;14:4.
15. National Center for Youth Law. *State minor consent statutes: a summary.* Cincinnati, OH: Center for Continuing Education in Adolescent Health; 1995.
16. Bourne R. Legal issues in pediatric and adolescent gynecology. In: Emans SJH, Goldstein DP, eds. *Pediatric and adolescent gynecology.* 3rd ed. Boston: Little, Brown; 1990:569.
17. Holder AR. *Legal issues in pediatrics and adolescent medicine.* 2nd ed. New Haven: Yale University Press; 1985.
18. Holder AR. Minors' right to consent to medical care. *JAMA* 1987;257:3400.
19. Torres A. Telling parents: clinic policies and adolescents' use of family planning and abortion services. *Fam Plann Perspect* 1980;12:284.
20. Demetriou E, Kaplan DW. Adolescent contraceptive use and parental notification. *American Journal of Diseases of Children* 1989;143:1166.
21. Zabin LS, Clark SD Jr. Why they delay: a study of teenage family planning clinics. *Fam Plann Perspect* 1981;13:205.
22. Zabin LS, Clark SD Jr. Institutional facts affecting teenagers' choice and reasons for delay in attending a family planning clinic. *Fam Plann Perspect* 1983;15:25.

23. Kenney AM, Forrest JD, Torres A. Storm over Washington: the parental notification proposal. *Fam Plann Perspect* 1982;14:185.

24. Harris L, and Associates. *American teens speak: sex, myths, TV, and birth control.* New York: Planned Parenthood Federation of America; 1986.

25. *Griswold v. Connecticut,* 381 U.S. 479 (1965).

26. *Carey v. Population Serv. Int'l,* 431 U.S. 693 (1977).

27. *Doe v. Irwin,* 615 F.2d 1162, (6th Cir. 1980), cert. denied, 101 S. Ct. 95.

28. Mahler K. Condom availability in the schools: lessons from the courtroom. *Fam Plann Perspect* 1996;28:75.

29. *Planned Parenthood Fed'n of America v. Heckler,* 712 f.2d 650 (D.C. Cir. 1983).

30. *N.Y. v. Heckler,* 719 F. 2d 1191 (2d Cir. 1983).

31. Centers for Disease Control and Prevention. Abortion surveillance: preliminary data—United States, 1993.*MMWR Morb Mortal Wkly Rep* 1996;45:235.

32. Henshaw SK, Kost K. Parental involvement in minors' abortion decisions. *Fam Plann Perspect* 1992;24:196.

33. Joyce TJ, Mocan NH. The impact of legalized abortion on adolescent childbearing in New York City. *Am J Public Health* 1990;80:273.

34. *Planned Parenthood of Central Missouri v. Danforth,* 428 U.S. 74 (1976).

35. *Bellotti v. Baird,* 424 U.S. 952 (1976).

36. *Bellotti v. Baird II,* 443 U.S. (1979).

37. *City of Akron v. Akron Center for Reproductive Health,* 462 U.S. 416 (1983).

38. *Planned Parenthood of Kansas City, Missouri v. Ashcroft,* 462 U.S. 476 (1983).

39. *H.L. v. Matheson,* 450 U.S. 398 (1981).

40. Strasburger VC, Eisner JM, Tilson JQ, et al. Teenagers, physicians, and the law in New England. *Journal of Adolescent Health Care* 1985;6:377.

41. *Hodgeson v. Minnesota,* 853 F.2d 1452 (1988).

42. *Ohio v. Akron Center for Reproductive Health,* (U.S.L.W. 2106, U.S. Aug. 12, 1988, No. 86-3664).

43. Greenhouse L. States may require girl to notify parents before having an abortion. *New York Times* 1990;June 26:00.

44. Henshaw SK. The impact of requirements for parental consent on minors' abortions in Mississippi. *Fam Plann Perspect* 1995;27:120.

45. Rogers JL, Boruch RF, Stoms GB, et al. Impact of the Minnesota parental notification law on abortion and birth. *Am J Public Health* 1991;81:294.

46. Committee on Adolescence, American Academy of Pediatrics. The adolescent's right to confidential care when considering abortion (policy statement). *Pediatrics* 1996;97:746.

SUGGESTED READING

Committee on Adolescence, American Academy of Pediatrics. The adolescent's right to confidential care when considering abortion (policy statement). *Pediatrics* 1996;97:746.

Council on Scientific Affairs, American Medical Association. Confidential health services for adolescents. *JAMA* 1993;269:1420.

English A. Overcoming obstacles to adolescent care: legal issues. *Adolescent Medicine: State of the Art Reviews* 1991;2:429.

English A. Changing health environments and adolescent health care: legal and policy challenges. *Adolescent Medicine: State of the Art Reviews* 1997;8(3):375.

Gans JE, ed. *Confidential health services for adolescents.* Chicago: American Medical Association; 1993.

Hofmann AD. A rational policy toward consent and confidentiality in adolescent health care. *Journal of Adolescent Health Care* 1980;1:9.

Hofmann AD. Consent and confidentiality: critical issues in providing contraceptive care. In: Strasburger VC, ed. *Basic adolescent gynecology: an office guide.* Baltimore: Urban & Schwarzenberg; 1990:9.

Holder AR. *Legal issues in pediatrics and adolescent medicine.* 2nd ed. New Haven: Yale University Press; 1985.

Holder AR. Minors' right to consent to medical care. *JAMA* 1987;257:3400.

Holder AR. Legal issues in adolescent sexual health. *Adolescent Medicine: State of the Art Reviews* 1992;3:257.

Mahler K. Condom availability in the schools: lessons from the courtroom. *Fam Plann Perspect.* 1996;28:75.

Morrissey JM, Hofmann AD, Thrope JC. *Consent and confidentiality in the health care of children and adolescents.* New York: Free Press; 1986.

National Center for Youth Law. *State minor consent statutes: a summary.* Cincinnati, OH: Center for Continuing Education in Adolescent Health; 1995.

Quinn MM, Dubler NN. The health care provider's role in adolescent medical decision-making. *Adolescent Medicine: State of the Art Reviews* 1997;8(3):415.

Weisz VP, Melton GB. Legal issues in adolescent health care. In: Wallander JL, Siegel LJ, eds. *Adolescent health problems: behavioral perspectives.* New York: Guilford Press; 1995:72.

Wibbelsman C. Confidentiality in an age of managed care: can it exist? *Adolescent Medicine: State of the Art Reviews* 1997;8(3):427.

Subject Index

Note: Page numbers followed by f indicate figures; those followed by t indicate tables.

A

Abdominal pain, chronic, diagnosis and management of, 420–422, 421t
Ability, academic, teen sexual activity and, 161
Abortion, 222–223, 223t, 498–499
　rate among adolescents, 151, 156
Abscesses, tuboovarian, 286
Abstinence, sexual
　as contraceptive method, 207
　reasonableness as goal, 162–163
Academic ability, teen sexual activity and, 161
Academic performance, chronic disorders and, 142
Access to care, 23–24
Acetoenhanced androscopy, 312
Achilles tendinitis, 356, 357t
Acidosis, in diabetes mellitus. *See* Diabetic ketoacidosis (DKA)
Acne, 29, 33–40
　classification of, 34, 35, 35t
　etiology of, 33–34, 34f, 34t, 35t
　factors contributing to, 34–35, 36t
　inflammatory, 34
　oral contraception and, 198, 198f
　treatment of, 35, 35t, 36–40
　　benzoyl peroxide for, 36–37
　　new developments in, 39
　　oral isotretinoin for, 38–39
　　systemic antibiotics for, 38
　　tips for, 39t, 39–40, 40t
　　topical antibiotics for, 37–38
　　tretinoin for, 36t, 37
Acquired immunodeficiency syndrome (AIDS). *See* Human immunodeficiency virus (HIV) infections/AIDS
Acromioclavicular separation, 360
Acting-out, by adolescents with chronic disorders, 147
Adapalene (Differin)
　for acne, 39, 40
　cost of, 40
Addiction. *See also* Substance use and abuse
　to narcotics, 480, 481t
Adenovirus infections, infectious mononucleosis associated with, 43t
Adipostat, 445–446
Adoption, 222
β₂-Adrenergic agonists, for asthma, 77–78
Adulthood, ambivalence about, 372

Advantage 24, 203–204
Alcohol use, 470–472, 471t
　inconsistent cultural attitude toward, 463–464, 470–471
　violence related to, 468t
Alkaline phosphatase, Tanner staging and, 2–3, 6f
Alpha₁-blockers, for hypertension, 132t
Alprazolam, for premenstrual syndrome, 245
Ambulatory care. *See* Office practice; Office visits
Amenorrhea, 238–242
　in anorexia nervosa, 432
　primary, 238–240
　　causes of, 239t, 239–240
　　indications for evaluation of, 238, 238t
　　sequential evaluation of, 238–239, 239t
　secondary, 240–242
　　causes of, 241t
　　sequential evaluation of, 241t, 241–242
Amitriptyline, for depression, 407t
Amlodipine, for hypertension, 133t
Amoxicillin
　for *Chlamydia trachomatis* vaginitis and cervicitis, 277, 277t
　cost of, 68t
Amoxicillin-potassium clavulanate (Augmentin)
　cost of, 68t
　for sinusitis, 71
Amphetamines
　abuse of, 476–477
　as ergogenic drugs, 362t
Ampicillin, for bacterial vaginosis, 265t
Anabolic steroids, as ergogenic drugs, 361–362, 362t
Androscopy, acetoenhanced, 312
Anger, parental, about chronic disorders, 146
Angiotensin-converting enzyme (ACE) inhibitors, for hypertension, 132t, 133t
Ankle injuries, 352–354, 353f, 354t, 355t
Anorexia nervosa, 430–435
　diagnosis of, 431–432, 433t, 434t
　epidemiology of, 431
　etiology of, 431
　prognosis of, 435
　treatment of, 432–435, 434t
Anterior drawer test, 346f
Antibiotics. *See also specific drugs and disorders*
　for acne, 37–38, 40
　cost of, 40
　for urinary tract infections, 105
Antidepressants, tricyclic, for depression, 407, 407t, 408t